Orthopedic Management of the Hip and Pelvis

Scott W. Cheatham, PT, DPT, OCS, ATC, CSCS

Assistant Professor
Director, Pre–Physical Therapy Program
Division of Kinesiology
California State University, Dominguez Hills
Carson, California
President and CEO
National Institute of Restorative Exercise, Inc.
Torrance, California

Morey J. Kolber, PT, PhD, OCS, Cert. MDT, CSCS*D

Associate Professor
Department of Physical Therapy
Nova Southeastern University
Fort Lauderdale, Florida
Director of Physical Therapy
Boca Raton Orthopaedic Group
Boca Raton, Florida

ELSEVIER

ELSEVIER

3251 Riverport Lane
St. Louis, Missouri 63043

ORTHOPEDIC MANAGEMENT OF THE HIP AND PELVIS ISBN: 978-0-323-29438-6

Notices

Knowledge and best practice in this field are constantly changing. As new research and experience broaden our understanding, changes in research methods, professional practices, or medical treatment may become necessary.

Practitioners and researchers must always rely on their own experience and knowledge in evaluating and using any information, methods, compounds, or experiments described herein. In using such information or methods, they should be mindful of their own safety and the safety of others, including parties for whom they have a professional responsibility.

With respect to any drug or pharmaceutical products identified, readers are advised to check the most current information provided (i) on procedures featured or (ii) by the manufacturer of each product to be administered, to verify the recommended dose or formula, the method and duration of administration, and contraindications. It is the responsibility of practitioners, relying on their own experience and knowledge of their patients, to make diagnoses, to determine dosages and the best treatment for each individual patient, and to take all appropriate safety precautions.

To the fullest extent of the law, neither the Publisher nor the authors, contributors, or editors assume any liability for any injury and/or damage to persons or property as a matter of products liability, negligence, or otherwise or from any use or operation of any methods, products, instructions, or ideas contained in the material herein.

Library of Congress Cataloging-in-Publication Data

Names: Cheatham, Scott W., editor. | Kolber, Morey J., editor.
Title: Orthopedic management of the hip and pelvis / [edited by] Scott W. Cheatham, Morey J. Kolber.
Description: St. Louis, Missouri : Elsevier, Inc., [2016]
Identifiers: LCCN 2015042030 | ISBN 9780323294386 (pbk. : alk. paper)
Subjects: | MESH: Hip Injuries–therapy. | Pelvis–injuries. | Orthopedic Procedures.
Classification: LCC RD549 | NLM WE 855 | DDC 617.5/81044–dc23
LC record available at http://lccn.loc.gov/2015042030

Executive Content Strategist: Kathy Falk
Professional Content Development Manager: Jolynn Gower
Senior Content Development Specialist: Courtney Sprehe
Publishing Services Manager: Catherine Jackson
Senior Project Manager: Douglas Turner
Designer: Ryan Cook

Printed in the United States of America

Last digit is the print number: 9 8 7 6 5 4 3 2

Working together
to grow libraries in
developing countries

www.elsevier.com • www.bookaid.org

I would like to dedicate this textbook to my family. They were very patient and supportive during this 2-year project. To my wife, Mille, for the dedication and strength she brings to our marriage and family. Thank you for being my best friend. To both my sons, Connor and Alex, thank you for all the great talks you have with me and the joy you bring to our family. Both of you will grow up to do great things.

I want to thank my mentor, Leza L. Hatch, PT, OCS, for all her support over the years. Her passion for physical therapy has been an inspiration to me. I also want to thank my patients who have taught me so much over the years. I wish them all the best in health. Last, I want to thank my Mom for always being there for me. Your supportive presence in my life is a true blessing.

Scott W. Cheatham

I dedicate this book to my parents, whose unwavering support for me as a teenager and young adult provided me with the unrelenting confidence and motivation to pursue my dreams. To my father, Alan Kolber, who has led by example and instilled an incredible work ethic in me. Your never-ending drive and sacrifices to ensure that I had the necessary support to pursue my education symbolizes the father that I can only hope to be. To my mother, Elaine Kolber, who has provided me unconditional love and support throughout my life and taught me to always bet on myself and seize opportunities before they pass. You both have taught me that, although one's path may be stormy, the road may still lead to sunshine.

I also dedicate this book to my family, Shakira, Jordann, and Khloe. To my loving wife, Shakira, I am thankful for your unwaivering support and understanding of the endless time I have spent writing, teaching, and pursuing my professional goals over the years. To my daughter, Khloe, the young lady who has truly taught me what is important in life. I will always remember our times sitting together at the dining room table as I wrote this book while you patiently colored and practiced spelling our names.

Morey J. Kolber

Preface

The hip joint and pelvis has emerged as an area of study for clinicians and researchers alike. The nonsurgical and surgical management of common hip and pelvic pathologies has grown tremendously. As the health professional seeks out information on these topics, they are challenged by the paucity of available up-to-date evidence-based information. While many sources provide commentary on pathologies or surgery, they often lack the necessary detail with respect to emerging discoveries. These discoveries have created the need for a comprehensive evidence-based text about the hip and pelvis. With input and contribution from numerous experts in the field, this book was developed to meet the demands of the clinician and researcher desiring such information.

The text is divided into two sections. The first section covers basic regional anatomy and kinesiology and the basic examination process for the hip and pelvic complex. The second section provides comprehensive coverage of common pathologies such as hip labral tears, femoral acetabular impingement, snapping hip syndrome, women's health, joint arthroplasty, the dancer's hip, and much more.

We sincerely hope that you will find this textbook to be a central and reliable source of information. Whether you are a beginning or advanced clinician, researcher, or academician, we trust that the content will be an invaluable tool in your reference armamentarium. We thank you for embracing this textbook and have strove to ensure that its presence on your bookshelf will in some way help you achieve success in the orthopedic management of the hip and pelvis.

Acknowledgments

We want to acknowledge all the contributing authors of this textbook for the masterful work they have done. This textbook could not be possible without their dedication and passion to this project. The textbook is strengthened by the expertise and knowledge that each coauthor has shared in writing their chapter. Each chapter blends the latest evidence with clinical expertise, which provides a unique perspective to the reader. We also want to thank the Elsevier team and reviewers for their support and guidance with this project.

Scott W. Cheatham
Morey J. Kolber

Foreword

It is exciting to offer a foreword for this innovative and cutting-edge textbook on the management of hip and pelvis disorders. Most hip problems are not due to a single entity. Numerous factors may come into play, creating a "perfect storm" that leads to joint damage and dysfunction. All contributing factors may not be recognized, but hopefully enough can be identified and corrected, both nonsurgically and surgically, to reach a critical mass for successful treatment. Femoroacetabular impingement (FAI) is the most evident example to explain how joint damage occurs, but many active individuals with this condition are lifelong compensators, never developing symptoms or disability in the face of evident radiographic abnormalities. Thus, numerous elements may be involved, and there is not one exclusive treatment strategy. These multifaceted disorders require a multidisciplinary approach. This text epitomizes this concept, providing a comprehensive compendium on our current understanding of hip disorders and detailed information on the latest methods of management. The editors have assembled an excellent cast of contributors to accomplish this goal. Read the pages thoroughly and thoughtfully, and you will come away with a remarkably greater depth of knowledge on this rapidly evolving area. Then you can come back to this as a valuable resource later in your patient care. The patients are what this is all about, and I congratulate all the authors on their efforts to make us all better at what we do.

J.W. Thomas Byrd, MD
Nashville Sports Medicine and Orthopaedic Center
Nashville, Tennessee

Foreword

Orthopedic Management of the Hip and Pelvis is a timely and much-needed compilation of the best available evidence-based management strategies for patients with hip and pelvic disorders. The editorial team, as well as the contributing authors, consist of well-know clinicians and researchers at both the national and international levels on the topic of management of hip and pelvis musculoskeletal disorders.

The text starts with a chapter that delves into the details of the complex anatomy and kinesiology of the pelvis and hip region. This chapter includes numerous colorful Netter images that capture the essence of human anatomy. The next chapter discusses the subjective and physical examination and educates the reader not only on potential sinister pathologies that may mimic as musculoskeletal pain but also on the essential items from the patient history. In addition, this chapter covers the physical examination components and the psychometric properties that will greatly assist the clinician in identifying an accurate differential diagnosis.

The remainder of the text is nicely divided into chapters that discuss potential diagnoses. These chapters examine pathologies likely to be encountered by any health care provider dealing with hip and pelvic pain, including extraarticular hip pathologies, hip labral tears/femoral acetabular impingement, sports hernia and abdominal injuries, the arthritic hip, the pediatric hip, the dancer's hip, the female hip and pelvis, lumbopelvic region, and traumatic injuries. Each condition is examined in extensive detail regarding the typical client presentation, common mechanisms for the injury, and details about the best available conservative management strategies and appropriate surgical procedures with postoperative rehabilitation protocols. Seldom does a text delve into both conservative and surgical management with postoperative recommendations, which is just another highlight for this text. Additionally,

the detail for every condition far exceeds that of any rehabilitation text. For example, the chapter on hip osteoarthritis goes into more detail relative to the exact surgical procedure for each technique, as well as appropriate and safe management strategies for postoperative rehabilitation. Each chapter includes an extensive list of references, further attesting to the effort and time the authors invested in ensuring that their recommendations are based upon the best available scientific evidence.

Another brilliant addition to this text is the case studies, which are incorporated at the end of each chapter. Case studies are invaluable for discussing the clinical decision-making process, management, and outcomes of patients with various clinical disorders. These case studies will assist clinicians in developing a framework that they can use to appropriately manage their own patient population with hip or lumbopelvic disorders.

To date, no text exists that compiles the depth and breadth of information for management of patients with hip and pelvis musculoskeletal-related disorders as *Orthopaedic Management of the Hip and Pelvis* has done. This text is a must read and important reference for all clinicians managing patients with hip or lumbopelvic pain.

The Editors, Dr. Cheatham and Dr. Kolber, and the authors are to be applauded for the time and effort that was devoted to developing this extraordinary resource that is going to make a terrific contribution to the literature for many years to come.

Joshua A Cleland, PT, PhD
Professor
Doctor of Physical Therapy Program
College of Graduate and Professional Studies
Franklin Pierce University
Manchester, New Hampshire

Contributors

Darla Bowen Cathcart, PT, DPT, WCS, CLT
Clinical Instructor I
Department of Physical Therapy
University of Central Arkansas
Conway, Arkansas
Vice President
Section on Women's Health
American Physical Therapy Association
Arlington, Virginia

Whitney Chambers, PT, DPT, OCS, SCS
U18 Sports Medicine
Joe DiMaggio Children's Hospital
Coral Springs, Florida

Scott W. Cheatham, PT, DPT, OCS, ATC, CSCS
Assistant Professor
Director, Pre–Physical Therapy Program
Division of Kinesiology
California State University, Dominguez Hills
Carson, California
President and CEO
National Institute of Restorative Exercise, Inc.
Torrance, California

Keelan Enseki, MS, PT, OCS, SCS, ATC, CSCS
Program Director, Orthopaedic Physical Therapy
   Residency Program
Centers for Rehab Services
UPMC Center for Sports Medicine
Adjunct Instructor
Department of Physical Therapy
Adjunct Faculty
Department of Sports Medicine and Nutrition
School of Health and Rehabilitation Sciences
University of Pittsburgh
Pittsburgh, Pennsylvania

Alicia Fernandez-Fernandez, PT, DPT, PhD
Associate Professor
Department of Physical Therapy
Nova Southeastern University
Fort Lauderdale, Florida

Fran Guardo, MEd, MPT, DPT
Director of Rehabilitation and Physical Therapy
Paley Institute
West Palm Beach, Florida
Department of Physical Therapy
Nova Southeastern University
Fort Lauderdale, Florida

William J. Hanney, DPT, PhD, ATC, CSCS
Assistant Professor
Department of Health Professions
College of Health and Public Affairs
University of Central Florida
Orlando, Florida

Aimie F. Kachingwe, PT, DPT, EdD, OCS, FAAOMPT
Professor
Department of Physical Therapy
College of Health and Human Development
California State University, Northridge
Northridge, California

Dave Kohlrieser, PT, DPT, SCS, OCS, CSCS
Orthopedic One
Columbus, Ohio

Morey J. Kolber, PT, PhD, OCS, Cert. MDT, CSCS*D
Associate Professor
Department of Physical Therapy
Nova Southeastern University
Fort Lauderdale, Florida
Director of Physical Therapy
Boca Raton Orthopaedic Group
Boca Raton, Florida

Peter Aaron Sprague, PT, DPT, OCS
Associate Professor
Department of Physical Therapy
Nova Southeastern University
Fort Lauderdale, Florida

Melissa Moran Tovin, PT, MA, PhD
Associate Professor
Department of Physical Therapy
Nova Southeastern University
Fort Lauderdale, Florida

Contents

1

Anatomy of the Lumbopelvic Hip Complex

SCOTT W. CHEATHAM AND WILLIAM J. HANNEY

CHAPTER OUTLINE

The health care professional must have an understanding of basic anatomic, physiologic, and biomechanical concepts to examine and treat common disorders of the lumbopelvic and hip region effectively. This chapter provides a review of the lumbar spine, pelvis, and hip joint with an emphasis on the anatomy and biomechanics of each region. The first section is a review of the lumbar spine, sacrum, and coccyx. The second section provides a review of the pelvis and hip joint, while the third section discusses the fundamental biomechanical movements of the lumbopelvic hip complex. This chapter is a brief overview and is not intended to be a comprehensive resource. The information presented includes foundational concepts that support content discussed in subsequent chapters.

LUMBAR SPINE, SACRUM, AND COCCYX

Lumbar Spine

The lumbar spine has an interdependent function with the pelvis and hip that may refer symptoms into the hip and groin region. Because of this interdependent nature, the lumbar spine is often included in a comprehensive hip and pelvis examination. This section provides a brief review of the relevant anatomy.

The lumbar spine is generally composed of five individual vertebrae, notwithstanding absent or supernumerary vertebra, as seen in sacralization and lumbarization cases, respectively. The vertebrae of the lumbar spine form a lordotic curve that is approximately 32 to 50 degrees in the standing position.[1,2] Each lumbar vertebra consists of a vertebral body, two pedicles, two laminae, two pars interarticularis, and two superior and inferior zygapophyseal joints (i.e., articular processes) as well as one spinous and two transverse processes (Fig. 1-1).[3] The vertebral body consists of compact (cortical) bone wrapped around less dense trabecular or spongy bone. This osseous architecture of the lumbar vertebral body provides a level of rigidity, particularly during axial loading.[4] The less dense center portion of the vertebral body may allow for greater flexibility, which is essential during compressive forces. Posteriorly, the pedicles and laminae form the transverse processes laterally and the spinous process posteriorly (see Fig. 1-1).[5] Along the superior and inferior aspects, the lamina form their respective superior and inferior articular processes.

Zygapophyseal Joints

The lumbar spine has two superior and inferior articular processes that form the zygapophyseal or "facet" joints. The first lumbar vertebra has superior articular processes (which articulate with the 12th thoracic vertebrae) located primarily in the frontal plane and inferior articular processes which orient largely in the sagittal plane. Orientation of the superior and inferior articular processes continues generally to be in the sagittal plane, with a moderate transition toward the frontal plane through L5, the lowest lumbar vertebra (see Fig. 1-1). The inferior articular processes of L5 articulate with the sacral isthmus.[3,6] The facet joints are true synovial joints, and therefore each joint has an independent joint capsule, articular cartilage, and synovial fluid.[3,5] The primary roles of the zygapophyseal joint are to guide and limit movement in the lumbar

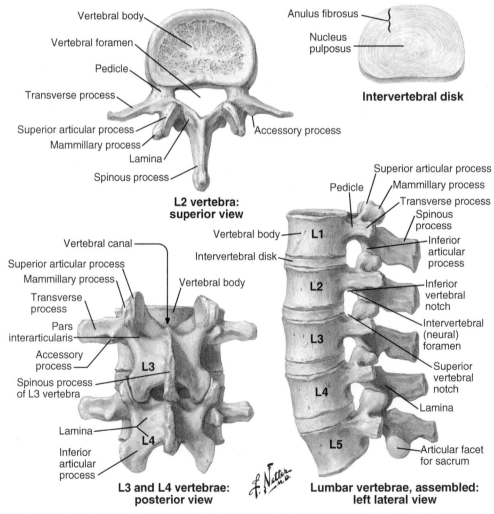

• **Figure 1-1** Lumbar Vertebrae. **A,** Lateral view. **B,** Superior view. (Netter illustrations from www.netterimages.com. © Elsevier Inc. All rights reserved.)

spine, as discussed further in the later section on lumbar biomechanics.

Intervertebral Foramen

The intervertebral foramen is formed by the posterior aspect of the vertebral body, the adjacent pedicle, and the anterior aspect of the articular process.[7] This space is further defined when two adjacent vertebrae come together, creating a space to allow the lumbar nerve roots to exit (Fig. 1-2). Because movement influences the intervertebral foramen space, persons with foraminal stenosis (i.e., narrowing of the intervertebral foramen) may experience symptom changes with positional variations.[8] As the cephalic vertebra flexes, the intervertebral foraminal space opens up approximately 12%; if the cephalic vertebra extends, this space will narrow (i.e., close down) approximately 11%.[5,8] The intervertebral foramen also narrows with lateral flexion to the same side and opens up with lateral flexion to the opposite side. Moreover, ipsilateral rotation narrows the foraminal space on the same side.[8] In addition, the posterolateral aspect of the intervertebral disk may encroach on this space, particularly if a defect exists in the annular fibers and subsequent herniation occurs (i.e., lateral directed herniation).

Vertebral Foramen

The vertebral foramen in the lumbar spine is a large, triangular space formed by the vertebral body anteriorly, the pedicles laterally, and the lamina posteriorly; it functions to protect the spinal cord and cauda equina (see Fig. 1-1).[3] Similar to the intervertebral foraminal space, the vertebral foramen is influenced by movement. The vertebral foramen space tends to increase during flexion movements and becomes narrower during movements such as extension.[5] In particular, changes in vertebral foramen space are often influenced by soft tissue changes (e.g., buckling of ligamentum flavum into the vertebral foramen with extension).

Intervertebral Disk and Vertebral End Plate

The intervertebral disks are located between the lumbar vertebral bodies (Fig. 1-3). The primary purposes of these disks are spinal mobility and shock absorption. The intervertebral disk has two primary parts: the annulus fibrosis and the nucleus pulposus.[3] The annulus fibrosis consists of rings of fibrocartilage lamellae, which create the outer portion of the intervertebral disk. Each lamella contains fibers that run obliquely from one vertebra to the other and in opposite directions to adjacent lamellae (see Fig. 1-3).[3] The outer third of the annulus is innervated by branches of the vertebral and sinuvertebral nerves that can transmit pain-related information to the brain in diskogenic-related conditions.[9-12] The most central portion of the intervertebral disk is referred to as the nucleus pulposus, which consists of dense mucoid material.[5] The nucleus pulposus is avascular and aneural, and it receives nutrition by diffusion from blood vessels at the periphery of the annulus and vertebral body end plates.[3] The vertebral end plates are cartilaginous structures located over the superior and inferior aspect of the articular disk. The end plates have both vascularity and nerve innervation.[13,14] They act as a structural transition between the nuclear material and the bone in the center of the vertebral body.[15] Abnormal changes in the vertebral end plate have been associated with intervertebral disk herniations.[16,17]

Ligaments

Ligamentous structures are extensive in the lumbosacral spine and contain numerous proprioceptors, mechanoreceptors, and free nerve endings.[12,18] These receptors play an important role in lumbopelvic sensory awareness, and some mechanoreceptors may contribute to pain perception.[19-23]

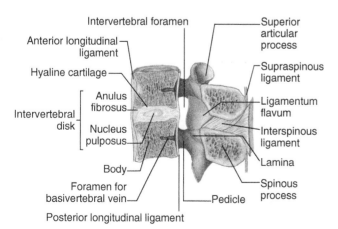

• **Figure 1-2** Table and Sagittal Cross-Sectional Area of the Lumbar Spine. (Waschke J, Paulsen F, eds. *Sobotta Atlas of Human Anatomy*. 15th ed. Munich: Elsevier GMbH, Urban & Fischer; 2013.)

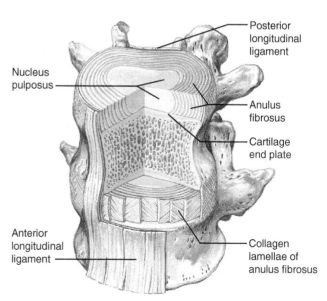

• **Figure 1-3** Lumbar Intervertebral Disk. (Netter illustration from www.netterimages.com. © Elsevier Inc. All rights reserved.)

Ligaments of the lumbosacral spine can be considered segmental or continuous. Segmental ligaments have local attachments between individual vertebrae. This segmental attachment suggests that the proprioceptive or nociceptive input will be localized.[24]

The five primary segmental ligaments classified in the lumbosacral spine are the interspinous ligament, supraspinous ligament, intertransverse ligament, iliolumbar ligament, and ligamentum flavum (Fig. 1-4). The interspinous ligament attaches to the adjacent spinous process by filling in the space between processes. The ligament fibers run diagonally and become taut during flexion and slack during extension.[25] The supraspinous ligament connects the tips of adjacent lumbar spinous processes. The supraspinous ligament is also taut during lumbar flexion and slack during extension. Both the supraspinous ligament and the interspinous ligament are the first posterior ligaments to fail with extreme flexion tension forces.[25,26] The intertransverse ligament attaches to the adjacent transverse process and becomes taut predominantly with lateral flexion to the opposite side and to a lesser degree with rotation.[5] The iliolumbar ligament is found in the lower lumbar segment and consists of a superior and inferior band. The superior band attaches from the transverse process of L4 to the ilium, and the inferior band connects the transverse process of L5 to the ilium. The iliolumbar ligaments become taut during spinal flexion and rotation because of their fiber orientation.[27] They also play a significant role in preventing anterior translation of L4 on L5 and of L5 on the sacral base by restricting motion.[5] The ligamentum flavum connects the lamina of adjacent vertebrae and receives the highest strain when it is stretched during flexion.[28] The ligament is under constant tension and creates a continuous compressive force to the intervertebral disks.[5]

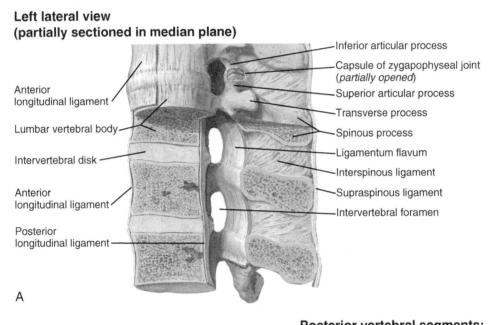

Left lateral view (partially sectioned in median plane)

Inferior articular process

Capsule of zygapophyseal joint (*partially opened*)

Superior articular process

Transverse process

Spinous process

Ligamentum flavum

Interspinous ligament

Supraspinous ligament

Intervertebral foramen

Anterior longitudinal ligament

Lumbar vertebral body

Intervertebral disk

Anterior longitudinal ligament

Posterior longitudinal ligament

A

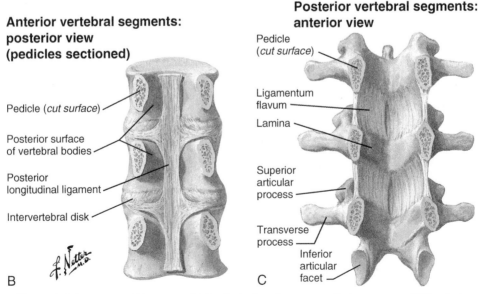

Anterior vertebral segments: posterior view (pedicles sectioned)

Pedicle (*cut surface*)

Posterior surface of vertebral bodies

Posterior longitudinal ligament

Intervertebral disk

B

Posterior vertebral segments: anterior view

Pedicle (*cut surface*)

Ligamentum flavum

Lamina

Superior articular process

Transverse process

Inferior articular facet

C

• **Figure 1-4** Lumbosacral Ligaments. (Netter illustrations from www.netterimages.com. © Elsevier Inc. All rights reserved.)

Continuous ligaments attach at multiple locations along the length of the lumbosacral spine. This multisegmental attachment and broader length suggest that injury to the continuous ligaments may contribute to diffuse symptoms.[24] The primary continuous ligaments include the anterior longitudinal ligament and the posterior longitudinal ligament (see Fig. 1-4). The anterior longitudinal ligament has attachments along the anterior portion of the vertebral bodies and extends down to the sacral base. The anterior longitudinal ligament tends to be a broad, thick ligament that increases in thickness and width from the lower thoracic area to L5 and S1. The ligament covers a large portion of the anterior lumbosacral vertebral bodies and helps to reinforce the anterolateral portion of the intervertebral disk.[5,29] The ligament is relaxed in flexion and taut in extension.[5] The posterior longitudinal ligament runs within the vertebral canal along the posterior aspect of the vertebral bodies. In the lumbar spine, the posterior longitudinal ligament narrows as it courses downward towards the sacrum. The narrowed ligament provides little support for the lumbar intervertebral joints, but it does reinforce the posterior surface of the intervertebral disk.[30] The ligament is taut in flexion and relaxed in extension.[5]

Sacrum and Coccyx

The sacrum consists of five fused vertebrae (Fig. 1-5).[3] The most cephalic sacral vertebra has superior articular facets referred to as the sacral isthmus. These processes articulate with the inferior facet joints of L5 and are largely present

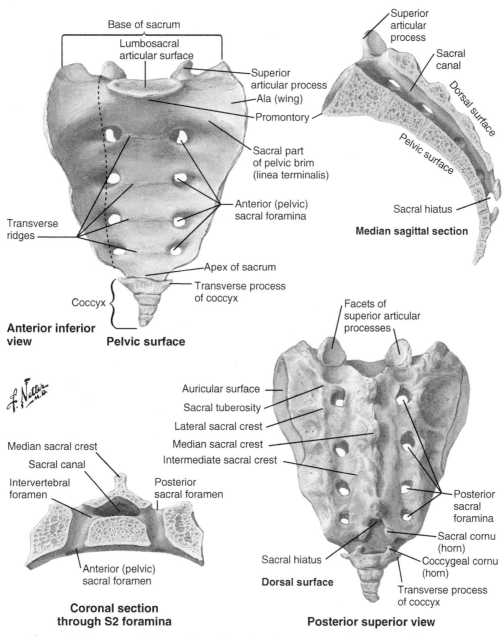

• **Figure 1-5** Sacrum and Coccyx. (Netter illustrations from www.netterimages.com. © Elsevier Inc. All rights reserved.)

in the frontal plane. The sacrum not only articulates with L5 superiorly but also articulates caudally with the coccyx and laterally with the ilia to form the sacroiliac (SI) joint.[5] The coccyx is a series of three to five fused vertebral rudiments that articulates with the inferior aspect of the sacrum (see Fig. 1-5).[3] The sacrum is discussed further later, in conjunction with the SI joint.

Nerves of the Lumbar Spinal Cord

The nerves from the lumbar spinal cord pass through the intervertebral foramen below the corresponding vertebra. These nerves subsequently divide into dorsal and ventral primary rami and contain both sensory and motor fibers.[3]

The lumbar plexus is a network of nerves composed of the ventral rami of L1 to L4 located anterior to the lumbar transverse processes and behind the psoas major muscle (Fig. 1-6).[31,32] The major branches of the plexus are discussed later. Table 1-1 also provides a summary of these nerves.[3]

Iliohypogastric and Ilioinguinal Nerves (T12 to L1)

The first lumbar nerve receives a branch from T12 and divides into upper and lower branches. The upper branch contains two divisions: the iliohypogastric nerve and the ilioinguinal nerve. The iliohypogastric nerve arises from

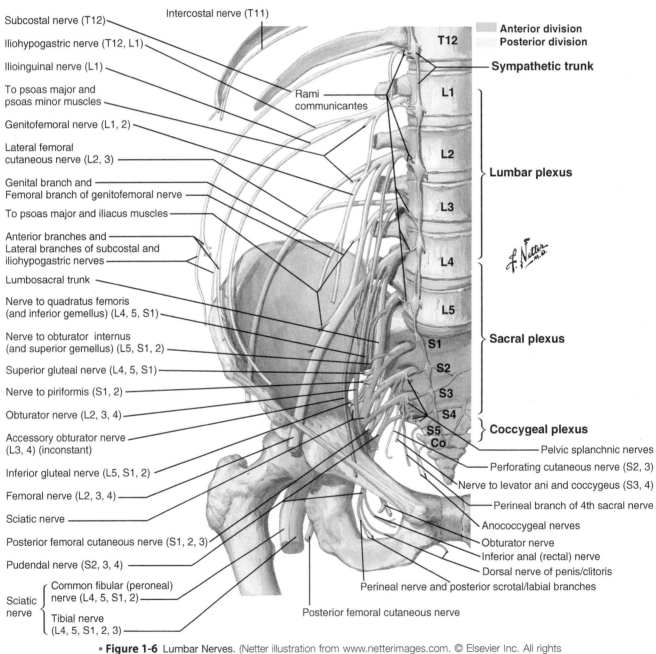

• Figure 1-6 Lumbar Nerves. (Netter illustration from www.netterimages.com. © Elsevier Inc. All rights reserved.)

the upper border of the psoas major muscle and crosses in an oblique direction to the iliac crest on the anterior quadratus lumborum muscle.[32] The nerve pierces the transversus abdominis muscle near the anterior superior iliac spine and splits into two cutaneous branches: lateral and anterior. The lateral branch passes through the internal and external abdominal oblique muscles to provide sensory innervation to the skin over the superolateral quadrant of the buttocks. The anterior branch continues to pass through the internal oblique abdominal muscle and fascia of the external oblique muscle to provide sensory innervation to the skin of the hypogastric region (superior to pubis).[3,32] The ilioinguinal nerve has the same anatomic course and relationship with the iliohypogastric nerve.

TABLE 1-1 Nerves of the Lumbopelvic Hip Region

Nerve	Origin	Distribution in Lumbopelvic Hip Region
Iliohypogastric nerve	T12 to L1	*Lateral branch:* sensory innervation to the skin over the superolateral quadrant of the buttocks *Anterior branch:* sensory innervation to the skin over the hypogastric region (superior to pubis)
Ilioinguinal nerve	T12 to L1	Sensory innervation to the skin over the proximal and medial parts of the thigh (femoral triangle), scrotum, and labia majora
Genitofemoral nerve	L2 to L3	*Genital branch:* sensory innervation to the scrotum and labia majora and motor innervation to the cremaster muscle *Femoral branch:* sensory innervation to the skin over the femoral triangle
Lateral cutaneous nerve of the thigh	L1 to L3	*Anterior branch:* sensory innervation to the skin over the anterolateral thigh *Posterior branch:* sensory innervation to the skin over the gluteal region and posterior thigh
Obturator nerve	L2 to L4	*Anterior branch:* motor innervation to the gracilis, adductor longus and magnus, and joining the saphenous nerve distally to provide sensory innervation to the inferomedial thigh near the knee joint *Posterior branch:* motor innervation to the obturator externus and adductor brevis *Articular branches:* sensory innervation to the hip joint
Femoral nerve	L2 to L4	*Anterior branch:* motor innervation to iliacus, sartorius, pectineus, and sensory innervation to the anterior and medial thigh *Posterior branch:* motor innervation to the quadriceps muscle and sensory innervation to the medial aspect of the lower leg through the saphenous nerve *Articular branches:* sensory innervation to the hip joint
Anterior femoral cutaneous nerve	L2 to L4	Branch of the femoral nerve that provides sensory innervation to the skin on the medial and anterior thigh
Sciatic nerve	L4 to S3	Sensory innervation to the posterior lower limb except for the medial side *Articular branches:* sensory innervation to the hip joint; two branches supplying motor innervation to the lower limb *Tibial nerve:* motor innervation to the hamstrings (except for short head of biceps femoris) and muscles of the lower leg and foot *Common peroneal (fibular) nerve:* motor innervation to the short head of the biceps femoris and sensory innervation to the posterior leg and knee joint through articular branches
Pudendal nerve	S2 to S4	Sensory innervation to the external genitalia and motor innervation to the perineal muscles, external urethral sphincter, and external anal sphincter
Superior gluteal nerve	L4 to S1	Motor innervation to the gluteus medius, minimus, tensor fasciae latae muscles, and sensory innervation to the hip joint
Inferior gluteal nerve	L5 to S2	Motor innervation to the gluteus maximus muscle
Nerve to quadratus femoris	L4 to S1	Sensory innervation to the hip joint and motor innervation to the quadratus femoris and inferior gemellus muscles
Nerve to obturator internus	L5 to S2	Motor innervation to the superior gemellus and obturator internus muscles
Nerve to piriformis	S1 to S2	Motor innervation to the piriformis muscle
Posterior cutaneous nerve of the thigh	S1 to S3	Sensory innervation to the skin over the buttocks, posterior thigh, and popliteal fossa

However; reports are mixed regarding whether the nerve originates solely from L1 or from both T12 and L1. The ilioinguinal nerve provides sensation to the skin over the proximal and medial parts of the thigh (femoral triangle), scrotum, and labia majora.[3,7,31,32]

Genitofemoral Nerve (L2 to L3) and Lateral Cutaneous Nerve of the Thigh (L1 to L3)

The second lumbar nerve receives the lower branch of the first lumbar nerve, which gives rise to two nerves. The genitofemoral nerve originates from the ventral rami of L2 to L3 and runs along the anterior aspect of the psoas major muscle deep to the psoas fascia and continues along the common and external iliac arteries. The nerve then divides into two branches: (1) a genital branch that passes through the inguinal ring to provide sensory innervation to the scrotum or labia major and motor innervation to the cremaster muscle and (2) a femoral branch that provides sensation to the skin over the femoral triangle.[32] The lateral cutaneous nerve of the thigh originates from the dorsal divisions of L1 to L3, emerges from lateral border of the psoas major, and crosses the iliacus, to the anterior superior iliac spine. The nerve then passes under the inguinal ligament and over the sartorius muscle and enters the thigh as the nerve divides into anterior and posterior branches. The anterior branch provides sensory innervation to the skin over the anterolateral thigh. The posterior branch provides sensory innervation to the skin over the gluteal region and posterior thigh.[33,34] The nerve may have a variable orientation in persons with different combinations of lumbar nerves originating from L1 to L3.[35] Entrapment of the anterior branch (i.e., meralgia paresthetica) can result in various sensory issues within the nerve distribution, as further discussed in Chapter 3.

Obturator and Femoral Nerves (L2 to L4)

The obturator nerve originates from the ventral divisions of the L2 to L4 ventral rami and emerges from the medial border of the psoas major, passes through the pelvis, and exits through the obturator foramen, where it divides into terminal and collateral branches. The terminal branch further divides into anterior and posterior branches. The anterior branch enters the medial thigh to provide motor innervation to the gracilis and adductor longus and magnus muscles and joins the saphenous nerve distally to provide sensory innervation to the medial thigh near the knee joint. The posterior branch travels through the obturator externus and adductor brevis muscles. This branch provides motor innervation to the obturator externus and adductor brevis muscles.[3,32] The collateral branches are two articular nerves that supply the hip joint and the obturator externus muscle.[32]

The femoral nerve originates from the dorsal divisions of the ventral rami of L2 to L4 and is the largest branch of the lumbar plexus. It emerges from the lateral border of the psoas major muscle and then passes deep to the inguinal ligament to the anterior thigh, where it ends with two ter-

minal divisions: anterior and posterior. The anterior division provides motor innervation to the iliacus, sartorius, and pectineus muscles and sensory innervation to the anterior and medial thigh. The posterior division provides motor innervation to the quadriceps muscle and sensory innervation to the medial aspect of the lower leg through the saphenous nerve.[3,32] The femoral nerve also has articular branches that provide sensory innervation to the hip joint. The anterior femoral cutaneous nerve is a branch of the femoral nerve that arises in the femoral triangle and pierces the tensor fasciae latae along the path of the sartorius muscle to provide sensation to the skin on the medial and anterior thigh.[3]

The autonomic nerves in the lumbar region include the vagus nerve and several splanchnic nerves that provide both presynaptic sympathetic and parasympathetic fibers to the nerve plexuses, as well as sympathetic ganglia along the abdominal aorta, vertebral bodies, and their extensions that reach the abdominal viscera.[3,7] A further discussion of the pelvic autonomic nerves is provided later in this chapter.

Blood Supply to the Lumbar Region

The abdominal aorta provides arterial blood supply to the lumbar region. The aorta begins at the aortic hiatus of the diaphragm at the approximate level of T12 and descends down the left side of the vertebral bodies to the L3 and L4 vertebrae (umbilicus region), where it bifurcates into right and left common iliac arteries.[3,7,36,37] The aorta lies anterior to the vertebral bodies of T12 to L4, and it supplies blood to the vertebrae through parietal branches called the lumbar arteries. The inferior vena cava provides venous return of deoxygenated blood from the legs and lumbopelvic region back to the heart. The inferior vena cava begins anterior to L5, ascends on the right side of the bodies of L5 to L3 up to caval foramen of the diaphragm, and passes through to the thorax.[3,7]

Muscles of the Trunk: Abdominal Core

The trunk or "abdominal core" is a general term that describes the structures of the lumbopelvic hip complex. The abdominal core can be described as a muscular box with four walls. The anterior wall consists of the abdominal muscles, the posterior wall is made up of the gluteal and spinal muscles, the superior wall would be represented by the diaphragm, and the inferior wall comprises the pelvic floor and hip girdle muscles.[38] The lumbopelvic hip complex has a total of 29 pairs of muscles that work together to perform patterns of functional movements.[38] This section discusses specific muscles in the lumbosacral region (anterior and posterior walls), followed by a classification system for the abdominal core. The subsequent sections discuss specific muscles of the pelvis and hip region.

Posterior Muscles

The posterior back muscles in the region of the thoracic and lumbopelvic spine have three layers. The superficial group

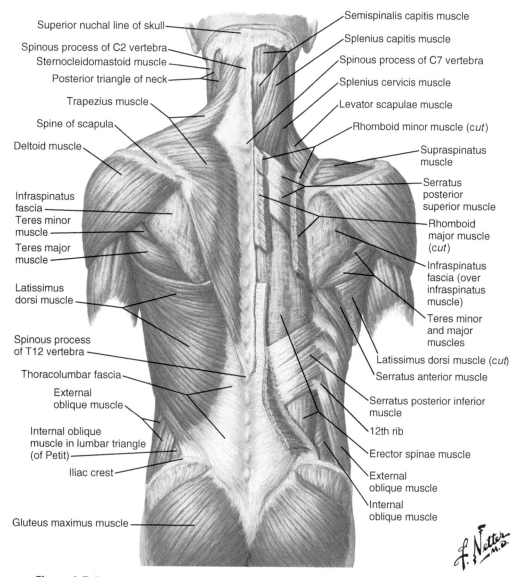

Superior nuchal line of skull

Spinous process of C2 vertebra

Sternocleidomastoid muscle

Posterior triangle of neck

Trapezius muscle

Spine of scapula

Deltoid muscle

Infraspinatus fascia

Teres minor muscle

Teres major muscle

Latissimus dorsi muscle

Spinous process of T12 vertebra

Thoracolumbar fascia

External oblique muscle

Internal oblique muscle in lumbar triangle (of Petit)

Iliac crest

Gluteus maximus muscle

Semispinalis capitis muscle

Splenius capitis muscle

Spinous process of C7 vertebra

Splenius cervicis muscle

Levator scapulae muscle

Rhomboid minor muscle (cut)

Supraspinatus muscle

Serratus posterior superior muscle

Rhomboid major muscle (cut)

Infraspinatus fascia (over infraspinatus muscle)

Teres minor and major muscles

Latissimus dorsi muscle (cut)

Serratus anterior muscle

Serratus posterior inferior muscle

12th rib

Erector spinae muscle

External oblique muscle

Internal oblique muscle

• **Figure 1-7** Posterior Back Muscles, Superficial. (Netter illustration from www.netterimages.com. © Elsevier Inc. All rights reserved.)

of muscles includes the latissimus dorsi and trapezius, which have an intimate attachment to the thoracolumbar fascia that covers the deep muscles of the back.[39] The thoracolumbar fascia spans laterally from the spinous processes with a narrow muscular overlay in the thoracic region and a thicker covering in the lumbar spine (Fig. 1-7).[7,39] The intermediate group of muscles includes the erector spinae group: iliocostalis (lateral), longissimus (intermediate), and spinalis (medial). The group has a common origin of attachment at the posterior iliac crest, posterior sacrum, SI ligament, and lower lumbar and sacral spinous processes. The muscles travel superiorly and attach to the various vertebrae of the lumbar, thoracic, and cervical spine. Because of their position, they are commonly classified by each region of the spine (e.g., iliocostalis lumborum or thoracis; Fig. 1-8). The deep layer of muscles includes the transversospinalis group: semispinalis (superficial), multifidus (middle), and rotatores (deep). The semispinalis muscle is also named by

its regional attachments in the spine (i.e., spinalis thoracis) (Fig. 1-9).[3]

Other posterior muscles include the quadratus lumborum, psoas major, and iliacus (Fig. 1-10). The quadratus lumborum spans distally from the iliolumbar ligament and iliac crest up to the twelfth rib and lumbar transverse processes.[3] The psoas major originates on the anterior bodies and intervertebral disks of T12 to L5 and inserts into the lesser trochanter of the femur. The iliacus originates with the iliac fossa, ala of the sacrum, and anterior SI ligament and distally joins the psoas major, inserting into the lesser trochanter of the femur.[7] Table 1-2 provides a summary of muscle groups involved in motion of the trunk.

Anterolateral Muscles

The anterolateral trunk region contains four muscles that help stabilize and control movement (Fig. 1-11). First, the

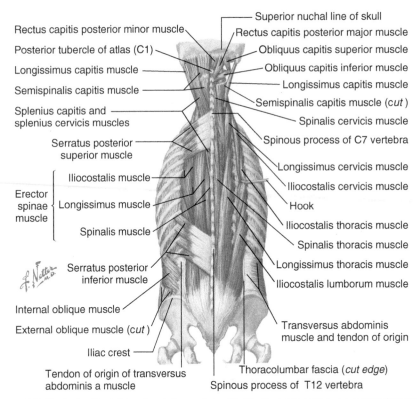

Rectus capitis posterior minor muscle

Posterior tubercle of atlas (C1)

Longissimus capitis muscle

Semispinalis capitis muscle

Splenius capitis and splenius cervicis muscles

Serratus posterior superior muscle

Iliocostalis muscle

Erector spinae muscle

Longissimus muscle

Spinalis muscle

Serratus posterior inferior muscle

Internal oblique muscle

External oblique muscle (*cut*)

Iliac crest

Tendon of origin of transversus abdominis a muscle

Superior nuchal line of skull

Rectus capitis posterior major muscle

Obliquus capitis superior muscle

Obliquus capitis inferior muscle

Longissimus capitis muscle

Semispinalis capitis muscle (*cut*)

Spinalis cervicis muscle

Spinous process of C7 vertebra

Longissimus cervicis muscle

Iliocostalis cervicis muscle

Hook

Iliocostalis thoracis muscle

Spinalis thoracis muscle

Longissimus thoracis muscle

Iliocostalis lumborum muscle

Transversus abdominis muscle and tendon of origin

Thoracolumbar fascia (*cut edge*)

Spinous process of T12 vertebra

• **Figure 1-8** Posterior Back Muscles, Intermediate. (Netter illustration from www.netterimages.com. © Elsevier Inc. All rights reserved.)

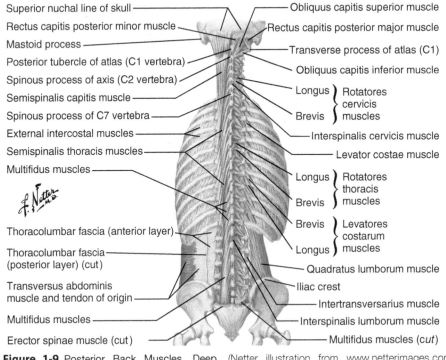

Superior nuchal line of skull

Rectus capitis posterior minor muscle

Mastoid process

Posterior tubercle of atlas (C1 vertebra)

Spinous process of axis (C2 vertebra)

Semispinalis capitis muscle

Spinous process of C7 vertebra

External intercostal muscles

Semispinalis thoracis muscles

Multifidus muscles

Thoracolumbar fascia (anterior layer)

Thoracolumbar fascia (posterior layer) (cut)

Transversus abdominis muscle and tendon of origin

Multifidus muscles

Erector spinae muscle (cut)

Obliquus capitis superior muscle

Rectus capitis posterior major muscle

Transverse process of atlas (C1)

Obliquus capitis inferior muscle

Longus } Rotatores
Brevis } cervicis muscles

Interspinalis cervicis muscle

Levator costae muscle

Longus } Rotatores
Brevis } thoracis muscles

Brevis } Levatores
Longus } costarum muscles

Quadratus lumborum muscle

Iliac crest

Intertransversarius muscle

Interspinalis lumborum muscle

Multifidus muscles (*cut*)

• **Figure 1-9** Posterior Back Muscles, Deep. (Netter illustration from www.netterimages.com. © Elsevier Inc. All rights reserved.)

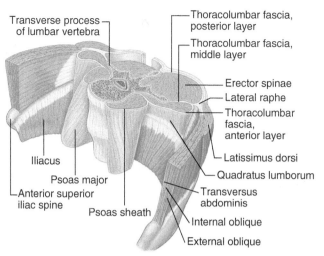

Transverse process of lumbar vertebra

Thoracolumbar fascia, posterior layer

Thoracolumbar fascia, middle layer

Erector spinae

Lateral raphe

Thoracolumbar fascia, anterior layer

Latissimus dorsi

Quadratus lumborum

Transversus abdominis

Internal oblique

External oblique

Iliacus

Psoas major

Anterior superior iliac spine

Psoas sheath

• **Figure 1-10** Posterior Abdominal Wall. (From Standring S. *Gray's Anatomy: The Anatomical Basis of Clinical Practice.* 41st ed. London: Churchill Livingstone; 2016.)

TABLE 1-2	Lumbopelvic Movements With Corresponding Muscles	
Movement	**Muscles**	
Rotation (unilateral)	Unilateral: rotatores, multifidus, external oblique, opposite internal oblique, semispinalis	
Side bending (unilateral)	Iliocostalis, longissimus, multifidus, external oblique, internal oblique, quadratus lumborum	
Flexion	Rectus abdominis, psoas major	
Extension	Erector spinae, multifidus, semispinalis	

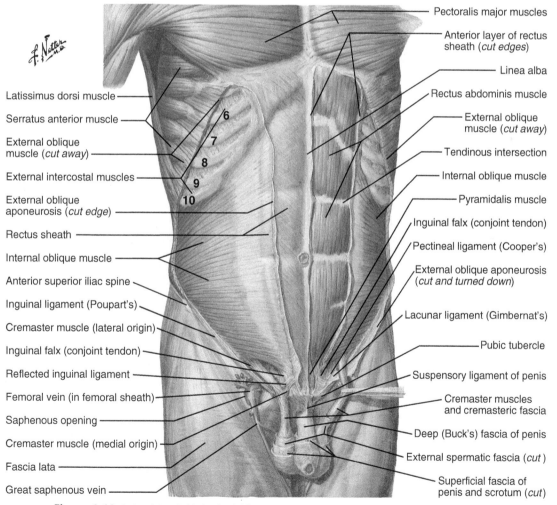

Latissimus dorsi muscle

Serratus anterior muscle

External oblique muscle (*cut away*)

External intercostal muscles

External oblique aponeurosis (*cut edge*)

Rectus sheath

Internal oblique muscle

Anterior superior iliac spine

Inguinal ligament (Poupart's)

Cremaster muscle (lateral origin)

Inguinal falx (conjoint tendon)

Reflected inguinal ligament

Femoral vein (in femoral sheath)

Saphenous opening

Cremaster muscle (medial origin)

Fascia lata

Great saphenous vein

6
7
8
9
10

Pectoralis major muscles

Anterior layer of rectus sheath (*cut edges*)

Linea alba

Rectus abdominis muscle

External oblique muscle (*cut away*)

Tendinous intersection

Internal oblique muscle

Pyramidalis muscle

Inguinal falx (conjoint tendon)

Pectineal ligament (Cooper's)

External oblique aponeurosis (*cut and turned down*)

Lacunar ligament (Gimbernat's)

Pubic tubercle

Suspensory ligament of penis

Cremaster muscles and cremasteric fascia

Deep (Buck's) fascia of penis

External spermatic fascia (*cut*)

Superficial fascia of penis and scrotum (*cut*)

• **Figure 1-11** Anterolateral Abdominal Muscles. (Netter illustration from www.netterimages.com. © Elsevier Inc. All rights reserved.)

rectus abdominis is a long, straplike muscle that originates on the pubic symphysis and pubic crest and inserts superiorly on the xiphoid process and costal cartilages of the ribs 5 to 7. Each side of the rectus abdominis is connected centrally by the linea alba, which is a vertical fibrous band that spans the length of the muscle.[3] It also has attachments with the oblique and transversus abdominis. Second, the external oblique originates on the external surface of ribs 5 to 12 and inserts into the linea alba, pubic tubercle, and anterior half of the iliac crest. Third, the internal oblique originates on the thoracolumbar fascia, anterior two thirds of the iliac crest, and lateral half of the inguinal ligament. The muscle inserts into the inferior border of ribs 10 to 12, linea alba, and pecten pubis (through the conjoint tendon).[3] Fourth, the transversus abdominis is the deepest of all the abdominal muscles (see Fig. 1-10). The fibers run in a transverse fashion, originating on the internal surface of the costal cartilage of ribs 6 to 12, thoracolumbar fascia, iliac crest, and lateral third of the inguinal ligament with insertion anteriorly onto the linea alba, aponeurosis of the internal oblique, pubic crest, and pecten pubis (through the conjoint tendon).[3,7] The transversus abdominis is a key muscle for local feed-forward stabilization and rehabilitation of the lumbosacral spine.[40,41] The anterolateral abdominal wall may be susceptible to hernias in the umbilical and inguinal region, as discussed further in Chapter 5. See Table 1-2 for a summary of muscle groups involved in motion of the trunk. Appendix A provides more information about the muscles.

Classifying the Abdominal Core

To understand the abdominal core fully, one must understand how all the structures work as a system. Clark and colleagues[42] created a system that classifies the structures of the lumbopelvic hip complex into two main systems: stabilization and movement. Each system has various subsystems that define the functional anatomy of that system (Fig. 1-12).

Stabilization System

The stabilization system is divided into two subsystems: local and global. The local muscle subsystem includes those structures that have direct influence on specific segments of the lumbosacral spine,[43] because of the proximal or distal attachment of a given muscle or the close proximity of these muscles to the vertebrae. These muscles are primarily composed of type I muscle fibers with a high density of muscle spindles.[1,42] The muscles work together to influence orientation of the individual vertebrae, increase segmental spinal stability through tension created in thoracolumbar fascia, decrease biomechanical forces (e.g., compression, shear), and assist with proprioception and postural control.[39,42,44] The muscles of the local system include the multifidus, internal oblique, pelvic floor muscles (see Chapter 9), and diaphragm.

The global subsystem includes muscles that influence several vertebral segments and often cross multiple joints

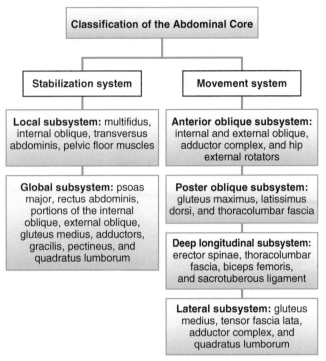

• **Figure 1-12** Classification of the Abdominal Core.

along the pelvis and spine.[43] These muscles help to transfer forces from the upper extremity to the lower extremity, provide stabilization, and promote eccentric control of the abdominal core during movement.[45] Because of the complex roles of these muscles, they may be involved with pathologic processes of the lumbosacral hip region. For example, trigger points have been identified in muscles of the global system.[46] These trigger points generally have distal referral patterns that may cross the lumbopelvic region and may be mistaken for pathologic conditions in other areas of the spine or hip.[47,48] The global system includes the following muscles: psoas major, rectus abdominis, portions of the internal oblique, external oblique, gluteus medius, adductors, gracilis, pectineus, and quadratus lumborum.[42,43]

Movement System

The movement system includes larger muscle that link the lumbopelvic region to the lower extremities. These muscles are responsible for both force production (concentric) and deceleration (eccentric) during multiplane dynamic movements.[42] This dynamic stability occurs from the muscles working in groups or subsystems, rather than in isolation. Efficient patterned movement is enhanced when these muscles are contracting synchronously. Four main subsystems comprise the movement system. First, the anterior oblique subsystem includes the internal oblique, external oblique, adductors, and hip external rotators. Second, the posterior oblique subsystem includes the gluteus maximus, latissimus dorsi, and thoracolumbar fascia. Third, the deep longitudinal subsystem includes the erector spinae, thoracolumbar fascia, sacrotuberous ligament, and biceps femoris. Fourth, the lateral subsystem includes the gluteus medius, tensor fasciae latae, adductor complex, and quadratus lumborum.

Thoracolumbar Fascia and Intraabdominal Pressure

The thoracolumbar fascia is a dense fascial network that has broad influence in functioning of the lumbosacral complex. This fascial network is interwoven throughout the anatomy of the lumbopelvic spine, contains several layers that separate the paraspinal and posterior abdominal wall muscles, and provides specific mechanical characteristics.[39,49] The thoracolumbar fascia plays a distinct role in helping to stabilize the lumbopelvic complex through its attachments to several muscles including the transversus abdominis, internal oblique, gluteus maximus, latissimus dorsi, quadratus lumborum, multifidus, and erector spinae.[3,42] Contraction of these muscles creates tension through the fascia that, in turn, may help create stability of the lumbopelvic region. Intraabdominal pressure also creates stability through this region by pushing the viscera upward and downward.[42] This movement raises the diaphragm and stimulates contraction of the pelvic floor assisting with intersegmental stability.[42]

Inguinal (Groin) Region

The inguinal region is a junction between the trunk and the lower limbs and is considered an area of weakness of the lower anterolateral abdominal wall.[3] The inguinal ligament spans the area from the anterior superior iliac spine to the pubic tubercle. Along with the pubic bones, the inguinal ligament marks the inferior border of the anterior abdominal wall and provides attachments for the transversus abdominis and internal oblique muscles.[3] The inguinal region is the most susceptible to hernias among all the areas of the anterolateral abdominal wall (see Chapter 5).[50]

The inguinal canal is a passage that houses the spermatic cord in males, the round ligament of the uterus in females, the blood and lymphatic vessels, and the ilioinguinal nerve (Fig. 1-13).[3,7,51] The deep (internal) inguinal ring is the entrance to the inguinal canal and is located superior to the inguinal ligament. The superficial (external) inguinal ring is the distal exit to the inguinal canal and is located between the fibers of the external oblique just superior lateral to the pubic tubercle. The superficial ring is the site that examiners often palpate to diagnose an indirect hernia.[52] The floor is formed by the superior surface of the inguinal ligament. The anterior wall formed by the aponeurosis of the external oblique and posterior wall is created by the transversalis fascia and medial part of the wall by the conjoint tendon. The conjoint tendon (aponeurotic falx) is a common tendon that connects the pubic attachments of the internal oblique and transversus abdominis aponeuroses.[3,51]

The femoral triangle is a fascial junctional inferior to the inguinal ligament. The femoral triangle is bound superiorly by the inguinal ligament, medially by adductor longus, and laterally by the sartorius. The roof of the femoral triangle is formed by the fascia lata, cribriform fascia, subcutaneous tissue, and skin.[53] The floor of the triangle is composed of the iliopsoas (laterally) and pectineus (medially). The contents of the femoral triangle include the femoral nerve (L2 to L4), arteries, and veins that are within the femoral fascial sheath, and each structure is housed within its own compartment (Fig. 1-14).[53] The lateral compartment contains the femoral artery, and the intermediate compartment contains the femoral vein, whereas the medial compartment contains the femoral canal. The femoral canal is the smallest of the compartments and contains lymph vessels, fat, and connective tissue. The femoral artery and vein bisect the triangle and enter the *adductor canal,* which is located in the middle third of the thigh between the vastus medialis and adductor muscles.[3]

THE PELVIC GIRDLE

Bones and Ligaments

The pelvis contains two innominate bones that are a fusion of the ilium, ischium, and pubis (Fig. 1-15). The female pelvis has a wider architecture and circular shape than the male pelvis (Fig. 1-16).[54] *Anteriorly,* the pubic bones form an amphiarthrodial, cartilaginous joint called the pubic symphysis with hyaline cartilage on the end of each pubic bone and an interpubic fibrocartilaginous disk that forms the joint.[3,55] The pubic symphysis is supported by four ligaments: the anterior pubic, posterior pubic, superior pubic, and inferior pubic.[56] This joint can be subject to overuse injury (e.g., osteitis pubis), as further discussed in Chapter 3. Along the lateral aspect of the innominate lies a deep socket called the acetabulum, which articulates with the femoral head to create the coxofemoral joint.[56] The hip joint is discussed later in this chapter.

Posteriorly, the ilium bones articulate at the sacrum to form the SI joint. The sacrum is shaped like an inverted triangle with the superior base (sacral promontory) formed by the first sacral vertebra, which contains two posterior facing facets that articulate with the inferior facets of the fifth lumbar vertebra to form the lumbosacral joint.[1] The articulation between L5 and S1 is supported by the iliolumbar ligaments, which connect L5 to the ilium.[3] The inferior apex is formed by the fifth sacral vertebra and contains small facets that articulate with the coccyx. The coccyx is a fusion of three to five vertebral rudiments and may be involved in trauma (i.e., fall) or may be a source of pain (i.e., coccydynia).[57] The precise anatomy and function of the coccygeal body and sacrococcygeal facet joints have been poorly studied and reported in the literature.[58] The articular surfaces of the SI joint (ilium and sacrum) are C shaped and covered with hyaline cartilage, with the sacral cartilage thicker than the ilial cartilage.[3,5]

The SI joint is a diarthrodial joint that possesses a unique combination of fibrocartilage and hyaline cartilage within a synovial capsule.[59,60] The joint is supported by the anterior and posterior SI ligaments (Fig. 1-17). The anterior SI ligament spans the anterior surface of the sacrum and ilium.[56] The posterior SI ligament spans the posterior surface between the sacrum and ilium and contains three regions: long, short, and interosseous.[3,56,60] The SI joint also receives support by the iliolumbar, sacrotuberous, and sacrospinous ligaments, respectively (see Fig. 1-17).[3] The SI joint is further supported by several abdominal core and hip muscles, including the latissimus dorsi, erector spinae, lumbar multifidus, rectus abdominis, internal oblique, external oblique, transversus abdominis, gluteus maximus, iliacus, piriformis, and biceps femoris.[1,5,60] These muscle work together to stabilize the SI joint.

Nerve Supply to the Pelvis

The pelvis is primarily innervated by the sacral plexus, coccygeal plexus, and pelvic region of the autonomic nervous system. All plexuses have both a sensory function and a motor function for a distinct area of the pelvis and lower extremities.[3] Each plexus and its corresponding nerves are discussed here.

Sacral Plexus

The sacral plexus resides on the posterior wall of the lesser pelvis close to the anterior surface of the piriformis muscle

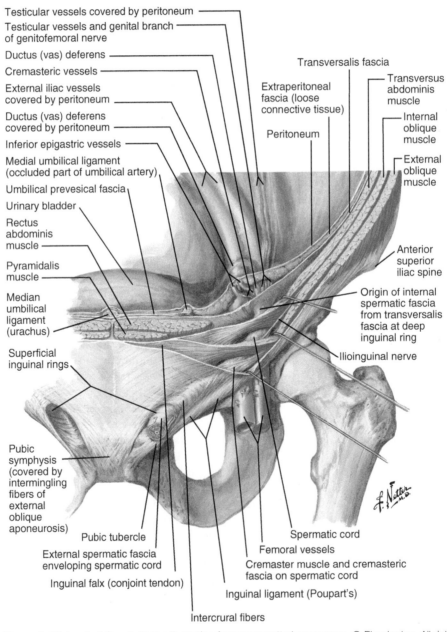

Testicular vessels covered by peritoneum
Testicular vessels and genital branch of genitofemoral nerve
Ductus (vas) deferens
Cremasteric vessels
External iliac vessels covered by peritoneum
Ductus (vas) deferens covered by peritoneum
Inferior epigastric vessels
Medial umbilical ligament (occluded part of umbilical artery)
Umbilical prevesical fascia
Urinary bladder
Rectus abdominis muscle
Pyramidalis muscle
Median umbilical ligament (urachus)
Superficial inguinal rings
Pubic symphysis (covered by intermingling fibers of external oblique aponeurosis)
Pubic tubercle
External spermatic fascia enveloping spermatic cord
Inguinal falx (conjoint tendon)
Intercrural fibers
Inguinal ligament (Poupart's)
Cremaster muscle and cremasteric fascia on spermatic cord
Femoral vessels
Spermatic cord
Ilioinguinal nerve
Origin of internal spermatic fascia from transversalis fascia at deep inguinal ring
Anterior superior iliac spine
External oblique muscle
Internal oblique muscle
Transversus abdominis muscle
Transversalis fascia
Extraperitoneal fascia (loose connective tissue)
Peritoneum

• **Figure 1-13** Inguinal Canal. (Netter illustration from www.netterimages.com. © Elsevier Inc. All rights reserved.)

(Fig. 1-18). Eight nerves emerge from the plexus, which include the sciatic, pudendal, superior gluteal, inferior gluteal, quadratus femoris, obturator internus, piriformis, and posterior cutaneous nerve of the thigh.

The sciatic nerve is formed by the ventral rami of L4 to S3 and provides motor and sensory innervation to the posterior lower limb, except for the medial side, which is innervated by the saphenous nerve.[61] The nerve passes through the greater sciatic foramen just below the piriformis muscle and descends down the posterior thigh to the popliteal fossa, where it bifurcates into the tibial and common peroneal (fibular) nerve. The tibial nerve provides motor innervation to the hamstrings (except for short head of biceps femoris) and muscles of the distal lower leg and foot. The nerve terminates at the foot as the medial and lateral plantar nerves. The common peroneal (fibular) nerve provides motor innervation to short head of biceps femoris and sensory innervation to the posterior leg and knee joint. The nerve further divides into the deep and superficial peroneal (fibular) nerves, which innervate the distal lower leg and foot.[3,61] In the proximal leg, the sciatic nerve contains articular branches that provide sensory innervation to hip joint.

The pudendal nerve is formed by the anterior divisions of the ventral rami of S2 to S4.[62] It passes with the pudendal artery through the greater sciatic foramen between the piriformis and coccygeus muscles. The pudendal nerve provides sensory innervation to the external genitalia and motor innervation to the perineal muscles, external urethral sphincter, and external anal sphincter.[3] *Entrapment of the pudendal nerve may be a cause of perineal pain.*[63,64] Chapter 9 provides a comprehensive discussion of this topic.

The superior gluteal nerve is formed by the posterior division of the ventral rami of L4 to S1 and exits the pelvis above the piriformis through the greater sciatic foramen, where it provides motor innervation to the gluteus medius, gluteus minimus, and tensor fasciae latae and sensory innervation to the hip joint.[3,65]

The inferior gluteal nerve is formed by the posterior divisions of the ventral rami of L5 to S2. It exits the pelvis

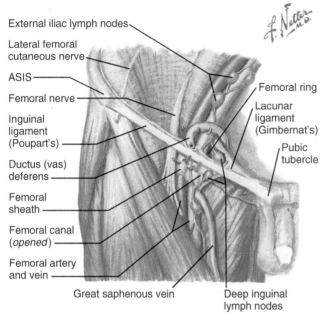

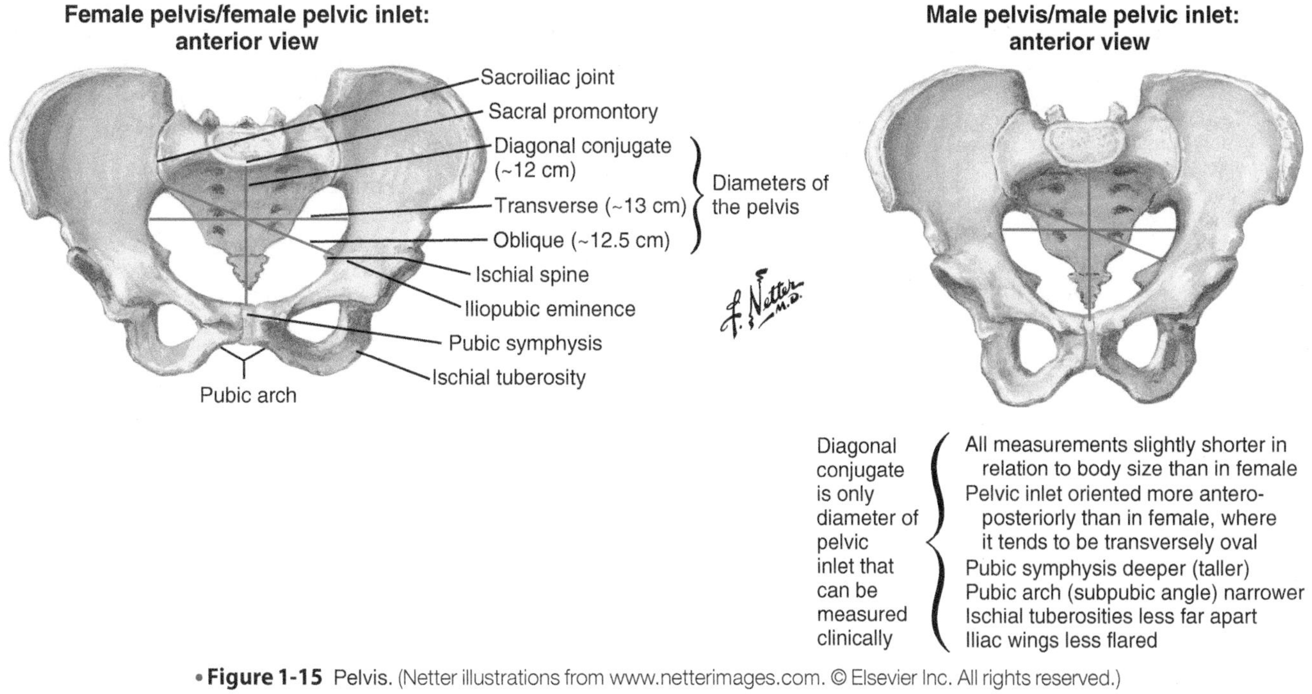

External iliac lymph nodes

Lateral femoral cutaneous nerve

ASIS

Femoral nerve

Inguinal ligament (Poupart's)

Ductus (vas) deferens

Femoral sheath

Femoral canal (*opened*)

Femoral artery and vein

Femoral ring

Lacunar ligament (Gimbernat's)

Pubic tubercle

Great saphenous vein

Deep inguinal lymph nodes

• **Figure 1-14** Femoral Triangle. *ASIS,* Anterior superior iliac spine. (Netter illustration from www.netterimages.com. © Elsevier Inc. All rights reserved.)

Female pelvis/female pelvic inlet: anterior view

Sacroiliac joint

Sacral promontory

Diagonal conjugate (~12 cm)

Transverse (~13 cm)

Oblique (~12.5 cm)

Diameters of the pelvis

Ischial spine

Iliopubic eminence

Pubic symphysis

Ischial tuberosity

Pubic arch

Male pelvis/male pelvic inlet: anterior view

Diagonal conjugate is only diameter of pelvic inlet that can be measured clinically

All measurements slightly shorter in relation to body size than in female
Pelvic inlet oriented more antero-posteriorly than in female, where it tends to be transversely oval
Pubic symphysis deeper (taller)
Pubic arch (subpubic angle) narrower
Ischial tuberosities less far apart
Iliac wings less flared

• **Figure 1-15** Pelvis. (Netter illustrations from www.netterimages.com. © Elsevier Inc. All rights reserved.)

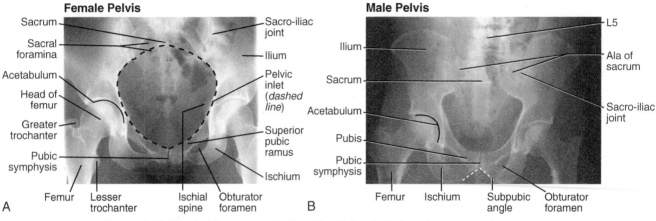

Female Pelvis

Sacrum
Sacral foramina
Acetabulum
Head of femur
Greater trochanter
Pubic symphysis
Femur
Lesser trochanter
Ischial spine
Obturator foramen
Sacro-iliac joint
Ilium
Pelvic inlet (*dashed line*)
Superior pubic ramus
Ischium

A

Male Pelvis

Ilium
Sacrum
Acetabulum
Pubis
Pubic symphysis
Femur
Ischium
Subpubic angle
Obturator foramen
L5
Ala of sacrum
Sacro-iliac joint

B

• **Figure 1-16** Female (**A**) versus male (**B**) pelvis. (Netter illustrations from www.netterimages.com. © Elsevier Inc. All rights reserved.)

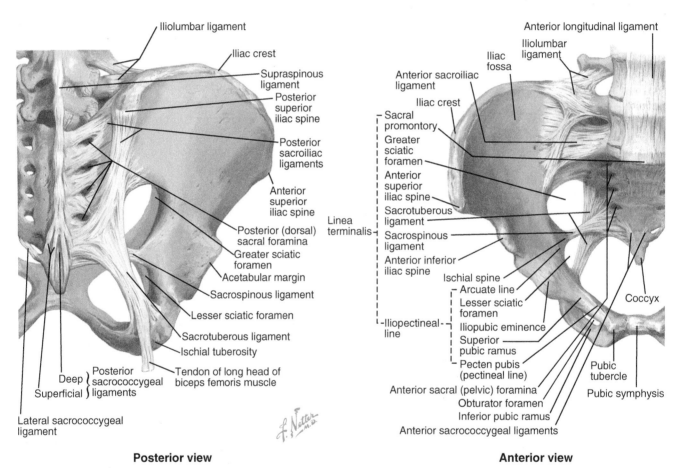

Posterior view

Iliolumbar ligament
Iliac crest
Supraspinous ligament
Posterior superior iliac spine
Posterior sacroiliac ligaments
Anterior superior iliac spine
Posterior (dorsal) sacral foramina
Greater sciatic foramen
Acetabular margin
Sacrospinous ligament
Lesser sciatic foramen
Sacrotuberous ligament
Ischial tuberosity
Deep / Superficial } Posterior sacrococcygeal ligaments
Tendon of long head of biceps femoris muscle
Lateral sacrococcygeal ligament

Anterior view

Anterior longitudinal ligament
Iliolumbar ligament
Iliac fossa
Anterior sacroiliac ligament
Iliac crest
Sacral promontory
Greater sciatic foramen
Anterior superior iliac spine
Sacrotuberous ligament
Sacrospinous ligament
Anterior inferior iliac spine
Ischial spine
Arcuate line
Lesser sciatic foramen
Iliopubic eminence
Superior pubic ramus
Pecten pubis (pectineal line)
Anterior sacral (pelvic) foramina
Obturator foramen
Inferior pubic ramus
Anterior sacrococcygeal ligaments
Linea terminalis
Iliopectineal line
Coccyx
Pubic tubercle
Pubic symphysis

• **Figure 1-17** Sacroiliac Ligaments. (Netter illustrations from www.netterimages.com. © Elsevier Inc. All rights reserved.)

below the piriformis, where it divides into several braches and provides motor innervation to the gluteus maximus muscle.

The **nerve to the quadratus femoris** is formed by the ventral rami of L4 to S1. It leaves the pelvis through the greater sciatic foramen to provide sensory innervation to the hip joint and motor innervation to the quadratus femoris and inferior gemellus muscles.[7]

The **nerve to the obturator internus** is formed by the ventral rami of L5 to S2. It enters the gluteal region through the greater sciatic foramen and lesser sciatic foremen to supply the superior gemellus and obturator internus muscles.

The **nerve to the piriformis** originates from the ventral divisions of S1 and S2. It enters the anterior surface of the piriformis muscle to provide motor innervation.[3]

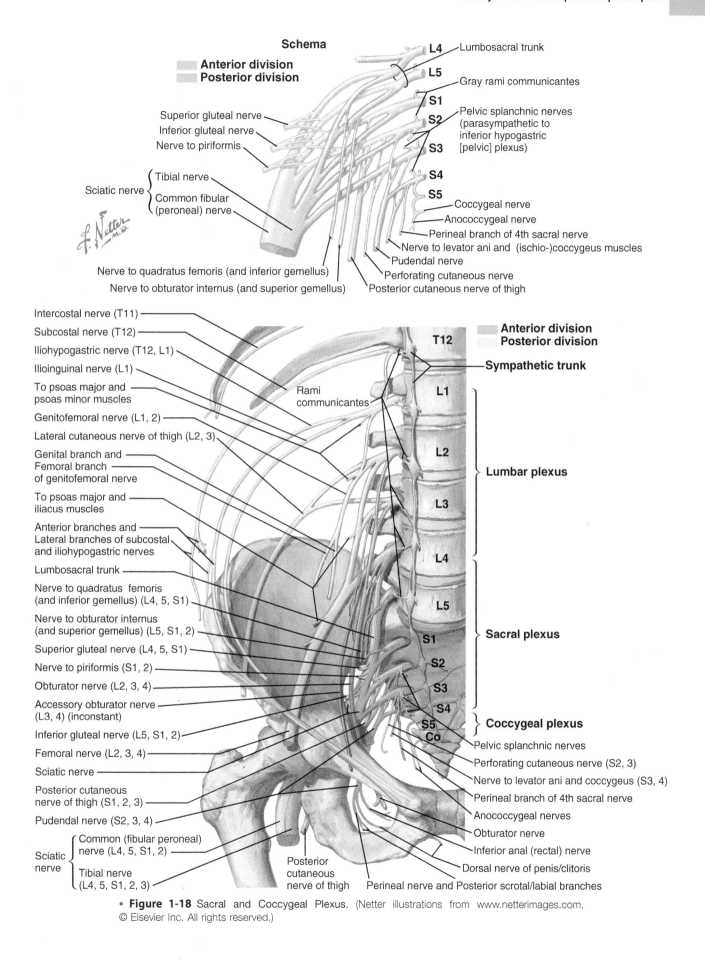

Schema

Anterior division
Posterior division

L4 — Lumbosacral trunk
L5
Gray rami communicantes
S1
S2 — Pelvic splanchnic nerves
(parasympathetic to
inferior hypogastric
[pelvic] plexus)
S3
S4
S5

Superior gluteal nerve
Inferior gluteal nerve
Nerve to piriformis

Sciatic nerve { Tibial nerve
Common fibular
(peroneal) nerve

Coccygeal nerve
Anococcygeal nerve
Perineal branch of 4th sacral nerve
Nerve to levator ani and (ischio-)coccygeus muscles
Pudendal nerve
Perforating cutaneous nerve
Posterior cutaneous nerve of thigh

Nerve to quadratus femoris (and inferior gemellus)
Nerve to obturator internus (and superior gemellus)

Intercostal nerve (T11)
Subcostal nerve (T12)
Iliohypogastric nerve (T12, L1)
Ilioinguinal nerve (L1)
To psoas major and
psoas minor muscles
Genitofemoral nerve (L1, 2)
Lateral cutaneous nerve of thigh (L2, 3)
Genital branch and
Femoral branch
of genitofemoral nerve
To psoas major and
iliacus muscles
Anterior branches and
Lateral branches of subcostal
and iliohypogastric nerves
Lumbosacral trunk
Nerve to quadratus femoris
(and inferior gemellus) (L4, 5, S1)
Nerve to obturator internus
(and superior gemellus) (L5, S1, 2)
Superior gluteal nerve (L4, 5, S1)
Nerve to piriformis (S1, 2)
Obturator nerve (L2, 3, 4)
Accessory obturator nerve
(L3, 4) (inconstant)
Inferior gluteal nerve (L5, S1, 2)
Femoral nerve (L2, 3, 4)
Sciatic nerve
Posterior cutaneous
nerve of thigh (S1, 2, 3)
Pudendal nerve (S2, 3, 4)
Sciatic
nerve { Common (fibular peroneal)
nerve (L4, 5, S1, 2)
Tibial nerve
(L4, 5, S1, 2, 3)

Rami
communicantes

T12
Anterior division
Posterior division
Sympathetic trunk
L1
L2
Lumbar plexus
L3
L4
L5
Sacral plexus
S1
S2
S3
S4
S5
Co
Coccygeal plexus
Pelvic splanchnic nerves
Perforating cutaneous nerve (S2, 3)
Nerve to levator ani and coccygeus (S3, 4)
Perineal branch of 4th sacral nerve
Anococcygeal nerves
Obturator nerve
Inferior anal (rectal) nerve
Dorsal nerve of penis/clitoris
Perineal nerve and Posterior scrotal/labial branches

Posterior
cutaneous
nerve of thigh

• **Figure 1-18** Sacral and Coccygeal Plexus. (Netter illustrations from www.netterimages.com.
© Elsevier Inc. All rights reserved.)

The posterior cutaneous nerve of the thigh (S1 to S3) is a branch of the sacral plexus. The nerve passes through the greater sciatic foramen to supply the skin over the buttocks, posterior thigh, and popliteal fossa. Table 1-1 provides a summary of the these nerves.[3]

Coccygeal Plexus

The coccygeal plexus is a small network of nerves formed by the ventral rami of S4 and S5 and the coccygeal nerves (see Fig. 1-18).[57] The network resides on the pelvic surface of the coccygeus and supplies this muscle, the levator ani, and sacrococcygeal joint.[3] The plexus also gives rise to the anococcygeal nerve, which pierces the sacrotuberous ligament to supply the subcutaneous tissue of the dorsal coccyx.[57] Woon and Stringer[57] conducted a cadaveric study of the coccygeal plexus with an interest in further studying its anatomy and potential role in coccyx pain or coccydynia. Their findings confirmed the role of the coccygeus plexus in providing nerve supply to the coccyx through the anococcygeal nerve and suggested that the plexus should be considered a potential source of pain in persons who suffer from coccydynia.[57] Further studies are needed to substantiate this theory. Chapter 10 provides more in-depth discussion of coccydynia.

Autonomic Nerves

The autonomic nerves that innervate the pelvis include the sacral sympathetic trunks, hypogastric plexus, and pelvic splanchnic nerves.[3] The primary role of the sacral sympathetic trunk is to provide sympathetic innervation to the lower limb, including vasomotor, pilomotor, and sudomotor. The hypogastric plexus provides autonomic innervation to the rectum, prostate, seminal vesicles, and inferolateral surface of the bladder in males. In females, the plexus provides innervation to the cervix and lateral fornices of the vagina, as well as to the inferolateral bladder.[3] The pelvic splanchnic nerves contain parasympathetic fibers derived from S2 to S4 spinal segments and visceral afferent fibers that merge with the hypogastric plexus to provide both parasympathetic and sympathetic innervation to the pelvic viscera.[3]

Blood Supply to the Pelvis

Arterial blood supply to the pelvis is provided by four main arteries: the internal iliac, gonadal, median sacral, and superior rectal arteries.[3,7] The abdominal aorta descends to approximately the level of L3 to L4 and bifurcates into the left and right common iliac arteries (Fig. 1-19). The internal iliac artery is a branch of the common iliac artery and supplies blood to the pelvis, buttocks, medial thigh, and perineum.[3] The internal iliac artery has an anterior division and posterior division. The anterior division includes eight branches: the umbilical, obturator, inferior vesical, middle rectal artery, vaginal, uterine, inferior gluteal, and internal

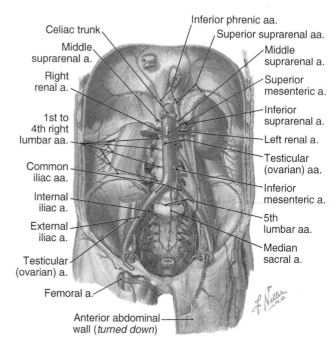

• **Figure 1-19** Pelvic Arteries. *a.,* Artery; *aa.,* arteries. (Netter illustration from www.netterimages.com. © Elsevier Inc. All rights reserved.)

pudendal arteries. The posterior division includes three branches: the superior gluteal, iliolumbar, and lateral sacral arteries. The ovarian artery arises from the abdominal aorta, supplies the ovary and uterine tubes, and is considered to be paired with the internal iliac artery. The median sacral artery arises from the posterior surface of the aorta above the bifurcation at L4.[3,7] This artery anastomoses with the lateral sacral arteries and the superior and inferior rectal arteries and supplies the posterior rectum.[3] The superior rectal artery is a continuation of the superior mesenteric artery, which arises from the anterior surface of the abdominal aorta. The artery bifurcates at the level of S3 and descends on each side to supply the rectum down to the internal sphincter. The superior rectal artery anastomoses with the middle and inferior rectal arteries.[3]

Venous return occurs primarily from the internal iliac veins and their corresponding branches. Blood is also drained by the ovarian, superior rectal, and median rectal veins. The internal iliac veins joins the external iliac veins to form the common iliac veins that unify to become the inferior vena cava at the L5 vertebral level.[3,7]

Muscles of the Pelvis

The muscles of the pelvis can be described based on their location in the anterior, lateral, posterior, and inferior aspects of the pelvis. The anterior pelvis contains no distinct muscles. The right and left lateral pelvis contains the obturator internus muscle, which is innervated by L5 with a main action of lateral femoral rotation. The posterior pelvis contains the piriformis muscles, which are innervated by the ventral rami of S1 and S2 and have main actions of lateral femoral rotation and abduction. The piriformis

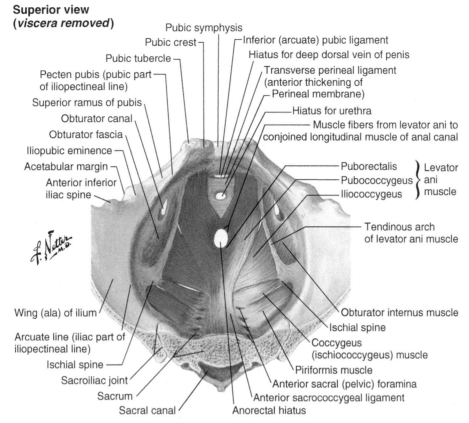

Superior view (*viscera removed*)

• **Figure 1-20** Pelvic Floor Muscles. (Netter illustration from www.netterimages.com. © Elsevier Inc. All rights reserved.)

muscle is also part of the deep external rotator group of the hip, as discussed in the next section. The inferior pelvis (i.e., pelvic floor) contains the pelvic diaphragm, which spans the pubis anteriorly, both lateral pelvic walls, and the coccyx posteriorly.[54] The pelvic diaphragm consists of the levator ani and coccygeus muscles (S2 to S4) (Fig. 1-20).[66] The levator ani group (pubococcygeus, puborectalis, and iliococcygeus) attaches to the internal surface of the lesser pelvis and forms most of the pelvic floor.[54,67] The coccygeus muscle has a proximal attachment on the ischial spine and a distal attachment to the inferior sacrum.[68] The pelvic diaphragm plays a large role in compressing the abdominal and pelvic content by raising the pelvic floor, an important action for forced expiration, urination, defecation, and fixation of the trunk during forceful lifting.[3,54,67] Pathologic conditions of the pelvic diaphragm can result from trauma or muscle weakness. Chapter 9 provides a comprehensive discussion of common pathologic conditions of this region, and Table 1-3 provides a summary of these muscles.

Hip Joint

The hip joint, or coxofemoral joint, is a diarthrodial ball and socket joint with a synovial capsule. It is composed of the acetabulum and the head of the femur and allows for three degrees of freedom.[3] Various congenital and development disorders may cause an abnormally shaped acetabu-

lum or malaligned hip joint (femur and acetabular alignment; see Chapter 7). The relevant hip joint anatomy is discussed here.

Acetabulum

The acetabulum (Fig. 1-21) is formed by the union of the ilium and ischium (75%) and the pubis (25%), which create a deep socket that is oriented laterally, inferiorly, and anteriorly.[1,69] The acetabulum commonly projects laterally with a certain degree of anterior and inferior tilt that is commonly called acetabular version. This tilt is measured by two methods. First, the center-edge angle is a measurement of the acetabular orientation in the frontal plane in relation to the pelvis and averages approximately 35 degrees in adults.[1] A decreased center-edge angle reduces acetabular coverage, thus increasing the risk for hip dislocation or other degenerative disorders.[70] Second, the angle of acetabular anteversion is a measurement of the acetabulum within the horizontal plane in relation to the pelvis. The average angle is approximately 20 degrees for both sexes (18.5 degrees for men and 21.5 degrees for women).[5] Excessive acetabular anteversion exposes the hip anteriorly and increases the risk of anterior dislocations or trauma to the anterior labrum.[1,70] Excessive acetabular retroversion has been linked to femoral acetabular impingement (FAI) and slipped capital femoral epiphysis.[71,72] The lunate surface of

TABLE 1-3 Muscles of the Pelvis

Muscle	Peripheral Nerve	Pelvic Region	Origin	Insertion	Action
Obturator internus	Nerve to Obturator (L5-S2)	Lateral pelvis	Ilium and ischium (pelvic surface), obturator membrane	Greater trochanter	Femoral lateral rotation
Piriformis	Nerve to piriformis (S1-2)	Posterior pelvis	Pelvic surface of sacrum and sacrotuberous ligament	Greater trochanter	Femoral lateral rotation
Levator ani (pubococcygeus, puborectalis, and iliococcygeus)	Nerve to levator ani (S4) and inferior rectal nerve and coccygeal plexus	Pelvic floor	Pubic body, tendinous arch of obturator fascia, and spine of ischium	Perineal body, coccyx, anococcygeal ligament, walls of prostate or vagina, rectum, and anal canal	Supports pelvic viscera and resists intraabdominal pressure
Coccygeus (ischiococcygeus)	Branches of S4 and S5	Pelvic floor	Ischial spine	Inferior sacrum	Forms small part of pelvic diaphragm. See above

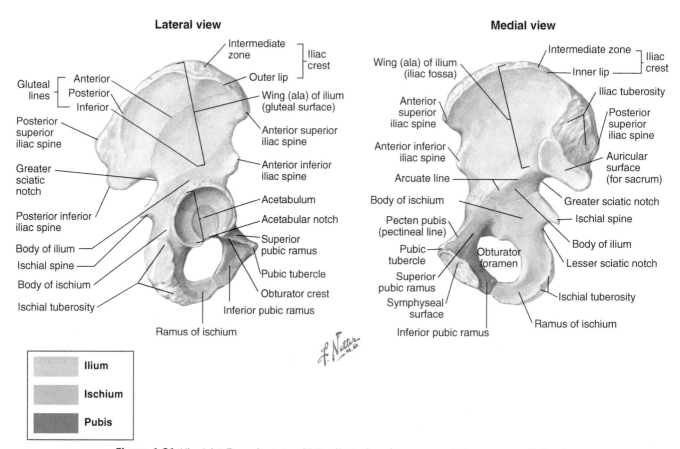

Lateral view

Medial view

• **Figure 1-21** Hip Joint Bony Anatomy. (Netter illustrations from www.netterimages.com. © Elsevier Inc. All rights reserved.)

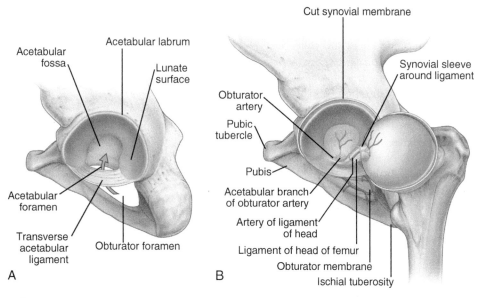

• **Figure 1-22** Acetabulum Anatomy. (From Drake R, Vogl AW, Mitchell AWM. *Gray's Anatomy for Students.* 4th ed. Philadelphia: Churchill Livingstone; 2015.)

the acetabulum articulates with the femur and is composed of hyaline cartilage (Fig. 1-22). Because the superior lunate surface is the primary weight-bearing surface of the acetabulum, it may be more susceptible to degenerative changes. The inferior region of the acetabulum contains the acetabular notch, as well as the transverse acetabular ligament.

The acetabular branch of the obturator artery provides arterial blood to the acetabulum through the acetabular notch, and the pubic branches supply the pelvic surface of the acetabulum. The deep branches of the superior gluteal artery supply the superior acetabular region, and the inferior gluteal artery supplies the posteroinferior region.[73] Venous return is accomplished by their corresponding veins.[5]

Acetabular Labrum

The acetabular labrum is a fibrocartilaginous ring that surrounds the edge of the acetabulum and is completed by the transverse acetabular ligament inferiorly over the acetabular notch (see Fig. 1-22).[3,69] The acetabular labrum can be divided into four distinct regions: superior, anterior, inferior, and posterior. The acetabular labrum is commonly triangular in cross section and is composed primarily of type I collagen fibers. These fibers are principally oriented parallel to the acetabular rim, with some fiber running obliquely.[74,75] In general, the labrum is 2 to 3 mm thick, and the anterior region is thinner and wider than the posterior region.[69,75,76] The acetabular labrum is believed to be primarily avascular, with only the outer periphery receiving blood supply from the obturator, superior gluteal, and inferior gluteal arteries.[69,77,78] The acetabular labrum does receive sensory nerve innervation. Haversath and associates[79] conducted a histologic investigation of the labrum and found pain-related free nerve endings in the inferior region of the labrum. Alzaharani and colleagues,[80] through an in vitro investigation, also found a high level of pain-related free nerve endings and nerve end organs in the anterosuperior and posterosuperior zones that play a role in pain and proprioception. The acetabular labrum creates a joint fluid seal and aids in joint stability, shock absorption, lubrication, load distribution, contact stress, increase in the surface area, and deepening of the acetabulum by approximately 28%.[69,74,75,81,82]

Different regions of the acetabular labrum can be subject to different forces or strains by certain hip motions. Safran and associates[83] examined strains across the acetabular labrum during various hip motions in cadaveric models. These investigators found that the greatest strain to the anterior labrum occurred in hip flexion with adduction. The anterolateral labrum had the greatest strain in full extension, followed by external rotation, and the least strain in neutral and internal rotation.[83,84] The posterior labrum undergoes the greatest strain in hip flexion, in adduction, or in neutral abduction and adduction. The lateral labrum undergoes the greatest strain at 90 degrees of flexion with abduction, external rotation, or neutral rotation.[83] Understanding how the labrum is strained during specific hip motions may provide a better understanding of the pathophysiology of labral tears and may therefore lead to more effective preventive strategies.

Several researchers also examined strains across the acetabular labrum during hip impingement test positions used to diagnose anterior or posterior labral disorders. In anterior disorders, the positions of flexion, adduction, and internal rotation caused the most strain to the anterolateral labrum and decreased posterior labral strain.[78,83] In posterior disorders, the positions of external rotation, full extension, and neutral flexion and extension caused the greatest strain to the posterior labrum while decreasing the anterolateral strain.[83,85]

Other factors such as pelvic position and posture have been associated with excessive loading of the hip joint and potential acetabular labral disorders. Ross and colleagues[86] found that dynamic pelvic anterior tilting is a predictor of earlier occurrences of FAI, whereas posterior pelvic tilt results in a later occurrence. These findings were also supported by Lewis and associates,[87-89] who found that anterior hip joint forces increase during gait with a swayback posture because the hip is in more extension. Pelvic position and posture may be potential causes of hip pain and disorders.

In the presence of acetabular labrum damage, joint destabilization may occur that eventually leads to degenerative changes and hip osteoarthrosis.[77,90] In particular, the anterior region of the labrum may be susceptible to damage from certain pathologic conditions such as FAI (see Chapter 4).[77] Tannast and colleagues[90] and McCarthy and associates[77] found, through retrospective, cadaveric, and surgical investigations, that the anterior portion of the labrum suffers the most damage when compared with other regions. This finding may reflect the inherent weakness of the anterior region, poor vascularity, or increased mechanical forces (i.e., torsional activities) in the anterior labrum.[69,75,77,89]

Femur

The femoral head is round, covered in hyaline cartilage, and articulates with the acetabulum.[3,5] The superior region is the primary weight-bearing surface; however, degenerative changes occur mostly to the periphery of the articular surface, around or below the fovea. The ligamentum teres connects the acetabulum to the femoral head through the fovea.[3,5] The femoral head transitions to the femoral neck, which is attached to the femoral shaft (see Fig. 1-21). The femoral head also contain the epiphysis, which encompasses a growth plate. Pathologic slippage of the epiphysis (i.e., slipped capital femoral epiphysis) can occur in adolescents (see Chapter 7).

The femoral head and neck form an angle of inclination that is approximately 150 degrees during infancy, decreases to 125 degrees in adulthood, and further decreases to 120 degrees in old age.[3,5] A pathologic increase in the angle (>125 degrees) of inclination is called coxa valga, and a pathologic decrease is termed coxa vara (<125 degrees) (Fig. 1-23).[5]

The femoral head and neck also form an angle of torsion, which is often called femoral anteversion or version (Fig. 1-24).[1,5,91,92] Anteversion refers to the more anterior position of the femur in relation to the transcondylar axis, and retroversion refers to the more posterior position. The angle of torsion has been described in two ways: (1) observed from above, it is the angle between an imaginary transverse line passing through the center of the femoral head and neck; and (2) it is the angular measurement of the axis of the femoral neck in relation to the condyles at the distal femur.[93,94] The angle of torsion is an average 31 degrees in the newborn and decreases with age.[94] The average angle of torsion in the adult ranges from 8 to 15 degrees but may

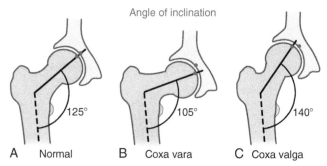

• **Figure 1-23 A** to **C,** Femur angle of inclination. (From Neumann DA. *Kinesiology of the Musculoskeletal System: Foundations for Rehabilitation.* 2nd ed. St. Louis: Mosby; 2010.)

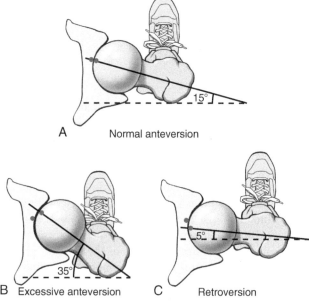

• **Figure 1-24 A** to **C,** Femur angle of torsion. (From Neumann DA. *Kinesiology of the Musculoskeletal System: Foundations for Rehabilitation.* 2nd ed. St. Louis: Mosby; 2010.)

vary.[5,93-95] A pathologic increase in the angle of torsion is often called excessive femoral anteversion, and a decrease is called retroversion.

The amount of femoral version may have an influence on femoral range of motion and the risk for FAI and labral tears. Excessive femoral anteversion has been related to higher degrees internal rotation, and excessive retroversion has been related to higher degrees of femoral external rotation range of motion.[70,91] Ejnisman and colleagues[91] found, through radiographic and intraoperative findings, that patients diagnosed with FAI and femoral anteversion greater than 15 degrees were 2.2 times more likely to have large tears (average, 38 mm) in the anterior labrum. Patients with hip anteversion of less than 5 degrees had smaller labral tears (average, 30 mm). Decreased femoral anteversion has also been associated with slipped capital femoral epiphysis in adolescents.[91]

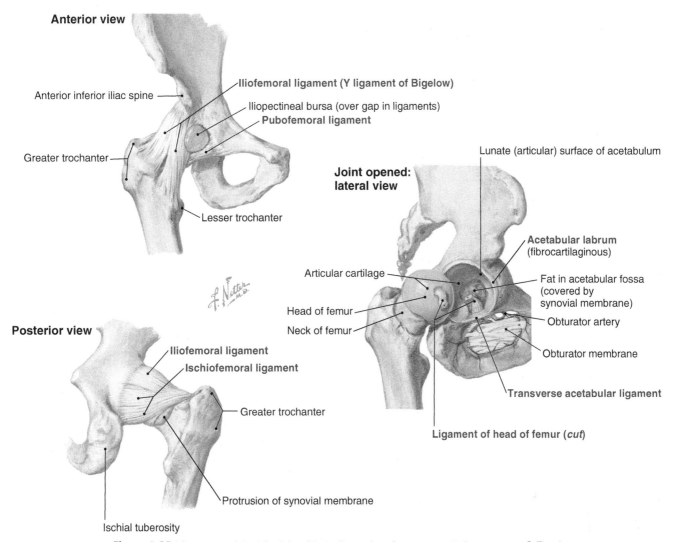

• **Figure 1-25** Ligaments of the Hip Joint. (Netter illustrations from www.netterimages.com. © Elsevier Inc. All rights reserved.)

Ligaments of the Hip Joint

The stability of the hip joint is also enforced by six ligaments. The most superficial ligaments include the iliofemoral (Y-ligament), ischiofemoral, and pubofemoral (Fig. 1-25). The iliofemoral ligament becomes taut with hip extension, external rotation, and adduction. Both the ischiofemoral and pubofemoral ligaments become taut during hip extension, abduction, and external rotation (Table 1-4).[1,3] Injury to these ligaments can occur with repetitive rotational activities such as dance (see Chapter 8). The acetabulum is attached to the head of the femur by the ligamentum teres, which runs beneath the transverse acetabular ligament to the head of the femur (fovea).[96] The ligamentum teres (ligament of head or femur) is taut during hip external rotation and lax during internal rotation and when the hip is in neutral.[96] The ligamentum teres has a role in hip stability, nociception, proprioception, and coordination of movement, as well as in providing blood supply to the femoral head.[96] The ligamentum teres can also

be damaged from trauma to the hip joint that could result in persistent pain.[97] It has been postulated that injury can occur from a combination of hip hyperabduction and excessive external or internal rotation.[96,97] The synovial joint also contains a capsular ligament that spans the neck of the

TABLE 1-4	Ligaments of the Hip Joint	
Ligaments	**Function**
Ligamentum teres	Tightens during external rotation, adduction, and flexion
Iliofemoral ligament	Tightens during external rotation, adduction, and extension
Ischiofemoral ligament	Tightens during external rotation, abduction, and extension
Pubofemoral ligament	Tightens during external rotation, abduction, and extension

femur to the acetabulum. The last ligament of interest is the transverse acetabular ligament that spans the lower portion of the acetabulum and creates a foramen for blood vessels that supply the femur.[56]

Blood Supply to the Hip Joint

As mentioned earlier, the abdominal aorta descends to approximately the level of L3 to L4 and bifurcates into the left and right common iliac arteries (see Fig. 1-19). The internal iliac artery is a continuation of the common iliac artery and supplies blood to the pelvis, buttocks, medial thigh, and perineum.[3,7] The external iliac artery is another branch of the common iliac artery that provides blood supply to the lower limb. The external iliac artery becomes the femoral artery as it enters the thigh through the superior femoral triangle.[3] The proximal femoral artery contains four branches that supply the hip joint and musculoskeletal structures: the deep artery of the thigh, obturator artery, medial circumflex femoral artery, and lateral circumflex femoral artery (Fig. 1-26). The deep artery of the thigh supplies the adductor magnus and hamstring muscles.[3,7] The retinacular, or circumflex, arteries contain two branches to supply blood to the femoral head and thigh. The medial circumflex artery may be a branch of either the deep artery of the thigh or the femoral artery. The artery supplies blood to the femoral head and neck and also supplies the posterior thigh.[3,7] The medial circumflex artery may be damage from trauma such as hip dislocations or fractures (see Chapter 11). The lateral circumflex artery, which may also be a branch of the deep or femoral artery, divides into branches that supply blood to the femoral head and lateral thigh region. If the retinacular arteries are damaged by trauma such as femoral fracture, avascular necrosis of the femoral head may result.[98] The femoral artery also enters the adductor canal, transcends distally, and exits the adductor hiatus to become the popliteal artery.[3]

The obturator artery may be a branch of the internal iliac artery or inferior epigastric artery and assists the deep artery (femoral branch) with supplying blood to the adductor muscles. The obturator artery also has a posterior branch that supplies blood to the femoral head. Finally, the ligamentum teres also provides blood supply to the head of the femur through a small artery (see Fig. 1-26).

Venous drainage of the lower limb occurs from several ascending superficial and deep vessels and their related tributaries. The main superficial vessels include the great and small saphenous veins. The main deep vessels include the iliac, epigastric, femoral, popliteal, peroneal, and tibial veins.[3,7] All the vessels and their tributaries help carry deoxygenated blood from the lower extremity back to the heart. At the level of L5, the external iliac veins receive blood from the lower extremity, pelvis, and lower abdomen and join the internal iliac vein, which drains the pelvic region. This union eventually forms the common iliac veins, which, in turn, unify to form the inferior vena cava that ascends to the heart.[3,7]

Nerve Supply to the Hip Joint

The anterior section of the hip joint capsule receives sensory nerve innervation from the articular branches of the femoral nerve, and the anteromedial joint capsule receives sensory innervation from the articular branches of the obturator nerve. The posterior and posteromedial hip joint capsule receives sensory innervation from the articular branches of

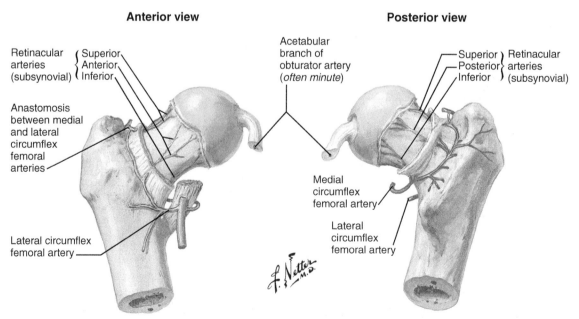

• **Figure 1-26** Arterial Supply to the Hip. (Netter illustrations from www.netterimages.com. © Elsevier Inc. All rights reserved.)

the sciatic nerve and the nerve to the quadratus femoris. The posterolateral joint capsule receives sensory innervation from the articular branches of the superior gluteal nerve.[3,99] The reader is referred to the earlier discussions on the lumbar and sacral plexuses to review nerves that innervate the hip joint. The reader is also referred to Table 1-1, which provides a summary of the major nerves.

Muscles of the Hip Joint

The hip joint contains many muscles that work together to move the joint in three planes of motion. The physiologic movements of the hip and corresponding muscles are discussed here. This section intends to provide a brief overview of the muscular anatomy, and the reader is referred to the reference list for more comprehensive discussions of these muscles.

The flexors of the hip are located along the anterior aspect of the hip joint (Fig. 1-27). The primary muscles involved in hip flexion include the iliopsoas, rectus femoris, tensor fasciae latae, pectineus, adductor longus, and sartorius. The adductor brevis, gracilis, and gluteus minimus (anterior fibers) muscles assist in hip flexion.[1,100] The ilio-

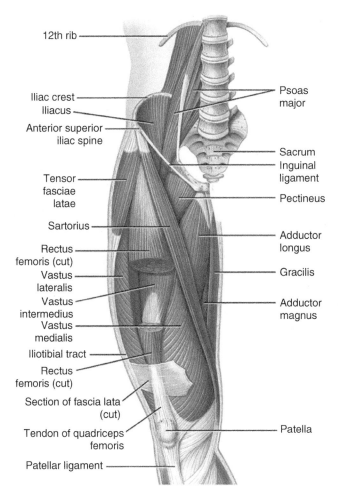

• Figure 1-27 Anterior Hip Muscles (Flexors). (From Tortora GJ, Derrickson BH. *Introduction to the Human Body.* 10th ed. Hoboken, NJ: John Wiley & Sons; 2015.)

psoas muscle can be involved in certain pathologic conditions such as internal snapping hip syndrome (i.e., coxa sultans) that could be a source of anterior hip pain (see Chapter 3).[101]

The extensors of the hip are located along the posterior aspect of the thigh and include the gluteus maximus, hamstrings (biceps femoris, semimembranosus, semitendinosus), and adductor magnus (posterior head). The adductor magnus (anterior head) and gluteus medius (posterior fibers) assist with hip extension (Fig. 1-28).[1,3,100] Injuries to the hamstrings are among the most common disorders in athletes and active persons that may result in severe functional deficits.[102] Chapter 3 discusses the management of proximal hamstring injuries.

The abductors of the hip are located along the lateral aspect of the thigh (Fig. 1-29). The primary muscles involved include the gluteus medius, gluteus minimus, and tensor fasciae latae, as well as the piriformis and sartorius.[1,100] The tensor fasciae latae and the tendon of the gluteus maximus merge distally into the iliotibial track or band. The iliotibial tract is a band of fibrous tissue that travels down the lateral thigh, over the femoral condyle, and attaches to the Gerdy tubercle on the anterolateral aspect of the tibia.[103] The iliotibial band has been linked to injuries in runners and is often classified as a source of lateral hip and thigh pain (knee pain), as discussed in Chapter 3.[104,105]

The adductors of the hip are located along the medial aspect of the thigh. The primary muscles involved include the adductor group (longus, brevis, and magnus), gracilis, and pectineus (see Fig. 1-29).[1,100] The biceps femoris (long head), gluteus maximus (lower fibers), and quadratus femoris assist with hip adduction.[1,3] Adductor-related groin pain is common in sports such as ice hockey and soccer (see Chapter 3), and it may be related to athletic pubalgia (see Chapter 5).[106]

The external rotators of the hip are located along the posterolateral aspect of the hip. The muscles involved include the gluteus maximus and six deep rotators: piriformis, obturator externus (origin: lateral pelvis), obturator internus, gemellus superior, gemellus inferior, and quadratus femoris (see Fig. 1-28).[1,3,100] The gluteus medius (posterior fibers), gluteus minimus (posterior fibers), sartorius, and biceps femoris (long head) assist with hip external rotation.[1,100] Weakness of the hip external rotators and abductors has been linked to several lower kinetic chain disorders such as chronic hip pain[107] and patellofemoral dysfunction.[108]

The internal rotators of the hip are located along the anterolateral aspect the hip. The muscles involved include the gluteus medius (anterior fibers), gluteus minimus (anterior fibers), and tensor fasciae latae. The adductor longus, adductor brevis, and pectineus assist with hip internal rotation.[1] Because force produced during external hip rotation is greater than that produced during internal rotation, rotational hip control is a focus of many rehabilitation programs. Table 1-5 provides a summary of the muscles and related movements.[1]

Superficial dissection   **Deeper dissection**

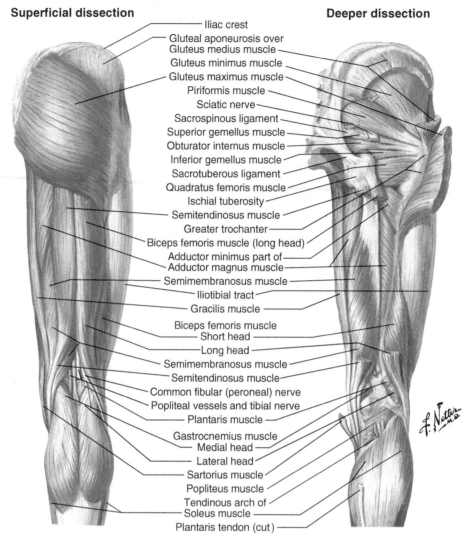

Iliac crest
Gluteal aponeurosis over
Gluteus medius muscle
Gluteus minimus muscle
Gluteus maximus muscle
Piriformis muscle
Sciatic nerve
Sacrospinous ligament
Superior gemellus muscle
Obturator internus muscle
Inferior gemellus muscle
Sacrotuberous ligament
Quadratus femoris muscle
Ischial tuberosity
Semitendinosus muscle
Greater trochanter
Biceps femoris muscle (long head)
Adductor minimus part of
Adductor magnus muscle
Semimembranosus muscle
Iliotibial tract
Gracilis muscle
Biceps femoris muscle
Short head
Long head
Semimembranosus muscle
Semitendinosus muscle
Common fibular (peroneal) nerve
Popliteal vessels and tibial nerve
Plantaris muscle
Gastrocnemius muscle
Medial head
Lateral head
Sartorius muscle
Popliteus muscle
Tendinous arch of
Soleus muscle
Plantaris tendon (cut)

• **Figure 1-28** Posterior Hip Muscles (Extensors). (Netter illustrations from www.netterimages.com.)

MOVEMENT OF THE LUMBOPELVIC HIP REGION

Lumbar Spine

The lumbar spine provides three planes of movement and has a primary role of weight-bearing support for the upper part of the body. The approximate range of motion for isolated flexion is 40 to 50 degrees, for extension is 15 to 20 degrees, for axial rotation is 5 to 7 degrees, and for lateral flexion is 20 degrees.[1] Because of facet orientation, the lumbar vertebrae are limited with rotation and lateral flexion from L1 to L4. The facets allow more movement with flexion and extension, with the greatest mobility occurring between L4 and S1.[109] The largest amount of lateral flexion and rotation occurs between L2 and L3.[5] Lumbar vertebral motion is often described as a coupled

motion, which was first introduced by Lovett in the early 1900s and was popularized by Freyette in the 1950s.[110] Freyette explained that when the lumbar spine is in neutral, side bending and rotation occur in opposite directions (type I). If the spine is flexed or extended, side bending and rotation will occur in the same direction because of the facets (type II). Since Freyette's publication of these motions, other researchers have conducted in vivo and in vitro investigations that have produced mixed results. To date, no consensus exists on lumbar spine–coupled motions in neutral, flexion, or extension.[110-113] The lumbar spine has an interdependence with the pelvis and the hip, and these structures are often examined together, as discussed later.

Pelvis and Sacroiliac Joint

The pelvis also provides several motions, including anterior tilting, posterior tilting, and right and left rotation. The SI joint's unique wedge shape allows small amounts of

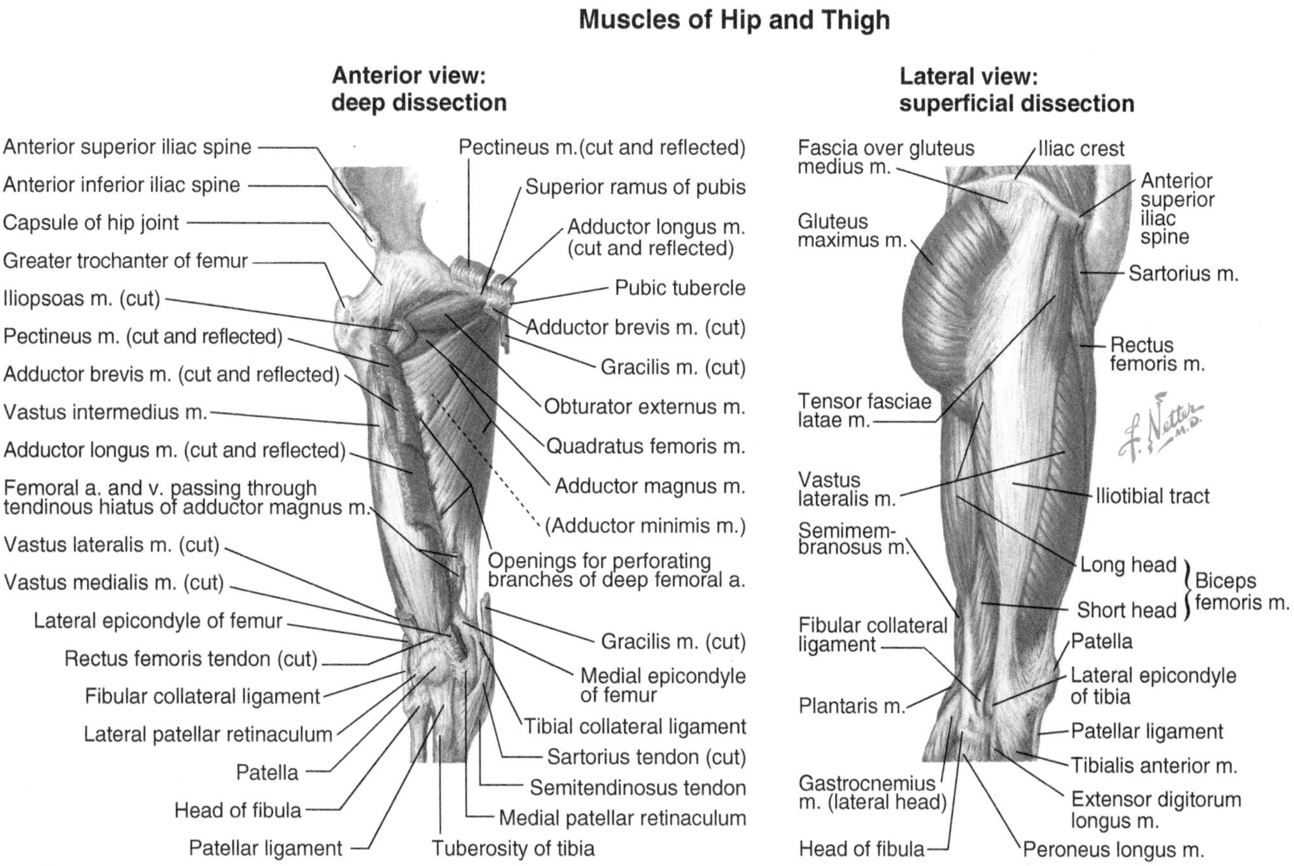

Muscles of Hip and Thigh

• **Figure 1-29** Lateral and Medial Thigh Muscles. *a.*, Artery; *m.*, muscle; *v.*, vein. (Netter illustrations from www.netterimages.com. © Elsevier Inc. All rights reserved.)

TABLE 1-5 Hip Muscles and Actions*

	Flexors	Adductors	Internal Rotators	Extensors	Abductors	External Rotators
Primary	Iliopsoas Sartorius Tensor fasciae latae Adductor longus Pectineus	Pectineus Adductor longus Gracilis Adductor brevis Adductor magnus	Not applicable	Gluteus maximus Biceps femoris (long head) Semitendinosus Adductor magnus (posterior head)	Gluteus medius Gluteus minimus Tensor fasciae latae	Gluteus maximus Piriformis Obturator internus Gemellus superior Gemellus interior Quadratus femoris
Secondary	Adductor brevis Gracilis Gluteus minimus (anterior fibers)	Biceps femoris (long head) Gluteus maximus (lower fibers) Quadratus femoris	Gluteus minimus (anterior fibers) Gluteus medius (anterior fibers) Adductor longus Adductor brevis Pectineus	Gluteus medius (posterior fibers) Adductor magnus (anterior head)	Piriformis Sartorius	Gluteus medius (posterior fibers) Obturator externus Sartorius Biceps femoris (long head)

From Neumann DA. *Kinesiology of the Musculoskeletal System: Foundations for Rehabilitation.* 2nd ed. St. Louis: Mosby; 2010.
*Each action assumes a muscle contraction that originates from the anatomic position. Several of these muscles may have a different action when they contract from a position other than the anatomic position.

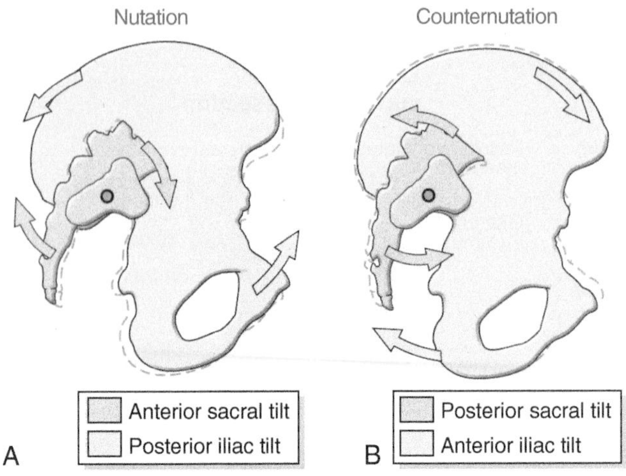

• **Figure 1-30 A** and **B,** Sacroiliac joint movement. (From Neumann DA. *Kinesiology of the Musculoskeletal System: Foundations for Rehabilitation.* 2nd ed. St. Louis: Mosby; 2010.)

rotational and translational motion. It has been reported that sacroiliac rotation occurs from 1 to 4 degrees and anteroposterior translation from 1 to 2 mm.[114] When the pelvis or innominate bones move in the sagittal plane, this motion causes the SI joint also to move. The two commonly used terms for movement of the sacrum in relation to the ilium are nutation and counternutation (Fig. 1-30). Nutation occurs when the sacral promontory moves anteriorly and inferiorly while the coccyx moves posteriorly. This motion is in relation to posterior tilting of the ilium.[1,5] The torque caused by nutation creates a stabilizing force to the SI joint as a result of gravity, passive tension from the stretched ligaments, and muscle activation (see the earlier section on the SI joint).[1,5] Nutation also reduces the anteroposterior diameter of the pelvic brim and increases the pelvic outlet. Counternutation occurs when the promontory moves posteriorly and superiorly while the coccyx moves anteriorly. This is in relation to anterior tilting of the ilium. This movement increases the anteroposterior diameter of the pelvic brim and decreases the pelvic outlet and stabilizing forces.[1,5]

Hip Joint

The hip joint also provides three degrees of freedom, which is described by six osteokinematic motions: flexion, extension, abduction, adduction, internal rotation, and external rotation (Fig. 1-31). The average passive range of osteokinematic motion in the sagittal plane includes flexion of 120 degrees (knee flexed), flexion of 70 to 80 degrees (knee straight), and extension of 20 degrees.[1] The average range of motion in the frontal plane includes abduction of 40 degrees and adduction of 25 degrees. The average range of motion in the transverse plane includes internal rotation to 35 degrees and external rotation to 45 degrees.[1,5] These values may vary depending on whether the hip is in a flexed

or extended position or is actively moved. Normal gait requires a minimum of 30 degrees of hip flexion, 10 degrees of extension, 5 degrees of abduction and adduction, and 5 degrees of internal and external rotation.[1,5]

The arthrokinematic properties of the hip joint are determined by the concave acetabular and convex femur. Motion occurs at the joint surface by spinning and gliding of the femur and acetabulum. The hip joint does contain small amounts of arthrokinematic movement in which joint mobilization may have an effect. Loubert and associates[115] looked at the amount of femoral translation glide during manual posteriorly directed joint mobilization at a force equal to 50% of the subject's body weight while concurrent ultrasound imaging was performed. The investigators found the translational gliding of the femur to be small. The average posterior femoral translation glide was 2.0 mm, and the average tangential glide required for hip flexion passive range of motion was 53.8 mm. Thus, the amplitude of glide is small for the hip joint.[115]

The hip joint's open packed position includes 30 degrees of flexion, 30 degrees of abduction, and 0 to 5 degrees of external rotation.[116] Hip posterior dislocations often occur in this position and are further discussed in Chapter 11. The closed packed position includes full extension, abduction, and internal rotation. The capsular pattern of the hip joint includes loss of flexion, internal rotation, and abduction, less extension, and little to no loss of adduction and external rotation.[116] Hip motion can also be influenced by the pelvis in all planes of motion. For example, anterior tilting of the pelvis increases hip flexion, whereas posterior tilting decreases hip flexion. This interdependent motion is discussed in the next section.

Lumbopelvic Hip Motion

The lumbar spine, pelvis, and hip all move together as a coordinated system, with each region contributing to the range of motion (Table 1-6).[5,100] For example, anterior tilting of the pelvis increases lumbar lordosis, whereas posterior tilting reduces lordosis.[1] When the composite movements of all three regions are performed in the sagittal plane, this motion is referred to as lumbopelvic rhythm. A normal lumbopelvic rhythm for flexion includes nearly simultaneous movements of lumbar flexion (40 degrees) and hip flexion (70 degrees; Fig. 1-32). A normal rhythm for extension occurs in three phases: (1) extension of the trunk begins by extension of the pelvis and femurs with strong activation from the hip extensors; (2) trunk extension continues by extension of the lumbar spine and activation of the lumbar extensors; and (3) completion of trunk extension occurs with less muscle action as the line of force from the body weight falls posterior to the hip joints (Fig. 1-33).[1] In pathologic conditions, these patterns of movements and ranges of movement can change.[1,116] Figure 1-32 summarizes normal and pathologic patterns of lumbopelvic rhythm for flexion.[1]

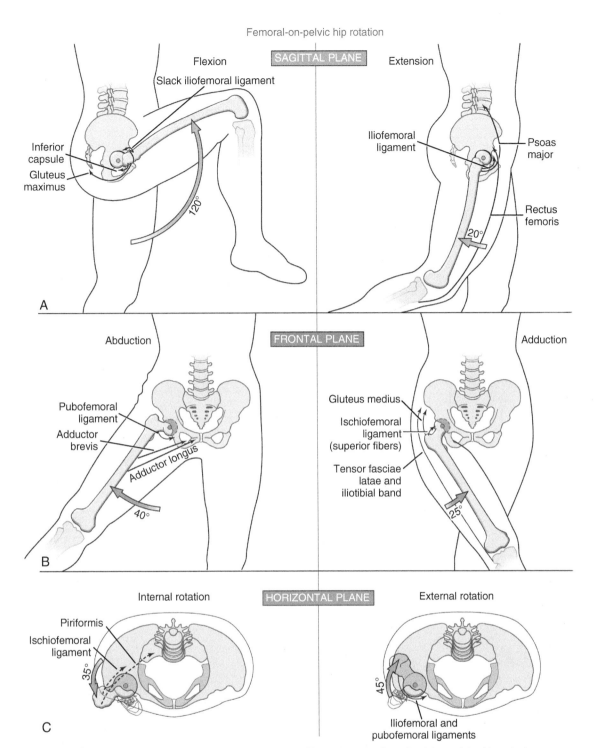

• **Figure 1-31 A** to **C,** Hip osteokinematic motions. (From Neumann DA. *Kinesiology of the Musculoskeletal System: Foundations for Rehabilitation.* 2nd ed. St. Louis: Mosby; 2010.)

TABLE 1-6	Composite Motions of the Lumbopelvic Hip Complex			
Pelvic Motion	**Lumbar Spine Motion**	**Right Hip Motion**	**Left Hip Motion**
Anterior tilt	Extension	Flexion	Flexion
Posterior tilt	Flexion	Extension	Extension
Right lateral tilt	Left lateral flexion	Abduction	Adduction
Left lateral tilt	Right lateral flexion	Adduction	Abduction
Right forward rotation	Left lumbar rotation	Internal rotation	External rotation
Left transverse rotation	Right lumbar rotation	External rotation	Internal rotation

Variations of lumbopelvic rhythms during trunk flexion: A kinematic analysis

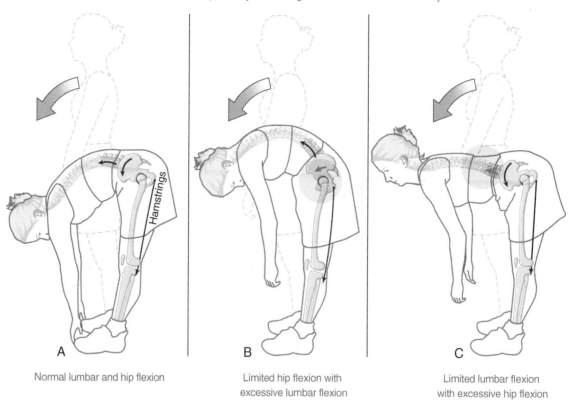

A
Normal lumbar and hip flexion

B
Limited hip flexion with excessive lumbar flexion

C
Limited lumbar flexion with excessive hip flexion

• **Figure 1-32 A** to **C,** Lumbopelvic rhythm, flexion. (From Neumann DA. *Kinesiology of the Musculoskeletal System: Foundations for Rehabilitation.* 2nd ed. St. Louis: Mosby; 2010.)

Lumbopelvic rhythm during trunk extension: A muscular analysis

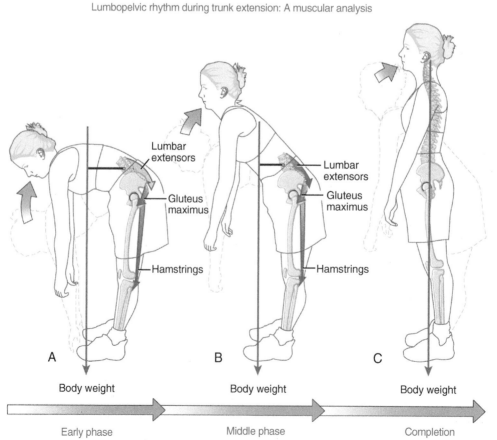

• **Figure 1-33 A** to **C,** Lumbopelvic rhythm, extension. (From Neumann DA. *Kinesiology of the Musculoskeletal System: Foundations for Rehabilitation.* 2nd ed. St. Louis: Mosby; 2010.)

Weight-Bearing Functions of the Lumbopelvic Hip Complex

The lumbopelvic hip complex architecture allows for transfer of weight efficiently down the spine, to the sacrum, through the pelvis, and down to the hip joint and femur. The trabecular bone lines up along columns of stress to create a bony system that meets the stresses placed on the lumbopelvic and lower extremity (Fig. 1-34). In standing, the primary weight-bearing surface of the acetabulum is the superior (lunate) surface and the superior surface of the femoral head. The femoral neck contains a zone of weakness because the trabeculae are thin and uncrossed, thereby increasing the risk for fractures in this area (see Chapter 11).[1] The bony architecture, extensive ligament structure, and muscles of the pelvis and hip joint demonstrate their roles in withstanding external forces.

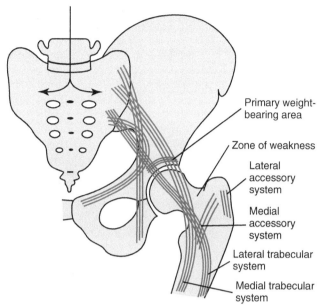

Primary weight-bearing area

Zone of weakness

Lateral accessory system

Medial accessory system

Lateral trabecular system

Medial trabecular system

• **Figure 1-34** Trabecular System of the Pelvis and Hip. (Redrawn from Levangie PK, Norkin CC. *Joint Structure and Function: A Comprehensive Analysis.* Philadelphia: F.A. Davis Company, 2011.)

Summary

This chapter provides a brief review of the anatomy and biomechanics of the lumbopelvic hip region. A foundational knowledge of the basic sciences is important to understanding pathologic conditions. All the concepts discussed in this chapter provide a general background for the disorders discussed in subsequent chapters. This chapter covers the most relevant concepts and is not meant to be a comprehensive resource. The reader is referred to the reference list for more comprehensive resources. Subsequent chapters provide brief discussions of these principles to remind the reader of the relevant anatomic structures involved with pathologic conditions.

References

1. Neumann DA. *Kinesiology of the Musculoskeletal System: Foundations for Rehabilitation.* 2nd ed. St. Louis: Mosby; 2010.
2. Salamh PA, Kolber M. The reliability, minimal detectable change and concurrent validity of a gravity-based bubble inclinometer and iPhone application for measuring standing lumbar lordosis. *Physiother Theory Pract.* 2014;30(1):62-67.
3. Moore KL, Dalley AF, Agur AMR. *Clinically Oriented Anatomy.* 7th ed. Baltimore: Lippincott Williams & Wilkins; 2014.
4. Bergmark A. Stability of the lumbar spine: a study in mechanical engineering. *Acta Orthop Scand Suppl.* 1989;230:1-54.
5. Levangie PK, Norkin CC. *Joint Structure and Function: A Comprehensive Analysis.* 5th ed. Philadelphia: F.A. Davis; 2011.
6. Varlotta GP, Lefkowitz TR, Schweitzer M, et al. The lumbar facet joint: a review of current knowledge. Part 1: anatomy, biomechanics, and grading. *Skeletal Radiol.* 2011;40(1):13-23.
7. Martini FH, Timmons MJ, Tallitsch RB. *Human Anatomy.* 8th ed. Boston: Pearson Benjamin Cummings; 2014.
8. Fujiwara A, An HS, Lim TH, et al. Morphologic changes in the lumbar intervertebral foramen due to flexion-extension, lateral bending, and axial rotation: an in vitro anatomic and biomechanical study. *Spine (Phila Pa 1976).* 2001;26(8):876-882.
9. Bogduk N. The lumbar disc and low back pain. *Neurosurg Clin North Am.* 1991;2(4):791-806.
10. Bogduk N, Aprill C, Derby R. Lumbar discogenic pain: state-of-the-art review. *Pain Med.* 2013;14(6):813-836.
11. Hurri H, Karppinen J. Discogenic pain. *Pain.* 2004;112(3):225-228.
12. Kuslich SD, Ulstrom CL, Michael CJ. The tissue origin of low back pain and sciatica: a report of pain response to tissue stimulation during operations on the lumbar spine using local anesthesia. *Orthop Clin North Am.* 1991;22(2):181-187.
13. Fields AJ, Liebenberg EC, Lotz JC. Innervation of pathologies in the lumbar vertebral end plate and intervertebral disc. *Spine J.* 2014;14(3):513-521.
14. Chandraraj S, Briggs CA, Opeskin K. Disc herniations in the young and end-plate vascularity. *Clin Anat.* 1998;11(3):171-176.
15. Paietta RC, Burger EL, Ferguson VL. Mineralization and collagen orientation throughout aging at the vertebral endplate in the human lumbar spine. *J Struct Biol.* 2013;184(2):310-320.
16. Rodrigues SA, Wade KR, Thambyah A, et al. Micromechanics of annulus-end plate integration in the intervertebral disc. *Spine J.* 2012;12(2):143-150.
17. Pouriesa M, Fouladi RF, Mesbahi S. Disproportion of end plates and the lumbar intervertebral disc herniation. *Spine J.* 2013;13(4):402-407.
18. Holm S, Indahl A, Solomonow M. Sensorimotor control of the spine. *J Electromyogr Kinesiol.* 2002;12(3):219-234.

19. Comerford MJ, Mottram SL. Movement and stability dysfunction: contemporary developments. *Man Ther*. 2001;6(1):15-26.

20. Saner J, Kool J, de Bie RA, et al. Movement control exercise versus general exercise to reduce disability in patients with low back pain and movement control impairment: a randomised controlled trial. *BMC Musculoskelet Disord*. 2011;12:207.

21. Paris SV. Anatomy as related to function and pain. *Orthop Clin North Am*. 1983;14(3):475-489.

22. Sekine M, Yamashita T, Takebayashi T, et al. Mechanosensitive afferent units in the lumbar posterior longitudinal ligament. *Spine (Phila Pa 1976)*. 2001;26(14):1516-1521.

23. Sakamoto N, Yamashita T, Takebayashi T, et al. An electrophysiologic study of mechanoreceptors in the sacroiliac joint and adjacent tissues. *Spine (Phila Pa 1976)*. 2001;26(20):E468-E471.

24. Bogduk N. *Clinical Anatomy of the Lumbar Spine and Sacrum*. 4th ed. New York: Churchill Livingstone; 2005.

25. Panjabi MM, Goel VK, Takata K. Physiologic strains in the lumbar spinal ligaments: an in vitro biomechanical study. 1981 Volvo award in biomechanics. *Spine (Phila Pa 1976)*. 1982;7(3):192-203.

26. Pizones J, Izquierdo E, Sanchez-Mariscal F, et al. Sequential damage assessment of the different components of the posterior ligamentous complex after magnetic resonance imaging interpretation: prospective study 74 traumatic fractures. *Spine (Phila Pa 1976)*. 2012;37(11):E662-E667.

27. Aihara T, Takahashi K, Yamagata M, et al. Biomechanical functions of the iliolumbar ligament in L5 spondylolysis. *J Orthop Sci*. 2000;5(3):238-242.

28. Olszewski AD, Yaszemski MJ, White AA 3rd. The anatomy of the human lumbar ligamentum flavum: new observations and their surgical importance. *Spine (Phila Pa 1976)*. 1996;21(20):2307-2312.

29. Prakash, Prabhu LV, Saralaya VV, et al. Vertebral body integrity: a review of various anatomical factors involved in the lumbar region. *Osteoporos Int*. 2007;18(7):891-903.

30. Ohshima H, Hirano N, Osada R, et al. Morphologic variation of lumbar posterior longitudinal ligament and the modality of disc herniation. *Spine (Phila Pa 1976)*. 1993;18(16):2408-2411.

31. Enneking FK, Chan V, Greger J, et al. Lower-extremity peripheral nerve blockade: essentials of our current understanding. *Reg Anesth Pain Med*. 2005;30(1):4-35.

32. Sforsini C, Wikinski JA. Anatomical review of the lumbosacral plexus and nerves of the lower extremity. *Tech Reg Anesth Pain Manage*. 2006;10(4):138-144.

33. Ivins GK. Meralgia paresthetica, the elusive diagnosis: clinical experience with 14 adult patients. *Ann Surg*. 2000;232(2):281-286.

34. Ropars M, Morandi X, Huten D, et al. Anatomical study of the lateral femoral cutaneous nerve with special reference to minimally invasive anterior approach for total hip replacement. *Surg Radiol Anat*. 2009;31(3):199-204.

35. Seror P, Seror R. Meralgia paresthetica: clinical and electrophysiological diagnosis in 120 cases. *Muscle Nerve*. 2006;33(5):650-654.

36. Beveridge TS, Power A, Johnson M, et al. The lumbar arteries and veins: quantification of variable anatomical positioning with application to retroperitoneal surgery. *Clin Anat*. 2015.

37. Bilhim T, Pereira JA, Fernandes L, et al. Angiographic anatomy of the male pelvic arteries. *AJR Am J Roentgenol*. 2014;203(4):W373-W382.

38. Akuthota V, Ferreiro A, Moore T, et al. Core stability exercise principles. *Curr Sports Med Rep*. 2008;7(1):39-44.

39. Willard FH, Vleeming A, Schuenke MD, et al. The thoracolumbar fascia: anatomy, function and clinical considerations. *J Anat*. 2012;221(6):507-536.

40. Hodges PW. Core stability exercise in chronic low back pain. *Orthop Clin North Am*. 2003;34(2):245-254.

41. Ferreira PH, Ferreira ML, Maher CG, et al. Changes in recruitment of transversus abdominis correlate with disability in people with chronic low back pain. *Br J Sports Med*. 2010;44(16):1166-1172.

42. Clark M, Sutton BG, Lucett S, eds. *NASM Essentials of Personal Fitness Training*. Burlington, Mass: Jones & Bartlett Learning; 2013.

43. Panjabi MM. The stabilizing system of the spine. Part I: function, dysfunction, adaptation, and enhancement. *J Spinal Disord*. 1992;5(4):383-389, discussion 397.

44. Panjabi MM, Cholewicki J, Nibu K, et al. Critical load of the human cervical spine: an in vitro experimental study. *Clin Biomech (Bristol, Avon)*. 1998;13(1):11-17.

45. Panjabi MM. The stabilizing system of the spine. Part II: neutral zone and instability hypothesis. *J Spinal Disord*. 1992;5(4):390-396, discussion 397.

46. Fryer G, Morris T, Gibbons P. Paraspinal muscles and intervertebral dysfunction: part two. *J Manipulative Physiol Ther*. 2004;27(5):348-357.

47. Travell JG, Simons DG. *Myofascial Pain and Dysfunction: The Trigger Point Manual*, Vol. 1. Baltimore: Williams & Wilkins; 1983.

48. Travell JG, Simons DG. *Myofascial Pain and Dysfunction: The Trigger Point Manual*, Vol. 2. Baltimore: Williams & Wilkins; 1992.

49. Bogduk N, Macintosh JE. The applied anatomy of the thoracolumbar fascia. *Spine (Phila Pa 1976)*. 1984;9(2):164-170.

50. Cabry RJ Jr, Thorell E, Heck K, et al. Understanding noninguinal abdominal hernias in the athlete. *Curr Sports Med Rep*. 2014;13(2):86-93.

51. Brandon CJ, Jacobson JA, Fessell D, et al. Groin pain beyond the hip: how anatomy predisposes to injury as visualized by musculoskeletal ultrasound and MRI. *AJR Am J Roentgenol*. 2011;197(5):1190-1197.

52. Tromp WG, van den Heuvel B, Dwars BJ. A new accurate method of physical examination for differentiation of inguinal hernia types. *Surg Endosc*. 2014;28(5):1460-1464.

53. Shadbolt CL, Heinze SB, Dietrich RB. Imaging of groin masses: inguinal anatomy and pathologic conditions revisited. *Radiographics*. 2001;21(Spec No):S261-S271.

54. Herschorn S. Female pelvic floor anatomy: the pelvic floor, supporting structures, and pelvic organs. *Rev Urol*. 2004;6(suppl 5):S2-S10.

55. Hamilton NP, Weimar W, Luttgens K. *Kinesiology: Scientific Basis of Human Motion*. New York: McGraw-Hill; 2012.

56. Behnke RS. *Kinetic Anatomy*. Leeds, United Kingdom: Human Kinetics; 2012.

57. Woon JT, Stringer MD. Redefining the coccygeal plexus. *Clin Anat*. 2014;27(2):254-260.

58. Woon JT, Stringer MD. Clinical anatomy of the coccyx: a systematic review. *Clin Anat*. 2012;25(2):158-167.

59. Forst SL, Wheeler MT, Fortin JD, et al. The sacroiliac joint: anatomy, physiology and clinical significance. *Pain Physician*. 2006;9(1):61-67.

60. Vleeming A, Schuenke MD, Masi AT, et al. The sacroiliac joint: an overview of its anatomy, function and potential clinical implications. *J Anat*. 2012;221(6):537-567.

61. Smoll NR. Variations of the piriformis and sciatic nerve with clinical consequence: a review. *Clin Anat*. 2010;23(1):8-17.

62. Shafik A, el-Sherif M, Youssef A, et al. Surgical anatomy of the pudendal nerve and its clinical implications. *Clin Anat*. 1995; 8(2):110-115.

63. Filler AG. Diagnosis and treatment of pudendal nerve entrapment syndrome subtypes: imaging, injections, and minimal access surgery. *Neurosurg Focus*. 2009;26(2):E9.

64. Popeney C, Ansell V, Renney K. Pudendal entrapment as an etiology of chronic perineal pain: diagnosis and treatment. *Neurourol Urodyn*. 2007;26(6):820-827.

65. Ray B, D'Souza AS, Saxena A, et al. Morphology of the superior gluteal nerve: a study in adult human cadavers. *Bratisl Lek Listy*. 2013;114(7):409-412.

66. Ghaderi F, Oskouei AE. Physiotherapy for women with stress urinary incontinence: a review article. *J Phys Ther Sci*. 2014; 26(9):1493-1499.

67. Wei JT, De Lancey JO. Functional anatomy of the pelvic floor and lower urinary tract. *Clin Obstet Gynecol*. 2004;47(1): 3-17.

68. Prather H, Dugan S, Fitzgerald C, et al. Review of anatomy, evaluation, and treatment of musculoskeletal pelvic floor pain in women. *PM R*. 2009;1(4):346-358.

69. Lewis CL, Sahrmann SA. Acetabular labral tears. *Phys Ther*. 2006;86(1):110-121.

70. Tönnis D, Heinecke A. Acetabular and femoral anteversion: relationship with osteoarthritis of the hip. *J Bone Joint Surg Am*. 1999;81(12):1747-1770.

71. Diaz-Ledezma C, Novack T, Marin-Pena O, et al. The relevance of the radiological signs of acetabular retroversion among patients with femoroacetabular impingement. *Bone Joint J*. 2013;95-B(7):893-899.

72. Bauer JP, Roy DR, Thomas SS. Acetabular retroversion in post slipped capital femoral epiphysis deformity. *J Child Orthop*. 2013;7(2):91-94.

73. Itokazu M, Takahashi K, Matsunaga T, et al. A study of the arterial supply of the human acetabulum using a corrosion casting method. *Clin Anat*. 1997;10(2):77-81.

74. Henak CR, Ellis BJ, Harris MD, et al. Role of the acetabular labrum in load support across the hip joint. *J Biomech*. 2011;44(12):2201-2206.

75. Groh MM, Herrera J. A comprehensive review of hip labral tears. *Curr Rev Musculoskelet Med*. 2009;2(2):105-117.

76. Seldes RM, Tan V, Hunt J, et al. Anatomy, histologic features, and vascularity of the adult acetabular labrum. *Clin Orthop Relat Res*. 2001;(382):232-240.

77. McCarthy JC, Noble PC, Schuck MR, et al. The Otto E. Aufranc award: the role of labral lesions to development of early degenerative hip disease. *Clin Orthop Relat Res*. 2001;(393): 25-37.

78. Kelly BT, Shapiro GS, Digiovanni CW, et al. Vascularity of the hip labrum: a cadaveric investigation. *Arthroscopy*. 2005;21(1): 3-11.

79. Haversath M, Hanke J, Landgraeber S, et al. The distribution of nociceptive innervation in the painful hip: a histological investigation. *Bone Joint J*. 2013;95-B(6):770-776.

80. Alzaharani A, Bali K, Gudena R, et al. The innervation of the human acetabular labrum and hip joint: an anatomic study. *BMC Musculoskelet Disord*. 2014;15:41.

81. Tan V, Seldes RM, Katz MA, et al. Contribution of acetabular labrum to articulating surface area and femoral head coverage in adult hip joints: an anatomic study in cadavera. *Am J Orthop (Belle Mead NJ)*. 2001;30(11):809-812.

82. Dwyer MK, Jones HL, Hogan MG, et al. The acetabular labrum regulates fluid circulation of the hip joint during functional activities. *Am J Sports Med*. 2014;42(4):812-819.

83. Safran MR, Giordano G, Lindsey DP, et al. Strains across the acetabular labrum during hip motion: a cadaveric model. *Am J Sports Med*. 2011;39(suppl):92S-102S.

84. Dy CJ, Thompson MT, Crawford MJ, et al. Tensile strain in the anterior part of the acetabular labrum during provocative maneuvering of the normal hip. *J Bone Joint Surg Am*. 2008; 90(7):1464-1472.

85. Signorelli C, Lopomo N, Bonanzinga T, et al. Relationship between femoroacetabular contact areas and hip position in the normal joint: an in vitro evaluation. *Knee Surg Sports Traumatol Arthrosc*. 2013;21(2):408-414.

86. Ross JR, Nepple JJ, Philippon MJ, et al. Effect of changes in pelvic tilt on range of motion to impingement and radiographic parameters of acetabular morphologic characteristics. *Am J Sports Med*. 2014;42(10):2402-2409.

87. Lewis CL, Khuu A, Marinko LN. Postural correction reduces hip pain in adult with acetabular dysplasia: a case report. *Man Ther*. 2015;20(3):508-512.

88. Lewis CL, Sahrmann SA. Effect of posture on hip angles and moments during gait. *Man Ther*. 2015;20(1):176-182.

89. Lewis CL, Sahrmann SA, Moran DW. Anterior hip joint force increases with hip extension, decreased gluteal force, or decreased iliopsoas force. *J Biomech*. 2007;40(16):3725-3731.

90. Tannast M, Goricki D, Beck M, et al. Hip damage occurs at the zone of femoroacetabular impingement. *Clin Orthop Relat Res*. 2008;466(2):273-280.

91. Ejnisman L, Philippon MJ, Lertwanich P, et al. Relationship between femoral anteversion and findings in hips with femoroacetabular impingement. *Orthopedics*. 2013;36(3):e293-e300.

92. Kudrna JC. Femoral version: definition, diagnosis, and intraoperative correction with modular femoral components. *Orthopedics*. 2005;28(suppl 9):S1045-S1047.

93. Fabry G, MacEwen GD, Shands AR. Torsion of the femur: a follow-up study in normal and abnormal conditions. *J Bone Surg Am*. 1973;55:1726-1738.

94. Cibulka MT. Determination and significance of femoral neck anteversion. *Phys Ther*. 2004;84(6):550-558.

95. Koerner JD, Patel NM, Yoon RS, et al. Femoral version of the general population: does "normal" vary by gender or ethnicity? *J Orthop Trauma*. 2013;27(6):308-311.

96. Cerezal L, Kassarjian A, Canga A, et al. Anatomy, biomechanics, imaging, and management of ligamentum teres injuries. *Radiographics*. 2010;30(6):1637-1651.

97. Byrd JW, Jones KS. Traumatic rupture of the ligamentum teres as a source of hip pain. *Arthroscopy*. 2004;20(4):385-391.

98. Barquet A, Mayora G, Guimaraes JM, et al. Avascular necrosis of the femoral head following trochanteric fractures in adults: a systematic review. *Injury*. 2014;45(12):1848-1858.

99. Birnbaum K, Prescher A, Hessler S, et al. The sensory innervation of the hip joint: an anatomical study. *Surg Radiol Anat*. 1997;19(6):371-375.

100. Floyd RT, Thompson C. *Manual of Structural Kinesiology.* New York: McGraw-Hill Education; 2014.

101. Lewis CL. Extra-articular snapping hip: a literature review. *Sports Health.* 2010;2(3):186-190.

102. Verrall GM, Esterman A, Hewett TE. Analysis of the three most prevalent injuries in Australian football demonstrates a season to season association between groin/hip/osteitis pubis injuries with ACL knee injuries. *Asian J Sports Med.* 2014;5(3):e23072.

103. Fairclough J, Hayashi K, Toumi H, et al. The functional anatomy of the iliotibial band during flexion and extension of the knee: implications for understanding iliotibial band syndrome. *J Anat.* 2006;208(3):309-316.

104. Louw M, Deary C. The biomechanical variables involved in the aetiology of iliotibial band syndrome in distance runners: a systematic review of the literature. *Phys Ther Sport.* 2014; 15(1):64-75.

105. Noehren B, Davis I, Hamill J. ASB clinical biomechanics award winner 2006 prospective study of the biomechanical factors associated with iliotibial band syndrome. *Clin Biomech (Bristol, Avon).* 2007;22(9):951-956.

106. Rossidis G, Perry A, Abbas H, et al. Laparoscopic hernia repair with adductor tenotomy for athletic pubalgia: an established procedure for an obscure entity. *Surg Endosc.* 2015;29(2): 381-386.

107. Harris-Hayes M, Mueller MJ, Sahrmann SA, et al. Persons with chronic hip joint pain exhibit reduced hip muscle strength. *J Orthop Sports Phys Ther.* 2014;44(11):890-898.

108. Van Cant J, Pineux C, Pitance L, et al. Hip muscle strength and endurance in females with patellofemoral pain: a systematic review with meta-analysis. *Int J Sports Phys Ther.* 2014;9(5): 564-582.

109. Panjabi MM, Oxland TR, Yamamoto I, et al. Mechanical behavior of the human lumbar and lumbosacral spine as shown by three-dimensional load-displacement curves. *J Bone Joint Surg Am.* 1994;76(3):413-424.

110. Legaspi O, Edmond SL. Does the evidence support the existence of lumbar spine coupled motion? A critical review of the literature. *J Orthop Sports Phys Ther.* 2007;37(4):169-178.

111. Cook C, Showalter C. A survey on the importance of lumbar coupling biomechanics in physiotherapy practice. *Man Ther.* 2004;9(3):164-172.

112. Huijbregts P. Lumbar spine coupled motions: a literature review with clinical implications. *Orthop Division Rev.* 2004;Sept/Oct:21-25.

113. Cook C. Lumbar coupling biomechanics: a literature review. *J Man Manip Ther.* 2003;11:137-145.

114. Goode A, Hegedus EJ, Sizer P, et al. Three-dimensional movements of the sacroiliac joint: a systematic review of the literature and assessment of clinical utility. *J Man Manip Ther.* 2008;16(1):25-38.

115. Loubert PV, Zipple JT, Klobucher MJ, et al. In vivo ultrasound measurement of posterior femoral glide during hip joint mobilization in healthy college students. *J Orthop Sports Phys Ther.* 2013;43(8):534-541.

116. Magee DJ. *Orthopedic Physical Assessment.* 6th ed. St. Louis: Saunders; 2013.

2

Examination of the Hip and Pelvis

SCOTT W. CHEATHAM

CHAPTER OUTLINE

Examination of the hip and pelvis can be very complex because of the many competing pathologic features that often lend uncertainty to the diagnosis. In fact, as many as 60% of patients undergoing hip arthroscopic procedures receive an initial misdiagnosis.[1,2] Traditional examination methods also use broad labels (i.e., groin pain) to describe a patient's problem, and this terminology makes it difficult to isolate the primary disorder. This chapter presents a systematic examination approach that focuses on the primary pathologic features observed in the hip and pelvis.

This chapter is divided into three main sections. The first section provides a clinical presentation of a common patient who is reporting hip pain. Specific subjective questions are discussed that help the reader to understand and prioritize the list of potential causes. The second section outlines a regional examination approach that focuses on the most common orthopedic problems of the hip and pelvic region. This section also discusses common imaging techniques. The third section discusses common patient-related outcome (PRO) measures used to gather more information about the patient. The main goal of this chapter is to provide the reader with an evidence-based examination approach for common hip and pelvic disorders discussed in subsequent chapters.

Client Profile

Patient History

Patients with hip pain may have trouble describing their symptoms. Therefore, the clinician must take a thorough history to make a differential diagnosis of the potential cause. Beginning the history with more general "open-ended" interview questions allows the patient to recount the potential mechanism or contributing events (i.e., traumatic versus insidious) related to the primary complaint (Box 2-1). A history of a traumatic event may be a good prognostic indicator of a correctable problem, and an insidious onset may be an indicator of a possible underlying degenerative disease or predisposing injury.[3] Based on the patient's answers, more specific questions should follow that focus on the region of injury (i.e., focal or diffuse), aggravating and relieving factors, types of pain, functional limitations (i.e., pain with sit to stand), and other symptoms (i.e., popping or clicking). Taking a regional approach to questioning may help the clinician to isolate potential disorders of the anterior, lateral, or posterior hip region.

Patients with hip pain may describe a cluster of symptoms that are both general and specific. General complaints

• BOX 2-1 Suggested Hip Examination Interview Questions

- Can you describe your hip pain and how it happened (e.g., trauma, insidious)?
- Can you point to the pain with your finger or hand (e.g., anterior, lateral, posterior hip)?
- Do you feel any other symptoms with your pain, such as "clicking and popping" or "numbness and tingling"? If yes, can you describe these symptoms?
- Can you describe any related events or activities that may have contributed to your pain?
- Can you describe what type of positions or activities increase your hip pain and which activities or positions help to relieve your pain?
- Can you rank your level of pain from lowest to highest and your average level of pain by using a scale from 0 to 10?
- Do you have any other medical conditions (e.g., low back pain) that may be related to your hip pain or that may affect your physical therapy program?
- Are you currently taking medications related to your hip pain?

may include increased pain with physical activity or sports, hip rotation or pivoting, transitional activities (e.g., sit to stand), walking up or down stairs, dressing (e.g., putting on shoes or socks), and dyspareunia.[3] Specific mechanical symptoms such as sharp stabbing, locking, catching, and popping may be good prognostic indicators of a correctable problem, as opposed to pain in the absence of mechanical symptoms that is often a poor prognostic indicator or suggestive of a more sinister cause.[3,4] More specifically, sharp pain with clicking and giving way may be related to an intraarticular pathologic condition such as an acetabular labral tear or cartilage defect (sensitivity, 100%; specificity, 85%).[5] Isolating the cause of the patient's symptoms may be difficult from the interview because of the many disorders that have similar clinical presentations. Ultimately, the clinician should determine whether the suspected pathologic process is intraarticular or extraarticular, and this distinction will help guide the rest of the examination process.

Anterior Hip Pain

Anterior hip pain is the most common regional complaint among patients and is often a diagnostic challenge because of the many potential pathologic conditions (Table 2-1).[6] Patients often describe a deep "anterior groin-related pain" and may point or cup their hand around the anterior hip region; this maneuver is often called the "C-sign" and is most indicative of intraarticular disease (Fig. 2-1).[3,7] Anterior groin pain that worsens with prolonged standing, sitting, and walking is often related to acetabular labral tears (sensitivity, 96% to 100%).[5] If the patient's pain is related to specific hip positions (e.g., flexion, adduction, and internal rotation) and sports activity (e.g., rotation and

pivoting), then femoral acetabular impingement (FAI), acetabular labrum tear, or other intraarticular disorder should be suspected.[8] The majority of anterior hip pain may originate from articular structures because the hip is primarily innervated by the femoral and obturator nerves, which innervate the anterior and medial hip joint.[6] These symptoms may be accompanied by lateral or posterior hip discomfort and mechanical symptoms such as clicking or popping.[3] Extraarticular hip problems such as internal snapping hip syndrome, iliopsoas tendinopathy, iliopectineal bursitis, or proximal quadriceps lesions may elicit a similar pain pattern and mechanical symptoms (e.g., snapping), but they may be described as more superficial.[9]

Given the close proximity of structures, pelvic disorders should also be considered as a source of anterior hip or "groin" pain. Primary pathologic conditions to consider include athletic pubalgia (sports hernia), adductor-related groin pain, inguinal hernia, osteitis pubis, pelvic floor dysfunction, and fractures of the femoral neck and pubic ramus. These disorders produce similar regional symptoms that are often mechanical and are exacerbated by sports or physical activity. Chapters 5, 8, and 11 provide comprehensive discussions of these disorders.

Lateral Hip Pain

Pain in the lateral hip is often more superficial, with the patient describing symptoms over the greater trochanter and surrounding lateral hip region.[3] The patient's symptoms may be mechanical or diffuse, depending on the pathologic process (see Table 2-1). The intraarticular disorders described in the foregoing section can also be a source of lateral hip pain and should be considered in the differential diagnosis. More commonly, extraarticular disorders such as external snapping hip syndrome, greater trochanteric bursitis, and gluteal tendon tears should be considered.[10] These disorders may elicit more focal mechanical symptoms that may be easily identified. Diffuse lateral hip and thigh symptoms may also originate from the lumbar spine or the sacroiliac joint or from entrapment of the lateral cutaneous nerve of the thigh (e.g., meralgia paresthetica).[1,2] Lumbar spine disorders should also be considered if symptoms travel distal to the knee.[2] Other injuries such as femoral head or neck fractures or hip pointer may result from a traumatic event.[10]

Posterior Hip Pain

Pain in the posterior hip is the least common region of complaint and is often caused by extraarticular disorders.[6] Pathologic conditions to consider include proximal hamstring tears, sacroiliac joint dysfunction, lumbar spine disorders, piriformis syndrome, and ischiogluteal bursitis (see Table 2-1). Lumbosacral disorders should be considered first because of all the nerves that course through the region.[6] Intraarticular disorders such as labral tears, FAI,

TABLE 2-1	Potential Causes of Hip Pain by Region

Anterior Hip (Groin)	Lateral Hip	Posterior Hip
Intraarticular • Labral tear • FAI • Chondral injuries • Dysplasia • Loose body • Ligamentum teres tear • Osteoarthritis • Osteonecrosis of femoral head • Septic hip arthritis • Slipped capital femoral epiphysis • Legg-Calvé-Perthes disease • Synovitis • Avulsion, fracture, or dislocation Extraarticular • Internal snapping hip syndrome • Iliopsoas tendinopathy • Adductor disorder • Iliopectineal bursitis • Proximal quadriceps lesions • Capsular laxity or adhesive capsulitis • Central iliopsoas impingement • Subspine impingement (anterior inferior iliac spine) • Postoperative scarring Nerve • Obturator, femoral, or genitofemoral nerve disorder Lumbopelvic • Athletic pubalgia • Inguinal hernia • Osteitis pubis • Lumbar spine disorder • Pelvic fracture • Postpartum symphysis separation • Pelvic floor dysfunction	Intraarticular • Labral tear • FAI • Osteoarthritis Extraarticular • Greater trochanteric-pelvic impingement • External snapping hip syndrome • Proximal iliotibial band syndrome • Greater trochanteric bursitis • Gluteal tendon dysfunction or tear • Avulsion, fracture, or dislocation • Hip pointer • Postoperative scarring Nerve • Lateral cutaneous nerve of the thigh (meralgia paresthetica) disorder Lumbopelvic • Lumbar spine disorder • Sacroiliac joint disorder • Pelvic fracture	Intraarticular • Labral tear • FAI • Osteoarthritis Extraarticular • Ischiofemoral impingement • Proximal hamstring tear • Hip extensor or rotator muscle disorder • Ischial bursitis • Avulsion, fracture, or dislocation Nerve • Sciatic nerve disorder Lumbopelvic • Lumbar spine disorder • Sacroiliac joint disorder • Pelvic fracture

FAI, Femoral acetabular impingement.

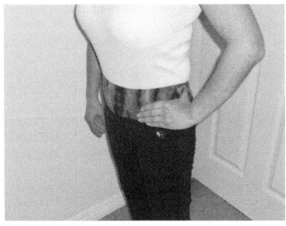

• **Figure 2-1** "C-Sign."

and osteoarthritis can refer mechanical pain into the posterior hip region and should be considered in the differential diagnosis.[3] If trauma to the posterior pelvic and hip occurred (e.g., a fall), then a possible proximal femur or pelvic fracture should be considered.

Red Flags

During the patient interview, the clinician should determine whether any medical "red flags" or contraindications to treatment are present. This determination can be accomplished through the standard medical screening questionnaire, systems review, and specific questioning of the patient. Table 2-2 provides a summary of nonmusculoskeletal causes of hip, pelvic, and groin pain.[2,11] Symptoms such as fever,

TABLE 2-2	Nonmusculoskeletal Causes of Hip and Groin Pain			
Genital or Reproductive	**Gastrointestinal**	**Vascular**	**Other**	
Epididymitis	Crohn disease	Abdominal aortic aneurysm	Lymphadenopathy	
Hydrocele/varicocele	Diverticular disease	Aortoiliac occlusive disease	Appendicitis	
Prostatitis	Inflammatory bowel disease		Intraabdominal abscess	
Testicular neoplasm or torsion			Rheumatic disease Hernia (e.g., inguinal, femoral, umbilical)	
Urethritis				
Ovarian cyst				
Pelvic inflammatory disease				
Urinary tract infection				

malaise, night sweats, weight loss, past or current diagnosis of cancer, immunocompromise, and history of trauma may indicate a medical red flag that necessitates further investigation and possible referral.[4] Ultimately, the clinician should determine whether the patient's condition is appropriate for physical therapy or requires further investigation and possible referral.

Summary

A systematic approach to the hip and pelvic examination begins with a comprehensive history. Taking a regional approach to questioning (e.g., anterior, lateral, or posterior) and determining whether the disorder is intraarticular or extraarticular will help the clinician to formulate a plausible hypothesis about what occurred and which anatomic structures are involved. This approach helps guide the objective portion of the examination.

Clinical Examination

The use of a systematic format for the clinical examination allows the clinician to perform the needed test and measures while the patient moves through the desired positions.[12] The patient's level of irritability should also be considered. Patients in acute pain may not be able to perform some of the clinical tests and may require the clinician to modify the examination. Continued testing in the presence of pain may produce a false-positive result, thus decreasing the diagnostic value of the clinical tests. The examination may also change depending on the patient's functional ability and suspected pathologic process. The examination format described in this chapter follows a specific sequence of standing, sitting, supine, side lying, and prone. The patient is dressed appropriately, with shoes off, if possible. The clinician is also observing the patient's demeanor, movements, and communication during all positions of testing. The suggested test and measures are described for each position.

Standing Examination

The standing examination may begin with a postural assessment to determine how the person holds himself or herself in a static posture. The clinician should take an organized approach to posture assessment with a focus on the lumbopelvis and lower extremities, with observation in all planes. It has been well documented in the literature that patients with hip disorders often demonstrate postural deviations. For example, patients with hip labral tears and anterior hip pain have been found to assume a swayback posture (Fig. 2-2) that affects their gait kinematics.[13,14] Anterior pelvic tilting has been associated with patients with cam-type FAI and acetabular dysplasia.[15] Patients with unilateral hip osteoarthritis may present with decreased lumbar lordosis and thoracic kyphosis with the body tilting forward.[16,17] The patient may also attempt to assume the position of least discomfort. For example, patients with synovitis or inflammation may position the hip in a flexed, abducted, and externally rotated position.[5] The clinician should attempt to identify any posture deviations (e.g., a swayback posture) that may be contributing to the patient's primary complaints.

The gait assessment should be conducted to determine how the hip pain and posture (e.g., swayback) affects the patient's function.[13] Sagittal and frontal plane motion should be observed to obtain a complete picture of the patient's gait pattern. Common gait parameters to assess include stance and swing phase, stride length, stride width, and pelvic motion.[7] The patient may develop a compensatory gait pattern as a result of hip pain, stiffness, decreased range of motion (ROM), and fear-based avoidance.[18-20] These impairments can lead to a slower gait pattern (cadence), decreased stride length, decreased stance, increased contralateral loading of the opposite hip (e.g., leaning toward the uninvolved hip), and decreased or abnormal pelvic motion.[20-25]

To obtain a better understanding of how the patient can perform activities of daily living, the patient should undergo

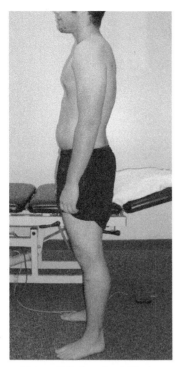

• **Figure 2-2** Swayback Posture.

functional testing. Suggested activities to test include sit to stand and stair ambulation to provide insight into the patient's current functional abilities. Patients with mild to moderate hip osteoarthritis often unload the involved hip during sit to stand transition movements.[26] For example, the patient may lean toward the uninvolved hip to unload or reduce the forces through the involved hip as he or she is rising from the seated position. In addition, patients with FAI may present with altered sagittal plane hip ROM during stair climbing and decreased hip flexion ROM during squatting activity.[25,27] The patient's level of pain and functional abilities should direct functional testing.

Athletes or active persons with higher functional levels can undergo *performance testing.* Often, such testing is used as a repeated measure to help determine whether the patient is ready to return to sport or physical activity. For example, the 30-second single leg stance test has a high sensitivity (100%) and specificity (97.3%) for detecting gluteus medius and minimus tendinopathy.[28] Performance testing may yield valuable information but can lead to increased pain and poor patient performance from the high demands of testing. The clinician must decide when is the best time to introduce such testing in the examination process. Appendix B provides a summary and normative values for common performance tests of the hip and lower extremity.[29]

Joint hypermobility testing can be conducted while the patient is in standing. Joint hypermobility has been recognized as a characteristic of various connective tissue disorders (Ehlers-Danlos and Marfan syndromes) and musculoskeletal disorders such hip FAI.[30] The Beighton score is a common test used to investigate the presence of hypermobility (Fig. 2-3).[30] The test measures hypermobility (1 is yes, 0 is no) at the lumbosacral spine, both thumbs, fifth metacarpophalangeal joints (little fingers), elbows, and knees. The Beighton score is calculated as follows: (1) one point if the patient can bend forward from a standing position and place the palms on the ground with legs straight, (2) one point for each thumb that touches the forearm when bent backward, (3) one point for each little finger that bends backward beyond 90 degrees, (4) one point for each elbow that bends backward, and (5) one point for each knee that bends backward. A score of 4 or higher out of 9 is considered to be positive for joint hypermobility.[31] The reproducibility of the test to diagnose both general joint hypermobility and benign joint hypermobility syndrome was found to be high (kappa, 0.74 to 0.84).[32,33] Benign joint hypermobility syndrome is another condition involving a cluster of subjective and objective findings including joint arthralgia, back pain, spondylosis, spondylolysis or spondylolisthesis, joint dislocation or subluxation, soft tissue rheumatism, marfanoid habitus, abnormal skin, eye signs, varicose veins, or hernia or uterine or rectal prolapse.[31] The Beighton score is a valid and reliable[34] measure in children,[35] women,[31] dancers,[36] and various ethnic groups.[31]

A general lumbar spine screen can be conducted at this phase if a potential concomitant pathologic process is suspected. Testing may include ROM and selected special tests to rule out any suspected disorder. Please see the later section on lumbosacral issues.

Seated Examination

The seated portion of the examination may include a seated posture assessment, ROM, neurologic screen, integument and vascular screen, and muscle performance evaluation. A seated posture assessment can be conducted that may provide some insight into how the hip symptoms affect sitting posture. Passive or active ROM measurements can be taken for the hip, knee, and ankle in this position. However, aggravating hip motions should be tested with caution. For example, seated internal rotation may aggravate the condition in a patient who is diagnosed with FAI, or hip flexion may aggravate a patient with low back pain and limited hip mobility.[27,37] Chapter 1 provides a description of hip ROM norms.

The neurologic screen should include testing of lower extremity motor, deep tendon reflex, and dermatome sensation.[38] Often, neurologic testing is done to screen for diskogenic or radicular disease. Motor testing from L3 to S1 has good specificity (100%) but weaker sensitivity (0% to 28%).[39] The Achilles deep tendon reflex (sensitivity, 87%; specificity, 89%) has stronger diagnostic accuracy than does the extensor digitorum brevis (sensitivity, 14%; specificity, 91%). Dermatome sensation testing of light touch or of sharp or dull has stronger specificity (100%) than sensitivity (50%).[40] Table 2-3 summarizes the components of the neurologic screen.

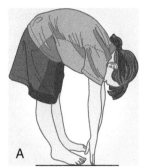

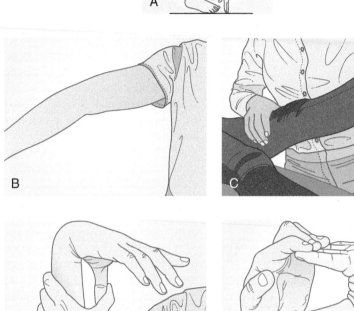

• **Figure 2-3** Beighton Score. **A,** Lumbar flexion. **B,** Elbow hyperextension. **C,** Knee hyperextension. **D,** Fifth metacarpophalangeal joint range. **E,** Wrist flexion. (From Evans AM. *Pocket Podiatry: Paediatrics.* Edinburgh: Churchill Livingstone; 2010.)

TABLE 2-3	Lower Extremity Neurologic Screen		
Level	**Myotome**	**Dermatome**	**Reflexes**
T12	None	Medial thigh and inguinal area	None
L1	None	Back, anterior thigh, as well as medial upper thigh	None
L2	Psoas and hip adductors	Back to anterolateral to proximal medial thigh	None
L3	Psoas and quadriceps	Back, upper buttock, to anterior and medial thigh to patella	Patellar reflex
L4	Tibialis anterior and extensor hallucis	Medial buttock, lateral thigh to medial lower leg and medial aspect of foot	Patellar reflex
L5	Extensor hallucis, peroneals, gluteus medius, and ankle dorsiflexors	Buttock, posterior and lateral thigh to anterolateral aspect of leg to the dorsum of foot	None
S1	Ankle plantar flexors and hamstrings	Buttock, thigh, and posterior leg and lateral foot	Achilles reflex

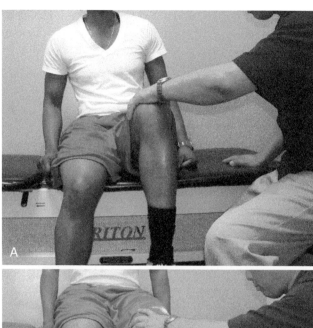
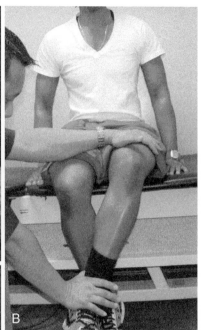
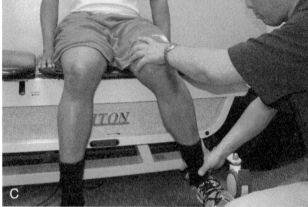

• **Figure 2-4** Examples of Seated Muscle Performance Tests. **A,** Hip flexion. **B,** Hip external rotation. **C,** Hip internal rotation.

Manual muscle testing (MMT), graded using a 0 to 5 scale, can also be done with the patient seated for the hip, knee, and ankle. Figure 2-4 provides an example of MMT for seated hip flexion and internal and external rotation.[38] Hip muscle deficits have been demonstrated in patients with FAI, hip osteoarthritis, and chronic hip pain.[41-43] MMT has proven to be a good clinical tool, but it may be enhanced by using a hand-held dynamometer to obtain a more quantitative and reproducible measurement.[44-46]

A general lower extremity integument inspection and vascular screen can also be conducted. Palpation of the femoral, popliteal, posterior tibialis, and dorsalis pedis pulses can determine whether the pulses are present or absent.[47]

Supine Examination

The supine examination can begin with standard goniometric hip ROM measurements for flexion (120 degrees with knee bent), abduction (40 degrees), adduction (25 degrees), internal rotation (35 degrees), and external rotation (45 degrees).[48,49] A digital inclinometer can also be used for enhanced accuracy.[48,50] For hip internal and external rotation, the hip and knee are flexed to approximately 90 degrees.

Care should be taken to avoid the impingement positions of flexion and adduction, which may cause pain during testing. Muscle length testing can be performed at this time to assess for any length deficits, bilaterally. Common muscle length tests include the 90-90 hamstring test, the straight leg raise test, and the modified Thomas test.

90-90 Hamstring Test

- Rationale: Assess for hamstring length.
- Patient position: The patient is supine on the table with both legs extended.
- Examiner position: The examiner is standing on the side of the test leg.
- Procedure: The examiner passively moves the ipsilateral hip to 90 degrees of flexion and maintains the position.[51,52] The knee is then passively extended to maximum range. The contralateral lower extremity is kept in full knee extension (Fig. 2-5).[51,52]
- Interpretation: A knee extension angle greater than 20 degrees indicates decreased hamstring length.[47,49]
- Reliability: Interrater reliability (intraclass correlation coefficient [ICC], 0.92 to 0.99).[51,53]
- Note: The clinician needs make sure the patient maintains a stable pelvis because an anterior or posterior pelvis

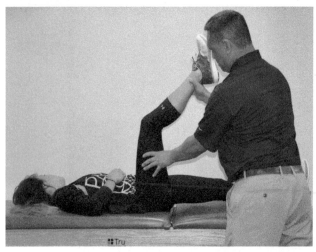

• **Figure 2-5** 90-90 Hamstring Test.

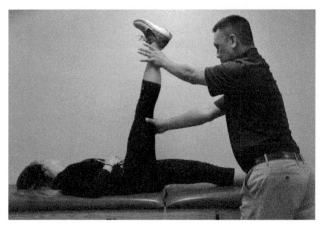

• **Figure 2-6** Straight Leg Raise Test.

can significantly affect the test results.[54] The contralateral extremity can also be fixed to the table by using a nylon strap to prevent movement.[52] A second examiner can also be used to take measurements.

Straight Leg Raise Test (Passive)

• Rationale: Assess for hamstring length.
• Patient position: The patient is supine on the table with both legs extended.
• Examiner position: The examiner is standing on the side of the test leg.
• Procedure: The examiner passively flexes the ipsilateral hip. The knee is fully extended throughout the test. The ankle is held in slight plantar flexion to avoid any neural tension.[51,55] At the end of the available ROM, the hip joint angle is measured. The contralateral lower extremity is kept in full knee extension (Fig. 2-6).[51,52,55]
• Interpretation: Straight leg raise of less than 80 degrees indicates hamstring tightness.[51]
• Reliability: Interrater reliability with inclinometer (ICC: >0.97).[51]
• Note: The straight leg raise test is also used to assess lumbar disk disease in patients who report "sciatic"

symptoms. The pelvis and contralateral extremity can be fixed on the table by using a nylon strap to prevent movement.[51] A second examiner can also be used to take measurements.

Modified Thomas Test

• Rationale: Assess anterior hip muscle length (iliopsoas and rectus femoris, tensor fasciae latae [TFL]).
• Patient position: The patient is supine at end of table with both knees bent over the edge of the table.
• Examiner position: The examiner is standing on the side of the test leg.
• Procedure: The patient maximally flexes the nontest hip, brings the knee to the chest, and holds the position.[56] The lumbar spine and pelvis are flat on table. The examiner can conduct three measurements of the test leg: (1) hip angle for iliopsoas length, (2) knee angle for rectus femoris length, (3) hip abduction angle for TFL/iliotibial band (ITB) flexibility.[56,57] The procedure can be repeated on the opposite side (Fig. 2-7).
• Interpretation: Normal muscle length is considered when the hip and posterior thigh are flat on the table, the hip is in line with the pelvis (not abducted), and the knee remains at a minimum of 90 degrees.[57,58] Decreased muscle length is considered when the hip is not flat on the table, or the hip is abducted, or the knee angle is less than 90 degrees (see Fig. 2-7). The hip and knee angles can be calculated and used as repeated measures or graded as a pass or fail.
• Modification: The examiner can actively stabilize the pelvis or passively stabilize it by using a strap. The hip and knee can also be passively moved into different positions to help isolate a muscle and assess its length (e.g., if the hip is not in full extension [flat on the table], passively extend the knee to relax the rectus femoris and further assess iliopsoas length). These test modifications are common in clinical practice but have not been fully studied.
• Reliability: Rectus femoris length goniometric measurements: intrarater (ICC, 0.67) and interrater (ICC, 0.50) reliability. Pass/fail criteria: intrarater (kappa = 0.040) and interrater (kappa = 0.50).[58] Active pelvic stabilization: intrarater (ICC, 0.99). Passive pelvic stabilization: intrarater (ICC, 0.98).[59]
• Note: A modified version of the Thomas test has also been used to assess the presence of intraarticular hip disorders. See Table 2-5 for a description of this test.

A secondary lower extremity integument inspection and palpation of suspected soft tissue structures can also be conducted. For palpation, a 0 to 4 scale is recommended to measure the patient's pressure pain threshold and reactivity level, which will help determine the patient's tolerance to further testing and treatment (Table 2-4).[60-75] Palpation should focus on the anatomic structures most proximal to the patient's region of complaint (e.g., the iliopsoas) because these structures are often involved in both intraarticular and extraarticular disorders.[5] Palpation should be part of a

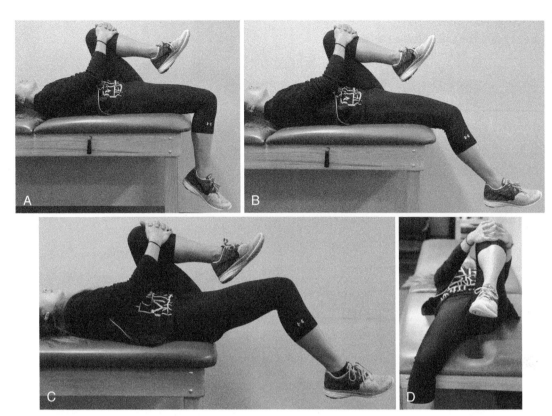

• **Figure 2-7** Modified Thomas Test. **A,** Normal muscle length. **B,** Decreased rectus femoris length. **C,** Decreased hip flexor length. **D,** Tensor fasciae latae and iliotibial band tightness (abducted hip).

TABLE 2-4	Palpation Pressure Pain Threshold Scale	
Grade	Interpretation	Criteria
0	No pain	No signs of pain or discomfort with pressure
I	Mild pain	Tenderness reported without flinching to pressure
II	Moderate pain	Wincing or flinching to pressure
III	Severe pain	Signs of severe pain such as verbal gestures and withdrawing of body part to pressure
IV	Noxious-intolerable pain	Unbearable pain; patient does not allow palpation to the specific area of pain

comprehensive examination; however; the research on anterior hip palpation is sparse and inconclusive. This should be considered when interpreting the findings of the clinical examination. Special testing can also be conducted in the supine position to rule in and rule out specific pelvic and hip disorders. Table 2-5 provides a description of special tests for various intraarticular and extraarticular hip disorders. The description and interpretation of these tests are

based on the investigations that described and reported the clinometric values of these tests. Other versions of the tests may exist or have been reported, but because their diagnostic value has not been studied, they are not included in this chapter.

Side-Lying Examination

The side-lying examination can begin with an integument inspection and palpation of the bony and soft tissue structures around the lateral hip. Specific regional structures that may be implicated in lateral hip disorders include the greater trochanter and bursa region, the posterior and anterior trochanter area, the proximal ITB, the TFL insertion into the ITB, and the gluteus medius muscle belly. Pain with palpation of the posterior trochanteric region may represent gluteus medius tendon involvement, whereas tenderness at the anterior trochanteric region may indicate gluteus minimus tendon involvement.[76] The absence of symptom reproduction with palpatory examination may lead the clinician to consider other sources of symptoms.[77] Martin and Sekiya[78] conducted a reliability study with 70 patients (mean age, 42 years; standard deviation, 15.4). Diagnoses in the hip region included FAI, capsular laxity, trochanteric bursitis, iliopsoas tendinitis, and adductor strains. The investigators found good interrater agreement for palpation of the greater trochanter for tenderness (kappa 0.66, 95% confidence interval 0.48 to 0.84).

| TABLE 2-5 | **Special Tests for the Pelvis and Hip** |

Clinical Tests	Pathologic Conditions	Procedures and Interpretation	Diagnostic Properties (Pooled)
Tests for Intraarticular Disorders			
Flexion-adduction-internal rotation test (FADIR)	FAI and labral tear	Patient position: Supine with legs extended onto the table Examiner position: Standing on the side of the test leg Procedure: The examiner passively moves the test hip into 90 degrees of hip and knee flexion; the hip is passively adducted with internal rotation and overpressure in both directions[62,63] Interpretation: A positive test result is reproduction of the patient's reported pain or mechanical symptoms	Accuracy (64% to 95%), sensitivity (75% to 100%), specificity (10% to 100%), positive predictive value (0.64 to 1.0), negative predictive value (0), positive likelihood ratio (0.86 to 2.4), negative likelihood ratio (0.04 to 2.2)[62,64,65]
Flexion internal rotation test	FAI and labral disorders	Patient position: Supine with legs extended onto the table Examiner position: Standing on the side of the test leg Procedure: The examiner passively moves the test hip into 90 degrees of hip and knee flexion; the hip is passively internally rotated with overpressure[62] Interpretation: A positive test result is reproduction of the patient's reported pain or mechanical symptoms	Accuracy (70% to 100%), sensitivity (100%), specificity (0%), positive predictive value (0.83 to 1.0), negative predictive value (NC), positive likelihood ratio (1.0)[63,66]
Thomas test	Intraarticular hip disorders	Patient position: Supine at the end of the table with both knees to the chest; the lumbar spine and pelvis are flat on the table Examiner position: Standing on the side of the test leg Procedure: The examiner passively lowers the test leg while stabilizing the ipsilateral side of the pelvis; the patient holds the nontest leg to the chest with both arms[62] Interpretation: A positive test result is reproduction of the patient's reported pain or mechanical symptoms such as a painful "click" Note: This is a modified version of the standard test that measures muscle length[62]	Sensitivity (89%), specificity (92%), positive likelihood ratio (11.1), negative likelihood ratio (0.12)[62]
Flexion-abduction-external rotation (FABER)	Intraarticular hip disorders, osteoarthritis, or sacroiliac joint disorders	Rationale: Assess for intraarticular hip disease or sacroiliac joint disorders Patient position: Supine with legs extended onto the table Examiner position: Standing on the side of the test leg Procedure: The examiner passively moves the test hip into hip flexion, abduction, and external rotation, followed by overpressure (downward); the opposite hand applies pressure to the contralateral iliac crest to stabilize the pelvis during testing Interpretation: A positive test result is reproduction of the patient's reported pain or mechanical symptoms[67]	Sensitivity (44% to 100%), specificity (57% to 100%), positive predictive value (46% to 100%), negative predictive value (9%), positive likelihood ratio (0.73), negative likelihood ratio (2.2)[64,67-70]

TABLE 2-5   Special Tests for the Pelvis and Hip—cont'd

Clinical Tests	Pathologic Conditions	Procedures and Interpretation	Diagnostic Properties (Pooled)
Impingement provocation test	Posterior labral tear	Patient position: Supine at the end of the table with both legs extended Examiner position: Standing on the side of the test leg Procedure: The examiner passively lowers the test leg into hyperextension, abduction, and external rotation with overpressure Interpretation: A positive test result is reproduction of the patient's reported pain	Accuracy (82%), sensitivity (100%), specificity (0%), positive predictive value (0.82), negative predictive value (NC), positive likelihood ratio (1.0), negative likelihood ratio (NC)[63]
Log roll test	Anterior capsular-ligamentous laxity of the hip joint	Patient position: Supine on the table with both legs extended Examiner position: Standing on the side of the test leg Procedure: The examiner grasps the patient's thigh and moves it into passive internal and external rotation; this maneuver is done several times Interpretation: A positive test result is a notable increase of external ROM in the test hip; pain or mechanical symptoms in the groin or anterior hip may indicate an intraarticular disorder	No diagnostics calculated, only interrater reliability (kappa 0.61)[64]
Resisted straight leg raise	Anterior capsule or acetabular labrum	Patient position: Supine on the table with both legs extended Examiner position: Standing on the side of the test leg Procedure: The patient actively flexes the straight leg to approximately 30 degrees; the patient is told to maintain the position while the examiner applies a downward force into extension Interpretation: A positive test result is reproduction of the patient's anterior hip or groin pain	Sensitivity (59%), specificity (32%), positive likelihood ratio (0.87), negative likelihood ratio (1.28)[69]
Scour test	Hip osteoarthritis	Patient position: Supine with legs extended onto the table Examiner position: Standing on the side of the test leg Procedure: The test hip is passively moved into 90 degrees of hip flexion, adduction, and internal rotation (toward opposite shoulder) with an axial load applied, followed by abduction and external rotation while slightly increasing flexion and maintaining an axial load Interpretation: A positive test result is reproduction of the patient's reported lateral hip or groin pain or mechanical symptoms	Sensitivity (62%), specificity (75%)[71]
Trendelenburg sign	Hip osteoarthritis	Patient position: Single leg stance on the affected leg by lifting the contralateral limb off the ground Examiner position: Standing next to the patient Procedure: The patient is asked to maintain this position for a total of 30 seconds Interpretation: A positive test result is a drop of the contralateral pelvis once the leg is lifted; a pelvic on femoral angle of 83 degrees or less is considered a positive sign	Sensitivity (55%), specificity (70%), positive likelihood ratio (1.83), negative likelihood ratio (0.82)[62,72]

Continued

TABLE 2-5   Special Tests for the Pelvis and Hip—cont'd

Clinical Tests	Pathologic Conditions	Procedures and Interpretation	Diagnostic Properties (Pooled)
Tests for Extraarticular Disorders			
Snapping hip maneuver	Internal snapping hip syndrome	Patient position: Supine on the table Procedure: The examiner grasps the affected hip and passively moves into hip flexion, external rotation, and abduction; then the hip is extended, internally rotated, and adducted; during this circumduction motion, the examiner's other hand is palpating the ipsilateral iliopsoas tendon Interpretation: A positive test result is reproduction of a "snapping" sensation between 30 and 45 degrees of hip flexion	No diagnostics calculated
Pelvic compression test	Meralgia paresthetica	Patient position: Side lying with the affected hip upward Examiner position: Standing behind the patient Procedure: The examiner grasps the pelvis over the anterior iliac spine, applies a downward compression force to the pelvic innominate, and maintains pressure for 45 seconds Interpretation: A positive test result is alleviation of symptoms	Sensitivity (95%), specificity (93%)[73]
Adductor squeeze test	Adductor-related groin pain, osteitis pubis	Patient position: Supine with the hip flexed to 45 degrees and the knees at 90 degrees, with feet flat Examiner position: Standing directly in front of the patient Procedure: The examiner places his or her "fist" or hands between the patient's flexed knees; the patient maximally contracts to squeeze the examiner's hands Interpretation: A positive test result is reproduction of the patient's pain	Accuracy (82%), sensitivity (43% to 55%), specificity (91% to 95%), positive predictive value (0.93), negative predictive value (0.34), positive likelihood ratio (4.8), negative likelihood ratio (0.63)[62,74]
30-second single leg stance test	Gluteal tendinopathy	Patient position: Single leg stance on the affected leg by lifting the contralateral limb off the ground Examiner position: Standing next to the patient Procedure: The patient is asked to maintain this position for a total of 30 seconds Interpretation: A positive test result is reproduction of the patient's pain over the lateral hip Note: This test is also called the Trendelenburg sign	Sensitivity (88% to 100%), specificity (97.3%)[62,72]
Resisted external de-rotation test	Gluteal tendinopathy	Patient position: Supine with the test hip and knee flexed to 90 degrees and in external rotation Examiner position: Standing on the side of the test hip Procedure: The examiner resists as the patient actively returns the hip to a neutral positon Interpretation: A positive test result is reproduction of the patient's pain Modification: If test result is negative, then the test is repeated with the patient prone, hip extended, and knee flexed to 90 degrees	Sensitivity (88%), specificity (97%), positive likelihood ratio (32.6), negative likelihood ratio (0.12)[62,72]

TABLE 2-5	Special Tests for the Pelvis and Hip—cont'd		
Clinical Tests	Pathologic Conditions	Procedures and Interpretation	Diagnostic Properties (Pooled)
Resisted hip abduction	Gluteal tendinopathy	Patient position: Side lying with affected hip upward Examiner position: Standing behind the patient Procedure: The patient abducts the hip to approximately 45 degrees; the patient resists a downward force applied by the examiner Interpretation: A positive test result is reproduction of the patient's symptoms	Sensitivity (71%), specificity (84%), positive likelihood ratio (6.83), negative likelihood ratio (0.25)
Flexion-adduction-internal rotation test (FAIR)	Piriformis syndrome	Patient position: Side lying with the affected hip upward; the hip is flexed to 60 degrees, and the knee is flexed between 60 and 90 degrees Examiner position: Standing in front of the patient Procedure: The examiner stabilizes the hip with one hand and internally rotates and adducts the hip by applying a downward force to the knee with the other hand Interpretation: A positive test result is reproduction of the patient's "sciatic" symptoms	Sensitivity (88%), specificity (83%)[75]
Tests for Suspected Hip Fractures			
Patella pubic percussion test	Femoral neck fracture	Patient position: Supine with the legs extended Examiner position: Standing at the side of the affected leg Procedure: The clinician places a stethoscope over the pubic tubercle, followed by tapping of the patella of the affected leg; the clinician assesses the quality of the sound Interpretation: A positive test result is diminished percussion noted when compared with the contralateral side Modification: A tuning fork can also be used for patellar percussion	Sensitivity (95%), specificity (86%), positive likelihood ratio (6.11), negative likelihood ratio (0.07)[62]
Fulcrum test	Femoral stress fracture	Patient position: Sitting at the side of the table with legs off the edge Examiner position: Standing at the side of the affected leg Procedure: The clinician places one arm under the test thigh, which is used as a fulcrum; the other hand provides a constant, mild downward pressure to the top of the thigh; the fulcrum arm is slowly moved from the distal to proximal thigh Interpretation: A positive test result is the patient's reporting pain with testing	Sensitivity (88% to 93%), specificity (13% to 75%), positive likelihood ratio (1.0 to 3.7), negative likelihood ratio (0.09 to 0.97)[62]

FAI, Femoral acetabular impingement; *NC,* not calculated; *ROM,* range of motion.

MMT of the hip abductors and adductors can be performed to assess lateral hip strength by using a 0 to 5 scale (Fig. 2-8).[38] Testing of the hip abductors should be conducted with the patient in the side-lying position with the hip in neutral position or internal rotation.[79,80] These positions have shown the highest activation levels in the gluteus medius.[79,80] The adductors can also be tested with the patient in the side-lying position.[81] Muscle length testing can be done at this time to assess for any length

deficits for the lateral hip region. A common test is the Ober (knee flexed) or modified Ober test (knee extended) (Fig. 2-9). Both versions have been found to produce different results among male and female patients and should be considered separate tests.[82] Special testing can also be conducted to rule in and rule out specific lateral hip disorders such as gluteal tendinopathy in greater trochanteric pain syndrome. Table 2-5 provides a description of these special tests.

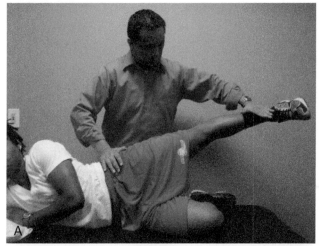

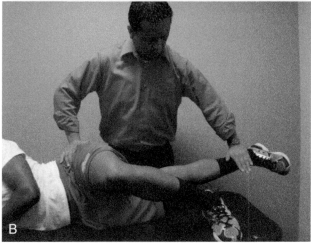

• **Figure 2-8** Hip Manual Muscle Testing. **A,** Hip abduction. **B,** Hip adduction.

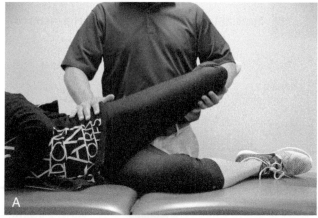

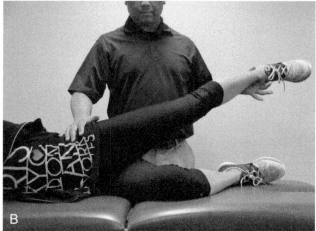

• **Figure 2-9 A,** Ober test. **B,** Modified Ober test.

Ober Test and Modified Ober Test

- Rationale: Assess for TFL/ITB tract length.
- Patient position: The patient is side lying with the test leg upward.
- Examiner position: The examiner is standing behind the patient.
- Procedure: The examiner passively abducts and extends the test hip with the knee flexed or extended (modified) above the hip level and in line with the trunk. The leg is kept in neutral to slight external rotation. The leg is passively lowered while the opposite hand stabilizes the pelvis (see Fig. 2-9).
- Interpretation: If the hip remains above the horizontal plane of the body or does not drop below the level of the greater trochanter (adduction), the test result is considered positive for decreased mobility.
- Reliability: Intrarater reliability using inclinometer for the Ober test (ICC, 0.90) and the modified Ober test (ICC, 0.91).[83]
- Note: The examiner should monitor for compensations through the pelvis. The hip should be held in extension

to neutral with slight external rotation as the test leg is passively lowered.

Prone Examination

The prone examination can also begin with an integument inspection and palpation of suspected anatomic structures. Common regions involved may include: the gluteals, deep hip rotators (e.g., piriformis syndrome), ischial tuberosity and proximal hamstring tendon (e.g., proximal hamstring tear, ischial bursitis), and sciatic notch (e.g., sciatic nerve involvement). Palpation of the posterior greater trochanter has some evidence showing its diagnostic utility for confirming a labral lesion (accuracy, 80%; sensitivity, 80%; specificity, not calculated; positive predictive value, 1.0; negative predictive value, 0).[84] MMT can also be done with the patient prone to assess strength of the gluteus maximus and hamstrings together (Fig. 2-10, *A*) or gluteus maximus (Fig. 2-10, *B*) by using a 0 to 5 scale.[38] Muscle length testing can be done to assess for any length deficits in the anterior hip musculature. A common test in this position is the prone knee flexion test or the Ely test for rectus femoris length (Fig. 2-11).[85] A description of the test is provided here. Special testing can also be conducted to rule in and rule out specific posterior hip and lumbosacral disorders.

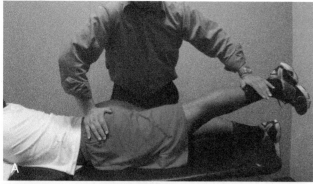

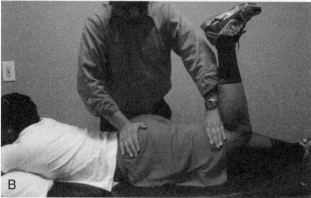

• **Figure 2-10** Manual Muscle Testing. **A,** Hip extension (knee straight). **B,** Hip extension (knee bent).

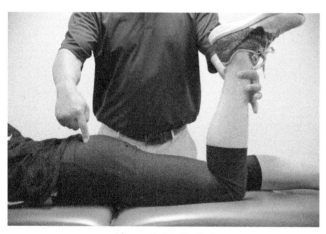

• **Figure 2-11** Ely Test.

Chapter 10 discusses various tests for common lumbosacral disorders.

Ely Test (Prone Knee Flexion)

• Rationale: Assess for rectus femoris length.
• Patient position: The patient is lying prone on the table with both legs extended.
• Examiner position: The examiner is standing at the side of the patient.
• Procedure: The examiner passively flexes the knee of the test leg while keeping the opposite knee fully extended (see Fig. 2-11).

• Interpretation: If the test hip rises as the knee is flexed, that indicates rectus femoris tightness.
• Modification: This test can be done passively by the clinician or actively by the patient.
• Reliability: Active motion by the patient: intrarater reliability (kappa = 0.52) and interrater reliability (kappa = 0.46).[85]
• Note: The examiner should monitor for compensations through the pelvis. This test is also used in the examination of patients with nonspecific low back pain[86] and cerebral palsy.[87,88]

Lumbosacral Screen

If lumbosacral involvement is suspected, then the examiner may need to test further for specific disorders, which can be integrated into the standard examination discussed earlier. Specific testing should be done in the most comfortable position for the patient, to avoid aggravating the condition. Chapter 10 provides a comprehensive discussion of the relationship between lumbosacral disease and hip pain. The chapter also provides clinical markers and examination strategies for common lumbosacral disorders that can refer symptoms into the hip region.

Summary of Clinical Tests

The clinical examination should be conducted in a standard sequence to allow the patient to transition easily between positions. Figure 2-12 details the proposed examination process, which may need to be modified according to the clinical findings or the patient's functional abilities. The clinician should develop a common set of evidence-based tests and measures that can be used in each position. This creates a systematic process that can be replicated with different patients. The clinical tests and measures detailed in this chapter are common to the hip and pelvic region and are not all inclusive. Results of special testing in this chapter may not enable the clinician to diagnose pathologic processes definitively. No cluster of tests has been developed to date. This must be considered when interpreting the results from the examination. The reader is encouraged to study these tests and measures further, to ensure good reproducibility. The examination process should always be based on evidence and should be structured to the individual patient.

Diagnostic Imaging

Diagnostic imaging is also part of a comprehensive examination process of the pelvis and hip. Common imaging includes radiographs, computed tomography (CT), bone scintigraphy, diagnostic ultrasound, magnetic resonance imaging (MRI), and magnetic resonance arthrography (MRA).[89] Imaging techniques, along with examples of their diagnostic abilities for detecting certain pathologic features, are discussed in this section.

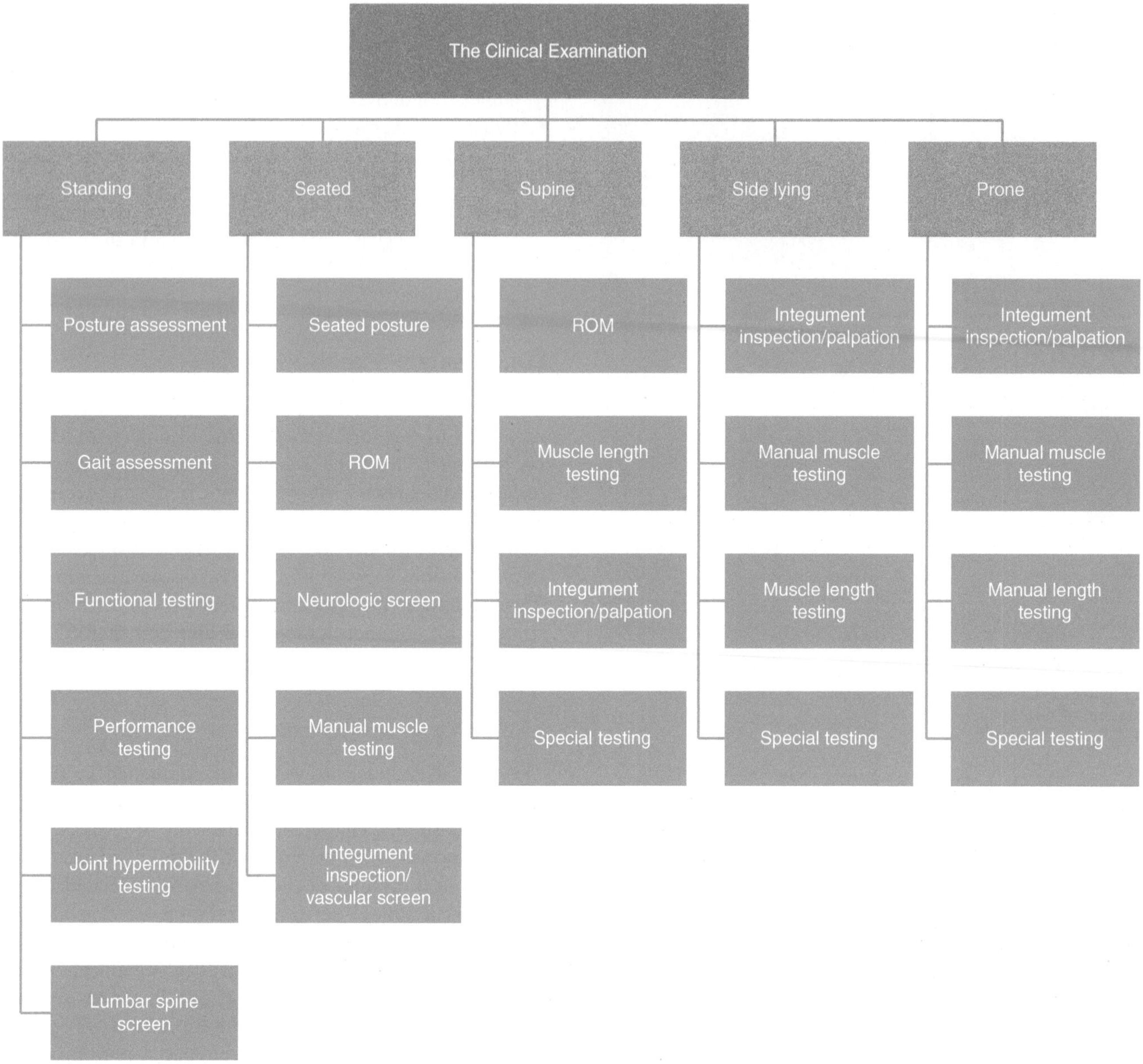

• **Figure 2-12** Hip Examination Process. *ROM,* Range of motion.

Radiographs are commonly taken to assess the bony architecture of the pelvis and hip for diagnosing various disorders such as fractures, abnormal hip morphology, and slipped capital epiphysis. Appendix C provides a comprehensive discussion of the various radiographic techniques involved in diagnosing the common pelvic and hip disorders discussed in subsequent chapters.

CT is a radiographic technique that combines many x-ray images combined with a computer to generate cross-sectional views of specific anatomic structures. **CT scans** are used to assess for bony (e.g., femoral head fractures, osseus abnormalities) and intraarticular (e.g., acetabular labral tears) disorders of the hip.[90] CT has shown good diagnostic accuracy for FAI and acetabular labral tears (sensitivity, 92% to 97%; specificity, 87% to 100%) and articular cartilage lesions (sensitivity, 88%; specificity, 82%).[3,91,92]

Bone scintigraphy, or **bone scan,** is a nuclear imaging test used to assess various bone disorders such as hip stress fractures, bone tumors, and osteoporosis. The bone scan has good diagnostic ability for detecting femoral neck and intertrochanteric fractures (sensitivity, 91%; specificity, 100%) and causes of low back pain in children (sensitivity, 94%; specificity, 100%), such as spondylolysis, bone tumors, infections (osteomyelitis), sacroiliitis, and fractures.[89,93]

Diagnostic ultrasound is an emerging test often used for soft tissue disorders such as muscle, tendon, and cartilage disease. Ultrasound examination sends sound waves into the specific tissues of the body through a transducer. The sounds waves reflect off the tissues and are recorded and converted into images.[94] Ultrasound is becoming more popular because it has no radiation and it costs less to administer than other diagnostic imaging methods. The

TABLE 2-6	Patient-Related Outcome Questionnaires	
Scale	**Content**	**Score Interpretation**
Hip and Groin Outcome Score (HAGOS)	6 subscales that measure pain, symptoms, physical function in daily living, physical function in sports and recreational activity, participation in physical activity, and hip or groin quality of life	Each subscale is scored separately; subscale scores are calculated, and raw scores are transformed to a 0 to 100 scale; this is interpreted as: (0) extreme hip/groin problems to (100) no hip/groin problems
Hip Outcome Score (HOS)	24 questions measuring activities of daily living and physical function during sports activity	Each subscale scores separately; the highest potential score for the activities of daily living scale is 68, and it is 38 for the sports subscale; scores are converted to a percentage; higher score represents a higher level of physical function
International Hip Outcome Tool-33 (IHOT-33) and IHOT-12 (short version)	IHOT: 33 questions that measure hip-related symptoms, function, sports, function with occupational activities, and quality of life IHOT-12: a modified version with 12 questions	Each question uses a visual analog scale grading format; scores are calculated transformed to a 0 to 100 scale, interpreted as: (0) worst to (100) best
Hip Disability and Osteoarthritis Outcome Score (HOOS)	5 subscales that measure pain, symptoms, function in activities of daily living, function in sport and recreation, and hip quality of life	Each subscale is scored separately; subscales scores are transformed to a 0 to 100 scale, interpreted as: (0) worst to (100) best
Western Ontario and McMaster Universities Osteoarthritis Index (WOMAC)	24 items with 3 subscales: pain, stiffness, and disability	Each subscale is scored separately; a higher score represents worse pain, and a lower score represents less pain
Harris Hip Score (HHS)	10 items; domains covered: pain, function, absence of deformity, and range of motion	Each item has a unique numeric scale, with 100 total points; scores are interpreted as follows: <70, poor result; 70 to 80, fair; 80 to 90, good; and 90 to 100, excellent result

diagnostic utility of ultrasound for the hip region is still emerging. The available studies have shown a sensitivity of 82% and a specificity of 60% for diagnosing acetabular labral tears and a sensitivity of 61% and a specificity of 100% in diagnosing gluteal tendinopathy in greater trochanteric pain syndrome.[94,95]

MRI and MRA are often used to assess the soft tissue structures of the hip. MRI uses magnetic fields and radio waves to form images of the body, whereas MRA uses the same technology to form images after injection of a contrast medium into the joint.[96] MRI and MRA are the preferred techniques for diagnosing intraarticular hip disorders. For example, MRI has a pooled sensitivity of 66% and specificity of 79% for diagnosing FAI, whereas MRA has a sensitivity of 91% and a specificity of 80%.[89,97] MRI and MRA have both shown moderate sensitivity (66%, 87%) and specificity (79%, 64%) for diagnosing acetabular labral tears.[97] For hip joint articular cartilage lesions, MRI has a pooled sensitivity of 59% and a specificity of 94%, whereas MRA has a sensitivity of 62% and a specificity of 86%.[96]

Diagnostic imaging is an important part of the examination process and is often used to diagnose or confirm a suspected pathologic process in lieu of the clinical examination findings. This section provides a brief discussion of the common types of diagnostic imaging with examples of their diagnostic accuracy. Subsequent chapters provide a more focused discussion on the preferred imaging techniques for the disorders discussed.

Patient-Related Outcome (PRO) Questionnaires

PRO questionnaires are often used to gain a better understanding of the patient's perceptions toward pain and function, as well as how their impairments affect their lives. Several PRO questionnaires are available to use for the hip and pelvic region (Table 2-6). Often, these questionnaires are used as repeated measures throughout the rehabilitation process to help determine the patient's progress during treatment. This section discusses selected questionnaires along with their statistical properties.

For pain assessment, the numeric pain rating scale (0, no pain; 10, worst pain) or visual analog scale are commonly used to assess a patient's level of pain and have been validated in the research.[98,99] For nonarthritic hip and groin disorders in young to middle-aged adults, the Copenhagen Hip and Groin Outcome Score (HAGOS), Hip Outcome Score (HOS), International Hip Outcome Tool-33

(IHOT-33), and IHOT-12 (short version) are recommended.[100] All questionnaires contain good clinometric properties including content validity (except HOS), test-retest reliability, responsiveness, construct validity, and interpretability.[100] The HAGOS contains six separate subscales that assess pain, symptoms, physical function in daily living, physical function in sports and recreational activity, participation in physical activity, and hip or groin quality of life.[101] The HOS contains 24 questions that measure both activities of daily living and physical function during sports activity.[89,100] The IHOT-33 contains 33 questions, and the IHOT-12 (short version) contains 12 questions. Both tools measure hip-related symptoms, function, sports, function with occupational activities, and quality of life.[102,103]

For adults with hip osteoarthritis, the Hip Disability and Osteoarthritis Outcome Score (HOOS), Western Ontario and McMaster Universities Osteoarthritis Index (WOMAC), and Harris Hip Score (HHS) are recommended.[104] All questionnaires contain good clinometric properties including content validity, test-retest reliability, responsiveness, construct validity, and interpretability.[104] The HOOS contains 5 subscales that measure pain, symptoms, function in activity of daily living, function in sport and recreation, and hip quality of life. The WOMAC is a 24-item index with 3 subscales that measure pain, stiffness, and disability.[105] The HOOS contains the same index and is considered an extension of the WOMAC.[104] The HHS is a 10-item instrument that measures pain, function, absence of deformity, and ROM.[104]

This section provides a brief discussion of commonly used PRO questionnaires for individuals with nonarthritic and arthritic hip pain. Many other questionnaires are available, and a comprehensive discussion of all available PRO questionnaires is beyond the scope of this text. Many of the PRO questionnaires mentioned here are discussed in subsequent chapters as related to the disorders discussed. The reader is encouraged to review the chapter reference list for the peer-reviewed sources used in this discussion.

Summary

This chapter provides a detailed description of the hip examination process. The suggested sequence and clinical tests for each position should be modified according to the patient's functional abilities. The reader is encouraged to develop a standardized evidence-based sequence to follow with every patient. This chapter provides foundational examination information for subsequent chapters.

References

1. Slipman CW, Jackson HB, Lipetz JS, et al. Sacroiliac joint pain referral zones. *Arch Phys Med Rehabil.* 2000;81(3):334-338.
2. Redmond JM, Gupta A, Nasser R, et al. The hip-spine connection: understanding its importance in the treatment of hip pathology. *Orthopedics.* 2015;38(1):49-55.
3. Byrd JW. Evaluation of the hip: history and physical examination. *N Am J Sports Phys Ther.* 2007;2(4):231-240.
4. O'Leary JA, Berend K, Vail TP. The relationship between diagnosis and outcome in arthroscopy of the hip. *Arthroscopy.* 2001;17(2):181-188.
5. Reiman MP, Mather RC 3rd, Hash TW 2nd, et al. Examination of acetabular labral tear: a continued diagnostic challenge. *Br J Sports Med.* 2014;48(4):311-319.
6. Frank RM, Slabaugh MA, Grumet RC, et al. Posterior hip pain in an athletic population: differential diagnosis and treatment options. *Sports Health.* 2010;2(3):237-246.
7. Martin HD, Shears SA, Palmer IJ. Evaluation of the hip. *Sports Med Arthrosc.* 2010;18(2):63-75.
8. Sink EL, Gralla J, Ryba A, et al. Clinical presentation of femoroacetabular impingement in adolescents. *J Pediatr Orthop.* 2008;28(8):806-811.
9. Tyler TF, Nicholas SJ. Rehabilitation of extra-articular sources of hip pain in athletes. *N Am J Sports Phys Ther.* 2007;2(4):207-216.
10. Grumet RC, Frank RM, Slabaugh MA, et al. Lateral hip pain in an athletic population: differential diagnosis and treatment options. *Sports Health.* 2010;2(3):191-196.
11. Dawson J, Linsell L, Doll H, et al. Assessment of the Lequesne index of severity for osteoarthritis of the hip in an elderly population. *Osteoarthritis Cartilage.* 2005;13(10):854-860.
12. Martin H, Palmer I. History and physical examination of the hip: the basics. *Curr Rev Musculoskelet Med.* 2013;6(3):219-225.
13. Lewis CL, Sahrmann SA. Effect of posture on hip angles and moments during gait. *Man Ther.* 2015;20(1):176-182.
14. Lewis CL, Khuu A, Marinko LN. Postural correction reduces hip pain in adult with acetabular dysplasia: a case report. *Man Ther.* 2015;20(3):508-512.
15. Ida T, Nakamura Y, Hagio T, et al. Prevalence and characteristics of cam-type femoroacetabular deformity in 100 hips with symptomatic acetabular dysplasia: a case control study. *J Orthop Surg Res.* 2014;9:93.
16. Truszczynska A, Drzal-Grabiec J, Rapala K, et al. Characteristics of selected parameters of body posture in patients with hip osteoarthritis. *Ortop Traumatol Rehabil.* 2014;16(3):351-360.
17. Weng WJ, Wang WJ, Wu MD, et al. Characteristics of sagittal spine-pelvis-leg alignment in patients with severe hip osteoarthritis. *Eur Spine J.* 2015;24(6):1228-1236.
18. Hurwitz DE, Hulet CH, Andriacchi TP, et al. Gait compensations in patients with osteoarthritis of the hip and their relationship to pain and passive hip motion. *J Orthop Res.* 1997;15(4):629-635.
19. Eitzen I, Fernandes L, Nordsletten L, et al. Sagittal plane gait characteristics in hip osteoarthritis patients with mild to moderate symptoms compared to healthy controls: a cross-sectional study. *BMC Musculoskelet Disord.* 2012;13:258.
20. Kokmeyer D, Strzelinski M, Lehecka BJ. Gait considerations in patients with femoroacetabular impingement. *Int J Sports Phys Ther.* 2014;9(6):827-838.
21. Watelain E, Dujardin F, Babier F, et al. Pelvic and lower limb compensatory actions of subjects in an early stage of hip osteoarthritis. *Arch Phys Med Rehabil.* 2001;82(12):1705-1711.
22. Constantinou M, Barrett R, Brown M, et al. Spatial-temporal gait characteristics in individuals with hip osteoarthritis: a systematic literature review and meta-analysis. *J Orthop Sports Phys Ther.* 2014;44(4):291-297.

23. Hunt MA, Guenther JR, Gilbart MK. Kinematic and kinetic differences during walking in patients with and without symptomatic femoroacetabular impingement. *Clin Biomech (Bristol, Avon)*. 2013;28(5):519-523.

24. Kennedy MJ, Lamontagne M, Beaule PE. Femoroacetabular impingement alters hip and pelvic biomechanics during gait walking biomechanics of FAI. *Gait Posture*. 2009;30(1):41-44.

25. Diamond LE, Dobson FL, Bennell KL, et al. Physical impairments and activity limitations in people with femoroacetabular impingement: a systematic review. *Br J Sports Med*. 2015;49(4):230-242.

26. Eitzen I, Fernandes L, Nordsletten L, et al. Weight-bearing asymmetries during sit-to-stand in patients with mild-to-moderate hip osteoarthritis. *Gait Posture*. 2014;39(2):683-688.

27. Lamontagne M, Kennedy MJ, Beaule PE. The effect of cam FAI on hip and pelvic motion during maximum squat. *Clin Orthop Relat Res*. 2009;467(3):645-650.

28. Lequesne M, Mathieu P, Vuillemin-Bodaghi V, et al. Gluteal tendinopathy in refractory greater trochanter pain syndrome: diagnostic value of two clinical tests. *Arthritis Rheum*. 2008;59(2):241-246.

29. Kivlan BR, Martin RL. Functional performance testing of the hip in athletes: a systematic review for reliability and validity. *Int J Sports Phys Ther*. 2012;7(4):402-412.

30. Naal FD, Hatzung G, Muller A, et al. Validation of a self-reported Beighton score to assess hypermobility in patients with femoroacetabular impingement. *Int Orthop*. 2014;38(11):2245-2250.

31. Remvig L, Jensen DV, Ward RC. Epidemiology of general joint hypermobility and basis for the proposed criteria for benign joint hypermobility syndrome: review of the literature. *J Rheumatol*. 2007;34(4):804-809.

32. Bulbena A, Duro JC, Porta M, et al. Clinical assessment of hypermobility of joints: assembling criteria. *J Rheumatol*. 1992;19(1):115-122.

33. Juul-Kristensen B, Rogind H, Jensen DV, et al. Inter-examiner reproducibility of tests and criteria for generalized joint hypermobility and benign joint hypermobility syndrome. *Rheumatology (Oxford)*. 2007;46(12):1835-1841.

34. Boyle KL, Witt P, Riegger-Krugh C. Intrarater and interrater reliability of the Beighton and Horan joint mobility index. *J Athl Train*. 2003;38(4):281-285.

35. Smits-Engelsman B, Klerks M, Kirby A. Beighton score: a valid measure for generalized hypermobility in children. *J Pediatr*. 2011;158(1):119-123, 123.e111-123.e114.

36. McCormack M, Briggs J, Hakim A, et al. Joint laxity and the benign joint hypermobility syndrome in student and professional ballet dancers. *J Rheumatol*. 2004;31(1):173-178.

37. Kim SH, Kwon OY, Yi CH, et al. Lumbopelvic motion during seated hip flexion in subjects with low-back pain accompanying limited hip flexion. *Eur Spine J*. 2014;23(1):142-148.

38. Cook C, Hegedus E. *Orthopedic Physical Examination Tests: An Evidence-Based Approach*. 2nd ed. New York: Pearson Education; 2012.

39. Kerr RS, Cadoux-Hudson TA, Adams CB. The value of accurate clinical assessment in the surgical management of the lumbar disc protrusion. *J Neurol Neurosurg Psychiatry*. 1988;51(2):169-173.

40. Peeters GG, Aufdemkampe G, Oostendorp RA. Sensibility testing in patients with a lumbosacral radicular syndrome. *J Manipulative Physiol Ther*. 1998;21(2):81-88.

41. Casartelli NC, Maffiuletti NA, Item-Glatthorn JF, et al. Hip muscle weakness in patients with symptomatic femoroacetabular impingement. *Osteoarthritis Cartilage*.2011;19(7):816-821.

42. Arokoski MH, Arokoski JP, Haara M, et al. Hip muscle strength and muscle cross sectional area in men with and without hip osteoarthritis. *J Rheumatol*. 2002;29(10):2185-2195.

43. Harris-Hayes M, Mueller MJ, Sahrmann SA, et al. Persons with chronic hip joint pain exhibit reduced hip muscle strength. *J Orthop Sports Phys Ther*. 2014;44(11):890-898.

44. Cuthbert SC, Goodheart GJ Jr. On the reliability and validity of manual muscle testing: a literature review. *Chiropr Osteopat*. 2007;15:4.

45. Stark T, Walker B, Phillips JK, et al. Hand-held dynamometry correlation with the gold standard isokinetic dynamometry: a systematic review. *PM R*. 2011;3(5):472-479.

46. Arnold CM, Warkentin KD, Chilibeck PD, et al. The reliability and validity of handheld dynamometry for the measurement of lower-extremity muscle strength in older adults. *J Strength Cond Res*. 2010;24(3):815-824.

47. Cournot M, Boccalon H, Cambou JP, et al. Accuracy of the screening physical examination to identify subclinical atherosclerosis and peripheral arterial disease in asymptomatic subjects. *J Vasc Surg*. 2007;46(6):1215-1221.

48. Bierma-Zeinstra SM, Bohnen AM, Ramlal R, et al. Comparison between two devices for measuring hip joint motions. *Clin Rehabil*. 1998;12(6):497-505.

49. Neumann DA. *Kinesiology of the Musculoskeletal System: Foundations for Rehabilitation*. St. Louis: Mosby; 2010.

50. Charlton PC, Mentiplay BF, Pua YH, et al. Reliability and concurrent validity of a smartphone, bubble inclinometer and motion analysis system for measurement of hip joint range of motion. *J Sci Med Sport*. 2015;18(3):262-267.

51. Davis DS, Quinn RO, Whiteman CT, et al. Concurrent validity of four clinical tests used to measure hamstring flexibility. *J Strength Cond Res*. 2008;22(2):583-588.

52. Fasen JM, O'Connor AM, Schwartz SL, et al. A randomized controlled trial of hamstring stretching: comparison of four techniques. *J Strength Cond Res*. 2009;23(2):660-667.

53. Fredriksen H, Dagfinrud H, Jacobsen V, et al. Passive knee extension test to measure hamstring muscle tightness. *Scand J Med Sci Sports*. 1997;7(5):279-282.

54. Herrington L. The effect of pelvic position on popliteal angle achieved during 90:90 hamstring-length test. *J Sport Rehabil*. 2013;22(4):254-256.

55. Ylinen JJ, Kautiainen HJ, Hakkinen AH. Comparison of active, manual, and instrumental straight leg raise in measuring hamstring extensibility. *J Strength Cond Res*. 2010;24(4):972-977.

56. Harvey D. Assessment of the flexibility of elite athletes using the modified Thomas test. *Br J Sports Med*. 1998;32(1):68-70.

57. Ferber R, Kendall KD, McElroy L. Normative and critical criteria for iliotibial band and iliopsoas muscle flexibility. *J Athl Train*. 2010;45(4):344-348.

58. Peeler JD, Anderson JE. Reliability limits of the modified Thomas test for assessing rectus femoris muscle flexibility about the knee joint. *J Athl Train*. 2008;43(5):470-476.

59. Kim GM, Ha SM. Reliability of the modified Thomas test using a lumbo-pelvic stabilization. *J Phys Ther Sci*. 2015;27(2):447-449.

60. Wolfe F, Smythe HA, Yunus MB, et al. The American College of Rheumatology 1990 criteria for the classification of fibromyalgia: report of the Multicenter Criteria Committee. *Arthritis Rheum*. 1990;33(2):160-172.

61. Cheatham SW, Kolber MJ. Rehabilitation after hip arthroscopy and labral repair in a high school football athlete. *Int J Sports Phys Ther.* 2012;7(2):173-184.

62. Reiman MP, Mather RC 3rd, Cook CE. Physical examination tests for hip dysfunction and injury. *Br J Sports Med.* 2015;49(6):357-361.

63. Leibold MR, Huijbregts PA, Jensen R. Concurrent criterion-related validity of physical examination tests for hip labral lesions: a systematic review. *J Man Manip Ther.* 2008;16(2):E24-E41.

64. Martin RL, Sekiya JK. The interrater reliability of 4 clinical tests used to assess individuals with musculoskeletal hip pain. *J Orthop Sports Phys Ther.* 2008;38(2):71-77.

65. Reiman MP, Goode AP, Cook CE, et al. Diagnostic accuracy of clinical tests for the diagnosis of hip femoroacetabular impingement/labral tear: a systematic review with meta-analysis. *Br J Sports Med.* 2015;49(12):811.

66. Santori N, Villar RN. Acetabular labral tears: result of arthroscopic partial limbectomy. *Arthroscopy.* 2000;16(1):11-15.

67. Troelsen A, Mechlenburg I, Gelineck J, et al. What is the role of clinical tests and ultrasound in acetabular labral tear diagnostics? *Acta Orthop.* 2009;80(3):314-318.

68. Mitchell B, McCrory P, Brukner P, et al. Hip joint pathology: clinical presentation and correlation between magnetic resonance arthrography, ultrasound, and arthroscopic findings in 25 consecutive cases. *Clin J Sport Med.* 2003;13(3):152-156.

69. Maslowski E, Sullivan W, Forster Harwood J, et al. The diagnostic validity of hip provocation maneuvers to detect intra-articular hip pathology. *PM R.* 2010;2(3):174-181.

70. Tijssen M, van Cingel R, Willemsen L, et al. Diagnostics of femoroacetabular impingement and labral pathology of the hip: a systematic review of the accuracy and validity of physical tests. *Arthroscopy.* 2012;28(6):860-871.

71. Sutlive TG, Lopez HP, Schnitker DE, et al. Development of a clinical prediction rule for diagnosing hip osteoarthritis in individuals with unilateral hip pain. *J Orthop Sports Phys Ther.* 2008;38(9):542-550.

72. Lequesne M, Mathieu P, Vuillemin-Bodaghi V, et al. Gluteal tendinopathy in refractory greater trochanter pain syndrome: diagnostic value of two clinical tests. *Arthritis Care Res.* 2008;59(2):241-246.

73. Nourae SA, Anand B, Spink G, et al. A novel approach to the diagnosis and management of meralgia paresthetica. *Neurosurgery.* 2007;60(4):696-700, discussion 700.

74. Verrall GM, Slavotinek JP, Barnes PG, et al. Description of pain provocation tests used for the diagnosis of sports-related chronic groin pain: relationship of tests to defined clinical (pain and tenderness) and MRI (pubic bone marrow oedema) criteria. *Scand J Med Sci Sports.* 2005;15(1):36-42.

75. Fishman LM, Dombi GW, Michaelsen C, et al. Piriformis syndrome: diagnosis, treatment, and outcome—a 10-year study. *Arch Phys Med Rehabil.* 2002;83(3):295-301.

76. Grumet RC, Frank RM, Slabaugh MA, et al. Lateral hip pain in an athletic population: differential diagnosis and treatment options. *Sports Health.* 2010;2(3):191-196.

77. Martin RL, Enseki KR, Draovitch P, et al. Acetabular labral tears of the hip: examination and diagnostic challenges. *J Orthop Sports Phys Ther.* 2006;36(7):503-515.

78. Martin RL, Sekiya JK. The interrater reliability of 4 clinical tests used to assess individuals with musculoskeletal hip pain. *J Orthop Sports Phys Ther.* 2008;38(2):71-77.

79. Otten R, Tol JL, Holmich P, Whiteley R. Electromyography activation levels of the 3 gluteus medius subdivisions during manual strength testing. *J Sport Rehabil.* 2015;24(3):244-251.

80. Widler KS, Glatthorn JF, Bizzini M, et al. Assessment of hip abductor muscle strength: a validity and reliability study. *J Bone Joint Surg Am.* 2009;91(11):2666-2672.

81. Hrysomallis C. Hip adductors' strength, flexibility, and injury risk. *J Strength Cond Res.* 2009;23(5):1514-1517.

82. Gajdosik RL, Sandler MM, Marr HL. Influence of knee positions and gender on the Ober test for length of the iliotibial band. *Clin Biomech (Bristol, Avon).* 2003;18(1):77-79.

83. Reese NB, Bandy WD. Use of an inclinometer to measure flexibility of the iliotibial band using the Ober test and the modified Ober test: differences in magnitude and reliability of measurements. *J Orthop Sports Phys Ther.* 2003;33(6):326-330.

84. Hase T, Ueo T. Acetabular labral tear: arthroscopic diagnosis and treatment. *Arthroscopy.* 1999;15(2):138-141.

85. Peeler J, Anderson JE. Reliability of the Ely's test for assessing rectus femoris muscle flexibility and joint range of motion. *J Orthop Res.* 2008;26(6):793-799.

86. Carlsson H, Rasmussen-Barr E. Clinical screening tests for assessing movement control in non-specific low-back pain: a systematic review of intra- and inter-observer reliability studies. *Man Ther.* 2013;18(2):103-110.

87. Lee SY, Sung KH, Chung CY, et al. Reliability and validity of the Duncan-Ely test for assessing rectus femoris spasticity in patients with cerebral palsy. *Dev Med Child Neurol.* 2015 Apr 6;[Epub ahead of print].

88. Kay RM, Rethlefsen SA, Kelly JP, et al. Predictive value of the Duncan-Ely test in distal rectus femoris transfer. *J Pediatr Orthop.* 2004;24(1):59-62.

89. Reiman MP, Thorborg K. Clinical examination and physical assessment of hip joint-related pain in athletes. *Int J Sports Phys Ther.* 2014;9(6):737-755.

90. Nepple JJ, Prather H, Trousdale RT, et al. Diagnostic imaging of femoroacetabular impingement. *J Am Acad Orthop Surg.* 2013;21(suppl 1):S20-S26.

91. Nishii T, Tanaka H, Sugano N, et al. Disorders of acetabular labrum and articular cartilage in hip dysplasia: evaluation using isotropic high-resolutional CT arthrography with sequential radial reformation. *Osteoarthritis Cartilage.* 2007;15(3):251-257.

92. Yamamoto Y, Tonotsuka H, Ueda T, et al. Usefulness of radial contrast-enhanced computed tomography for the diagnosis of acetabular labrum injury. *Arthroscopy.* 2007;23(12):1290-1294.

93. Alkhawaldeh K, Ghuweri AA, Kawar J, et al. Back pain in children and diagnostic value of (99m)Tc MDP bone scintigraphy. *Acta Inform Med.* 2014;22(5):297-301.

94. Kong A, Van der Vliet A, Zadow S. MRI and US of gluteal tendinopathy in greater trochanteric pain syndrome. *Eur Radiol.* 2007;17(7):1772-1783.

95. Fearon AM, Scarvell JM, Cook JL, et al. Does ultrasound correlate with surgical or histologic findings in greater trochanteric pain syndrome? A pilot study. *Clin Orthop Relat Res.* 2010;468(7):1838-1844.

96. Smith TO, Simpson M, Ejindu V, et al. The diagnostic test accuracy of magnetic resonance imaging, magnetic resonance arthrography and computer tomography in the detection of chondral lesions of the hip. *Eur J Orthop Surg Traumatol.* 2013;23(3):335-344.

97. Smith TO, Hilton G, Toms AP, et al. The diagnostic accuracy of acetabular labral tears using magnetic resonance imaging and

magnetic resonance arthrography: a meta-analysis. *Eur Radiol.* 2011;21(4):863-874.

98. Hjermstad MJ, Fayers PM, Haugen DF, et al. Studies comparing numerical rating scales, verbal rating scales, and visual analogue scales for assessment of pain intensity in adults: a systematic literature review. *J Pain Symptom Manage.* 2011;41(6):1073-1093.

99. Breivik EK, Bjornsson GA, Skovlund E. A comparison of pain rating scales by sampling from clinical trial data. *Clin J Pain.* 2000;16(1):22-28.

100. Thorborg K, Tijssen M, Habets B, et al. Patient-reported outcome (PRO) questionnaires for young to middle-aged adults with hip and groin disability: a systematic review of the clinimetric evidence. *Br J Sports Med.* 2015;49(12):812.

101. Thorborg K, Holmich P, Christensen R, et al. The Copenhagen Hip and Groin Outcome Score (HAGOS): development and validation according to the COSMIN checklist. *Br J Sports Med.* 2011;45(6):478-491.

102. Mohtadi NG, Griffin DR, Pedersen ME, et al. The development and validation of a self-administered quality-of-life outcome measure for young, active patients with symptomatic hip disease: the International Hip Outcome Tool (iHOT-33). *Arthroscopy.* 2012;28(5):595-605, quiz 606-510 e591.

103. Griffin DR, Parsons N, Mohtadi NG, et al. A short version of the International Hip Outcome Tool (iHOT-12) for use in routine clinical practice. *Arthroscopy.* 2012;28(5):611-616, quiz 616-618.

104. Nilsdotter A, Bremander A. Measures of hip function and symptoms: Harris Hip Score (HHS), Hip Disability and Osteoarthritis Outcome Score (HOOS), Oxford Hip Score (OHS), Lequesne Index of Severity for Osteoarthritis of the Hip (LISOH), and American Academy of Orthopedic Surgeons (AAOS) Hip and Knee Questionnaire. *Arthritis Care Res.* 2011;63(S11):S200-S207.

105. Bellamy N, Buchanan WW, Goldsmith CH, et al. Validation study of WOMAC: a health status instrument for measuring clinically important patient relevant outcomes to antirheumatic drug therapy in patients with osteoarthritis of the hip or knee. *J Rheumatol.* 1988;15(12):1833-1840.

3

Hip Disorders: Extraarticular

KEELAN ENSEKI AND SCOTT W. CHEATHAM

CHAPTER OUTLINE

The differential diagnosis of conditions of the hip can be challenging because of the many possible intraarticular and extraarticular pathologic processes. In fact, up to 60% of patients who undergo arthroscopic surgical procedures of the hip have misdiagnosed conditions.[1] This chapter discusses common extraarticular hip disorders, whereas Chapter 4 discusses the common intraarticular disorders. Some of the common pathologic conditions described in this chapter include snapping hip syndrome (SHS), meralgia paresthetica (MP), adductor-related groin pain, greater trochanteric pain syndrome (GTPS), and proximal hamstring injuries.

Snapping Hip Syndrome

SHS or coxa saltans is a condition characterized by a palpable or audible "snapping" that occurs around the hip with movement.[2] This condition is commonly classified as either internal SHS (ISHS) or external SHS (ESHS). With ISHS, the "snapping" is often felt in the anterior hip region, and with ESHS, the sensation is felt over the lateral hip region.[3]

The epidemiologic data are sparse, with few studies reporting prevalence. According to the available data, SHS occurs in 5% to 10% of the population and most often in persons 15 to 40 years old; it affects female patients more than male patients.[4-6] SHS is often related to repetitive activity and is common in sports such as running, track, football, soccer, golf, weightlifting, and dance (see Chapter 8).[5-11] SHS is often not considered a secondary diagnosis when compared with the more common diagnoses such as femoral acetabular impingement (FAI) and is often ruled out during the differential diagnosis of hip pain.[12]

Patient Profile and Mechanism of Injury

For both ISHS and ESHS, patients may first report a "non-painful" sensation or audible snapping, clicking, or popping with activity, which may eventually lead to discomfort. With ISHS, the sensation may be provoked during deep flexion (e.g., >90 degrees) and hip external rotation movements.[3,13] Specific movements that may be difficult include getting into or out of a car, sitting to standing, and running.[3] SHS is primarily caused by snapping of the iliopsoas tendon over the iliopectineal eminence, anterior hip capsule, femoral head, or iliofemoral ligament.[9,13,14] With ESHS, the sensation may be provoked during hip flexion or during external or internal rotation.[3] Specific movements that may be difficult include carrying heavy loads, climbing stairs, playing golf, and running.[3] The sensation may be caused by snapping of the iliotibial band (ITB) or gluteus maximus tendon over the greater trochanter or subluxation of the proximal hamstring over the ischial tuberosity during rotational movements.[3,4,15-17]

Clinical Examination

SHS is often diagnosed from the patient's history and provocation testing during the clinical examination. This section discusses the common special tests for ISHS and ESHS. The reader is referred to Chapter 2 for a comprehensive discussion of the hip examination.

For both conditions, very few special tests have been described in the literature. For ISHS, the only special test described in the literature is called the snapping hip maneuver, which attempts to reproduce the snapping sensation through a contraction of the iliopsoas.[3,18] The examiner palpates the iliopsoas tendon on the affected hip. The hip is brought into flexion, external rotation, and abduction by the examiner. Then the hip is passively extended, internally rotated, and adducted. The test result is positive if it reproduces the "snapping" sensation reported by the patient between 30 and 45 degrees of hip flexion and may be decreased with manual pressure to the iliopsoas tendon (Fig. 3-1).[2,5] Currently, no investigations have measured the clinometric properties of this test. The clinician will need to consider this when using this test in clinical practice.

For ESHS, the ITB complex is often involved and is typically the focus of clinical testing if this condition is suspected. Movement tests often include femoral rotation of a flexed hip, rotation of an extended and adducted hip, or flexing and extending the hip.[3,18] No specific test is mentioned in the literature. In addition, with these movements, no reports have measured the clinometric properties of these movements. Other tests that may yield information include the Thomas test and the Ober test.

Currently, no specific patient outcome tools are related to SHS. The clinician may have to use related hip outcome

questionnaires (e.g., Lower Extremity Function Scale) that will yield valuable information related to the patient's function, preferred activity, and rehabilitation goals.

Differential Diagnosis

Differential diagnosis often involves a good patient history to determine whether the "snapping sensation" is felt in the anterior hip (ISHS) or lateral hip (ESHS), followed by reproduction of the sensation. This is considered one of the most important diagnostic indicators for differentiating SHS from other potential disorders.[3] For ISHS, other disorders that should be considered include iliopectineal bursitis, rectus femoris tendinitis, and, to a lesser extent, intraarticular disease (e.g., FAI). For ESHS, other pathologic processes to consider include trochanteric bursitis and gluteus medius tendinitis. These pathologic conditions may accompany SHS and should be ruled out during the examination.

Imaging

Different types of imaging are commonly used to rule out other disorders and to confirm involved structures. Radiographic findings are often normal in patients with SHS but may be used to check for fractures, small femoral neck angle (coxa vara), or developmental dysplasia, which have been linked to SHS.[3,5,19] Radiographic imaging often includes anteroposterior and frog-lateral views.[5]

Magnetic resonance imaging (MRI) is often used to evaluate possible intraarticular causes such as FAI, acetabular labral tears, osteochondral fractures, and loose bodies. MRI can also be used to evaluate possible extraarticular causes including iliopsoas tendon disorders (ISHS), trochanteric bursitis (ESHS), and soft tissue tumors.[3,5]

Ultrasound is also used to detect tendinopathy, bursitis, and synovitis. Dynamic ultrasound has been used to detect the pathologic movement of the iliopsoas tendon in ISHS and the gluteus maximus and ITB in ESHS during provocation movements.[3,5]

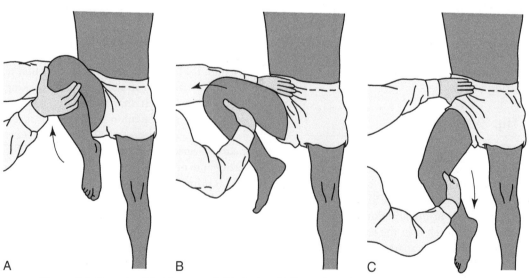

• Figure 3-1 Snapping Hip Maneuver. **A,** Hip flexion. **B,** External rotation and abduction. **C,** Extension, internal rotation, and adduction.

Postinjury Considerations

As mentioned earlier, SHS may have an insidious onset and may eventually worsen with prolonged repetitive movements. These patients may seek medical consultation if the condition begins to reduce their ability to function or becomes painful. The physician may impose activity restrictions, prescribe oral medications, administer a cortisone or anesthetic injection, and order imaging as needed (e.g., MRI, ultrasound).[3,4] Physical therapy is often prescribed with a focus on decreasing pain with modalities (e.g., ice) and restoring myofascial mobility, muscle length, strength, and function of the lower kinetic chain.[3,4]

Rehabilitation Considerations

Patient Education

Patient education should include education to avoid painful movements, proper training techniques, early injury recognition, and restorative techniques after activity (e.g., stretching, foam rolling). These patients may tend to ignore the "snapping" sensation, which could eventually lead to discomfort during activity. The patient should be symptom free with activity. Proper warmup and cool-down activity should be reinforced, especially stretching after activity.

Rehabilitation Programming

Rehabilitation interventions must address the musculoskeletal impairments that are contributing to the syndrome. The literature on SHS rehabilitation is sparse, containing only case studies and clinical commentaries.[2-7,10,14,17,20] The primary strategies that are discussed are manual therapy, myofascial release, stretching, and strengthening exercises.

Manual Therapy

Each type of SHS may have specific soft tissue restrictions that contribute to the problem. For ISHS, the iliopsoas is often tight and is the primary muscle involved.[3] Soft tissue mobilization may be used to release the iliopsoas muscle (Fig. 3-2).[10] Mobilization or manipulative treatment of the pelvis has also been cited as an effective intervention.[5,10,20] For ESHS, similar soft tissue mobilization techniques targeting the gluteus maximus, tensor fasciae latae (TFL), and ITB complex may be effective interventions. Secondary soft tissue restrictions in the hamstrings, hip external rotators, and adductors may be present and will need to be addressed during treatment.

Stretching and Self-Myofascial Release

For ISHS, stretching of the iliopsoas and rectus femoris muscles has been found to be an effective intervention, along with self-myofascial release techniques such as foam rolling to the anterior hip muscles.[10,14,17,21] For ESHS, the gluteals, hip abductors, and external rotators may need stretching and myofascial release techniques.[3,22] Specific stretching techniques, such as static stretching and proprioceptive neuromuscular facilitation (PNF), stretching may be effective in achieving increased muscle length.[23,24] Dynamic stretching may also be beneficial but should be done with caution.[23,25] Certain dynamic stretching patterns require multiplane hip movements that could elicit the "snapping" sensation of the inner or outer hip. It is recommended that the client perform symptom-free activity.

During the initial postinjury phase, consistent daily stretching should be emphasized, to promote tissue lengthening. The stretching and myofascial mobility program should first address the tight tissues and then progress to a global maintenance program once the desired mobility is obtained.

Strengthening and Functional Activity

For both ISHS and ESHS, specific strengthening exercises should be prescribed that help restore proper strength and control. As mentioned earlier, early hip control appears to have a strong influence on lower kinetic chain alignment. For the internal snapping hip, strengthening of the gluteals, hip external rotators, and iliopsoas should be the focus, with the other major muscles of the hip strengthened as needed. For the external snapping hip, the gluteals, external rotators, hip abductors, and adductors should be the focus, with strengthening of other muscle groups as needed. Clients with SHS should be progressed slowly to avoid any discomfort. Any activity that elicits the "snapping" should be avoided. Basic closed kinetic chain progression is advised, beginning with sagittal plane movement, then frontal plane movements, and last transverse or multiplane movements. Caution should be taken with multiplane movements because they can elicit an internal or external snapping. As the patient improves, more advanced movements can be performed. Table 3-1 provides some examples of closed kinetic chain activities in various planes of motion.

Surgical Intervention

If conservative management fails, then surgical intervention is an option for both ISHS and ESHS. For ISHS, an arthroscopic or open iliopsoas tendon release is conducted

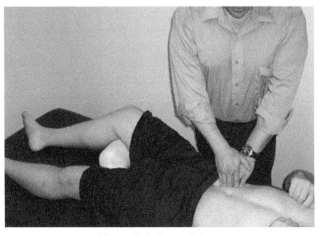

• **Figure 3-2** Psoas Release.

TABLE 3-1	Suggested Closed Kinetic Chain Progression for the Lower Extremity	
Plane of Motion	**Exercise Progression (Easy → Difficult)**	
Sagittal plane	Leg press machine → wall squats with ball → forward lunges → stair walking → bilateral squats on foam → bilateral squats on air-filled disk or BOSU → single leg squats on ground → single leg squat on foam → single leg squats on air-filled disk or BOSU	
Frontal plane	Side stepping on level surface → side stepping up onto a step → side stepping with bands → side stepping (fast) with ball passing → slide board	
Combined planes	Multidirectional lunges → single leg balance with multidirectional toe touch → Single leg cone reach → multidirectional hops (bilateral) → multidirectional hops (single leg)	

BOSU, BOSU Balance Trainer (BOSU, Ashland, Ohio).

at the level of the hip joint or at the insertion at the lesser trochanter.[26] Khan and colleagues[13] conducted a systematic review looking at the success rate of both open and arthroscopic procedures for ISHS. These investigators found that 100% of patients reported a resolution of symptoms after arthroscopic release, and 77% had a resolution of symptoms after open procedures. The complication rate was 21% for the open procedure compared with 2.3% for the arthroscopic.[13] For ESHS, the arthroscopic or open technique is meant to release the ITB by producing a diamond-shaped defect lateral to the greater trochanter that allows the trochanter to move freely without snapping, or a Z-plasty is conducted to lengthen the ITB.[26-28] The research on outcomes of both procedures is still emerging. Preliminary investigations of the Z-plasty for ESHS have shown good short-term outcomes.[27-30] A comprehensive discussion on these surgical interventions is beyond the scope of this chapter. The reader is referred to the reference list for related articles on this topic.

Summary

Both ISHS and ESHS are commonly caused by repetitive overuse activity and are usually diagnosed through the clinical examination. Imaging is often used to rule out other potential pathologic processes. The management of SHS frequently includes a multimodal program consisting of patient education (e.g., reducing risk factors), manual therapy, therapeutic exercise, and modalities.

Meralgia Paresthetica

MP is a nerve entrapment resulting in any combination of pain, paresthesias, and sensory loss within the distribution of the lateral femoral cutaneous nerve or lateral cutaneous nerve of the thigh (LCNT).[31,32] The reported incident rate is 4.3 cases per 10,000 patient-years in the general population and 247 cases per 100,000 patient-years in patients with diabetes mellitus.[33-35] MP is most prevalent in 30- to 40-year old persons and in male patients more commonly than female.[32,36] MP has been associated with various sports and physical activities including gymnastics, baseball, soccer, body building, and strenuous exercise.[32,37-42]

Anatomic Review

The LCNT is part of the lumbar plexus and functions primarily as a sensory nerve that innervates the anterolateral thigh. The nerve may have a variable orientation among persons with several different combinations of lumbar nerves that originate from L1 to L3.[31] The LCNT emerges from the lumbar plexus at the lateral border of the psoas major muscle and crosses the iliacus, to the anterior superior iliac spine. The nerve then passes under the inguinal ligament and over the sartorius muscle and enters the thigh as it divides into anterior and posterior branches.[37,44] Individual variations may be seen in the anatomic course of the nerve as it exits the pelvis. Five different types of variations have been reported through cadaveric investigations (Table 3-2).[44-46] This variation is important for clinical practice because compression of the LCNT most commonly occurs as it exits the pelvis. Patients may present with different signs and symptoms that reflect their own unique anatomy.[47]

Patient Profile

Patients diagnosed with MP may present with one or more of the following symptoms: pain, burning, numbness, muscle achiness, coldness, lightning pain, or buzzing (like a cell phone) in their anterolateral thigh.[31,48,49] Patients may experience a mild onset with spontaneous resolution or more severe symptoms that limit function.[31,48] Prolonged standing and walking may also cause pain, and sitting may alleviate pain as a result of hip flexion, which theoretically reduces or changes the tension in the LCNT.[32,48,50]

Each patient has a unique clinical presentation and distribution of symptoms. Seror and Seror[51] conducted an investigation using neurophysiologic studies in a sample of 120 patients diagnosed with MP. These investigators found that the lateral thigh was solely involved in 88 (73%) cases, and the anterolateral thigh was involved in 32 (26%) cases. The right thigh was involved in 62 (51.6%) cases and the left in 58 (48.3%) of cases.[51] Thus, patients may have unilateral or bilateral symptoms that occur in the lateral or anterolateral thigh.

TABLE 3-2 Variations in Anatomy of the Lateral Cutaneous Nerve of the Thigh

Types*	Percentage (%)	Anatomic Location
A	4	Posterior to the anterior superior iliac spine, across the iliac crest
B	27	Anterior to the anterior superior iliac spine and superficial to the origin of the sartorius muscle but within the substance of the inguinal ligament
C	23	Medial to the anterior superior iliac spine, ensheathed in the tendinous origin of the sartorius muscle
D	26	Medial to the origin of the sartorius muscle located in an interval between the tendon of the sartorius muscle and thick fascia of the iliopsoas muscle, deep to the inguinal ligament
E	20	Most medial and embedded in loose connective tissue, deep to the inguinal ligament, overlying the thin fascia of the iliopsoas muscle, and contributing to the femoral branch of the genitofemoral nerve

Data from Aszmann OC, Dellon ES, Dellon AL. Anatomical course of the lateral femoral cutaneous nerve and its susceptibility to compression and injury. *Plast Reconstr Surg.* 1997;100(3):600-604.
*Types A, B, and C are most susceptible to mechanical trauma.

neuropathic pain scores; visual analog scale (VAS), to quantify pain; 12-Item Short Form Health Survey (SF-12), to quantify overall health; University of California Los Angeles (UCLA) activity scale, to quantify activity level; and the Western Ontario and McMaster Universities Osteoarthritis Index (WOMAC), to quantify pain, stiffness, and physical function. The investigators found that 170 patients (81%) had reported LCNT neurapraxia with a mean severity score of 2.32 out of 10 and a mean neuropathic pain score of 2.42 out of 10 1 year postoperatively. Despite the presence of severity and pain, the subjects reported an absence of functional limitations with the SF-12, UCLA activity scale, and WOMAC.[64] Patients who underwent anterior approach hip resurfacing (91%) had a higher incidence than those who had anterior approach THA (67%).[32] Bhargava and colleagues[65] reported similar findings in a retrospective case review of 81 patients who underwent anterior approach THA. These investigators also found similar symptoms among patients with no apparent functional deficits.

MP has also been reported as a complication in patients after surgical procedures of the spine. Gupta and colleagues[66] reported on the incidences of MP in 110 patients (66 male and 44 female; 15 to 81 years old; mean age, 46.9 years) who underwent posterior lumbar spine operations.[32] Thirteen patients (12%) had MP postoperatively. The investigators hypothesized that when the patient is prone, the anterior hip becomes compressed from the surgical equipment during surgical procedures, and this leads to the onset of MP.[66] Other investigators have reported equipment-related incidents in patients who underwent direct lateral and posterior lumbar spinal surgery.[67-70] MP has also been reported as a postsurgical complication in iliac bone harvesting, open and laparoscopic appendectomy, cesarean section with epidural analgesics, and other obstetric and gynecologic surgical procedures.[71-75]

Clinical Examination

Patients with MP may present with a cluster of symptoms that can mimic the more common hip and lumbar disorders. Diagnosis of MP often includes a clinical examination and, if necessary, neurophysiologic and imaging tests. The clinical examination often includes common test and measures such as active range of motion (AROM), passive range of motion (PROM), palpation, strength testing, function, and special clinical tests. This section discusses special clinical tests that are commonly used to diagnose MP. The reader is also referred to Chapter 2, which provides a comprehensive discussion of the hip examination.

Pelvic Compression Test

The pelvic compression test is based on the premise that the LCNT is compressed by the inguinal ligament and that a downward force to the innominate will slack the ligament and temporarily alleviate the patient's symptoms.[76] Thus, a positive test result consists of alleviation of symptoms. With testing, the patient is positioned in the side-lying position

Prevalence and Mechanism of Injury

MP can be classified as either idiopathic or iatrogenic.[48] Idiopathic MP is often related to mechanical factors that result in the compression of the LCNT along its anatomic course as it exits the pelvis. Related mechanical factors include direct trauma, obesity (body mass index ≥ 30 kg/m^2), tight garments such as jeans, military and police uniforms, pregnancy, seat belts, muscle spasm, spinal scoliosis, leg length changes, and iliacus hemotoma.[34,52-63] MP has been linked to several metabolic factors such as diabetes mellitus, alcoholism, and lead poisoning.[48]

MP has also been reported as an iatrogenic complication after hip joint replacement. Goulding and associates[64] examined the occurrences of injury to the LCNT in 192 patients, 85 of whom underwent anterior-approach total hip arthroplasty (THA) and 107 of whom had hip resurfacing.[32,64] As their outcomes measures, these investigators used self-administered questionnaires including the following:

with the symptomatic side facing upward. The examiner applies a downward, compression force to the pelvis (Fig. 3-3) and maintains pressure for 45 seconds. If the patient reports an alleviation of symptoms, the test result is considered positive.[32,76] The test has a sensitivity of 95% and a specificity of 93.3% for diagnosing the condition as MP when compared with electromyography (EMG).[76]

Tinel Sign

The Tinel sign test is based on the premise that tapping over the LCNT as it exits the inguinal ligament region will elicit symptoms reported by the patient.[77] Currently, no published studies have investigated the diagnostic utility of this test. The Tinel sign has primarily been used in the diagnosis of upper extremity disorders such as carpel tunnel syndrome.[78,79]

Neurodynamic Testing

Neurodynamic testing is based on the premise that adverse mechanical tension of the LCNT is a contributor to the

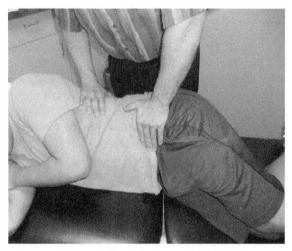

• **Figure 3-3** Pelvic Compression Test.

patient's reported symptoms.[80] With testing, the patient is in the side-lying position with the symptomatic side upward and the bottom knee bent.[80,81] The examiner stabilizes the pelvis with the cranial hand and grasps the lower extremity at the knee with the caudal hand. The examiner then bends the knee and adducts the hip to tension the LCNT (Fig. 3-4).[80,81] A positive test result consists of reproduction of the patient's neurologic symptoms versus feeling tension in the soft tissue structures of the hip. Neurodynamic testing of the LCNT has not been assessed in the literature for its diagnostic ability.[32] This lack of evidence should be considered when using this test as part of the clinical examination.

Differential Diagnosis

MP is often a considered a potential pathologic condition once the more common hip disorders have been excluded. MP can be challenging to diagnose because it has neurologic symptoms (e.g., numbness, paresthesias) similar to those that accompany the more common causes of anterolateral thigh pain such as lumbar stenosis, disk herniation, and nerve root radiculopathy.[82-85] One clinical method of differential diagnosis is the nerve block test that is commonly done by physicians. With this test, the physicians injects an anesthetic (e.g., 1% lidocaine) at the site where the LCNT exits the pelvis at the inguinal ligament to see whether the patient's symptoms change.[81,82] The test is considered successful if the patient has immediate symptom relief that lasts 30 to 40 minutes after injection.[81,82] This is often a more economical confirmatory test before ordering more expensive neurophysiologic tests or imaging. The nerve block may also be used as a treatment.

Neurophysiologic Studies and Imaging

Physicians may also order neurophysiologic tests or imaging to confirm or deny their clinical diagnoses further. Common neurophysiologic studies include somatosensory evoked potentials and sensory nerve conduction tests, which are

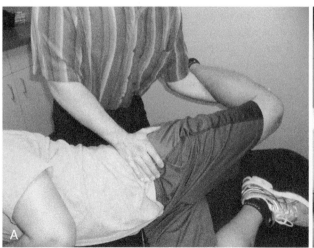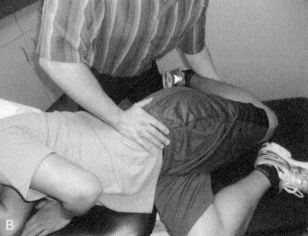

• **Figure 3-4 A** and **B,** Neurodynamic testing of the lateral femoral cutaneous nerve or lateral cutaneous nerve of the thigh (LCNT).

often considered the gold standard in diagnosing MP and may be less expensive than imaging studies.[86-88]

Magnetic resonance neurography (MRN) has been used to capture direct images of the nerves of the body (Fig. 3-5). MRN produces a detailed image of the nerve from the resonance signals that come from the nerve itself.[89] Chhabra and colleagues[90] investigated the intrarater reliability between two blinded raters in the diagnosis of MP using MRN in a sample of 38 persons (11 with MP, 28 controls). The sensitivity, specificity, positive predictive value, and negative predictive value of MRN for MP diagnosis were 71% or higher and 94% or higher for both raters, and the diagnostic accuracy was 90% or higher for both raters.[90] The physician may elect to order either neurophysiologic testing or MRN to confirm the diagnosis of MP further.

Postinjury Considerations

Postinjury management often includes a period of conservative nonsurgical care. If the condition is recalcitrant to treatment, then surgical interventions are an option. Nonsurgical and surgical interventions for MP are currently underinvestigated. Khalil and associates[91,92] conducted a systematic review in 2008 with a follow-up in 2012 and found no quasi-controlled or randomized controlled trials for either nonsurgical or surgical interventions. The weakness in the literature must be considered by the clinician when integrating these techniques into the plan of care.

Nonsurgical Interventions

Nonsurgical treatments may include medications (e.g., nonsteroidal antiinflammatory drugs [NSAIDs]), protection of the area, avoidance of compression activities, and rehabilitation.[31,48] Rehabilitation interventions for MP are underreported in the literature, with only case reports and a few

clinical trials.[38,42,58,74,93-97] To date, no comprehensive study has assessed the efficacy of physical therapy interventions for the treatment of MP. The available literature on rehabilitation interventions is discussed later in this section.

Manual Therapy

The available literature on manual therapy is sparse, with only two chiropractic case studies describing the management of patients with chronic MP and one chiropractic case study describing the management of a pregnant patient with MP.[93,97,98] The treatments reported among the three case studies included active release techniques, mobilization or manipulation for the pelvis, myofascial therapy for the rectus femoris and iliopsoas, transverse friction massage of the inguinal ligament, stretching exercises for the hip and pelvic musculature, and pelvic stabilization or abdominal core exercises.[93,97,98] Based on the successful outcomes reported, the combination of interventions described may be effective in treating MP. However, the clinician must keep in mind that case studies fail to offer a high level of evidence. More controlled trials are needed to validate these interventions further. As for negative outcomes, only one previous study cites a case in which chiropractic manual treatment of the hip and pelvis resulted in MP.[99]

Kinesio Taping

The effectiveness of kinesio (Kinesio Precut, Albuquerque, NM) taping for various orthopedic conditions has seen a growing amount of evidence. Currently, only one pilot study is investigating the effects of kinesio tape on relieving symptoms of MP. Kalichman and colleagues[94] investigated the effects of kinesio taping (Fig. 3-6) in a group of 10 patients (6 men and 4 women; mean age, 52 years) with a clinical and neurophysiologic diagnosis of MP over a 4-week period (8 treatment sessions). The investigators used the VAS, VAS global quality of life (QOL) instrument, and the

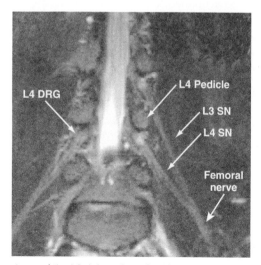

• **Figure 3-5** Normal anatomy of the L3, L4, and proximal L5 nerve roots and lumbar spinal nerves as they exit the spine and travel in essentially linear fashion. *DRG,* Dorsal root ganglion; *SN,* spinal nerve. (From Filler AG, Maravilla KR, Tsuruda JS. MR neurography and muscle MR imaging for image diagnosis of disorders affecting the peripheral nerves and musculature. *Neurol Clin.* 2004;22:643.)

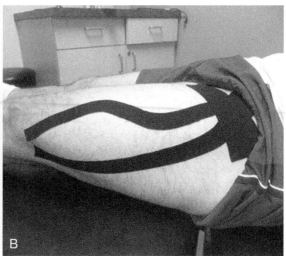

• **Figure 3-6 A** and **B,** Kinesio taping technique for meralgia paresthetica.

size of the symptomatic area as their outcome measures. On conclusion, the investigators found significant improvements in all measures, including a decrease in the patients' reported symptoms and symptomatic area after kinesio taping.[94] Despite the small sample size, this pilot study suggests that kinesio taping may be a good intervention in the treatment of MP. Further studies will be needed to confirm these findings.

Acupuncture

Acupuncture treatment (e.g., needling and cupping) for MP has elicited interest among Eastern and European researchers, although most of the publications are in Eastern journals. A systematic review found 21 studies on acupuncture treatment for MP that have been published in Eastern journals since 1956.[100,101] Among the case studies, one particular case report from German researchers described the successful treatment of MP with acupuncture in two patients who did not respond well to conventional physical therapy.[102] Another study, by Wang and colleagues,[103] reported the successful acupuncture treatment of 43 patients diagnosed with MP who underwent an intervention of needling and cupping. The available literature suggests that acupuncture may be effective in the treatment of MP. However, the exact physiologic mechanisms are still under investigation.[104,105] Further studies are needed in general to develop a broader understanding of the efficacy of acupuncture in the treatment for MP.

Other Nonsurgical Interventions

Pulsed radiofrequency ablation is an emerging treatment for MP when conservative treatment fails. Pulsed radiofrequency uses a high-frequency alternating current. The heat generated from the high-frequency alternating current ablates the nerve fibers or dysfunctional tissues without damaging the surrounding tissue.[106] Currently, no clinical trials have been conducted, and only case reports describing the intervention have been published.[106-108]

As mentioned in the previous section, physicians may also use a nerve block as a diagnostic test or as nonsurgical treatment. For treatment, LCNT blocks use a combination of lidocaine and corticosteroids.[65] Tagliafico and associates[50] reported their experience conducting an ultrasound-guided nerve block in 20 patients (7 male, 13 female; age range, 23 to 66 years) with a diagnosis of MP confirmed by EMG. These investigators used the pain VAS and VAS QOL scales as their outcome measures. At 1 week after injection, 16 patients (80%) experienced progressively decreased symptoms, and 4 patients (20%) required a second injection for continued pain. At the 2-month follow-up, all patients experienced complete resolution of symptoms and significant improvements on the QOL scale.[50] Other researchers have found similar outcomes.[109,110]

Surgical Interventions

If nonsurgical interventions fail, then surgical interventions may be an option. LCNT neurolysis and resection are optional interventions. Neurolysis is destruction of the nerve, and a resection is removal of the nerve or a section of nerve. Neurolysis has shown favorable outcomes in patients up to 4 years postoperatively, and resection has also shown favorable results despite the complete loss of sensation in the anterolateral thigh that occurs after the surgical procedure.[111-114] The overall consensus on which procedure is the best is still unknown.[111] Emamhadi[115] compared neurolysis with resection in the treatment of 14 patients diagnosed with MP, with a follow-up within 18 months. This investigator found that the resection group (n = 9) reported complete relief, whereas the neurolysis group (n = 5) reported a recurrence of symptoms within 1 to 9 months.[115] de Ruiter and colleagues[111] also found higher success rates with resection than with neurolysis.[111] These comparison studies suggest that LCNT resection produces better outcomes; however; both procedures are still under-investigated. The success of LCNT resection may be caused by the complete resolution of symptoms and the acceptance of permanent changes (e.g., numbness) by the patient.[111] Neurolysis may provide symptom relief, but with a proba-bility of recurrence.[115] Thus, neurolysis procedures may be considered first and resection considered if the nerve has been severely damaged.[115]

Summary

MP is challenging to diagnose and should be considered once the more common diagnoses are excluded. The diag-nosis and nonsurgical and surgical management of MP are currently underinvestigated. The available evidence does provide some guidance for clinical practice. These limita-tions should be considered when using the information for clinical practice.

Adductor-Related Groin Injuries

Groin pain in the athlete has traditionally been classified as a pathologic condition of the adductor muscle group.[116,117] Most often, the adductor longus is involved as a single source of groin pain or in combination with abdominal injury (sports hernia) or intraarticular hip disorders.[118,119] Despite the traditional definition, the recent literature examining sports-related injuries has expanded the defini-tion of "groin pain" to other disorders such as FAI, sports hernia, osteitis pubis, inguinal hernia, and obturator neuropathy.[120-123] For this section, *adductor-related groin pain* is used to differentiate adductor muscle injury from other potential pathologic conditions.[124]

Anatomic Review

Among all the groin muscles, the adductor group (brevis, longus, and magnus) has a unique role in stabilizing the hip during sports activity.[125,126] This muscle group is susceptible to injury resulting from the demands it undergoes with both open-chain and closed-chain hip movements, with the adductor longus the most involved.[116] The anatomic archi-tecture of the adductor longus and its relationship with athletic pubalgia (see Chapter 5) have garnered interest among researchers. Athletic pubalgia is commonly classified as a distal rectus abdominis injury at the pubic symphysis, conjoint tendon injury, and injury to the proximal adductor longus.[116,120,127] Norton-Old and colleagues[128] investigated the anatomic relationship of the adductor longus with this

disorder by using cadaveric dissection. The investigators found that the adductor longus attached to the anteroinfe-rior aspect of the pubis, with the superficial fibers tendinous and the deep fibers muscular.[128] Other researchers have con-firmed this anatomic variation.[129,130] Norton-Old and asso-ciates[128] also found that the adductor longus had secondary communications with the following structures: contralateral distal rectus sheath, pubic symphysis, anterior capsule, ilio-inguinal ligament, and contralateral proximal adductor longus tendon. The investigators also simulated a mechani-cal load across one of the adductor longus muscles and measured the strain in the ipsilateral and contralateral rectus sheath with a strain gauge. They found that the strain expe-rience was varied among cadavers and concluded that the proximal attachment of the adductor longus plays a role in withstanding high forces across the pubic symphysis during multidirectional athletic activity. These investigators con-cluded that this finding may explain the vulnerability of the anatomic relationship of the rectus abdominis and adductor longus.[128]

Biomechanical Considerations

The actions of the adductor longus muscle during lower extremity motions such as kicking and skating has been a topic of interest because of the high prevalence of injuries among soccer and ice hockey players. Charnock and col-leagues[131] examined adductor muscle length and activation during a soccer kick in male collegiate soccer players. Their investigation revealed the following: maximum hip exten-sion occurred near 40% of swing phase, the maximum rate of stretch of the adductor longus occurred at 65% of the swing phase, activation of the adductor longus occurred between 10% and 50% of the swing phase, and maximum hip abduction occurred at 80% of swing phase. The inves-tigators concluded that the adductor longus could be at risk for injury during the transition from hip extension to flexion.[131]

Chang and associates[132] examined the role of the hip adductors during forward skating in ice hockey players. These investigators used surface EMG to measure adductor muscle activity at three different skating velocities: slow, medium, and fast. They investigators found that with increased skating velocity, the adductor magnus exhibited an extremely large increase in peak muscle activation and prolonged activation.[132] They also found that with increased skating velocity, lower extremity stride rate and stride length increased despite a lack of significant increases in hip, knee and ankle total range of motion (ROM). To accommodate for the increased stride rate with higher skating speeds, the rate of hip joint abduction and adduc-tors muscle activation increased together, a finding indicat-ing a substantial eccentric contraction.[132]

The available research suggests that the adductor muscle group may be susceptible to injury because of the unique anatomy and high demands experienced during various sports such as soccer and ice hockey. In the presence of pain, adductor muscle activation may be inhibited, resulting in weakness and a potential risk for further injury. Crow and colleagues[133] found decreased adductor muscle strength with the onset of groin pain or injury in Australian football players. Tyler and associates[134] also found that adduction strength was 78% of abduction strength in injured ice hockey players compared with 95% adduction strength in uninjured players.

Prevalence and Mechanism of Injury

The prevalence of groin injuries represents 2% to 5% of all sports-related injuries and 5% to 9% of high school injuries in the United States, with the adductor group most commonly involved.[135,136] The incidence of groin injuries in soccer can be as high as 10 to 18 injury incidents per 100 players.[135,137,138] Hagglund and colleagues[139] found that 56% of adductor injuries occurred in the kicking leg in a sample of professional soccer players from 2001 to 2010. In professional ice hockey players, 10% to 11% of all injuries are groin related.[116] Previous data from the National Hockey League (NHL) showed that groin and abdominal injuries occurred at a rate of 12.99 injuries per 100 players per year during the 1991 to 1992 season, with an increase to 19.87 injuries per 100 players per year during the 1997 to 1997 season; 90% of injuries were not contact related.[140] Adductor-related groin pain has also been reported in other sports such as rugby, swimming, water polo, and cricket.[141-145] Among all the sports, adductor-related groin injuries are most prevalent in ice hockey and soccer and may occur in 10% to 20% of players.[116]

Common mechanisms associated with adductor-related groin pain have been reported in the literature.[127,141,146-148] Athletes who participate in sports involving repetitive kicking and multidirectional movements such as ice hockey may be susceptible to adductor-related groin injuries.[149] The most common reported risk factors include hip muscle weakness, abdominal core muscle weakness, delayed transversus abdominis recruitment, poor off-season conditioning, years of experience, age, and earlier groin injury.* Other risk factors include decreased hip ROM,[151,152] adductor strength less than 80% of abductor strength,[126,134] reduced muscle activation of the abductors and adductors with groin pain,[133,153] poor preseason lower extremity flexibility,[154] pelvic instability,[155] and poor adductor flexibility.[156]

Patient Profile

Patients may report a general "groin pain" that is mechanical in nature. Adductor-related groin pain is typically localized along the adductor longus belly, the proximal musculotendinous junction, or the origin at the inferior pubic ramus.[157] The pain often is exacerbated with physical activity or contraction of the muscle, depending on the extent of the

injury. With mild adductor strains, the proximal pain may slightly decrease initially with activity, but if the injury is untreated, the pain may persist during activity.[143] With more severe strains, the pain may affect function. If groin pain is recalcitrant and fails to resolve with conservative treatment, then further differential diagnosis should be conducted. Other common musculoskeletal disorders such as FAI, osteitis pubis, obturator neuropathy, hip or pelvic fracture, lumbar injury, inguinal hernia, and athletic pubalgia should be excluded.[120-123,158,159] Although they are less common, proximal adductor longus ruptures can occur. Several published case reports have described the recognition and management (e.g., surgical and nonsurgical) of adductor longus trauma in equestrian,[160] soccer,[161-163] rugby,[164] and football athletes.[165,166] The clinician needs to consider this injury during the differential diagnosis because it can be mistaken for another pathologic condition such as inguinal hernia.[167]

If a nonmusculoskeletal cause is suspected, then the clinician should consider other conditions such as genitourinary (e.g., prostatitis or urinary tract infection), neurologic (e.g., genitofemoral nerve entrapment), gastrointestinal (e.g., Crohn disease), and vascular (e.g., abdominal aortic aneurysm).[168] Chapter 2 provides a more comprehensive discussion of the differential diagnosis process.

Clinical Examination

The clinical examination often includes common tests and measures such as AROM, PROM, palpation, strength testing, function, and special clinical tests. Special testing is an important part of the differential diagnostic process. Because adductor-related groin pain is mechanical, provocation testing should include contraction of the musculotendinous unit. Few special tests exist for assessing adductor-related groin pain. The gold standard used by clinicians and researchers is the adductor squeeze test.[169,170] In this test, the patient is supine, with the examiner isometrically testing hip adduction at three different hip flexion angles: 0, 45, and 90 degrees (Fig. 3-7).[171] Researchers have found that the highest EMG muscle activity occurs at 45 and 0 degrees.[171,172] Thus, testing should occur at different hip flexion angles to test the adductor muscle fully. The adductor squeeze test has been shown to have good intra-rater reliability when a sphygmomanometer is used to measure pressure (intraclass correlation coefficient: 0.89 to 0.92).[169] The test also has a sensitivity of 55%, specificity of 95%, positive predictive value of 93%, and a negative predictive value of 34% when compared with MRI findings.[173] Other relevant clinical tests that may be used in the examination process include palpatory pain of the adductor muscle origin at the pubis and tests for flexibility such as the bent knee fall out test.[118,174]

Imaging

Radiographs, ultrasound, and MRI are typically used with the clinical examination in the differential diagnosis of

---

*References 64, 116, 138, 139, 141, 148, 150.

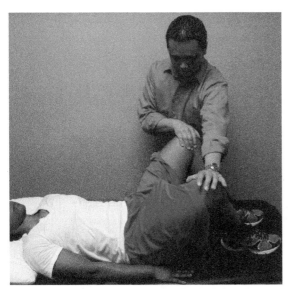

• **Figure 3-7** Adductor Squeeze Test.

groin pain. Conventional radiographs are used to examine both the bony and articular structures of the region, whereas ultrasound is used to take real-time images of tendons and muscles in the groin region.[175] Ultrasound has become more popular because of its portability, absence of radiation, and low cost.[176] Ultrasound has been found to have high accuracy, sensitivity, specificity, and positive and negative predictive values for diagnosing groin hernias, but the research for adductor-related pain is still emerging.[177-179] MRI is often used in the further differential diagnosis of competing causes of groin pain such adductor-related pain, osteitis pubis, and athletic pubalgia.[175,180] Zoga and associates[181] investigated the clinometric properties of MRI and found a sensitivity of 86% and specificity of 89% for adductor tendon injury in athletes diagnosed with athletic pubalgia.

Currently, no standard MRI evaluation protocol exists for adductor-related groin pain; however; the literature has shown good outcomes, with MRI an effective tool for diagnosing the condition.[182-184] Branci and colleagues[182] introduced the Copenhagen standardized protocol, which is a newer 11-element MRI evaluation protocol used to diagnose pubic symphysis and adductor disorders. In this investigation, the intrarater reliability of 2 radiologists was tested with 86 male athletes who underwent standard MRI.[182] The protocol demonstrated moderate to good intrarater agreement (kappa = 0.45 to 0.67) in identifying pubic symphysis disorders and weak agreement (kappa = 0.05 to 0.06) with diagnosing adductor-related pathologic conditions. Further studies are needed to determine the clinometric properties of the protocol as it relates to the clinical examination. The ability of MRI to predict future pathologic conditions of the groin has also been examined in both soccer and ice hockey players. Several investigations looked at the correlation of pathologic MRI finding in asymptomatic athletes and future injuries over a 4-year follow-up period. None of the studies found any predictive value of MRI in identifying future injuries in these athletes.[185-187]

Postinjury Considerations

Postinjury management often includes a period of conservative nonsurgical care. The physician may prescribe medications (e.g., NSAIDs), restrict activity, and refer the patient for rehabilitation. A trial of conservative rehabilitation is often recommended for a 2-month period. If the patient's condition is recalcitrant to treatment, then surgical intervention is an option.[188]

Rehabilitation Programs

Studies of nonsurgical interventions for adductor-related groin pain have been reported in the literature. The available research has shown favorable outcomes, but a lack of consensus for optimal intensity, frequency, and duration still exists.[189,190] The evidence from randomized controlled trials is also lacking, and this must be considered for clinical practice.[191] This section discusses the current literature for interventions and rehabilitation programs.

Common Exercises

One challenge for rehabilitation is finding the most optimal exercise for the patient. A study by Delmore and associates[192] examined six common adductor exercises by using EMG analysis to determine which exercises created the highest muscle activity. The investigators ranked the six exercises from highest to lowest: side-lying hip adduction, ball squeezes, side lunges, standing adduction on a Swiss ball, rotational squats, and sumo squats.

Another study, by Jensen and colleagues,[193] investigated the effects of an 8-week progressive hip adduction program, using an elastic band, on eccentric adductor strength. The investigators randomly assigned a group of 32 soccer players into experimental and control groups. The control group did not perform exercises. The experimental subjects performed standing hip adduction using a combination of muscle contractions (3 seconds concentric, 2 seconds isometric, and 3 seconds of eccentric) for each repetition. Each week, the band resistance was progressed, or an extra band was used. The exercise program was as follows: *weeks 1 to 2* (2 training sessions, 3 times 15 repetitions maximum), *weeks 3 to 6* (3 training sessions, 3 times 10 repetitions maximum), *weeks 7 to 8* (3 training sessions, 3 times 8 repetitions maximum). At the conclusion of the study, the investigators found that the experimental group experienced a 30% increase in eccentric muscle strength compared with 17% in the control group after the 8-week intervention period.[193,194] Research by Serner and associates[195] also found the highest EMG activity with hip adduction using elastic bands. Based on the available research, hip adduction may provide the most benefit in the side-lying or standing position and with resistance.

Manual Therapy

The research on manual treatment for groin disorders is sparse; only one study investigated a single manual treatment as the primary intervention. Weir and colleagues[196] did a retrospective study that examined the effects of the Van Den Akker manual therapy technique and a home exercise program in the treatment of 33 athletes with chronic adductor-related groin pain. The manual technique was described as manually tensioning the adductor muscles with one hand and then using the other hand to move the hip into abduction and external rotation, knee fully extended, which created a circular motion to stretch the adductors. The movement was repeated 3 times for approximately 25 seconds in one to two treatment sessions. After the manual intervention, athletes were given a home program that included a 5-minute warmup with slow jogging or cycling, adductor stretching, and a 10-minute warm bath for 2 weeks.[196] The outcomes measures were patient satisfaction, return to activity, and numeric pain scores. At the conclusion of the study, 83% (25 of 30) of the athletes reported good to excellent satisfaction, and 90% (27 of 30) resumed sports at (15 of 30) or below (12 of 30) their previous activity level; the average pain score decreased significantly from 8.7 before treatment to 2.2 after the treatment.[196] To date, this is the first investigation to use a manual therapy technique as a primary intervention for treating adductor-related groin pain. Despite these positive outcomes, the study contains several limitations, including the retrospective design, lack of control group, questionable intervention parameters (unsupervised home program), and inclusion criteria. These factors need to be considered before using this intervention in clinical practice. Other investigations have found favorable results with manual therapy as part of a multimodal rehabilitation program, as discussed later.[197,198]

Compression Garments

One emerging area of research is the use of clothing to decrease the muscular demands on the lower extremity. In a preliminary investigation, Chaudhari and associates[199] looked at the effects of compression shorts on adductor contractions. These investigators used EMG to measure the amount of adductor activity in 29 healthy persons wearing compression shorts, during unanticipated 45-degree run-to-cut maneuvers. The investigators found a significant ($P < .04$) decrease in adductor activity in the stance limb when compared with the control side. Most of the research on the use of compression garments has focused on their ability to reduce fatigue,[200] facilitate recovery after high intensity exercise,[201,202] and enhance balance.[203] These preliminary studies suggest that compression shorts may help in the recovery of a groin strain, but further investigation is necessary to validate these findings.

Exercise Programs

Investigators have examined the effects of formal exercise programs for treating adductor-related groin pain. Holmich and colleagues[124] conducted two studies: (1) an initial investigation and (2) a long-term follow-up investigation. The initial investigation examined the effects of an 8- to 12-week supervised active exercise program in a group of

TABLE 3-3	Exercise Program of Holmich and Colleagues*
Module 1 (0-2 weeks)	Isometric adduction against soccer ball placed between feet in supine (30 sec,10 repetitions)
	Isometric adduction against soccer ball placed between knees in supine (30 sec,10 repetitions)
	Sit-ups (straight and oblique direction) (5 sets,10 repetitions each)
	Combined sit-up and hip flexion from supine and with soccer ball placed between knees (folding knife exercise) (5 sets, 10 repetitions)
	Balance training with wobble board (5 min)
	One-legged exercises on sliding board, with parallel feet as well as with 90-degree angle between feet (5 sets of 1 min bilaterally in both positions)
Module 2 (3 weeks and beyond)	Side-lying hip abduction and adduction exercises (5 sets, 10 repetitions for each exercise)
	Lumbar extension exercises prone over end of couch (5 sets, 10 repetitions)
	Standing hip abduction/adduction with weighted pulley (5 sets, 10 repetitions for each leg)
	Sit-ups (straight and oblique direction) (5 sets,10 repetitions each)
	One-legged synchronous exercise flexing and extending knee and swinging arms (cross-country skiing on one leg) (5 sets, 10 repetitions for each leg)
	Coronal plane training using the "Fitter"† balance system (5 min)
	Balance training on wobble board for (5 min)
	Skating movements on sliding board (5 sets, 1 min)

Modified from Holmich P, Uhrskou P, Ulnits L, et al. Effectiveness of active physical training as treatment for long-standing adductor-related groin pain in athletes: randomised trial. *Lancet*. 1999;353(9151):439-443.
*All exercises were done twice at each training session.
†Fitter balance system, Fitterfirst (Fitter International Inc, Calgary, Canada).

68 athletic male patients with a history of groin pain who were randomly assigned to an experimental or control group. The experimental group underwent a supervised exercise program (three times per week for 90 minutes) that targeted the muscles of the pelvis and adductor group and home program on the nontreatment days (Table 3-3).[124] The exercise program ran for a minimum of 8 weeks to a maximum of 12 weeks, with the participants completing their treatment once they were pain free or decided to stop treatment. The control group underwent conventional physical therapy twice per week for 90 minutes that included the following: cross-friction massage (10 minutes) to the proximal adductors; stretching of the adductors, hamstrings, and hip flexors (three times 30 seconds); laser

treatment; and transcutaneous electric nerve stimulation (30 minutes). The control group performed prescribed stretches on nontreatment days.[124] On conclusion, 59 participants finished the study. The investigators found that 29 (79%) participants in the experimental group had complete resolution of symptoms and returned to their earlier level of sports activity compared with 27 (14%) participants in the control group. The experimental group also achieved significantly higher adductor strength gains when compared with the control group.[124]

In the second study, Holmich and associates[204] conducted an 8- to 12-year follow-up on 47 (80%) of the original 59 participants. All participants underwent the same initial examination protocol for diagnosis from the original study using a blinded physician who was unaware of the earlier study. On completion of the study, the investigators found a lasting significant effect ($P = .047$) from the original exercise program in all participants at the 8- to 12-year follow-up.[204] Therapeutic exercise investigations have shown some positive outcomes for both short-term and long-term periods. Despite these positive outcomes, few published investigations exist, and this lack needs to be considered when interpreting the results for clinical practice.

Multimodal Programs

Researchers have also investigated the effects of multimodal treatment programs. Weir and colleagues[205] compared a multimodal treatment program consisting of heat, manual therapy, stretching, and a return to running program with a home-based exercise program consisting of a return to running program with instruction on three occasions from a physical therapist. Fifty-four participants with a diagnosis of adductor-related groin pain were randomly assigned into the two groups. The primary outcome measure was time to return to full sports participation, and the secondary outcome measures were objective outcome scores and VAS scores during sports activities. Outcomes were assessed at 0, 6, 16, and 24 weeks. On completion, the investigators found that the multimodal treatment group returned to sports more quickly (12.8 weeks, SD 6.0) than the active home-based exercise group (17.3 weeks, SD 4.4) but only 50% to 55% of all athletes made a full return to sports. Moreover, no difference was noted between groups with the secondary outcome measures.[205]

Weir and colleagues[206] conducted a second investigation measuring the short-term and midterm effects of a five-phase multimodal program consisting of joint mobilization, abdominal core exercise, and agility or sports drills in a sample of 44 athletes with long-standing adductor-related groin pain (Table 3-4). The investigators used a criterion-based progression for subjects to progress through each phase. The main outcome measures were return to the earlier level of sport, restrictions in sports, and recurrence of injury. At the conclusion of the study, the investigators found that 86% (38 of 44) athletes successfully returned to their earlier level of play. At the midterm follow-up (median, 22 months; range, 6.5 to 51 months), 26% (10 of 38) experienced a recurrence of groin pain.

TABLE 3-4	Five-Phase Rehabilitation Program by Weir and Colleagues
Phase I	Clinical milestones: normal physical findings on hip range of motion and sacroiliac joint dysfunction (Gillet test), selective transversus abdominis recruitment without abdominal bracing Patient education: advice and information Joint mobilization: hip and sacroiliac joints and lumbar spine Muscle reeducation: transversus abdominis recruitment
Phase II	Clinical milestones: normative values for core stability endurance exercises, low-load hip adduction exercise without pain Core strengthening: transversus abdominis recruitment with core stabilization exercises (prone bridge, lateral bridge, oblique, and straight sit-up) Hip strengthening: low-load hip adduction exercises (seated adduction machine, one-leg pulley in standing)
Phase III	Clinical milestones: no pain during the squeeze test and modified Thomas test and bent knee fallout test, running for 15 min without pain General strengthening: general whole body stabilizing exercises (wobble board, Swiss ball) Hip strengthening: increase in hip adduction strength exercise intensity with decreased number of repetitions while experiencing no adduction pain (begin with 3 times 15 repetitions and then progress program) Cardiovascular: Begin running if biking or swimming is pain free
Phase IV	Clinical milestones: 80% of subjectively estimated performance capacity Agility drills and sport-specific exercises (begin at 30% intensity and then progress program)
Phase V	Return to sport

Modified from Weir A, Jansen J, van Keulen J, et al. Short- and mid-term results of a comprehensive treatment program for longstanding adductor-related groin pain in athletes: a case series. *Phys Ther Sport.* 2010;11(3):99-103.

The current research on multimodal programs is not very robust. The available studies have shown mixed results, with the best evidence supporting positive short-term results. This ambiguity needs to be considered when interpreting the outcomes of these studies.

Injury Prevention

The prevention of lower extremity and groin injuries has become a focus for various sports such as soccer and ice hockey. The current research has produce mixed results that make it a challenge to develop a consensus on which programs are the best for a specific sport. This section covers the most relevant research for soccer and hockey.

One of the more notable programs for soccer is the Fédération Internationale de Football Association program (FIFA 11), which is a prevention program consisting of 10 exercises that focus on lower extremity strengthening, core stability, balance, and dynamic stabilization.[207] Several clinical trials using the FIFA 11 have shown favorable results by reducing lower extremity injuries in youth, amateur, and collegiate soccer players.[208-211] Steffen and associates[209] found that players with high compliance (1.5 sessions per week; mean, 49.2 sessions per season; range, 33 to 95 sessions per season) with the program reduced their risk of seasonal injuries by 35% compared with players with low compliance (0.7 sessions per week; mean, 23.4 sessions per season; range, 15 to 32 sessions per season). Grooms and colleagues[210] also found that players who had high compliance with the program had a 72% lower risk of seasonal injury compared with a control group.

Holmich and colleagues[150] also examined the effects of a single season exercise-based injury prevention program for the adductors and pelvic muscles in a group of 977 soccer players who were randomly assigned to experimental and control groups. The program consisted of six exercises that included strengthening, balance or coordination, and core stability. At the conclusion of the study, the experimental group had a 31% reduced risk of injury when compared with the control group. The investigators also discovered that earlier groin injury doubled the risk for reinjury, and high levels of play (e.g., professional) tripled the risk.[150] Despite the positive results of the FIFA 11 program and the program of Holmich and associates, other investigators have found no significant difference in injury reduction with these types of programs when compared with matched controls.[212-214] The mixed results need to be considered before initiating such programs for all levels of soccer.

Ice hockey players experience a higher level of adductor-related groin injuries when compared with participants in other sports. The high incidence has created an interest in injury prevention programs. Tyler and associates[215] examined the effects of a 6-week preseason injury prevention program focusing on improving adductor strength. The 33 NHL players were identified as "at risk," based on their ratio of adduction to abduction strength of less than 80%, and participated in the program. Surveillance of the players was conducted over two seasons. The results of the study were promising, with only 3 adductor strains in 2 seasons compared with 11 in the previous 2 seasons (0.71 versus 3.2 per 1000 player-game exposures).[215] These preliminary findings suggest that ice hockey injury prevention programs may reduce the risk of adductor-related groin injuries, but further investigations are needed. Further studies are still required to validate this program and establish a global consensus on the most effective program.

Surgical Interventions

If patients fail to respond to conservative treatment (>2 months), then surgery may be an option.[188,205] The most common surgical approach is the adductor tenotomy, which is often used as an intervention for both adductor-related groin pain and sports hernias (see Chapter 5).[216] Robertson and colleagues[217] described the following four-level pain grading system to determine the need for surgical intervention: level 1, pain-free optimal performance; level 2, performance affected by pain; level 3, training or playing limited by pain; and level 4, inability to train or play. Through their investigation, they found that athletes with maximal discomfort (levels 3 and 4) preoperatively benefited the most from the surgical treatment. This grading system may be a good way to clinically assess the need for surgical intervention. The several versions of the adductor tenotomy are discussed in the following subsection, along with postsurgical rehabilitation.

Adductor Longus Tenotomy: Complete, Partial, and Bilateral

With the adductor longus tenotomy procedure, the surgeon fully releases the adductor longus from its pubic attachment, thereby freeing the tendon.[218] The tenotomy is an emerging procedure for treating both adductor-related groin pain and athletic pubalgia. Mei-Dan and associates[188] reported the outcomes of adductor tenotomy and hernioplasty in a group of 155 soccer players with long-term groin pain between 2000 and 2006. Ninety-six patients were treated with adductor tenotomy, and 59 were treated with the combined tenotomy and hernioplasty. The main outcome was return to play. The investigators found that athletes were able to return to their sport at a mean time of 11 weeks (range, 4 to 36 weeks) postoperatively. The investigators concluded that athletes with adductor-related groin pain and accompanying sports hernia may benefit from adductor tenotomy. Other researchers have found similar results with adductor tenotomy alone or combined with sports hernia repair.[217-222]

Some surgeons are studying the effects of a partial versus a complete adductor longus tenotomy. Schilders and colleagues[223] investigated the effects of a partial adductor longus release in 43 professional athletes with chronic adductor-related groin pain. The outcomes were time to return to sport and pain measured with the VAS. The average follow-up time was 40.2 months (range, 25 to 72 months). Ninety-eight percent (42 of 43) of the athletes returned to their preinjury level of sport at an average of 9.21 weeks (range, 4 to 24 weeks), and all subjects had significant improvement on their VAS scores from preoperatively to postoperatively.[223]

Other surgeons are investigating the bilateral adductor tenotomy in treating unilateral adductor longus groin pain. Maffulli and associates[224] investigated the effects of bilateral minimally invasive adductor tenotomy in 29 athletes from 2004 to 2007. The outcomes measures were return to training and sport, the Hip Disability and Osteoarthritis Outcome Score (HOOS), the Short Form Health Survey (SF-36), and the European Quality of Life Five-Dimensions scale (EQ-5D). The median follow-up after the surgical procedure was 36 months.[224] At the last follow-up, the investigators found that 69% (20 of 29) patients returned to the preinjury level of sport, 7% (2 of 29) returned to a higher level, 14% (4 of 29) returned to a lower level of sport, and 10% (3 of 29) did not return to sport. All questionnaires showed significant improvement from preoperatively to postoperatively, and the median return to training was 11 weeks and 18 weeks to return to sports. The investigators concluded that bilateral adductor tenotomy may be an effective treatment for unilateral adductor-related groin pain.[224] Research on the different versions of adductor tenotomy is still emerging. The preliminary studies show positive outcomes, but more controlled long-term investigations are needed using matched control groups.

Pubic Symphysis Curettage and Adductor Reattachment

Some patients with adductor-related groin pain may also have pubic pain. Investigators have shown some interest in the effects of surgically treating both issues. Hopp and colleagues[225] investigated the effects of a pubic symphysis curettage (e.g., scraping or scooping) and adductor reattachment in five nonprofessional soccer players with chronic osteitis pubis and adductor-related groin pain. The outcome measures were time to return to sport, VAS scores, and sports activity with pain. At the conclusion of the study, all patients return to their earlier sports activity at an average of 14.4 weeks. VAS and sports activity pain scores improved significantly from preoperatively to postoperatively. No patients developed pubic instability at follow-up.[225] Other investigators have found success with surgical interventions to the pubic symphysis for pubic and groin pain.[226-230] The investigation by Hopp and associates[225] of this combined procedure further supports the finding by Mens and associates[155] that pubic instability may be a risk factor for adductor-related groin pain. Further investigations are needed to understand the role of pubic instability and adductor function.

Postsurgical Rehabilitation

Given the emergence of these surgical procedures, the research on postoperative rehabilitation is underreferenced. The current literature focuses on surgical interventions with adjunctive rehabilitation, with reporting of the overall outcomes.[218,230] Gill and colleagues[218] described an 8-week postsurgical rehabilitation program after adductor tenotomy that focused on returning the athletes to their earlier sporting activity. The rehabilitation program is outlined in Table 3-5.

Summary

Adductor-related groin pain is a potential pathologic process that should be considered in the differential diagnosis of anterior hip pain. This disorder is common among soccer and hockey players and has a direct relationship with athletic pubalgia. Although the available current evidence is weak, it shows moderate support for prevention, rehabilita-

TABLE 3-5	Eight-Week Rehabilitation Program by Gill and Colleagues
Phase I (week I)	Goals: wound healing, preventing reattachment of the tendon Patient positioning: keep legs abducted first 3 days, sleep with pillow between leg to maintain hip abduction Stretching: day 3 and beyond, abduction stretch every 2 hours
Phase II (weeks II-V)	Goal: keep adductors stretched, prevent scarring, improve flexibility Stretching: standing bilateral abduction, standing unilateral adduction, standing hamstring stretch, and supine quadriceps stretch (20-sec hold, 10 repetitions, 2-3 days per week) Strengthening (begin week 3): standing single leg abduction, supine stretch leg raise, standing single leg circumduction, and straight leg sit-ups (20 repetitions, 2-3 times per day)
Phase III (week VI-beyond)	Goals: complete wound healing, full hip range of motion, pain-free adductor muscle activity, resolution of presurgical groin pain Week 6: gradual return to running Week 7: sports-specific activity resumed Week 8: return to sports activity Week 12: return to full competition

Modified from Gill TJ, Carroll KM, Makani A, et al. Surgical technique for treatment of recalcitrant adductor longus tendinopathy. *Arthrosc Tech.* 2014;3(2):e293-e297.

tion, and surgical intervention. The clinician must have a comprehensive understanding of these factors to manage this condition effectively.

Osteitis Pubis

Osteitis pubis is potential pathologic condition causing groin-related pain and is often part of the differential diagnosis. Osteitis pubis is often described as an overuse condition caused by a biomechanical overloading of the pubic symphysis and adjacent parasymphyseal bone and soft tissue.[231] The four classifications of osteitis pubis are as follows: (1) sports-related or athletic osteitis pubis; (2) degenerative or rheumatologic osteitis pubis; (3) noninfectious osteitis pubis associated with urologic procedures, gynecologic procedures, and pregnancy; and (4) infectious osteitis pubis associated with local or distant infections.[232] This section focuses on sports-related osteitis pubis.

Prevalence and Mechanism of Injury

Sports-related groin injuries have been reported to range from 0.5% to 6.2% and up to 5% to 15% in soccer players.[233] Rodriguez and associates[234] reported that osteitis pubis represented 3% to 5% of all injuries sustained by a professional soccer team between 1989 and 1997.[234] Osteitis pubis is increasingly recognized in other sports such as ice hockey, rugby, football, and running sports.[7,233-235] More cases of osteitis pubis have been reported in male than in female athletes, but that may not be accurate because female athletes may be underreported in the literature.[233] Predisposing factors that may contribute to this condition include increased athletic participation, forceful running, repetitive kicking, repetitive cutting or pivoting, repetitive acceleration or deceleration, trauma, pregnancy, degenerative or rheumatologic disease, and urologic and gynecologic procedures.[233,236] Osteitis pubis has also been associated with athletic pubalgia,[181,237] adductor-related groin injury,[238] and FAI.[239,240]

Among athletes, the possible etiologic factors include muscle imbalance, pelvic instability, and chronic overuse injury to the bone and joint.[232] The primary etiologic factor suggested is a muscle imbalance between the rectus abdominis and the hip adductors (e.g., adductors, gracilis). The symphysis pubis is a central attachment site for both muscle groups and may be subject to extreme forces and microtrauma as a result of their antagonistic action.[232] This condition may be caused by the repetitive kicking motion seen in soccer, hockey, and rugby.[232]

Patient Profile

The onset of a patient's pain may be acute after an event such as kicking or insidious. Patients commonly present with a primary complaint of pain at the symphysis pubis, superior pubic rami, or proximal adductors. The patient may also report pain in the lower abdominal, anteromedial groin, hip, perineum, inguinal region, and scrotal region, thus making the diagnosis challenging.[232,234] Because the swing phase of gait may be painful, walking and running may be difficult.[241]

The clinician must be aware that osteomyelitis of the pubic symphysis can also occur to a lesser extent. The patient reports a sudden onset accompanied by a fever.[242] The osteomyelitis can be caused by *Staphylococcus aureus*, *Pseudomonas aeruginosa*, *Escherichia coli*, *Salmonella* species, and anaerobic bacteria. The diagnosis may include imaging studies, pubic symphysis aspirate, and blood cultures.[233]

Clinical Examination

The clinical examination often includes a comprehensive history, physical examination, and possible imaging. The history may reveal strong correlation with the athlete's sport, onset, and current symptoms. As part of the clinical examination, special tests are performed to help differentiate the cause of the reported pain. Several published clinical tests are used to help diagnose osteitis pubis and other types of groin-related pain. Several investigators have described using an isometric adductor squeeze test in various positions (90, 45, and 0 degrees) to provoke a patient's symp-

toms.[171,173,234-243] The previous section on adductor-related groin pain discusses these tests and their clinometric properties (see Fig. 3-7). Despite current research, a reference standard test for this region has not been established because of the variability in methodology among studies.[244] This issue must be considered when integrating these tests into the clinical examination.

Imaging

After a comprehensive clinical examination, radiographs and MRI may be ordered to diagnose osteitis pubis more precisely. Common radiographic findings may include widening of the pubic symphysis, marginal irregularity, symmetrical bone reabsorption, reactive sclerosis along the rami, and sacroiliac joint irregularities.[232,245] If pubic symphysis instability is suspected, then an anteroposterior radiograph is obtained with the patient in the single leg standing (flamingo view) to assess the alignment of the pubic symphysis under load. Vertical displacement of more than 2 mm and a symphyseal gap wider than 7 mm is considered abnormal.[232,245] The radiographic abnormalities seen on radiographs can also be grading based on the severity. A four-point grading scale is used: 0, no bony changes; 1, slight bony changes; 2, intermediate changes; and 3, advanced changes.[246]

MRI is also used and may reveal specific bone and soft tissues changes at the pubic symphysis.[247] Kunduracioglu and colleagues[245] correlated MRI findings and clinical features of osteitis pubis in 22 collegiate athletes with groin pain. The investigators found that the most reliable MRI findings for patients with recent symptoms (symptoms for <6 months) included subchondral bone marrow edema, fluid in the pubic symphysis joint, and periarticular edema.[245] The most reliable findings for patients with chronic osteitis pubis (>6 months) included subchondral sclerosis, subchondral resorption, osteophytes, and bony margin irregularities.[245] MRI with contrast has also been used to assess osteitis pubis further. The finding of a "secondary cleft sign" or a peel-back periosteal stripping tear of the anterior capsule of the symphysis is revealed by the contrast material and indicates a pathologic process of the pubic symphysis.[248] The "secondary cleft sign" has a sensitivity and specificity of 100% in diagnosing osteitis pubis.[248] This sign has also been used to diagnose adductor disorders.[175,238] Diagnostic ultrasound can also be used to assess the soft tissue (e.g., tendons) structures involved, and computed tomography can be used to rule out other conditions such as pelvic and hip stress fractures, pelvic abscesses, and avulsion fractures.[232,249]

Postinjury Considerations

Osteitis pubis may have a prolonged clinical course of 4 to 9 months that makes it challenging for the rehabilitation team.[232] Conservative nonsurgical treatment is often prescribed first and may include pubic symphysis injections (e.g., corticosteroid), prolotherapy, oral antiinflammatory medications, activity modification, and rest.[232] Physical therapy is also prescribed, as discussed in the next section. If conservative management fails, then surgical intervention may be an option.[233]

Rehabilitation

Physical therapy is commonly prescribed as part of the conservative management of osteitis pubis. Of particular interest are the outcomes of nonoperative rehabilitation programs focused on returning the athletes to preinjury levels of participation. The most recent systematic review to date (2011) examined the spectrum of treatments for osteitis pubis and found only level 4 (case report or case series) evidence with varying approaches to treatment.[233] Six case reports described successful outcomes when nonoperative rehabilitation was combined with oral antiinflammatory medication. The investigators found no randomized controlled trials, and this lack of high-level evidence makes it a challenge for the clinician to compare or interpret the findings of these case reports accurately for clinical practice.[233]

Since the last systematic review, the available evidence has not changed, with only case reports (level 4 evidence) and no randomized controlled trials. The available evidence suggests that an individualized nonoperative multimodal program may help athletes diagnosed with osteitis pubis return to their preinjury level of activity. The descriptive nature of the case reports makes it difficult to make a direct comparison of rehabilitation programs. All case reports used return to preinjury activity as the main outcome measure.[235,241,250,251] Only one case report[241] used patient-related outcome measures (Lower Extremity Function Scale, VAS), and two case reports[235,241] conducted a follow-up at 6 months. All case reports described a structured multimodal program (range, 4 to 14 weeks) that consisted of strengthening, flexibility, sports specific exercises, and manual therapy.[235,241,250,251] One case study described an addition of aquatic exercises to the program.[251] Despite the positive outcomes described in the case reports, further high-level research is needed to determine the optimal rehabilitation program for the athlete diagnosed with osteitis pubis.

Surgical Interventions and Postsurgical Rehabilitation

If the patient's condition is recalcitrant to conservative treatment, then surgical intervention is an option. Several surgical procedures are available, including plate arthrodesis augmented with cortical bone graft (stabilization), wedge or total resection of the symphysis, extraperitoneal retropubic synthetic mesh, and arthroscopic curettage of the fibrocartilage disk.[225-227,229,232,252] Reporting of long-term outcomes of these procedures has been limited.[229] A systematic review found that the best evidence to date included case studies (level 4 evidence) and no randomized controlled trials.[233] The patients in these case reports had

TABLE 3-6	Return to Sport After Conservative and Surgical Rehabilitation for Osteitis Pubis	
Intervention	Return to Sport (Weeks)
Rehabilitation	9.55
Corticosteroid injection	8
Prolotherapy	9
Curettage of pubic symphysis	22.4
Extraperitoneal retropubic synthetic mesh	7.2
Pubis stabilization	26.4

prolonged osteitis pubis (average, 17 months) that was recalcitrant to conservative measures. The best success rates for return to sport reported came from curettage of the pubic symphysis (72%), synthetic mesh (92%), and pubic symphysis stabilization (100%). The synthetic mesh provided the fastest return to sport, averaging 7.2 weeks.[233] To date, postsurgical rehabilitation programs have not been investigated or detailed in the literature. They have been mentioned only as part of postsurgical management in surgical investigations.

Summary

Osteitis pubis is a source of groin pain that should be part of the differential diagnosis. Osteitis pubis has been associated with adductor-related groin pain, athletic pubalgia, and FAI. The research on both conservative nonsurgical and surgical treatment is weak, with only level 4 evidence and no controlled comparison trials. This situation makes it difficult to compare interventions directly. Despite the weakness of evidence, with both conservative management and surgical interventions patients were reported to have a successful return to their earlier level of sports activity between 7 and 27 weeks (Table 3-6).[233] These results are from patients with various levels of the disorder, which must be considered for clinical practice.

Lateral Hip Pain and Greater Trochanteric Pain Syndrome: Bursitis, Proximal Iliotibial Band Syndrome, and Gluteal Tendon Disorders

Lateral hip pain is a common complaint of patients that covers a wide range of potential diagnoses. The term *greater trochanteric pain syndrome (GTPS)* is frequently used to represent the clinical presentation of symptoms in this region, but it is nonspecific in regard to identifying specific causes of symptoms.[253] Although pain in the greater trochanteric region is fairly common, it is difficult to estimate prevalence because of the somewhat broad definition of

GTPS. Strauss and associates[254] estimated the condition to occur in 10% to 25% of the general population. Conversely, Williams and Cohen[255] estimated prevalence at 1.8 per 1000 patients per year. GTPS was once thought to be primarily caused by trochanteric bursa disease, but more recent inquiry revealed additional causes of pain in this region.[254] Despite these advances, the literature on the diagnosis and treatment protocols for various causes of lateral hip pain remains scant. This section discusses common causes of and treatment concepts for lateral hip pain.

When evaluating patients with pain in the lateral hip region, clinicians must consider a large spectrum of etiologic factors. This broad span of diagnoses may necessitate an examination approach that considers localized soft tissue sources, hip joint involvement, and referred or radicular influences. The patient's history and intake findings may guide the clinician to employ a more global lower quarter screening approach or a more specific localized examination.

Common causes of GTPS include greater trochanteric bursitis, ITB syndrome, and gluteus medius tendinopathy or strain.[253] Although more commonly associated with groin pain, intraarticular involvement can manifest as lateral hip symptoms.[256] Clinical tests to determine hip joint involvement may be necessary to rule out intraarticular influences in patients with lateral hip pain (see Chapter 2). Radicular influences of the lumbosacral spine and sciatic nerve involvement must also be considered as potential causes of lateral hip symptoms. The most common spinal nerve levels of involvement that may cause symptoms in this region are L3 to S1.[257] Additionally, it is not uncommon for nonarticular lateral hip structures, intraarticular disorders, and lumbosacral involvement to occur in some combination, thus further complicating the process of differential diagnosis in this population of patients.[257,258]

Patient Profile

The history and profile of patients with lateral hip pain are highly variable because of the multitude of potential underlying causes. Even so, careful delineation of the events and factors that contributed to the current presentation will allow efficient evaluation and appropriate treatment. Although less common than gradual development, traumatic onset is possible. Falls directly onto the trochanteric region may result in inflammation of the trochanteric bursa or the proximal ITB.[259] As with any traumatic mechanism, the potential for fracture (greater trochanter) must always be considered and excluded. Noncontact sudden-onset lateral hip pain caused by snapping of the ITB over the greater trochanter is possible. This occurrence is often accompanied by an audible snapping sensation (see the earlier discussion of SHS.).

Patient-specific factors may also assist in determination of underlying causes of lateral hip pain. The patient's age may be helpful in diagnosing the cause of symptoms. Women are thought to experience a higher rate of GTPS.[254]

A higher incidence of the conditions encompassed by GTPS is observed in the 40- to 60-year age range.[260] Current or past musculoskeletal conditions may also predispose a person to GTPS. Low back pain, knee osteoarthritis, and obesity in the patient's history have been identified as risk factors for developing GTPS.[255]

The patient should be asked to identify the focal point of maximal discomfort and describe the entire distribution of symptoms. This is particularly important because the general term "hip pain" carries many variable interpretations. Pain distribution is typically focused in the lateral hip, potentially radiating down the side of the thigh toward the knee and, at times, below the knee.[255,261] Numerous activities may be noted to increase the patient's primary symptoms: lying on the affected side, standing for prolonged periods of time, sitting with legs crossed, walking, ascending and descending stairs, and running.

Mechanism of Injury

Multiple mechanisms of injury are recognized for the various causes of lateral hip pain. When possible, identifying the specific mechanism helps clinicians verify the diagnosis and aids in developing a treatment plan of care. Common mechanisms in the development of trochanteric bursitis, proximal ITB syndrome, and gluteal tendon disorders are discussed in this section. Trochanteric bursitis and proximal ITB syndrome are discussed together, whereas gluteal tendon injury is described separately.

Trochanteric Bursitis and Proximal Iliotibial Band Syndrome

Greater trochanter bursitis and proximal ITB syndrome are commonly cited sources of lateral hip pain. True trochanteric bursitis is an inflammatory condition. By this definition, many cases of GTPS are not truly generated from the trochanteric bursa, but rather arise from other tissues in the region, including the proximal ITB.[262] As mentioned, a direct fall onto the trochanteric region may result in the development of trochanteric bursitis.[259] However, repetitive activity is a much more common mechanism for the development of the trochanteric bursitis and proximal ITB syndrome. Repetitive friction of the proximal ITB over the trochanter with repetitive movement may result in inflammation of the bursa or irritation of the proximal ITB.[253] Distance running is a commonly described factor in the development of trochanter bursitis. Nielsen and associates[263] found that novice-level runners who increased their distance by more than 30% over a 2-week period were more likely to experience injuries, including ITB syndrome and trochanteric bursitis. True trochanteric bursitis is often self-limiting, and it typically responds well to conservative treatment.[253]

Gluteal Tendon Disorders

Gluteal tendon injuries are increasingly recognized as a cause of recalcitrant lateral hip pain. Cases that previously would have been diagnosed as trochanteric bursitis or under the general GTPS category are now known to have a specific relationship with gluteal tendon disorders. Most often, the gluteus medius tendon is affected. The gluteus minimus may be involved as well.[264] Tears can range from partial to full thickness, with partial thickness the more common finding.[253] Gluteal tendinopathy can also be associated with trochanteric bursitis.[265]

Most gluteal tendon injuries stem from overuse mechanisms similar to the mechanisms described for trochanter bursitis and proximal ITB syndrome. Rare cases of acute-onset tears have been reported.[266,267] The limited literature on acute-onset ruptures mostly describes a condition with spontaneous, noncontact onset in the older population.[268] Ruptures of this nature are generally thought to occur when tendons that have already experienced degenerative changes become overloaded to the point of complete tearing.[268] Gluteal tendon tears have also been described in patients after THA or procedures to address femoral neck fractures.[269] Although a specific reason for this association has not been described, it is often thought that these patients experience signs of lateral hip pain before undergoing surgical treatment.[270] Tyler and colleagues[271] described a mechanism in athletes in which the person lacks strength to control excessive movement that is beyond the physiologic limits of the kinetic chain, with resulting eventual damage to the gluteus medius or minimus tendons.

Clinical Examination

A complete, well-structured approach to examination is crucial when attempting to delineate the cause or causes of lateral hip pain. ROM, flexibility, and strength of the regional hip and pelvic musculature should routinely be evaluated. In many cases, clinical tests to determine potential involvement of the hip joint should be performed as well. A more detailed description of the general approach to hip and pelvic examination is described in Chapter 2. This section reviews the clinical examination components that are of specific interest when evaluating patients with lateral hip pain.

Palpation

Patients with symptoms originating from structures of the lateral hip should most often exhibit reproduction of symptoms with palpation. Clinicians should palpate the following structures as part of their standard examination: greater trochanter and bursa region, posterior and anterior trochanter area, proximal ITB, TFL insertion into the ITB, and gluteus medius muscle belly. Pain with palpation of the posterior trochanteric region may represent gluteus medius tendon involvement, whereas tenderness at the anterior trochanteric region may indicate gluteus minimus tendon involvement.[253] The absence of symptom reproduction with palpatory examination may lead the clinician to consider other sources of symptoms.[258] Martin and Sekiya[272] conducted a reliability study with 70 patients (mean age, 42

years; SD = 15.4). Diagnoses in the hip region included FAI, capsular laxity, trochanteric bursitis, iliopsoas tendinitis, and adductor strains. These investigators found palpation of the greater trochanter for tenderness to a kappa value of 0.66 (95% confidence interval: 0.48 to 0.84), a finding indicating good agreement.

Clinical Tests

Because of the broad definition of GTPS and the spectrum of conditions that may manifest as lateral hip pain, clinical tests to identify these conditions are not supported by a substantial body of evidence.[273] The literature does not clearly define a gold standard clinical test. As a better understanding of the clinical entities that manifest as lateral hip pain is developed, stronger evidence to support clinical tests for diagnosis should follow. Currently, pain provocation tests are the primary means of defining GTPS.[274]

Ober Test and Modified Ober Test

The Ober test (knee flexed to 90 degrees) and modified Ober test (knee extended) are performed to assess potential tightness of the ITB tract and also can be used to examine patients for symptom provocation (see Chapter 2 for details on performance and interpretation of the Ober test). Reese and Bandy[275] conducted a study to determine the reliability of measuring ITB flexibility. Sixty-one subjects with a mean age of 24.2 years (SD = 4.3) were assessed over 2 sessions with the Ober test and modified Ober test. These investigators calculated intraclass correlation coefficient values of 0.90 for the Ober test and 0.91 for the modified Ober test, thus indicating that the tests were reliable.

30-Second Single Leg Stance

The 30-second single leg stance test has been described as an assessment method to determine whether someone is experiencing GTPS, as defined by the presence of greater trochanteric bursitis or gluteal tendon lesions.[274] The presence of a Trendelenburg sign (indicating gluteus medius weakness) may also be observed. However, this is not described or considered part of the test when evaluating specifically for GTPS.

Procedure: The patient is asked to stand on one leg and maintain this position for 30 seconds.
Interpretation: If pain is reported in the region of the greater trochanter when assuming the single limb stance position, this result is considered positive for GTPS.

Resisted External Derotation Test

The resisted external derotation test (Fig. 3-8) has been described as an assessment method to determine whether someone is experiencing GTPS, as defined by the presence of greater trochanteric bursitis or gluteal tendon lesions.[274]

Procedure: The patient assumes a supine position and flexes the knee and hip to a 90-degree angle. The hip is placed in external rotation as tolerated. The patient is asked to

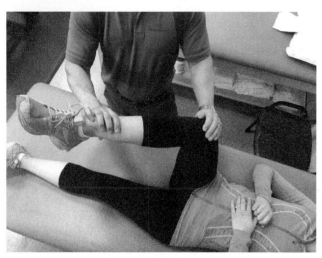

• **Figure 3-8** Resisted Derotational Test.

rotate the hip internally against resistance back to neutral rotation.

Interpretation: Reproduction of pain in the region of the greater trochanter is considered positive for GTPS.

A few studies examined the measurement properties of the 30-second single leg stance and resisted external derotational tests as they relate to the diagnosis of GTPS. Lequesne and colleagues[274] evaluated both tests for determining the presence of GTPS in 17 patients with refractory lateral hip pain (average of 13 months). A matched control population was used with the same tests. The investigators defined GTPS as the presence of MRI-confirmed greater trochanteric bursitis or gluteal tendon lesions. They found a sensitivity and specificity of 100% and 97.3%, respectively, for the 30-second single leg stance test and a sensitivity and specificity of 88% and 97.3%, respectively, for the resisted external derotation test. Most study subjects were older adults (mean age, 68 years). In a systematic review with meta-analysis, Reiman and associates[273] found that of all the clinical tests that were studied for gluteal tendinopathy, only the resisted external derotation test demonstrated the ability to modify the posttest probability of the diagnosis.

Imaging

Diagnostic imaging may be useful in differentiating specific causes of lateral hip pain. The lack of evidence supporting clinical tests for GTPS[273] may justify the use of imaging modalities in refractory cases that are not responsive to a course of rehabilitation. However, evidence supporting imaging options for GTPS is also limited.[276] Other than ruling out bony involvement, such as fractures, plain radiography is not typically useful in evaluation of GTPS. Chowdhury and colleagues[277] suggested diagnostic ultrasound as the best choice of initial imaging secondary to availability, low cost, dynamic nature, and ability to guide treatments such as steroid injections. Diagnostic ultrasound can be used to identify gluteus medius and minimus tendon thickening and excessive fluid.[278] Dynamic ultrasound can assess movement of the ITB over the greater trochanter, associated bursitis, and gluteal tendinopathy. When gluteal tendinopathy or bursitis is confirmed, diagnostic ultrasound may be useful in guiding injections as treatment.[279] These investigators also suggested that MRI be used when further delineation of structure involvement was needed in patients with refractory cases who were likely to be referred to an orthopedic specialist. When evaluating clinical tests for GTPS, Lequesne and associates[274] used MRI as the gold standard in confirming the presence of greater trochanteric bursitis and gluteal tendon lesions. Bewyer and Bewyer[280] recommended MRI to assess for tendon rupture versus tendinopathy in patients with no strength improvements after 4 to 6 weeks of rehabilitation. Additional imaging options may be considered if localized imaging results are negative, and structures outside the lateral hip region are thought to be responsible for the patient's symptom presentation.

Treatment

Injection

Although cortisone injection is commonly used as a treatment for GTPS, no consensus on specific indications for this treatment in patents with GTPS exists. Furthermore, reported results of injection in this population of patients are mixed. In a study of 120 patients (18 to 80 years old), Brinks and colleagues[281] found that when compared with a group receiving rest and oral analgesics as needed, patients receiving corticosteroid injections showed significantly less pain at 3-month follow-up. However, no difference was observed between groups at 12-month follow-up, a finding suggesting that corticosteroid injections may give short-term relief in patients with GTPS. Sayegh and associates[282] reported long-term (time not specified) relief of symptoms from trochanteric bursitis in female patients with coexisting sciatica and low back pain when these patients had injections of glucocorticoids mixed with 2% lidocaine.

Rehabilitation

Conservative treatment is most often the initial approach to lateral hip pain classified as GTPS. At this time, no evidence-supported treatment algorithms are available to apply to this population of patients. Intervention is based on acuity, impairments identified during physical examination, and the patient's functional limitations and goals. In patients not responsive to rehabilitation, a comprehensive reevaluation should be performed, considering other regions of the body. When the condition is unresponsive to conservative treatment and no other body regions can be implicated, clinicians should consider referral for further diagnostic testing.

The goals of the initial stage of treatment for GTPS are comparable to those of many other soft tissue conditions. Measures should be taken to decrease the acuity of the patient's presentation. In cases of trauma or when the presence of inflammation is expected, NSAIDs, massage, and certain modalities may be theoretically useful. Potential modalities include cold-based treatment,[271] ultrasound, transcutaneous electrical stimulation (TENS), and iontophoresis.[280] Clinicians should consider the use of these modalities based on the principles of inflammation and the theoretical ability of such treatment options to affect the inflammatory process.

Factors that subject the structures of interest (ITB, tendons, or bursa) to excessive loads must be moderated to allow healing and prevent further aggravation of the condition.

Initial activity modifications are typically intended to reduce gluteal muscle use or decrease the total amount of tension placed on the lateral tissue structures.[280] In very acute cases, assistive devices may be used to decrease total use and strain of the gluteal muscles. Assistive devices may also serve to encourage a normal gait pattern. If a cane or crutch is to be used in a unilateral fashion, then it should be held on the asymptomatic side. Use of the device in this manner can provide substantial load reduction for the gluteus medius muscle.[280] Patient education regarding activity modification should be a consistent part of the initial treatment program. Potential activity modifications include sleeping with a pillow between the knees to decrease tension on the lateral structures of the hip and standing with even weight distribution.[280] Any patient-specific activities that are determined as aggravating during the evaluation should also be modified when possible.

After acuity of presentation is diminished, passive intervention should be used only as needed, and impairments identified during the physical examination should be addressed. Flexibility deficits of the hip and pelvic muscles must be addressed. Patients experiencing symptoms that are caused by trochanteric bursitis or proximal ITB-TFL syndrome, in which friction resulting from a tight ITB-TFL complex causes localized irritation, should use stretching techniques for the ITB.[253] Numerous variations of ITB-TFL complex stretching are possible. Clinicians can manually apply tension to the ITB-TFL complex by emphasizing the adduction component of the Ober test position or by moving the test hip into adduction while in the Thomas test position. Patients can independently stretch the ITB by standing upright, crossing (adducting) the target leg behind the noninvolved limb, and side bending the upper body away from the target leg.

A progressive strength program is usually a fundamental component of the rehabilitation program.[253,254,264,271] Clinicians must be cautious to progress strengthening exercises in a manner that does not supersede the patient's symptomatic threshold. The patient's tolerance and reaction to strengthening exercises should consistently be assessed before progressing resistance or volume. Tyler and colleagues[271] suggested that, as with other tendinopathies, a program that emphasizes progression toward eccentric training may be beneficial to the patient. They also noted, at this time, no literature is available to confirm the benefits of eccentric training specifically in the GTPS population. Activities that maximize use of the gluteal muscles while

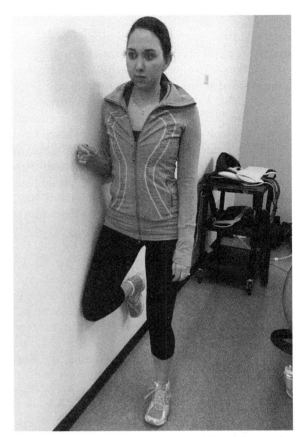

• **Figure 3-9** Standing Isometric Gluteal Muscle Contraction.

minimizing TFL activation are often preferred as part of the rehabilitation program. The goal is to strengthen the larger gluteal stabilizer without TFL predominance, which is associated with internal rotation and flexion tendencies. Selkowitz and associates[283] examined commonly prescribed rehabilitation components to determine the rationale of gluteal-to-TFL activity. They performed EMG assessment on 20 healthy subjects who completed 11 commonly prescribed exercises for the hip and pelvic region. Gluteal-to-TFL ratio values were calculated for each exercise. The exercises with the greatest gluteal-to-TFL activation ratio were the band-resisted clamshell exercise, resisted sidestep, unilateral bridge, and quadruped hip extension activities.

The treatment program should be progressed to include weight-bearing exercises as tolerated by the patient. These exercises more closely simulate the positions that are often symptomatic and provide the greatest functional challenge to patients. Stabilization of the pelvis in the frontal plane should be emphasized. Figure 3-9 shows an exercise that uses isometric abduction of both hips in single leg stance. Of particular concern are the demands created by the stance phase of gait and other activities that require a component of single leg loading. Bolgla and Uhl[284] compared EMG activity of 16 healthy subjects when performing non–weight-bearing and weight-bearing hip exercises. These investigators found that the weight-bearing exercises required greater activation of the gluteus medius when compared with non–weight-bearing exercises. These findings support the functional progression to weight-bearing exercises when tolerated by the patient.

When the patient demonstrates minimal symptoms and has achieved restoring appropriate strength and flexibility, he or she should be progressed in a manner that emphasizes return to function. This final stage of rehabilitation may be highly variable in time and content because it is based on the patient's specific activity goals.[271] Activities that represent the demands of the patient's preferred activities should be used. Patients should be monitored to ensure that they do not experience a recurrence of symptoms and that they do not demonstrate incorrect form or compensatory patterns that may predispose them to re-injury.

Surgery

As the role of gluteal tendon tears in the presentation of GTPS becomes better understood, the interest in surgical options has increased. When conservative treatment fails, several surgical options have been described in the literature. Surgical approaches that have been described include open procedures involving bone anchors or sutures, similar endoscopic approaches, and tendon augmentation to reinforce repairs.[285] Although the literature on outcomes after gluteal tendon procedures is relatively limited, early case series show promising results. Domb and colleagues[286] reported the results of 14 women and 1 man who underwent endoscopic gluteus medius repair. These investigators obtained at least a 2-year follow-up of each patient; 14 of 15 patients reported significant improvement in hip outcome scores, and patient satisfaction was rated from good to excellent. McCormick and associates[287] reported similar success in 9 of 10 patients. Additionally, they noted that all patients demonstrated significantly improved hip abductor strength. It was also noted that younger patients (age range, 60 to 74 years) reported better postoperative outcomes.

When recurrent trochanteric bursitis does not respond to conservative treatment, bursectomy procedures may be used. Lustenberger and colleagues[265] performed a systematic review that examined treatment of trochanteric bursitis. They concluded that bursectomy was an effective treatment for refractory cases of trochanteric bursitis. In a 12-subject retrospective case series review by Van Hofwegen and associates,[288] the investigators found that patients undergoing arthroscopic bursectomy reported a notable decrease of pain. At an average of 36-month follow-up, patients reported an average decrease of pain from 9.3 to 3.3 (11-point scale); 62% of patients were able to use their hip without pain, and 10 patients noted that they would undergo the procedure again secondary to their level of symptom improvement.

Summary

Lateral hip region pain is often a challenging entity to diagnose and treat. It is often collectively called the greater trochanteric pain syndrome (GTPS) because it was once thought that the trochanteric bursa was the primary cause of symptoms. Lesions of the gluteus medius and minimus tendons are now recognized as commonly observed components of the clinical presentation. Although few studies specifically examining rehabilitation for GTPS exist, conservative treatment is often described as effective in treating lateral hip region pain. When symptoms do not sufficiently resolve with conservative treatment, surgical repair of lesioned gluteal tendons and bursectomy are potential options.

Proximal Hamstring Injuries

Hamstring injuries are some of the most common injuries experienced by active persons and athletes at all levels of participation. Verrall and colleagues[289] found hamstring injuries to be the most prevalent disorders among Australian football players. Hamstring injuries are the most commonly reported injury among professional soccer players.[290] Proximal hamstring injuries can pose a particular challenge to rehabilitation and achievement of full return to earlier functional status. In a study of 83 athletes with hamstring injuries, Verrall and associates[291] found that the most common site of injury was the myotendinous junction of the biceps femoris and that proximal and midsubstance injuries were more common than those occurring in the distal third of the complex. Evaluation and treatment of persons suspected of having injuries to the hamstring complex must be structured, based on the best available evidence, and must take adjacent structures into consideration. Depending on severity, treatment often is conservative. However, in patients with severe or chronic cases who do not respond to noninvasive approaches, surgical intervention may be warranted.

Prevalence

The prevalence of hamstring injuries has been reported for various sports and athletic groups such as sprinters (29%) and Australian rules football players (8% to 25%).[290,292] The rate of injury for competitive soccer players ranges from 12% to 16%.[293] The prevalence differences observed between male and female athletes in the literature may be attributed to the sampling of various athletic groups that often have biased gender participation rates.[292]

Recurrence of injury is a significant concern for patients with hamstring disorders. Even though this is a major topic of interest, particularly in the active population, clinicians have not been able to decrease the recurrence rate dramatically.[294] Approximately one third of active patients in this population experience recurrence within a year.[295] Recurrent hamstring injury has also been shown to result in a greater loss of function and a greater amount of time for returning to activity than with the initial injury.[296] Feeley and colleagues[297] conducted a 10-year study of National Football League (NFL) players and injury occurrence in preseason training camps. The investigators found hamstring injuries to be the second most common injuries during training camp. The high rate of recurrence for proximal hamstring injuries challenges the current rehabilitation approaches commonly used in these patients.[295]

Patient Profile

The clinical presentation of a person experiencing a proximal hamstring injury varies depending on the severity of involvement. The spectrum of damage ranges from minor disruption of fibers in the muscle belly to complete rupture of the muscle or tendon from the ischial tuberosity. The initial occurrence is typically characterized by posterior buttock pain that has developed suddenly through a mechanical stretch injury. However, the clinician should consider the high prevalence of recurrent cases, and therefore a patient may report an acute or traumatic onset or a chronic onset, as well as recurring injuries.[295] Patients with chronic cases may demonstrate apprehension or report the impending feeling of injury when the hamstring is lengthened. Hamstring injuries can be graded on a scale of I to III.[295] Grade I (strain) is the mildest form, representing minor muscle tissue damage. Grade II (partial tear) is considered moderate damage. Grade III (complete disruption) represents rupture of the muscle or avulsion of the tendon. Higher grades of injury are associated with increased levels of pain and impaired function. The grading system for hamstring injury helps the clinician determine prognosis and aggressiveness of treatment. Most grade I or II hamstring injuries are treated conservatively. Grade III tears may be treated conservatively or considered for surgical intervention. The mechanism of injury, severity of damage, and location along the musculotendinous structures affect the patient's prognosis and plan of care.

Mechanism of Injury

Various mechanisms of proximal hamstring injuries have been described in the literature. In many cases, an acute mechanism may be reported. However, overuse and slower onset are possible. Proximal hamstring strains may often occur secondary to stretching of the muscle at extreme joint positions comprising a combination of hip flexion and knee extension. Examples of such activities include sprinting, hurdling, kicking, and movements associated with dancing. This stretching mechanism often compromises the proximal semimembranosus muscle fibers.[298] Askling and associates[299] found that runners and sprinters had a more traumatic onset with a more marked initial loss of flexibility and strength. Although dancers were often injured in a slow, stretching maneuver, they had fewer initial impairments compared with runners, but they took a significantly longer time to recover. When severity of tissue damage is relatively equal, proximal hamstring injuries tend to demand a longer recovery time when compared with distal hamstring injuries.[299] Proximity of injury to ischial tuberosity has been suggested to correlate with extent of injury and time for

return to activity.[298] Injuries occurring closer to the ischial tuberosity require a great period of rehabilitation. Both length and cross-sectional area of muscle involvement have been correlated with healing and functional return times.[300] When the motion of hip flexion and knee extension is rapidly produced and unopposed, a condition of passive insufficiency occurs within the hamstring complex. This rapid loss of available muscle length can result in avulsion of the tendinous insertion from the ischial tuberosity. Tendon rupture injuries in this area carry concerns about the mobility and function of the sciatic nerve secondary to the potential for formation of excessive scar tissue.[301]

Risk Factors

Numerous risk factors have been identified for the development of proximal hamstring injuries. The evidence to support suggested risk factors varies. Many of the suggested risk factors are modifiable and can be altered by preventive measures or modified rehabilitation strategies in the case of attempting to avoid recurrence. Box 3-1 lists suggested risk factors for hamstring injuries. As previously mentioned, recurrence of hamstring injuries is frequent.[294,295] Engebretsen and colleagues[302] found previous hamstring injury to be the strongest predictive factor in male soccer players. These investigators found that players with previous injury were twice as likely to have another occurrence compared with any other factors that were examined. Factors intrinsic to the actual hamstring structure, such as decreased flexibility and strength, have been associated with injury.[294,303] Particular emphasis has been placed on lack of eccentric strength.[303] Sugiura and associates[304] found that patients with hamstring injuries demonstrated eccentric weakness of the hamstrings and concentric weakness of general hip extension when tested at 60 degrees/second. Consequently, these investigators also found that a decreased hamstring-to-quadriceps and hamstring-to–hip extensor ratio was associated with a higher rate of injury.[304] This finding supports the suggestion of an imbalance between eccentric hamstring strength and concentric quadriceps strength as a contributing factor in the mechanism of injury.[305]

Additional factors related to the lower extremities and lumbopelvic complex have been reported as risk factors for

---

• BOX 3-1 Risk Factors Associated With Hamstring Injuries

- Prior hamstring injury
- Strength deficits
- Muscle fatigue
- Poor lumbopelvic stability
- Poor lumbar posture
- Earlier significant knee joint injury
- Sacroiliac dysfunction
- Leg length discrepancy
- Proprioceptive deficits
- Lack of warmup before physical activity

the occurrence of hamstring injuries. Small and colleagues[306] noted that soccer players demonstrated time-dependent changes (indicating fatigue) of sprint performance that may be related to shortened hamstring length and therefore could predispose such persons to an increased risk for hamstring injury. Poor lumbar posture and insufficient lumbopelvic stability are additional factors associated with an increased risk of injury.[307] The relationship of sacroiliac dysfunction with hamstring injury occurrence has been examined. Of particular interest is the association between anterior pelvic tilt and hamstring tightness.[308] Additional suggested risk factors include lack of a warmup program before physical activity, presence of a leg-length discrepancy, and proprioceptive deficits.[303,309]

Clinical Examination

To diagnose, determine prognosis, and administer efficient intervention in patients with hamstring tears, a structured approach based on current evidence must be used. This approach will allow clinicians to determine the location and severity of injury and to identify functional limitations associated with the injury. Additionally, competing differential diagnoses or concurrent conditions that ultimately may affect prognosis can be identified. Two variations of examination may be performed: acute or "on-field" examination and the subacute or chronic examination approach. The following sections describe the acute and subacute or chronic examination approaches to evaluation of persons with suspected proximal hamstring injuries.

Acute Injury Examination

The goals of acute or on-field examination in patients with suspected proximal hamstring injuries are to confirm the diagnosis, estimate level of involvement, and identify any associated injuries. The acuity of patient presentation may preclude the clinician from performing the battery of clinical tests that have been described in the literature. On conclusion of the on-field examination, the clinician should determine whether immediate referral for additional diagnostic testing is required.

The mechanism of injury should be confirmed. Often, the attending clinician witnesses the injury's occurrence. If contact occurs before injury, the clinician should monitor for findings that indicate involvement of other structures. In the case of avulsion from the ischial tuberosity, an audible "pop" may be reported or heard by those in proximity to the patient at the time of injury.

Visual inspection is particularly useful when evaluating a suspected hamstring injury in the acute setting. In more involved cases, swelling and ecchymosis may develop in the gluteal region and proximal thigh. Additionally, avulsion or significant muscle belly disruption may result in a visible defect. Grade II or III injury may result in altered gait patterns and decreased ability or willingness to bear weight through the extremity. The patient may also demonstrate a preferred position. In such cases, the patient may choose to

decrease tension on the hamstring complex by resting the hip in slight extension or knee flexion.

Palpation is necessary to confirm the presence, location, and potential severity of the injury. Effective palpation allows the clinician to confirm specific location and total area of involvement. Even with appropriate technique, it may be difficult to distinguish a proximal muscle belly rupture from an ischial tuberosity avulsion.[301] The entire hamstring complex should be palpated. This is typically performed with the patient in the prone position. AROM or gentle resistance may allow the clinician to identify specific muscle or tendinous structures. The muscle belly should be examined for specific defects or reproduction of pain. The tendinous insertions should be evaluated, with the ischial tuberosity the primary focus for proximal hamstring injuries.

ROM assessment helps to determine the level of involvement. Secondary to the biarticular span of the hamstring complex, positions of hip flexion or knee extension, particularly when combined, may be limited or increase symptoms. Flexibility testing may be performed if tolerated by the patient. To protect damaged tissue, flexibility testing should be deferred for persons with suspected grade II or III injuries.

The performance of strength assessment in the acute setting is determined by the patient's tolerance and suspected level of involvement. Initially, the ability of the patient to move the hip through the entire level of available extension and the knee through flexion should be determined. If the patient is unable or unwilling to complete full AROM of the hip and knee, further strength testing should be deferred. If deemed appropriate (suspected grade I and selected grade II injuries), formal isometric manual muscle testing (MMT) can be performed. The results provide an estimate not only of strength, but also severity of involvement: strong and painless (minimal disruption or irritation), strong and painful (minor disruption and irritation), weak and painful (more significant disruption, musculotendinous complex intact), and weak and painless (potential for complete disruption of the musculotendinous complex).

The course of care after on-field evaluation is dictated by the estimated severity of involvement. The patient may be immediately referred for further diagnostic imaging when avulsion or rupture is suspected. Grade II injuries will likely require a period of relative rest with treatment intended to control pain, control the inflammatory process, and allow initiation of the healing process. Patients with suspected grade I injuries should undergo a more thorough clinical examination.

Subacute and Chronic Injury Examination

Examination of the subacute or chronic patient allows for a more detailed approach. Although overlapping components exist between the acute and subacute or chronic examination, the expansion of evaluative measures in the subacute or chronic examination scheme allows the clinician to determine more precisely the level of severity, determine prognosis, and develop the rehabilitation plan of care. In many cases, the clinician performing the examination was not present at the time of onset and did not perform an acute examination. In such cases, it is important that a detailed history and visual inspection are conducted before the physical examination.

History

A thorough history is the initial step in efficient evaluation of patients suspected of experiencing a proximal hamstring injury. If previously unknown, the mode of onset should be established early in the evaluation process.

The mode of onset and mechanism of injury are important for determining prognosis and, in some cases, the need for referral for medical testing. An acute onset is common with proximal hamstring injuries and is described in this chapter. Participation in activities associated with a higher risk for proximal hamstring injury such as sprinting should be noted.[310] Identifying a potential complete muscle rupture or tendon avulsion is a priority. These more severe injuries may manifest with a combination of concerning findings: inability to tolerate weight bearing, loud "pop" sounds (more common with proximal tendon injury),[298] complete inability to contract muscle, or severe ecchymosis or a large palpable defect (muscle belly rupture). If these findings are present, particularly in combination with each other, additional referral should be considered. Additionally, known risk factors such as previous hamstring injury and factors that affect prognosis such as specific location of injury should be identified as part of the patient's history. As mentioned, the mode of onset can be gradual. However, this is rarer and strongly warrants consideration of other potential causes of the patient's symptoms.

Visual Inspection

Visual inspection may give the clinician further information regarding acuity and severity. In some cases, the clinician may have performed an immediate examination of the patient at the time of initial injury. In such situations, the clinician can compare the status of the patient at both points in time. The components of visual examination described in the section of this chapter regarding acute injury examination also apply in the subacute or chronic injury situations. Depending on severity and specific location of injury, sitting may be symptomatic because it produces compression of the proximal musculotendinous structures against a firm surface while the hip is flexed. The patient may demonstrate an unwillingness to bear weight through the extremity or to use the hip through normal ROM for gait. This may result in an antalgic and asymmetrical gait pattern. In more involved cases, ecchymosis in the posterior gluteal region and proximal third of the posterior thigh may be observed. Any visual signs of discoloration may indicate the extent of muscle damage. Clinicians should be aware that the location of discoloration does not always overlap with the most painful or damaged region.

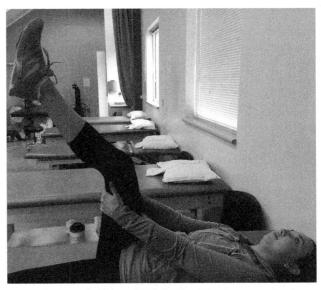

• **Figure 3-10** Popliteal Angle.

Physical Examination

ROM assessment and flexibility testing are routinely performed. These elements should be evaluated for both the hip and the knee to account for the biarticular nature of the hamstring complex. PROM assessment may also be useful when considering alternative conditions. Pain that occurs in areas other than the posterior thigh may indicate involvement of structures other than the hamstrings.

Tests for hamstring flexibility include the passive straight leg raise and popliteal angle tests.[295] The passive straight leg raise test is performed by assessing available hip flexion with the knee fully extended while the patient is in the supine position. A normal value is 80 degrees or greater. The popliteal angle (Fig. 3-10) or active knee extension test is performed by measuring active knee extension while the patient (in supine) holds the hip at 90 degrees of flexion. A knee flexion angle of 20 degrees or less is considered normal. Insufficient ROM measurements on the passive straight leg raise test or popliteal angle test may indicate hamstring muscle tightness. Testing is done bilaterally also to make comparisons with the uninjured side. The patient should also be asked whether posterior thigh symptoms are reproduced with the flexibility tests.

If tolerated, the strength of the hamstring and adjacent pelvic muscles should be measured. When appropriate, clinicians may perform MMT or testing with dynamometry. When available, isokinetic testing can provide additional information on muscle strength at variable speeds. This is most appropriate for patients who have a grade I injury or for cases that are considered chronic.

MMT provides information on strength and the source of symptoms. Hip extension should be assessed with the patient in a prone position. The patient should maintain knee extension to emphasize the hamstrings and flex the knee to 90 degrees to emphasize the gluteus maximus.[311]

While the tester stabilizes the pelvis, the patient is asked to extend the hip to end range (as determined by the PROM assessment). If the patient can achieve this position, he or she is then asked to resist pressure from the examiner into the direction of hip flexion. Side-to-side comparisons are made to determine strength and symptom provocation.

Knee flexion should be assessed with the patient in the prone position. Heiderscheit and associates[295] recommended performing strength testing of the hamstrings at the knee in 15 and 90 degrees of flexion. The therapist should stabilize the pelvis as the patient is asked to resist pressure into knee extension. The clinician can attempt to bias medial (semimembranosus and semitendinosus) or lateral hamstring involvement by rotating the lower leg internally or externally, respectively. Side-to-side comparisons are made to determine strength and symptom provocation.

Additional testing of other hip and lumbopelvic muscles should be performed as tolerated. Because poor pelvic stability and sacroiliac dysfunction have been noted as risk factors for injury, muscles that can affect the lumbopelvic complex must be considered when developing a comprehensive rehabilitation program.[307] Muscles of interest include the gluteus medius, internal and external rotators of the hip, adductors, lower abdominals, and lumbar extensors.

Palpatory examination helps the clinician verify the findings of ROM, flexibility, and strength testing. As described in the earlier section of this chapter on acute injury examination, the entire complex should be palpated to examine for specific defects and to determine the total area of involvement. The point of maximum pain in relation to the ischial tuberosity can be determined. As previously discussed, the distance of maximal pain from the ischial tuberosity has been correlated with length of recovery, with more proximal points indicating a longer recovery period.[295,298,299] Other structures in proximity to the hamstrings may also be palpated for purposes of differential diagnosis. Structures of interest include the piriformis, adductor, and ischial bursa.

Imaging

Imaging studies may be useful when the clinical examination yields ambiguous results or when concerns exist about the severity of injury. Imaging is not routinely used for grade I or grade II strains. Plain radiographs do not give detailed information on muscle or tendon structures and therefore are often not useful. However, in the case of suspected ischial tuberosity avulsion injuries, plain radiographs may be used to confirm the presence and severity of bone detachment from the tendinous origin.[310]

When the actual hamstring complex tissues are of specific interest, ultrasound and MRI are thought to give more detailed information[312] MRI is typically reserved for cases in which determination of partial versus complete rupture is desired, concerns exist about tendon retraction, and surgical treatment is being considered.[295] Connell and colleagues[300] suggested that ultrasound is as effective as MRI and is more cost effective for acute hamstring injuries.

Additional imaging may be considered for the purpose of differential diagnosis. Plain radiography or MRI of the spine may be used to rule out radicular influences. Imaging of the pelvis can provide details of the bursae, lymph nodes, and reproductive and other organs. Although not a standard differential diagnosis for proximal hamstring disorders, if the hip joint is of concern, plain radiography, MRI, or MRI with contrast can be performed.[313]

Differential Diagnosis or Concurrent Issues

Numerous conditions can closely resemble the clinical presentation of proximal hamstring strains. When the history and clinical examination do not strongly support the primary diagnosis, other sources should be considered. If a specific point of onset cannot be determined, suspicion of other structures' involvement should be increased. Clinicians should also consider that these conditions may coexist with a proximal hamstring injury. Identification of alternative or concurrent sources of symptoms aids the clinician in developing a comprehensive treatment plan. Ischial bursitis is an uncommon source of gluteal region test. The clinical presentation of ischial bursitis often shares similar findings with proximal hamstring injuries.[314] However, acute onset is much less common with ischial bursitis. Fortunately, many overlapping treatment strategies exist for the two diagnoses.

Other musculotendinous structures should be considered as well. The adductor group and piriformis muscle attach or span in proximity to the proximal hamstring tendons. Involvement of the adductors may be difficult to differentiate from medial hamstring involvement, and injuries of both structures can occur simultaneously.[298] Like many proximal hamstring injuries, adductor injuries are often traumatic. However, they are more often associated with a quick change of direction.[315] Accurate palpation and specific MMT should help to differentiate between hamstring and adductor structures as the source of symptoms.

Radicular influences and neural tension issues should also be considered in the differential diagnosis or as a concurrent condition. If spinal nerve roots are a source of symptoms, the clinician will typically see an S1 or S2 distribution. When the sciatic nerve is irritated or hypomobile, it can produce symptoms that mimic or coincide with hamstring symptoms distribution. In such cases, neural tension testing positions such as the slump test should reproduce symptoms. Investigators have suggested that severe and recurrent injuries are more likely to create sciatic nerve irritation resulting from decreased mobility associated with adhesions.[312]

Treatment

Numerous conservative treatment protocols for hamstring injuries have been discussed in the literature. Programs are often described in stages or phases based on expected healing times. Worrell[309] described a five-stage program based on level of acuity and stages of tissue healing. Sherry and Best[307] compared two treatment programs, both consisting of two phases. One program emphasized progressive agility and trunk stabilization. The other program emphasized hamstring stretching and strengthening. The investigators found that the program focusing on agility and trunk strengthening was more effective at promoting return to sports and prevention of reinjury.[307] Schmitt and associates[294] designed a program that emphasized eccentric training of the hamstrings in a lengthened state. Heiderscheit and colleagues[295] described a three-stage rehabilitation program that includes specific criteria for progression and return to sport. In the next section, a multistaged conservative treatment program is described, based on current concepts discussed in the literature (Box 3-2).

Stage 1: Initial Postinjury Rehabilitation

The goals of immediate postinjury rehabilitation (from approximately 0 to 4 weeks after injury for conservative treatment) are to control pain and edema,[309] protect tissue to allow initiation of healing, minimize loss of strength and ROM, prevent fiber adhesions,[309] and normalize gait. The time required to achieve each of these goals depends on the severity of injury, as well as on patient-intrinsic factors.

Immediate control of pain and moderation of inflammation are priorities. The traditional application of principles of rest, ice, compression, and elevation (RICE) continue to be used. Various cold-based modalities are applicable and should be used several times per day to help moderate

---

• BOX 3-2 Conservative and Postoperative Rehabilitation for Hamstring Injuries

Stage 1: Initial Postinjury Conservative Rehabilitation (2 to 4 Weeks*)

Goals
- Pain and edema control
- Tissue protection
- Minimizing of ROM and strength deficits
- Prevention of fiber adhesions
- Normalization of gait

Intervention
- Rest, ice-based modalities, compression, elevation
- Gentle soft tissue mobilization
- AROM exercises for the hip and knee
- Gentle strength activities
- Gait training

Criteria for Advancement
- Full PROM and AROM of hip and knee
- Symmetrical gait pattern
- Tolerance to all therapeutic exercises

Stage 1: Initial Postoperative Rehabilitation (12 Weeks*)

Goals
- Pain and edema control
- Protection of healing tissue
- Maintenance of joint mobility
- Normalization of gait

Intervention
- Protected weight bearing with assistive devices (variable time frame)
- Protected ROM, minimizing tensile strain
- Gentle, general lower body strength exercises
- Exercises emphasizing lumbopelvic stability
- Gentle hamstring strengthening (>6 weeks)
- Low-impact aerobic activities (>8 weeks)

Criteria for Advancement
- Full PROM and AROM of hip and knee
- Symmetrical gait pattern
- Tolerance to all therapeutic exercises

Stage 2: Intermediate Level Rehabilitation (2 to 4 Weeks*)

Goals
- Restoration of flexibility
- Increased endurance
- Improved pelvic stability and neuromuscular control

Intervention
- Progression of strengthening exercises
  - Progress to end-range strengthening
  - Consideration of initiating eccentric strengthening
- Exercises emphasizing lumbopelvic stability
- Balance and neuromuscular control activities
- Endurance activities

Criteria for Advancement
- Full and symmetrical hamstring flexibility
- Full and symmetrical hamstring strength with MMT
- Appropriate neuromuscular control
- Jogging without pain or asymmetry of form

Stage 3: Functional Restoration (2 to 4 Weeks*)

Goals
- Full restoration of strength and flexibility
- Full restoration of neuromuscular control and endurance (matching patient's activity demands)
- Return to labor- or sport-specific activities

Intervention
- Strength progression to meet patient's demands
  - Emphasis on strengthening with the muscle in a lengthened state
- Progress balance and neuromuscular control activities
- Labor- or sport-specific training
  - Consideration of plyometric exercises

Criteria for Advancement†
- Full strength in all joint positions
- Full flexibility
- Performing all sport- or labor-specific activities at maximal speed without symptoms

---

AROM, Active range of motion; *MMT,* manual muscle testing; *PROM,* passive range of motion; *ROM,* range of motion.
*Estimation of time spent in a particular stage of rehabilitation; stages 2 and 3 may require a longer time frame for postoperative rehabilitation.
†Criteria for return-to-sport are not well defined in the literature.

inflammation and pain.[309,310] The addition of compression and elevation is useful to contain swelling. Numerous machines and devices are available that can provide cold water compression in both static and intermittent delivery modes. A compression wrap may be used for the patient's comfort. Numerous other modalities such as various electrical stimulation applications, pulsed ultrasound, and cold-laser treatment protocols have been recommended, but they lack strong evidence.[295] Soft tissue mobilization and massage to decrease potential for adhesion development have also been recommended, with the support of relatively weak evidence.[294,295,309] Soft tissue mobilization in this stage should be considered only as the level of injury acuity decreases and the patient is preparing to transition into stage 2 of rehabilitation. A short period of immobilization may be appropriate.[310,316]

NSAIDs have often been recommended for controlling pain and inflammation associated with hamstring injuries. However, the efficacy of regular use of NSAIDs for such injuries has been debated. Long-standing concerns about the potential of NSAIDs to slow the healing process, which includes an inflammatory component, have been expressed.[317]

Therapeutic rehabilitation activities should be started early for patients with grade I and II hamstring strains.[316] Early passive hip and knee ROM can help to avoid muscle stiffness and adhesion formation. These activities should be performed in a manner that does not place excessive stress across the healing hamstring tissue. However, controlled tension may encourage healing with tissue of better quality and justifies early initiation of gentle strength activities. Schmitt and associates[294] recommend pain free submaximal isometrics of knee flexion at multiple angles as soon as 48 hours after injury, to aid scar tissue quality. Pelvic alignment correction (if an anterior innominate rotation is present) has been recommended on the basis of observations of pelvic position on hamstring characteristics such as strength, although the cumulative evidence to support this notion is not strong.[318] Examples of early therapeutic exercises include multiple angle, submaximal, isometric hamstring contractions (heel-digs, machine-based isometrics); hip extension isometric exercises; and active motion of the hip and knee, as tolerated.

Another priority early in rehabilitation should be normalization of gait. To achieve protection of the injured muscle, assistive devices such as crutches may be used in more uninvolved cases.[309] The aquatic environment may also allow gait training in a deweighted environment, as well as more comfortable PROM.

Criteria to progress to the next stage of rehabilitation include full AROM and PROM, minimal swelling, symmetrical gait pattern, and tolerance to all prescribed rehabilitation activities. If the patient is not achieving these objectives, he or she should be reevaluated and the plan of care modified. The time frame for this stage of rehabilitation often ranges from 2 to 4 weeks, depending on injury severity and the individual patient's characteristics.

Stage 2: Intermediate-Level Rehabilitation Progression

After the patient has progressed through the acute and initial subacute stages of recovery (approximately 4 to 6 weeks after injury for conservative treatment and 12 to 14 weeks after surgical repair), the aggressiveness of rehabilitation increases. The goals of this stage are to restore preinjury flexibility of the hamstrings and other proximal muscles, increase general endurance, and improve pelvic stability and neuromuscular control.[307] Progressive controlled mechanical force aiding in the healing of the injured tissue continues in this stage and encourages muscle collagen alignment.[309] The clinician may consider neural mobilization techniques (slump position or "flossing" techniques) if the patient is presenting with symptoms representative of sciatic nerve irritation.[318]

Progressive strengthening should be emphasized in this stage. During this period of increased loading, the patient should be monitored for any increase of symptoms. Pain and other signs of inflammation indicate that the current level of activity is excessive and must be adjusted to the patient's tolerance.[309] Isometric exercises should be performed with increasing force and progressed to activities with a concentric and eccentric emphasis. Initially, exercises should be performed actively in midrange. Progression to exercises that incorporate end ranges is important in achieving functional goals. Examples of exercises that can be incorporated in this stage include resisted hip extension and knee flexion in prone and standing positions, as well as squat or leg press activities.

The importance of eccentric strengthening in hamstring injuries has been comprehensively discussed in the literature.[294,295,305,307,309] Activities such as running and other athletic endeavors require eccentric strength. In a systematic review, Goode and colleagues[319] found that patients who were compliant with programs containing eccentric strengthening activities experienced a lower rate of hamstring injuries. Askling and associates[320] found that eccentric training resulted in fewer injuries for elite soccer players. Eccentric strength training may also play a role in reducing the risk of reinjury.[295] Initial eccentric activities can be based on a progression of hip extension and knee flexion exercises and single leg bridging with an emphasis on control of lowering the body to the starting position. Clinicians should consider the additional demand that eccentric exercise places on the musculotendinous unit when compared with typical isotonically based programs. Therefore, patients should not be progressed to exercises with a heavy eccentric emphasis until they have minimal baseline pain and do not report an increase of symptoms with the rehabilitation exercises that they have been performing from the earlier portion of the program. Schmitt and colleagues[294] recommend not progressing to the stage in rehabilitation that focuses on eccentric progression until the patient has obtained at least 50% of the hamstring strength of the unaffected extremity.

Exercises that focus on lumbopelvic control should be included as part of the rehabilitation program to treat proximal hamstring injuries. Strengthening of the hip, low back, and abdominal muscles should be incorporated as indicated by physical examination.

Sherry and Best[307] found that a program that included progressive agility and trunk stabilization exercises was more effective in preventing injury occurrence than a program that promoted only hamstring stretching and strengthening activities.[307]

As the patient establishes proficiency in performing basic and intermediate level hamstring strength exercises, activities that incorporate balance and neuromuscular control should be introduced. Balance activities should initially be predictable and static (e.g., single leg stance) and then should be progressed to tasks that involve multisegmental movement on unstable surfaces (e.g., throwing a ball while maintaining balance on a destabilization board). Activities that involve maintaining a stable position while an external perturbation force is applied to the patient can be added to increase task difficulty.

Endurance-based exercise should be introduced in a manner that does not excessively stress healing tissue. Having the patient ride the stationary bicycle with consistent resistance at a constant speed allows the clinician to determine the patient's initial tolerance to endurance activity. Slow jogging can be introduced as tolerated. Caution should be used when attempting to increase speed and stride length because this will place greater tension demands and require greater eccentric control of the hamstring muscles.

Criteria to progress from the intermediate to functional restoration stage of rehabilitation include full and symmetrical flexibility (compared with the uninvolved side), full and symmetrical hamstring strength (compared with the uninvolved side) with MMT, no obvious deficits in balance or neuromuscular control, and jogging without pain or asymmetries. The time frame for this stage of rehabilitation often ranges from 2 to 4 weeks, depending on injury severity and the individual patient's characteristics.

Stage 3: Progression to Function Restoration

The final stage of rehabilitation (approximately 6 to 8 weeks after injury for conservative treatment and more than 14 weeks after surgical repair) should lead to a full return to activity. The goals of this stage of rehabilitation are full restoration of flexibility and strength in all planes and the entire ROM, appropriate neuromuscular control and endurance for the patient's activities of interest, and tolerance to all sport- or labor-specific activities of interest.

Strengthening activities tailored to meet the demands of strenuous labor- and sport-specific activities should be continued. A continued emphasis should be placed on progressing eccentric strengthening. Schmitt and colleagues[294] described a rehabilitation approach using eccentric strength exercises in a lengthened state (hip flexed, knee extended) to reduce the potential for reinjury. Examples of strength exercises that may be used at this stage include resisted single leg Romanian deadlifts (RDLs; Fig. 3-11) and Nordic hamstring exercises (Fig. 3-12).

Endurance and neuromuscular control exercises should represent the demands of the patient's required physical demands. Proprioceptive activities that were initiated in the previous stage of rehabilitation can now be progressed in level of difficulty. Running can be incrementally progressed toward sprinting. Interval training can be initiated to recreate the athletic activities in which many patients participate. Multidirectional drills that involve cutting and pivoting can be introduced in a progressive manner.

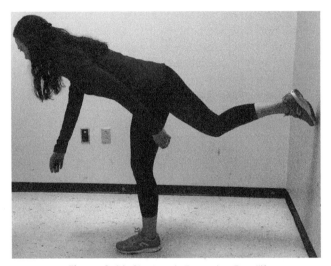

• **Figure 3-11** Single Leg Romanian Deadlift.

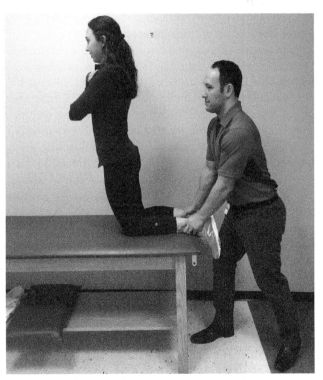

• **Figure 3-12** Nordic Hamstring Exercise.

Power can be regained through plyometric exercises. These activities are key components in developing the explosiveness required to participate in competitive athletic events. The emphasis on increasing force over short periods of time to improve performance increases demands on the hamstring and other muscle groups. The patient should be continuously reevaluated for any adverse reaction to the increased demand on the extremity.

The criteria to complete the final stage of rehabilitation and return to sport are not explicitly defined in the literature. Minimal criteria should be full strength at all positions, full flexibility, and performing all sport-specific activities at maximal effort and full speed with no symptoms. Isokinetic strength testing can provide objective information on concentric and eccentric strength.[295] Clinicians should educate patients that the time required for return to full activity after involved proximal hamstring injuries may be long. Fredericson and associates[321] estimated recovery time for conservative treatment to be as long as 8 to 12 weeks following the initial injury.

Surgical Intervention and Postoperative Considerations for Proximal Hamstring Injuries

Although most proximal hamstring injuries respond well to conservative treatment, some patients with complete muscle ruptures or tendon avulsions and some patients with chronic injuries will require surgical treatment. The most common condition requiring surgical intervention is complete tendon avulsion from the pelvic attachment. Occasionally, excessive scar tissue develops that can affect the function of the hamstring muscle complex and irritate the sciatic nerve. Surgical intervention to remove the scar tissue may decrease symptoms in such cases.

Candidates Versus Noncandidates

Candidates for surgical treatment are typically determined based on severity of injury or, in selected cases, chronicity with failure of conservative care. Pedersen and colleagues[301] recommended strong consideration of surgical treatment in active patients with avulsion of the hamstring and suggested that it be performed within 2 to 3 weeks to avoid complications such as excessive scarring and sciatic nerve involvement. Klingele and Sallay[322] recommended waiting no longer than 4 weeks. For the same reasons, Domb and associates[323] suggested that young and active patients with complete hamstring tendon avulsions do not respond well to conservative treatment and should undergo surgical treatment to maximize functional recovery. These investigators cited several indications for surgical repair: complete osseous avulsion with 2-cm retraction, complete tears of all three hamstring tendons with or without retraction, and partial tears that remain symptomatic after failed conservative treatment.[312,323] Patients with chronic pain and symptoms that represent sciatic nerve irritation, in whom conservative care has failed, may require scar tissue release around the proximal hamstring and sciatic nerve.[321]

Surgical Procedure

Surgical repair of the proximal hamstring complex has been described in the literature.[312 323] Typically, the patient is in the prone position during the operation.[323] The surgical procedure involves creation of an incision in the gluteal crease, mobilization of the ruptured tendon, and reattachment to the ischial tuberosity with the use of various mechanisms of fixation.[312] An area of the ischial tuberosity is exposed to allow bleeding before reattachment. Retracted tendons must be mobilized back to the proximal origin. Care must be taken to avoid damaging the sciatic nerve during the procedure.[323]

When scar tissue and adhesions form in the region of the proximal hamstring and affect the mobility of the sciatic nerve, surgical treatment may be performed to release and débride this excessive tissue. Caution must be employed to avoid damage of the sciatic nerve during the procedure.[323] Additionally, the posterior femoral cutaneous nerve must be recognized and protected during the surgical procedure.

Postoperative Rehabilitation

Postoperative rehabilitation following proximal hamstring repair procedures has been described in the literature, with no consensus on specific guidelines. The reader is directed to review Box 3-2 for a summary of the postoperative rehabilitation guidelines described in this section. Protection of the tissues affected by the surgical procedure is the initial priority. Reduced weight bearing by using crutches is typically recommended. The postoperative weight-bearing status may range from non–weight bearing to partial weight bearing. Cohen and Bradley[312] suggested toe-touch weight bearing for 10 to 14 days, with progression to 25% weight bearing over 3 weeks. Domb and associates[323] recommended 20 pounds of weight bearing for 6 weeks in most cases. Lefevre and colleagues[324] allowed immediate partial weight bearing with forearm crutches and initiation of walking 1 to 2 days postoperatively. Most protocols progress to full weight bearing by 6 weeks postoperatively. A postoperative brace may be prescribed to keep the knee in flexion or prevent hip flexion. The purpose of the brace is to prevent excessive tension from being placed across the healing tissue. No consensus exists on specific settings of braces after proximal hamstring repair operations, and recommendations often vary with the degree of mobilization required to approximate retracted tendons back to their insertion.

Early, protected ROM of the hip and knee is typically recommended. The amount and progression of ROM activities often vary according to the amount of tendon retraction and subsequent mobilization required during the surgical procedure. Particular care must be taken not to move the surgical limb past the limits of hip flexion and knee extension as determined by the attending surgeon. Cohen and Bradley[312] recommended beginning PROM at 2 weeks and progressing to AROM at 4 weeks. AROM of the knee for flexion is often not allowed or is significantly limited for up to 6 weeks.[324]

Early exercises focus on minimizing loss of general lower extremity strength. In most cases, submaximal isometric quadriceps and gentle ankle strength exercises can be initiated immediately.[324] By 6 weeks postoperatively, the patient is allowed to start gentle strengthening of the hamstring, typically beginning with active knee flexion and avoiding end-range extension. The patient can slowly progress the exercises in terms of resistance and with a comfortable ROM. Weight bearing (bodyweight), lumbopelvic stabilization and balance activities should be initiated within tolerable limits. Light, low-impact aerobic exercise such as use of the stationary bicycle can slowly be initiated after 8 weeks. This stage of rehabilitation typically persists until approximately 12 weeks postoperatively. By the end of this postoperative stage, patients should be ambulating with a symmetrical gait pattern, demonstrate minimal baseline pain, have full passive knee and hip joint ROM (not necessarily full hamstring flexibility), and tolerate all prescribed exercises without increasing symptoms.

Approximately 12 weeks after the surgical procedure, if the patient has met the foregoing criteria, he or she should now be able to progress to stage 2 (intermediate level rehabilitation progression) of the previous section that discussed conservative treatment of rehabilitation for proximal hamstring injuries. As is the case with conservative treatment of proximal hamstring injuries, the length of time spent in this stage varies among patients postoperatively. Stages 2 (4 to 6 weeks after injury) and 3 (6 to 8 weeks after injury) from the previous section describing conservative treatment are the same as stages 2 (12 to 14 weeks after surgery) and 3 (>14 weeks after surgery) for postoperative treatment. This progression allows the postoperative patient who underwent proximal hamstring repair to progress back to full activity and provide objective criteria on which to base such a progression.

Surgical Outcomes

The literature examining clinical outcomes after proximal hamstring repair is fairly limited and often involves mixed cohorts of patients with both acute and chronic injuries.[323] Average follow-up for studies varies from 12 months to more than 7 years.[312] Most of the available evidence is at the level of case series. Cohen and Bradley[312,325] reported that 58% to 85% of patients returned to function and sports activity with nearly normal strength and less pain.

Summary

Proximal hamstring injuries are a relatively common occurrence, particularly in the athletic population. The spectrum of injury can range from minor tissue disruption and irritation to full rupture or avulsion from the tendon origin. Conservative treatment is typically prescribed for injuries that do not completely disrupt the function of the musculotendinous complex. Patients with avulsion or complete muscle rupture injuries, as well as partial disruption injuries that have not responded well to rehabilitation, may be candidates for surgical intervention. Although no definitive consensus exists on conservative and postoperative rehabilitation, numerous concepts have been emphasized in the literature.

Hip Flexor Injuries and Iliopsoas Bursitis

The list of potential causes of anterior hip and groin pain can be extensive.[258,271] Many conditions in this region manifest with similar symptoms, including involvement of articular hip structures, musculotendinous tissues, the pelvic floor, bursae, internal organs, and lymphatic structures. Clinicians must also consider potential involvement of the peripheral nerves and spinal nerve roots. Involvement of hip flexor structures and the iliopsoas bursa can be verified by thorough examination. Muscles that can produce flexion of the hip include the iliopsoas complex, rectus femoris, TFL, gracilis, and sartorius. Among these muscles, the iliopsoas produces the greatest proportion of hip flexion strength. The rectus femoris is a two-joint muscle crossing the hip and knee. Therefore, the relative contribution of the rectus femoris in producing hip flexion depends on the knee being flexed. One of several bursae in the hip and pelvic region, the iliopsoas bursa (or iliopectineal bursa) is the largest and is located between the iliopsoas muscle complex (anterior boundary) and the hip joint capsule (posterior boundary). This section focuses on iliopsoas tendinopathy (not related to SHS), iliopsoas bursitis, proximal rectus femoris injuries, and TFL conditions. Hip flexor tendinopathy is often the result of an overuse mechanism in athletes. This mechanism has been described in athletes participating in running, cycling, football, hockey, and soccer.[326-330] Traumatic-onset injuries, including avulsion or rupture injuries, are possible. This is more common in injuries of the rectus femoris.

Iliopsoas Strain and Bursitis

Conditions related to the iliopsoas complex often result in anterior groin pain. Potential conditions related to the iliopsoas complex may include tendinopathy, snapping tendon, and avulsion injuries.[331] The incidence of iliopsoas-related disorders is, for the most part, unknown.[271] However, specific populations that are at higher risk to develop iliopsoas-related issues have been identified and include dancers,[332] runners, American football players, and soccer players.[333,334] The reader is encouraged to review the earlier section on SHS for specific details of the diagnosis and treatment of iliopsoas disorders related to SHS. Although this chapter focuses on mechanical causes of iliopsoas complex conditions, the condition has been shown to occur at a higher rate in patients with rheumatoid arthritis and those who have undergone THA and hip arthroscopy procedures.[331,335,336]

Mechanism of Injury

Iliopsoas tendinopathy and bursitis can occur through numerous, often overlapping, mechanisms. Acute or repetitive overuse mechanisms are possible.[135] Most often, overuse and repetitive movements of the hip in the sagittal plane are associated with development of the condition. The mechanical results of these repetitive movements are excessive friction and eventually irritation of the structures comprising the iliopsoas complex. Sports that have been associated with the development of iliopsoas tendinopathy and bursitis include soccer, ballet, uphill running, hurdling, and jumping.[135] As mentioned, iliopsoas bursitis can also be observed as an inflammatory manifestation of the synovial lining that occurs with rheumatic arthritis.[335]

Clinical Examination

Iliopsoas involvement can be confirmed through a detailed history and by flexibility and strength testing. Identification of participation in any of the activities associated with the development of psoas-related conditions should be noted. Because of the depth of the structures of interest and their overlapping locations, palpatory examination may be of limited use to the clinician. Palpation deep into the femoral triangle region may elicit pain. The Thomas test can be used to identify tightness of the iliopsoas complex. The reader is encouraged to review Chapter 2 for detailed information on the Thomas test. Flexibility and strength of other hip potential flexors such as the rectus femoris and TFL should also be assessed to determine the potential involvement of these structures in the patient's presentation. General and specific hip muscle strength should also be assessed. The reader is encouraged to review Chapter 2 for the details of clinical examination of the hip region. Resisted testing of hip flexion combined with external rotation may more specifically emphasize the iliopsoas complex (resisted straight leg raise with the lower leg turned outward).[337] Because of the potential role it may have in postural stabilization, Tyler and colleagues[271] recommended that clinicians consider using components of static and dynamic assessment of lumbopelvic influences.

Treatment

Because the cause and specific nature of pain related to the iliopsoas complex is not well understood, treatment of this group of disorders is also not well defined.[330] Most patients with iliopsoas complex disorders respond well to conservative treatment. Minimal evidence is available that compares different conservative treatment approaches for iliopsoas-related disorders. Intervention is heavily driven by impairments found during the clinical examination and activity modification. Johnston and associates[338] used a home program emphasizing exercises that strengthened the hip rotators and stretching to treat nine patients (mean age, 35.6 years; eight women and one man) who were diagnosed with iliopsoas syndrome. These patients reported a significant decrease in pain levels, and 77% of patients returned to their previous level of function. Ingber[339] reported significant decreases in pain, improved hip and spine extension, and a return to normal activity in six

patients with iliopsoas impairments and low back pain when treatment used dry needling techniques to address iliopsoas trigger points. Tyler and colleagues[271] recommended using a foundation of core stabilization with progressive hip strengthening activities (emphasis on hip flexors) performed in multiple positions to treat patients with iliopsoas syndrome.

Rectus Femoris Injuries

The rectus femoris has two proximal originations: the straight head arises from anterior inferior iliac spine, and the reflected head originates from the superior acetabular region. The muscle crosses the hip and knee joint and then inserts at the base of the patella as a portion of the quadriceps tendon. Being a two-joint muscle, it is susceptible to influences from both the hip and knee. The injury spectrum of the rectus femoris ranges from minor strains to full rupture or avulsion. Additionally, the proximal rectus region is a potential area where apophysitis can occur in persons who have not reached skeletal maturity.

Mechanism of Injury

Proximal rectus femoris rupture or avulsion is relatively rare.[340] The injury is typically associated with a traumatic onset. The straight head is the most common location of avulsion.[341] Kicking and jumping mechanisms are commonly reported. In a case series of four professional soccer players with complete rectus proximal rectus femoris avulsion injuries, Ueblacker and associates[342] noted that all subjects incurred the injury while kicking with the dominant affected leg. Immediate pain and a popping sensation are often reported. Palpable tenderness at the proximal origin, visual deformity, swelling, and discoloration are often observed.

Strains of the rectus femoris are more common in the middle or distal part of the muscle. When proximal strains occur, they typically occur through the same mechanisms described for avulsion injuries, but with less damage. Hughes and colleagues[343] described a series of 10 athletes with intrasubstance injuries occurring at the proximal muscle-tendon junction. The most common mechanism of injury in this series of patients was kicking or sprinting activity.

Clinical Examination

Rectus femoris injuries can be confirmed through observation, palpation, ROM, flexibility, and strength testing. Clinicians should recognize that physical examination may be limited in acute cases, secondary to the patient's tolerance and the potential for avulsion of the proximal tendon. When complete avulsion or rupture is suspected, the patient should be considered for referral or imaging studies to confirm the severity of injury. The presence of significant swelling or discoloration may be correlated with a more acute, and potentially more involved, injury.

Palpatory examination may help to confirm the severity and specific location of injury. The proximal attachment region of the anterior inferior iliac spine should be palpated. The myotendinous junction and muscle belly should be palpated. A mass that may be tender may be found in the intramuscular substance.[343] Proximal musculotendinous structures that should be palpated to rule out their involvement include the TFL, sartorius, pectineus, adductor longus, and other quadriceps muscles.

In subacute or chronic cases, flexibility testing can confirm sources of symptoms as well as residual flexibility deficits. Clinicians can use the modified Thomas test or the Ely test to assess rectus femoris flexibility. The reader is encouraged to review Chapter 2 for detailed information on the modified Thomas test. The Ely test is performed with the patient in the prone position. The examiner passively flexes the subject's knee until the heel touches the buttocks. If the patient's heel does not reach the buttocks or the hip simultaneously flexes, lifting the pelvis off the table, the test result is considered positive for rectus femoris tightness. Peeler and Anderson[344] conducted a study with 54 healthy persons (18 to 54 years old), to determine intrarater and interrater reliability of the Ely test. They found only moderate agreement levels for intrarater (kappa = 0.52) and interrater (kappa = 0.46) reliability.

Strength testing can identify residual weakness and confirm the location of injury. Formal strength testing should be deferred if rupture or avulsion injury is suspected. The ability of a patient to perform a straight leg raise procedure may be useful to determine the ability to lift the hip against gravity. Formal muscle testing should attempt to use the positions of relative hip extension and knee flexion to maximize tension on the rectus femoris. Performing a test for knee extension strength with the patient in the prone position and the knee flexed to 90 degrees can achieve this objective.

Treatment

Treatment of proximal rectus femoris avulsion injuries is often nonoperative.[345] Gamradt and colleagues[345] described nonoperative treatment of rectus femoris avulsion injuries in 11 NFL players. These investigators found that all included subjects returned to play in 6 to 12 weeks, with a mean of 69.2 days. When surgical treatment was performed, most athletes are able to return to preinjury levels of activity within 5 to 10 months.[340] Ueblacker and associates[342] reported a case series of four professional soccer players who underwent proximal rectus femoris repair (suture anchor fixation) after complete avulsion. These investigators reported that all subjects returned to their preinjury level of competition by 16 weeks postoperatively. The success reported in case series for nonoperative and operative treatment of proximal rectus femoris avulsion injuries does not allow for a consensus on the best standard of care in treating patients with these injuries.

Conservative treatment of rectus femoris strains is comparable to that of strains of other lower extremity muscles. The intervention approach described to treat iliopsoas strains is applicable in the acute stages of treatment for rectus femoris strains. The initial goals are to decrease symptoms, control inflammation, and promote early healing with controlled mobility.

Several structure-specific concerns exist when progressing patients with rectus femoris strains through the subacute stages and back to full function. Stretching and strengthening interventions should take into account that the muscle crosses both the hip and knee joints. Initially, treatment may be directed at emphasizing movement at each joint separately. As tolerated, activities should be progress to place the patient in positions that require simultaneous hip extension and knee flexion.

Tensor Fasciae Latae Injuries

Tendinopathy of the TFL has been identified as a potential cause of anterior groin pain.[346] It has been suggested that underactivity or inhibition of the primary stabilizers, such as the gluteus medius, may result in overactivity and eventual pain from the TFL.[347] Symptomatic TFL conditions may also be indicative of other underlying pathologic processes. Sutter and associates[348] examined 35 patients undergoing MRI for hip abductor pain. These investigators found that in patients with hip abductor tears (n = 16), a significant proportion showed hypertrophy of the TFL when compared with the healthy side. TFL conditions are often part of the spectrum of ITB syndrome.

Mechanism of Injury

Running is a commonly reported mechanism for development of TFL injuries and other overuse conditions of the lower extremity.[263] Hip abductor, flexor, and adductor weakness has been associated with lower extremity overuse injuries in runners.[349] When this occurs, the TFL may play a significant role in frontal plane stabilization, as opposed to being a secondary stabilizer. Because of the anatomic relationship between the TFL and the ITB, their associated mechanisms of injury often overlap.

Clinical Examination

Palpation can be useful for verifying TFL involvement and determining acuity of symptoms. Clinicians should evaluate the proximal origins at the anterior superior iliac spine, anterior iliac crest, and insertions into the fibrous proximal ITB. Additionally, proximal structures such as the sartorius, gluteus medius, and trochanteric bursa should be palpated to rule out additional tissue involvement. Assessment of relative TFL muscle size (compared with the noninvolved side) may be useful to the clinician. Bass and Connell[346] found that in a group of athletes (n = 12) with anterior groin pain, the TFL was enlarged up to 2.5 times the normal size.

Flexibility testing of the TFL-ITB complex should also be performed. Useful clinical tests for tightness include the Ober test and the modified Thomas test. For specific details of the Ober test and the modified Thomas test, the reader is encouraged to review Chapter 2.

Strength testing of all hip and pelvic muscles should be performed when evaluating a patient with pain that is potentially originating from the TFL. Of particular interest is the gluteus medius muscle. MMT may also be used to reproduce pain, thus confirming contractile tissue involvement. For specific details on MMT of the hip muscles, the reader is encouraged to review Chapter 2.

Treatment

Activity modification is part of the initial treatment for TFL conditions. Relative rest should be used when the patient's presentation is acute. With runners commonly affected by TFL injuries, modification of the patient's running program may be justified. Nielsen and colleagues[263] found that novice runners who increased their mileage more than 30% over a 2-week period experienced a greater risk of distance-related injuries when compared with runners who increased their distance less than 10% over the same period of time.

Treatment of TFL injuries is primarily based on impairments identified during the clinical examination. As mentioned, TFL injuries are often part of or associated with ITB syndrome. Stretching of the ITB-TFL complex may be indicated. Any other flexibility deficits identified during clinical examination should be addressed to promote normal mechanical function during repetitive activities.

Muscle weakness found during clinical examination should be addressed. Providing frontal plane stabilization with the gluteal muscles can theoretically decrease the cumulative stress experienced by the TFL muscles. An attempt should be made to provide selective strengthening of the gluteal muscles while attempting to minimize TFL activation. Selkowitz and associates[283] analyzed EMG data on 20 healthy subjects to determine activity of the gluteal muscles (gluteus medius and superior portion of the gluteus maximus) and TFL during common rehabilitation exercises. These investigators found the highest gluteal-to-TFL activation ratio for band-resisted sidestep, unilateral bridge, and both quadruped hip extension exercises.

Numerous manual therapy techniques to address soft tissue dysfunction have been anecdotally recommended for treatment of TFL-related disorders. Such techniques include massage, trigger point therapy, acupressure, and dry needling techniques. Although clinicians report improvements in their patients with these interventions, literature investigating the specific use of such treatments in patients with TFL injury is minimal.

Summary

Hip flexor injuries are a potential cause of anterior hip and groin pain. Iliopsoas tendinopathy and bursitis are most often produced through overuse or repetitive activity in the sagittal plane. The most common rectus femoris injury is a strain in the middle or distal muscle belly, whereas proximal avulsion is a rarer occurrence. TFL injuries most often manifest as anterior and lateral hip region pain and may be the result of insufficient use of the primary movers and stabilizers of the hip joint. Most patients with hip flexor injuries that do not significantly disrupt form or function of the musculotendinous unit respond well to conservative treatment. Accurate clinical diagnosis of various hip flexor conditions depends on skilled palpation and appropriate performance of strength and flexibility tests, as well as on effectively ruling out intraarticular causes of pain.

Piriformis Syndrome

Piriformis syndrome is an entrapment condition of the sciatic nerve from an abnormal condition of the piriformis muscle. It is estimated that 6% to 36% of patients diagnosed as having low back pain actually have piriformis syndrome.[350] Piriformis syndrome is considered a controversial diagnosis and can be difficult to identify because it can mimic sacral dysfunction, lumbar disk disorders, lumbar radiculopathy, and trochanteric bursitis.[350,351]

Anatomic Review and Mechanisms of Injury

The piriformis muscle (S1 to S2) originates on the anterior surface of sacrum at the second to fourth sacral levels and inserts into superior medial aspect of the greater trochanter through the round tendon.[352] The piriformis muscle actions include hip external rotation, weak abduction, and posture stability during standing and ambulation.[350] In most persons, the sciatic nerve passes deep to the piriformis muscles, but in up to 22% of the population, the sciatic nerve passes through the muscle, splits the muscle, or both, and this predisposes the patient to piriformis syndrome.[350]

Two types of piriformis syndrome are described in the literature. Primary piriformis syndrome is related to an anatomic cause such as a split sciatic nerve, split piriformis muscle, or sciatic nerve with an irregular path. This condition is rarer, and a comprehensive differential diagnosis should be made to rule out more common pathologic conditions.[353] Secondary piriformis syndrome is more common and may result from macrotrauma or microtrauma. Macrotrauma may include traumatic injury to the buttocks that results in soft tissue injury, inflammation, and muscle spasm and causes in sciatic nerve compression. Microtrauma may result from overuse of the muscle (e.g., from prolonged walking or running) or from direct compression (e.g., sitting on a hard surface), which may compress the sciatic nerve. Piriformis syndrome may also be related to sacral dysfunction.[350]

Patient Profile

Piriformis syndrome occurs most frequently in the fourth or fifth decade of life and affects women more than men.[350] This sex difference may reflect the biomechanics of the wider female pelvis and hip.[354] Piriformis syndrome can occur in persons of all occupations and activity levels.

Patients may complain of radiating pain and or paresthesia from the sacral region down the posterior thigh to the knee, pain with sitting or standing more that 15 to 20 minutes, pain with moving from sitting to standing, tying shoes, ipsilateral muscle weakness in lower extremity, difficulty walking, and sensory abnormalities in the foot.[350,355] Pain may be improved with ambulation. Other symptoms that may occur include abdominal, pelvic, or inguinal pain and pain with bowel movements, as well as dyspareunia in women.[350]

Clinical Examination

The clinical examination often includes a comprehensive history and special testing to differentiate piriformis syndrome from other pathologic conditions. Common findings include palpable tenderness over the piriformis, region of the sacroiliac joint, and greater sciatic notch. Limited internal rotation of the affected limb may be present in patients with sacroiliac joint disorders (e.g., rotated sacrum) and compensatory lumbar rotation.[350] Results of clinical tests may be positive, as discussed in the following subsections.

Lasègue Sign

Procedure: With the Lasègue sign or straight leg raise test, the examiner passively flexes the hip while the knee is in full extension.
Interpretation: A positive test result is reproduction of the patient's symptoms.

This test has been validated as an assessment for lumbar disk herniation.[356] No studies have investigated its utility for assessing piriformis syndrome; it has been detailed only in clinical commentaries.[350]

Freiberg Test

Procedure: With this test, the examiner passively internally rotates the extended hip with the patient supine.
Interpretation: Reproduction of the patient's symptoms is considered a positive test result.[354]

The clinometric properties of this test have not been examined. The test has been described only in the literature.[350]

FAIR (Flexion, Adduction, and Internal Rotation) Test

Procedure: With this test, the patient is side lying with the affected side up, the hip is flexed to 60 degrees, and the knee is flexed between 60 to 90 degrees. The examiner stabilizes the hip with the cranial hand and internally rotates and adducts the knee by applying a downward force to the knee with the caudal hand.[350] Alternative positions include the patient supine or seated with the hip and knee flexed, with the hip internally rotated, while the patient resists the examiner's attempts to externally rotate and abduct the hip.[350]
Interpretation: Reproduction of the patient's sciatic symptoms is considered a positive test result.[350]

This test has been found to have a sensitivity of 0.88 and specificity of 0.83.[357]

Beatty Test

Procedure: With this test, the patient is side lying with the affected leg upward. The hip is flexed, followed by the patient's lifting and holding the knee approximately 4 inches above the table.
Interpretation: Reproduction of the patient's symptoms is considered a positive test result.

This test was first described in 1994, but its clinometric properties have not been investigated since its introduction.[358] The test has been described only in clinical commentaries.[350,359]

Imaging and Testing

Radiographs have limited application in diagnosing piriformis syndrome.[350] Neurophysiologic testing such as EMG is commonly used to help diagnose the presence of sciatic entrapment by the piriformis muscle.[357,360] MRN has been used to successfully diagnose patients with piriformis syndrome (specificity of 93% and sensitivity of 64%).[361,362] MRI and computed tomography can reveal pathologic processes of the piriformis muscle but are often used to rule out lumbar disk or vertebral disorders pathology.[350,363,364]

Postinjury Management and Rehabilitation

Nonsurgical conservative treatment is often done first in the treatment of piriformis syndrome. If the condition is recalcitrant to conservative measures, then surgery is an option. Conservative treatment often includes a multimodal approach that comprises therapeutic exercise, stretching, modalities (e.g., ultrasound, electrical current), manual therapy (e.g., mobilization or manipulation), oral antiinflammatory medication, acupuncture, prolotherapy, and injections (local anesthetic, corticosteroids, and botulinum toxin).[350,365,366] Fishman and colleagues[357] found that the FAIR special test coupled with injection and physical therapy and/or surgery was an effective means of diagnosing and treating piriformis syndrome in a sample of 918 patients (1014 legs). With conservative treatment, 79% (514 of 655) of subjects with a positive FAIR test improved 50% or more from injection and physical therapy at a mean follow-up of 10.2 months.[357] With surgery, 65% of subjects (28 of 43) with a positive FAIR test showed 50% or greater (68% average improvement) at a mean follow-up of 16 months.[357] Fishman and associates[365] found successful results combining botulinum toxin (Botox) with rehabilitation in a randomized controlled trial. Botox injection are becoming an emerging treatment with favorable outcomes in the literature but does lead to atrophy and degeneration of the piriformis muscle, which may have long-term consequences.[367,368] Besides these two investigations, there have been no other controlled trials specifically measuring the effectiveness of conservative rehabilitation for piriformis syndrome. One other case study (level 4) reported successful outcomes with a nonsurgical multimodal progam.[369]

The research on nonoperative rehabilitation programs for piriformis syndrome is understudied. Currently, there is no consensus on the optimal rehabilitation program. This must be considered when interpreting these results for clinical practice.

Surgical Intervention

If conservative treatment is unsuccessful, then surgical intervention is an option. The surgical option is to release the piriformis tendon and sciatic neurolysis in order to decompress the sciatic nerve.[370] Several investigations have reported successful short-term outcomes in patient satisfaction, recurrence of symptoms, and quality of life with this procedure.[357,364,370,371] To date, there are no clinical trials investigating postsurgical rehabilitation programs.

Summary

Piriformis syndrome remains a controversial diagnosis because it can mimic other common pathologic conditions of the lumbopelvic region. The research findings on the clinical examination are inconclusive, with no consensus on the best clinical tests and diagnostic imaging. The research findings on both conservative and postsurgical rehabilitation are also sparse, with no consensus on the best rehabilitation programs. Further controlled trials are needed for both the examination and management of this disorder, to develop a consensus to guide clinical practice.

Entrapment Neuropathies of the Hip and Pelvis

The differential diagnosis of hip and pelvic pain must consider the possibility of nerve entrapment to the major peripheral nerves that innervate the pelvic and lower extremity. This section discusses four common nerve entrapments: femoral nerve, obturator nerve, sciatic nerve, and LCNT.

Femoral Neuropathy

The femoral nerve originates from the dorsal divisions of L2 to L4 and is the largest branch of the lumbar plexus. It emerges from the lateral border of the psoas major muscle where it supplies the iliacus and then passes deep to the inguinal ligament (lateral to the femoral artery and vein) to the anterior thigh, where it ends with four terminal braches: the internal and external musculocutaneous nerves, the deep branch to the quadriceps, and the saphenous nerve. The femoral nerve provides motor innervation to the psoas, iliacus, and quadriceps group.[352,372]

The femoral nerve is most commonly injured within the retroperitoneal space or under the inguinal ligament. The most common cause (60% of femoral nerve lesions) is

iatrogenic injury resulting from intraabdominal, pelvic, gynecologic, and urologic surgical procedures.[372-374] Surgical procedures of the hip that use the anterior and anterolateral approaches may cause injury by direct compression of the nerve by the self-retaining retractors or the position of the hip (e.g., flexion, abduction, and external rotation [FABER]) during the operation.[372,373] Femoral neuropathy secondary to iliacus hematoma is less frequent but can occur in patients receiving anticoagulation therapy or who have clotting disorders. In rare cases, traumatic iliacus hematoma has been reported as a sports-related injury in younger persons (12 to 24 years of age).[375] These conditions need to be considered during the differential diagnosis of possible femoral neuropathy.

Patients with femoral neuropathy present with unilateral weakness of hip flexion (e.g., lesion above the inguinal ligament) or knee extension (lesion below the inguinal ligament) with impaired function related to the weakness. The patellar reflex is diminished, and pain may be elicited with extension of the hip. Electrodiagnostic testing is often used to confirm the diagnosis.[376]

Obturator Neuropathy

The obturator nerve originates from the L2 to L4 nerve roots, emerges from the medial border of the psoas major muscle, and passes through the pelvis, where it divides into terminal and collateral branches.[352] The terminal branch further divides into anterior and posterior branches. The anterior branch enters the medial thigh to supply motor fibers to the gracilis and adductor longus and magnus muscles and joins the saphenous nerve distally to provide cutaneous distribution to the medial thigh near the knee joint. The posterior branch travels through the obturator externus and adductor brevis muscles.[352,372] This branch supplies the obturator externus, adductor brevis, and hip joint. The collateral branches are two articular nerves that supplying the hip joint and the obturator externus muscle.

Damage to the obturator nerve is less frequent and may result from trauma such as pelvic fractures or iatrogenic injury from hip positions during THA, pelvic surgical procedures, and femoral artery procedures.[372,374] Nerve fascial entrapment can occur as the nerve enters the adductor canal and is related to exercise and sports activity.[372]

Patients may present with medial thigh or groin pain, adductor weakness, and sensory loss in the middle thigh. The patient may walk with a circumduction gait as a result of weakness of hip adduction and internal rotation. Electrodiagnostic testing is also conducted to diagnose obturator neuropathy more definitively.[377]

Sciatic Neuropathy

The sciatic nerve is formed by the ventral rami of L4 to S3 and supplies the posterior lower limb.[378] The nerve passes through the greater sciatic foramen just below the piriformis muscle and descends down the posterior thigh until the popliteal fossa, where it bifurcates into the tibial and common peroneal (fibular) nerve.

The sciatic nerve can be damaged at the pelvis or gluteal region by trauma such as hip joint fractures, derangement of the sacroiliac joint, and posterior hip dislocations. Iatrogenic injury can also occur after hip replacement. The nerve can suffer entrapment by the piriformis muscle in a condition called *piriformis syndrome,* discussed earlier.

Patients with sciatic neuropathy may present with radiating pain from the sacrum down the posterior leg and weakness in the hamstrings (hip extension, knee flexion) and muscles in the peroneal and tibial nerve distribution.[350] Sensory abnormalities of the lower leg may be seen in the peroneal and tibial distribution and distribution of the posterior femoral cutaneous nerve.[372] The Achilles and hamstring reflexes are diminished or absent, with an unaffected patellar reflex.[372] The patient may have difficulty walking because of weakness and sensory loss and pain with sitting or squatting.[350] Electrodiagnostic testing is also performed to diagnose sciatic neuropathy more precisely.[377]

Lateral Cutaneous Nerve of the Thigh

The reader is referred to the earlier section on MP, which is entrapment of the LCNT.

Treatment

Depending on the severity of nerve entrapment, postinjury management may first include conservative treatment and then surgical intervention if no regeneration occurs 3 to 6 months after injury.[374] In general, conservative treatment may include rest, modalities, manual therapy, strengthening exercise, stretching, oral antiinflammatory medication, and corticosteroid injections.[375,377] Conservative treatment often varies by patient, and this requires constant attention to the patient's response to treatment. If treatment fails, then a surgical procedure such as neurolysis or resection may be performed.[379]

Nerve entrapments of the hip and pelvis should be considered in the differential diagnosis once the more common pathologic conditions have been excluded. This section discussed four common nerve entrapments of this region. Chapter 9 discusses other nerve entrapments (i.e., pudendal) of the pelvic region.

Case Studies

Examples of hip disorders are provided in Case Studies 3-1 and 3-2.

CASE STUDY 3-1

Nonoperative Treatment of a Patient With a Proximal Hamstring Strain

Patient History

A 28-year-old male patient reported to physical therapy in an outpatient clinic with a complaint of sudden-onset posterior thigh and gluteal region pain. The patient was self-referred in a state that allows direct access for physical therapy treatment. He noted a sudden onset of pain while sprinting downfield during the second half of a club-level soccer game 3 days before the initial physical therapy consultation. At the time of injury, he immediately quit playing and rested on the sidelines. He was resting for the last 3 days and applying ice to the injured area. He subjectively noted minor swelling and discoloration from the gluteal fold down to the middle of the posterior thigh. He could bear weight and ambulate, but this was often uncomfortable if walking more than 30 feet. He noted soreness if seated on relatively firm surfaces for more than 15 minutes. He was also taking over-the-counter nonsteroidal antiinflammatory drugs (NSAIDs) as directed for the past several days. The patient noted that he believed the NSAIDs and ice were helpful in controlling discomfort and swelling. He was a graduate student at the local university and currently was between semesters. The patient noted that in addition to regular participation in club soccer, he also enjoyed yoga once a week. Other than a minor sprained ankle more than 5 years ago, the patient denied any other significant medical history. At the time of his initial physical therapy evaluation, the patient rated his pain range as 2 to 6 out of 10, depending on his level of activity. The greatest amount of pain at the time of evaluation occurred with negotiating relatively high stairs and prolonged periods of walking.

Systems Review

Observation yielded a 28-year-old, 6-foot tall, 200-pound man in minimal distress. His standing posture showed a relative anterior tilt of the pelvis in static standing. He was unremarkable for any other deviations of the spine or lower extremities. The patient's gait pattern was asymmetrical with a slightly flexed knee throughout stance and decreased time spent on the involved extremity. He was not using any assistive devices at the time of evaluation. When standing, he kept the knee of the affected extremity slightly flexed. An area of blue and yellow discoloration was noted on the proximal one third of his thigh. No notable swelling was observed at the time of evaluation.

Tests and Measures

The patient completed and scored 40 points on the Lower Extremity Function Scale (LEFS). The LEFS was chosen because it is a validated, self-reported functional assessment tool for lower extremity conditions.[380] The maximal score is 80 points, indicating no difficulty with any of the described activities.

Next, a physical examination of the patient was completed. Knee and hip range of motion (ROM) were assessed. The patient reported posterior thigh and gluteal pain when the hip was flexed to 90 degrees or more with the knee in a relatively flexed position to avoid excessive tension on the hamstring structures. Flexibility testing of the lower extremity was deferred secondary to the acuity of the injury. The patient was able to flex the knee to 90 degrees actively while standing;

Continued

CASE STUDY 3-1

Nonoperative Treatment of a Patient With a Proximal Hamstring Strain—cont'd

125 degrees of passive knee flexion was available. Pain increased to 5 out of 10 when attempting this motion. He was able to extend the hip 5 degrees off the table in the prone position and was limited secondary to pain; 15 degrees of passive hip extension was available. Pain levels increased to 6 out of 10 when attempting to do this. The patient was able to produce at least 3/5 strength in all other planes of motion at the hip. Formal manual muscle testing was deferred because of the acuity of the patient's symptoms. Palpation of the proximal thigh in the area of the myotendinous junction of the hamstring and inferior portion of the ischial tuberosity was painful, rated at 3 out of 10. Other than the presence of the previously mentioned anterior pelvic tilt position, no other significant findings involving the lumbopelvic complex were observed.

Evaluation, Diagnosis, and Prognosis

Based on the patient's history, observation, and physical examination, it was determined that the cause of the patient's pain and dysfunction was highly likely to be a grade II proximal hamstring strain. The patient demonstrated strength, flexibility, and palpation deficits that have been suggested to occur with this patient population. The traumatic mode of onset also was consistent with a strain of the proximal hamstring. The patient was able to extend the hip and flex the knee partially against gravity, thus decreasing suspicion of complete muscle rupture or avulsion of the hamstring from the ischial tuberosity. That the injury location was fairly close to the ischial tuberosity indicated the potential for a relatively longer period of rehabilitation when compared with distal hamstring injuries of comparable magnitude.

Intervention

A multimodal approach was used for this patient. Initially, ice, compression, and elevation helped to minimize the amount of inflammation in the area of injury. Gentle passive ROM, active ROM, and hip muscle isometric exercises were initiated as tolerated by the patient. Gentle massage was initiated with the objectives of assisting fluid mobility and discouraging formation of scar tissue in the area of injury. The patient was educated on application of a compression wrap for use on days when he was going to be very active, with use of the lower extremities.

Gentle isometrics of the hamstrings ("heel-dig" exercises) were performed with the knee in multiple positions of flexion. Hip extension isometric exercises in the supine position were also used. Active ROM exercises for hip extension and knee flexion were performed as tolerated. These exercises were initially performed in standing and then progressed to the prone position to increase difficulty. Gentle strengthening exercises for the quadriceps, hip abductors, and adductors were also prescribed.

Lumbopelvic exercises were introduced to address the presence of an anterior pelvic tilt. The patient was taught to perform isometric contraction of the transverse abdominis muscle, as well as posterior pelvic tilt maneuvers in the supine position. These activities would later be progressed to similar exercises in standing and combined with other therapeutic exercises. The overall objective was to incorporate appropriate pelvic control into activities of daily living.

The foregoing program was to be followed for a total of 3 weeks. During this time, the patient would attend physical therapy for six visits. He performed the home exercise program and applied ice daily.

Reexamination After 3 Weeks

After 3 weeks of the initial program, the patient was reevaluated. He reported a pain level of 1 to 3 out of 10, with the majority of pain occurring after walking or sitting on firm surfaces for more than 25 minutes. His LEFS score improved to 68 points. This was considered a significant improvement because the minimal clinically important difference for the LEFS is 9 points.[380] He had minimal palpable tenderness, no swelling, and very minor yellow discoloration in the proximal one third of the posterior thigh. The patient was able to extend the hip (with the knee in both the flexed and extended positions) actively and flex the knee through the entire ROM with minimal discomfort. Gentle application of the popliteal angle test for hamstring tightness resulted in 25 degrees of flexion at end range and a feeling of stiffness. This result indicated residual diminished flexibility of the involved hamstring muscle. Manual muscle testing showed a 4/5 grade for the hamstrings when tested at 15 degrees and 90 degrees of flexion. Hip extension also tested at 4/5. Minor soreness (1 out of 10) was reported with manual muscle testing. Additionally, the hip adductors on the involved side were tested at 4/5 with no reproduction of symptoms. The patient no longer exhibited an anterior pelvic tilt during postural examination. No gait deviations or asymmetries with stair negotiation were observed.

Intervention Progression

Progressive resistance exercises for the hamstrings were advanced. Straight leg raise exercises in prone and side lying for hip adduction were initiated. Weights were added for these exercises as tolerated over a period of 3 weeks. Bridging exercises were introduced. The bridge exercise was progressed from using two legs to one leg over a period of 3 weeks. Single leg Romanian deadlifts (RDLs) were added within a nonsymptomatic range. Single leg RDLs require the patient to maintain pelvic stabilization in the frontal plane, maintain balance, and use the hamstring muscles in a lengthened position. Squatting exercises were incorporated with a focus on even weight distribution and appropriate form. The patient was educated on the use of resistance equipment to supplement all exercises prescribed in rehabilitation sessions. As part of the patient's home exercise program, the exercises used included hamstring curl, knee extension, leg press, and gluteal press machines.

Balance activities were introduced in this period of rehabilitation. These activities were progressed from double to single leg stance. Additionally, less stable surfaces and perturbation through the addition of external forces were used to increase task difficulty.

The patient was allowed to initiate gentle stretching of the hamstring tissues. He achieved this by using a strap to assist in a straight leg raise maneuver and active extension of the knee while the hip was stabilized at 90 degrees of flexion (popliteal angle position). All stretches were kept within a subsymptomatic range, and the patient was instructed to monitor for any adverse reaction to the activities.

In addition to the foregoing, a gradual progression of endurance activities was initiated. Use of the stationary bicycle was the first endurance activity performed. The elliptical

Nonoperative Treatment of a Patient With a Proximal Hamstring Strain—cont'd

machine and gentle jogging (self-regulated at 50% effort) were initiated at 5 and 6 weeks, respectively, after the beginning rehabilitation. The total time for this stage of rehabilitation was 3 weeks, ending at 6 weeks after the initiation of physical therapy. A total of six formal clinic visits were conducted during this period.

Reexamination After 6 Weeks

After 6 weeks of physical therapy and compliance with an independent home exercise program, the patient was formally reevaluated. At the time of reevaluation, the patient scored a 78 out of 80 on the LEFS, a result indicating close to full function of daily activities and general exercise activities (not sport-specific activities). Manual muscle testing showed full strength of the hamstring and other hip muscles, symmetrical to the uninvolved side. The patient's knee reached 10 degrees of flexion in the popliteal angle position. This measurement is considered normal and was symmetrical to the uninvolved side. He had no palpable tenderness at any point of the hamstring complex. At this point, the patient was deemed appropriate to begin sport-specific training. After completion of the next phase of rehabilitation, the patient could be released back to full physical activity, contingent on completing all appropriate testing.

Treatment Progression and Return to Sport Preparation

Sport-specific training involved plyometric exercises, a running progression, and cutting and pivoting exercises, as well as activities that re-created the demands of soccer. During this time period, the patient slowly returned to weekly yoga, with the understanding that all activities should cause no more than 1 out of 10 pain. The speed and intensity of exercises were increased as tolerated. This final stage of rehabilitation lasted 3 weeks, with the patient attending five visits of formal physical therapy. During the last week, the patient attended two soccer

practice sessions and performed unopposed drills with the team. The patient tolerated the program progression well, with no more than 1 out of 10 pain at any point, no swelling, and only minor general fatigue. After 9 cumulative weeks of rehabilitation, the patient was deemed appropriate for testing to confirm readiness for discharge and return to soccer.

Termination of Physical Therapy

To confirm appropriateness for return to sport, the patient underwent full physical reevaluation, isokinetic strength testing, and physical activity assessment. No deficits were observed for manual muscle strength or flexibility testing. Isokinetic testing showed a 5% deficit in hamstring strength and no difference when comparing quadriceps strength of the involved and uninvolved limbs. The difference in hamstring strength was deemed acceptable. The ratio of hamstring to quadriceps strength was approximately 70%, which was also considered appropriate. The test results were consistent among variable testing speeds.

The physical activity assessment consisted of numerous tests to challenge the integrity of the hamstring and adjacent muscle structures of the lower extremity. Additionally, such tests can help a clinician assess the athlete's perceived readiness for such activity. The patient completed a 1-mile run in 7 minutes. He also completed measurements of distance for double leg long jumps, single leg hops, and vertical jumps. He was able to achieve 90% or greater distance when compared with the uninvolved side for all the listed tests. The patient's final LEFS score was 80 out of 80, indicating a self-reported full level of function.

After performing at a satisfactory level for the described criteria, the patient was discharged from formal physical therapy and was allowed to return to soccer at an unrestricted level of play. A home exercise and gym program was issued. The patient was instructed to contact the physical therapist if any significant return of symptoms was experienced.

Anterior Hip Pain in a Female Recreational Runner

History and Mechanism

A 25-year-old female recreational runner (e.g., 10 to 20 miles per week) with a mixed endomorphic-mesomorphic build (mass, 58.96 kg; height, 165.1 cm; body mass index, 21.6) initially underwent left ankle arthroscopic surgery in September 2008 for débridement and excision of a left nonunion distal fibular fracture caused by a fall and that resulted in poor healing of the fibula. After the surgical procedure, the patient underwent physical therapy with good success and full return to pain-free physical activity including running and resistance exercises. Nine months later, the patient suffered a recurrence of left hip pain with no known mechanism. She saw an orthopedic surgeon for symptoms of anterior hip pain, occasional clicking and popping, and pain with hip internal rotation. Results of radiographs and a magnetic resonance arthrogram (Tesla 3T from Philips) were negative for any soft

tissue (e.g., hip labral tears) or bony abnormalities (e.g., femoral acetabular impingement [FAI]). The patient was diagnosed with a hip flexor strain and continued with her own exercise program. For the next 3 years, the patient continued to have intermittent left hip pain, which was exacerbated by a fall on her mountain bike in February 2012. The patient saw her primary care physician for symptoms of anterior hip pain after the traumatic event. The physician diagnosed the patient as having acute on chronic left hip pain and referred her to physical therapy.

Test and Measures

At the initial visit, the patient was given the Lower Extremity Functional Scale (LEFS) to obtain a better understanding of her functional abilities. The minimal detectable change and minimal clinically important difference comprise 9 scale points. The

Continued

Anterior Hip Pain in a Female Recreational Runner—cont'd

patient scored a 61 out of 80 (76%) scaled points and reported the most difficulty with her usual hobbies, recreational or sporting activities, squatting, and sitting longer than 1 hour.

For pain, an 11-point numeric pain rating scale (0 [no pain] to 10 [worst pain imaginable]) was used to elicit an objective ranking of the patient's pain level. The patient reported a 3 out of 10 pain with athletic activity (e.g., yoga), squatting, prolonged sitting (>1 hour), and rotational hip motions. The patient's pain was decreased to a 2 out of 10 pain with medication. When asked about the location of pain, the patient verbally reported anterior hip pain and demonstrated the "C sign" in which she cupped her hands in a "C" shape above the greater trochanter, which has been reported as a common sign of hip pain.

Posture, Gait, and Range of Motion

A general postural screen was conducted in standing that revealed an anterior tilted pelvis and a mild right trunk shift. Observational gait analysis revealed decreased left hip motion (e.g., step length) and lateral weight bearing of the foot during the stance phase when compared with the right. The patient's hip, knee, and ankle range of motion (ROM) was tested both actively and passively. Bilateral measurements were within normal limits and symmetrical, with the exception of the left hip, because of the patient's discomfort and apprehension. Passive ROM of the left hip revealed the following: flexion 90 degrees, internal rotation 25 degrees (pain), external rotation 30 degrees, abduction 25 degrees, adduction 10 degrees, and hip extension 0 degrees.

TABLE 3-7	Case Study 3-2: Muscle Performance Testing	
Muscle Groups Tested	**Right**	**Left**
Hip flexors	5/5	3/5
Hip extensors	5/5	3+/5
Hip abductors	5/5	3+/5
Hip adductors	5/5	3+/5
Hip external rotators	5/5	3+/5
Hip internal rotators	5/5	3+/5
Knee extensors	5/5	5/5
Knee flexors	5/5	4/5
Ankle dorsiflexors	5/5	4/5
Ankle plantarflexors	5/5	4/5
Ankle inverters	5/5	4/5
Ankle everters	5/5	4/5

Muscle Performance and Muscle Length

The patient's bilateral hip, knee, and ankle strength was measured using manual muscle testing in the available pain-free ROM (Table 3-7). Both the left hip and ankle demonstrated strength deficits when compared with the right side. Muscle length was tested on the patient's lower extremities. The patient's left lower extremity tested positive for the following: Ober test, 90/90 hamstring test, Thomas test, and Ely test for rectus femoris length. The patient's right lower extremity tested positive for the following: Ober test for iliotibial band length and 90/90 test for hamstring muscle length.

Palpation and Special Testing

Palpation of the left hip musculature was assessed using a five-point pain scale (grade 0 to 4) (Table 3-8). Palpation revealed grade II (moderate) tenderness along the left common iliopsoas tendon, tensor fasciae latae hip abductors, and external rotators. A contralateral hip assessment revealed no significant findings. Postural stability was assessed using the single limb balance test with shoes off for a period of 30 seconds with eyes open and closed.[19] Testing revealed poor postural stability with the left lower extremity for both conditions (eyes open and closed) when compared with the right lower extremity. The flexion-adduction-internal rotation (FADIR) test was also conducted to assess for the presence of an FAI. The test result was positive, with immediate reproduction of the patient's anterior hip pain, and FADIR was used as a comparable test throughout the rehabilitation process.

Summary of Assessment

The results from the examination were as follows: poor posture and gait, decreased ROM and muscle length throughout the left hip region, general weakness of the left hip and foot when compared with the right, palpable tenderness in the anterior and lateral hip musculature, and a positive FADIR test result.

Rehabilitation

The patient attended rehabilitation two times a week for 4 weeks. Table 3-8 provides a further description of the patient's rehabilitation program with a midterm reassessment. A review of the patient's history revealed no current or earlier medical issues that would have impeded rehabilitation.

Discharge and Follow-Up

The patient was discharged after completing 4 weeks of physical therapy with 0 out of 10 pain with activities of daily living (e.g., sitting), weight training, and sports activity (e.g., jogging). Her posttreatment LEFS scores were 80 out of 80 scaled points or 100%. The left hip had full pain-free motion, normal muscle length except for mild hip flexor tightness, normal strength (5 out of 5), and adequate neuromuscular control with single leg activity, multidirectional activity, and light treadmill jogging. This was demonstrated by little compensatory movement at the hip, knee, and ankle. At the 1 month follow-up, the patient was contacted by phone and reported pain-free jogging and gym activity with no recurrence of hip pain.

CASE STUDY 3-2

Anterior Hip Pain in a Female Recreational Runner—cont'd

TABLE 3-8 Case Study 3-2: Rehabilitation Program

Timeline	Rehabilitation Program
Week 1	Focus: restore muscular symmetry across the hip and pelvis; begin strengthening of the abdominal core and left ankle Strengthening/balance: core strengthening (e.g., abdominal bracing) and ankle exercises (e.g., resistance bands); single limb balance activity on a stable surface Manual therapy/stretching: soft tissue management of the surrounding hip musculature with emphasis on the iliopsoas, rectus femoris, iliotibial band complex, and hamstrings; graded joint mobilization using a belt for general distraction of the hip; static stretching focusing on the iliopsoas, quadriceps, gluteals, hip external rotators, hamstrings, and iliotibial band complex Cardiovascular/ROM: stationary biking for up to 20 minutes with light to moderate resistance Home program: stretching, core strengthening, ankle strengthening, and stationary biking
Week 2	Focus: begin basic strengthening, functional movements, and progress core strengthening Strengthening/balance: Side-lying hip abduction, clams, double leg bridges, and leg press; core strengthening and balance activity progressed with the addition of planks and single leg stance on the foam pad Manual therapy/stretching: soft tissue management continued with emphasis on the iliopsoas and rectus femoris; joint mobilization including graded anterior to posterior glides and long-axis distraction; stretching activities continued with the addition of self-myofascial release with the foam roll Cardiovascular: stationary biking for up to 20 minutes with light to moderate resistance Home program: week 1 activity with the addition of the foam roll and cardiovascular conditioning with the elliptical trainer
Reassessment	Formal reassessment conducted between weeks 2 and 3 ROM: pain-free left hip internal rotation of 35 degrees (10-degree increase) MMT: all hip and knee manual muscle tests graded 4/5 Special testing: FADIR test of the left hip negative (no pain) Function: poor eccentric control with lunge, single leg squat, and multidirectional toe touching
Week 3	Focus: continue strengthening and introduce functional movements Strengthening/balance: continuation of basic stretching, self-myofascial release, core and lower extremity strengthening with the addition of CKC functional activity; CKC exercises including lunges, side steps, and single leg squats; balance further progressed with activity on the BOSU trainer Manual therapy/stretching: continuation of soft tissue management of the hip musculature and graded joint mobilization to maintain joint mobility; stretching activities continued with the addition of self-myofascial release with the foam roll Cardiovascular: cardiovascular activity progressed with light treadmill jogging Home program: week 1 and week 2 activity with the addition of CKC activity and light treadmill jogging
Week 4	Focus: return to pain-free running and gym activity Strengthening/balance: sports-specific activity including multidirectional agility drills (e.g., ladder drills), and movements on the TRX suspension training system including single leg squats and side lunges; advanced balance activity introduced including single leg balance and bilateral squats on air-filled disks Manual therapy/stretching: continuation of soft tissue and joint mobilization as needed to maintain adequate soft tissue and joint mobility; dynamic warmups introduced before activity and stretching, and foam roll techniques continued after physical activity Cardiovascular: progressive jogging on the treadmill and outdoor track Home program: week 2 to week 4 activity

BOSU, BOSU Balance Trainer (BOSU, Ashland, Ohio); *CKC,* closed kinetic chain; *FADIR,* flexion-adduction-internal rotation; *MMT,* manual muscle testing; *ROM,* range of motion; *TRX suspension training system,* TRX suspension training system (Fitness Anywhere, LLC, San Francisco, Calif.).

References

1. Domb BG, Brooks AG, Byrd JW. Clinical examination of the hip joint in athletes. *J Sport Rehabil.* 2009;18(1):3-23.

2. Allen WC, Cope R. Coxa saltans: the snapping hip revisited. *J Am Acad Orthop Surg.* 1995;3(5):303-308.

3. Lewis CL. Extra-articular snapping hip: a literature review. *Sports Health.* 2010;2(3):186-190.

4. Byrd JWT. Snapping hip. *Oper Tech Sports Med.* 2005;13(1):46-54.

5. Idjadi J, Meislin R. Symptomatic snapping hip: targeted treatment for maximum pain relief. *Phys Sportsmed.* 2004;32(1):25-31.

6. Winston P, Awan R, Cassidy JD, Bleakney RK. Clinical examination and ultrasound of self-reported snapping hip syndrome in elite ballet dancers. *Am J Sports Med.* 2007;35(1):118-126.

7. Henning PT. The running athlete: stress fractures, osteitis pubis, and snapping hips. *Sports Health.* 2014;6(2):122-127.

8. Wettstein M, Jung J, Dienst M. Arthroscopic psoas tenotomy. *Arthroscopy.* 2006;22(8):907.e901-907.e904.

9. Ilizaliturri VM Jr, Villalobos FE Jr, Chaidez PA, et al. Internal snapping hip syndrome: treatment by endoscopic release of the iliopsoas tendon. *Arthroscopy.* 2005;21(11):1375-1380.

10. Konczak CR, Ames R. Relief of internal snapping hip syndrome in a marathon runner after chiropractic treatment. *J Manipulative Physiol Ther.* 2005;28(1):e1-e7.

11. Gruen GS, Scioscia TN, Lowenstein JE. The surgical treatment of internal snapping hip. *Am J Sports Med.* 2002;30(4):607-613.

12. White RA, Hughes MS, Burd T, et al. A new operative approach in the correction of external coxa saltans: the snapping hip. *Am J Sports Med.* 2004;32(6):1504-1508.

13. Khan M, Adamich J, Simunovic N, et al. Surgical management of internal snapping hip syndrome: a systematic review evaluating open and arthroscopic approaches. *Arthroscopy.* 2013;29(5):942-948.

14. Keskula DR, Lott J, Duncan JB. Snapping iliopsoas tendon in a recreational athlete: a case report. *J Athl Train.* 1999;34(4):382-385.

15. Shur N, Dandachli W, Findlay I, et al. A pain in the backside: a case report of coxa saltans occurring at the proximal hamstring origin. *Hip Int.* 2014;24(3):302-305.

16. Rask MR. "Snapping bottom": subluxation of the tendon of the long head of the biceps femoris muscle. *Muscle Nerve.* 1980;3(3):250-251.

17. Scillia A, Choo A, Milman E, et al. Snapping of the proximal hamstring origin: a rare cause of coxa saltans—a case report. *J Bone Joint Surg Am.* 2011;93(21):e1251-e1253.

18. Margo K, Drezner J, Motzkin D. Evaluation and management of hip pain: an algorithmic approach. *J Fam Pract.* 2003;52(8):607-617.

19. Larsen E, Johansen J. Snapping hip. *Acta Orthop Scand.* 1986;57(2):168-170.

20. Tufo A, Desai GJ, Cox WJ. Psoas syndrome: a frequently missed diagnosis. *J Am Osteopath Assoc.* 2012;112(8):522-528.

21. Sullivan KM, Silvey DB, Button DC, Behm DG. Roller-massager application to the hamstrings increases sit-and-reach range of motion within five to ten seconds without performance impairments. *Int J Sports Phys Ther.* 2013;8(3):228-236.

22. Faraj AA, Moulton A, Sirivastava VM. Snapping iliotibial band: report of ten cases and review of the literature. *Acta Orthop Belg.* 2001;67(1):19-23.

23. Behm DG, Chaouachi A. A review of the acute effects of static and dynamic stretching on performance. *Eur J Appl Physiol.* 2011;111(11):2633-2651.

24. O'Hora J, Cartwright A, Wade CD, et al. Efficacy of static stretching and proprioceptive neuromuscular facilitation stretch on hamstrings length after a single session. *J Strength Cond Res.* 2011;25(6):1586-1591.

25. Kallerud H, Gleeson N. Effects of stretching on performances involving stretch-shortening cycles. *Sports Med.* 2013;43(8):733-750.

26. Ilizaliturri VM Jr, Camacho-Galindo J. Endoscopic treatment of snapping hips, iliotibial band, and iliopsoas tendon. *Sports Med Arthrosc.* 2010;18(2):120-127.

27. Nam KW, Yoo JJ, Koo KH, et al. A modified Z-plasty technique for severe tightness of the gluteus maximus. *Scand J Med Sci Sports.* 2011;21(1):85-89.

28. Provencher MT, Hofmeister EP, Muldoon MP. The surgical treatment of external coxa saltans (the snapping hip) by Z-plasty of the iliotibial band. *Am J Sports Med.* 2004;32(2):470-476.

29. Polesello GC, Queiroz MC, Domb BG, et al. Surgical technique: endoscopic gluteus maximus tendon release for external snapping hip syndrome. *Clin Orthop Relat Res.* 2013;471(8):2471-2476.

30. Zini R, Munegato D, De Benedetto M, et al. Endoscopic iliotibial band release in snapping hip. *Hip Int.* 2013;23(2):225-232.

31. Ivins GK. Meralgia paresthetica, the elusive diagnosis: clinical experience with 14 adult patients. *Ann Surg.* 2000;232(2):281-286.

32. Cheatham SW, Kolber MJ, Salamh PA. Meralgia paresthetica: a review of the literature. *Int J Sports Phys Ther.* 2013;8(6):883-893.

33. van Slobbe AM, Bohnen AM, Bernsen RM, et al. Incidence rates and determinants in meralgia paresthetica in general practice. *J Neurol.* 2004;251(3):294-297.

34. Parisi TJ, Mandrekar J, Dyck PJ, Klein CJ. Meralgia paresthetica: relation to obesity, advanced age, and diabetes mellitus. *Neurology.* 2011;77(16):1538-1542.

35. Harney D, Patijn J. Meralgia paresthetica: diagnosis and management strategies. *Pain Med.* 2007;8(8):669-677.

36. Martinez-Salio A, Moreno-Ramos T, Diaz-Sanchez M, et al. Meralgia paraesthetica: a report on a series of 140 cases. *Rev Neurol.* 2009;49(8):405-408. [in Spanish].

37. Standring S. *Gray's Anatomy: The Anatomical Basis of Clinical Practice.* 40th ed. London: Churchill Livingstone; 2008.

38. Kho KH, Blijham PJ, Zwarts MJ. Meralgia paresthetica after strenuous exercise. *Muscle Nerve.* 2005;31(6):761-763.

39. Macgregor J, Moncur JA. Meralgia paraesthetica: a sports lesion in girl gymnasts. *Br J Sports Med.* 1977;11(1):16-19.

40. Szewczyk J, Hoffmann M, Kabelis J. Meralgia paraesthetica in a body-builder. *Sportverletz Sportschaden.* 1994;8(1):43-45. [in German].

41. Ulkar B, Yildiz Y, Kunduracioglu B. Meralgia paresthetica: a long-standing performance-limiting cause of anterior thigh pain in a soccer player. *Am J Sports Med.* 2003;31(5):787-789.

42. Otoshi K, Itoh Y, Tsujino A, Kikuchi S. Case report: meralgia paresthetica in a baseball pitcher. *Clin Orthop Relat Res.* 2008;466(9):2268-2270.

43. Reference deleted in review.

44. Uzel M, Akkin SM, Tanyeli E, Koebke J. Relationships of the lateral femoral cutaneous nerve to bony landmarks. *Clin Orthop Relat Res.* 2011;469(9):2605-2611.

45. Majkrzak A, Johnston J, Kacey D, Zeller J. Variability of the lateral femoral cutaneous nerve: an anatomic basis for planning safe surgical approaches. *Clin Anat.* 2010;23(3):304-311.

46. Ropars M, Morandi X, Huten D, et al. Anatomical study of the lateral femoral cutaneous nerve with special reference to minimally invasive anterior approach for total hip replacement. *Surg Radiol Anat.* 2009;31(3):199-204.

47. Sunderland S. Anatomical features of nerve trunks in relation to nerve injury and nerve repair. *Clin Neurosurg.* 1970; 17:38-62.

48. Grossman MG, Ducey SA, Nadler SS, Levy AS. Meralgia paresthetica: diagnosis and treatment. *J Am Acad Orthop Surg.* 2001;9(5):336-344.

49. Williams PH, Trzil KP. Management of meralgia paresthetica. *J Neurosurg.* 1991;74(1):76-80.

50. Tagliafico A, Serafini G, Lacelli F, et al. Ultrasound-guided treatment of meralgia paresthetica (lateral femoral cutaneous neuropathy): technical description and results of treatment in 20 consecutive patients. *J Ultrasound Med.* 2011;30(10): 1341-1346.

51. Seror P, Seror R. Meralgia paresthetica: clinical and electrophysiological diagnosis in 120 cases. *Muscle Nerve.* 2006;33(5): 650-654.

52. Beresford HR. Meralgia paresthetica after seat-belt trauma. *J Trauma.* 1971;11(7):629-630.

53. Blake SM, Treble NJ. Meralgia paraesthetica: an addition to 'seatbelt syndrome'. *Ann R Coll Surg Engl.* 2004;86(6): W6-W7.

54. Fargo MV, Konitzer LN. Meralgia paresthetica due to body armor wear in U.S. soldiers serving in Iraq: a case report and review of the literature. *Mil Med.* 2007;172(6):663-665.

55. Goel A. Meralgia paresthetica secondary to limb length discrepancy: case report. *Arch Phys Med Rehabil.* 1999;80(3):348-349.

56. Haim A, Pritsch T, Ben-Galim P, Dekel S. Meralgia paresthetica: a retrospective analysis of 79 patients evaluated and treated according to a standard algorithm. *Acta Orthop.* 2006; 77(3):482-486.

57. Jiang GX, Xu WD, Wang AH. Spinal stenosis with meralgia paraesthetica. *J Bone Joint Surg Br.* 1988;70(2):272-273.

58. Korkmaz N, Ozcakar L. Meralgia paresthetica in a policeman: the belt or the gun. *Plast Reconstr Surg.* 2004;114(4):1012-1013.

59. Mondelli M, Rossi S, Romano C. Body mass index in meralgia paresthetica: a case-control study. *Acta Neurol Scand.* 2007; 116(2):118-123.

60. Moscona AR, Sekel R. Post-traumatic meralgia paresthetica: an unusual presentation. *J Trauma.* 1978;18(4):288.

61. Park JW, Kim DH, Hwang M, Bun HR. Meralgia paresthetica caused by hip-huggers in a patient with aberrant course of the lateral femoral cutaneous nerve. *Muscle Nerve.* 2007;35(5): 678-680.

62. Sax TW, Rosenbaum RB. Neuromuscular disorders in pregnancy. *Muscle Nerve.* 2006;34(5):559-571.

63. Yi TI, Yoon TH, Kim JS, et al. Femoral neuropathy and meralgia paresthetica secondary to an iliacus hematoma. *Ann Rehabil Med.* 2012;36(2):273-277.

64. Goulding K, Beaule PE, Kim PR, Fazekas A. Incidence of lateral femoral cutaneous nerve neurapraxia after anterior approach hip arthroplasty. *Clin Orthop Relat Res.* 2010;468(9): 2397-2404.

65. Bhargava T, Goytia RN, Jones LC, Hungerford MW. Lateral femoral cutaneous nerve impairment after direct anterior approach for total hip arthroplasty. *Orthopedics.* 2010;33(7): 472.

66. Gupta A, Muzumdar D, Ramani PS. Meralgia paraesthetica following lumbar spine surgery: a study in 110 consecutive surgically treated cases. *Neurol India.* 2004;52(1):64-66.

67. Mirovsky Y, Neuwirth M. Injuries to the lateral femoral cutaneous nerve during spine surgery. *Spine (Phila Pa 1976).* 2000; 25(10):1266-1269.

68. Cho KT, Lee HJ. Prone position-related meralgia paresthetica after lumbar spinal surgery: a case report and review of the literature. *J Korean Neurosurg Soc.* 2008;44(6):392-395.

69. Yang SH, Wu CC, Chen PQ. Postoperative meralgia paresthetica after posterior spine surgery: incidence, risk factors, and clinical outcomes. *Spine (Phila Pa 1976).* 2005;30(18): e547-e550.

70. Knight RQ, Schwaegler P, Hanscom D, Roh J. Direct lateral lumbar interbody fusion for degenerative conditions: early complication profile. *J Spinal Disord Tech.* 2009;22(1):34-37.

71. Yamamoto T, Nagira K, Kurosaka M. Meralgia paresthetica occurring 40 years after iliac bone graft harvesting: case report. *Neurosurgery.* 2001;49(6):1455-1457.

72. Kavanagh D, Connolly S, Fleming F, et al. Meralgia paraesthetica following open appendicectomy. *Ir Med J.* 2005;98(6): 183-185.

73. Polidori L, Magarelli M, Tramutoli R. Meralgia paresthetica as a complication of laparoscopic appendectomy. *Surg Endosc.* 2003;17(5):832.

74. Paul F, Zipp F. Bilateral meralgia paresthetica after cesarian section with epidural analgesia. *J Peripher Nerv Syst.* 2006; 11(1):98-99.

75. Peters G, Larner AJ. Meralgia paresthetica following gynecologic and obstetric surgery. *Int J Gynaecol Obstet.* 2006; 95(1):42-43.

76. Nouraei SA, Anand B, Spink G, O'Neill KS. A novel approach to the diagnosis and management of meralgia paresthetica. *Neurosurgery.* 2007;60(4):696-700, discussion 700.

77. Parmar MS. Hiphuggers' tingly thighs. *CMAJ.* 2003;168(1): 16.

78. El Miedany Y, Ashour S, Youssef S, et al. Clinical diagnosis of carpal tunnel syndrome: old tests-new concepts. *Joint Bone Spine.* 2008;75(4):451-457.

79. MacDermid JC, Doherty T. Clinical and electrodiagnostic testing of carpal tunnel syndrome: a narrative review. *J Orthop Sports Phys Ther.* 2004;34(10):565-588.

80. Butler D. *The Neurodynamic Techniques: A Definitive Guide From the Noigroup Team.* Adelaide City West, South Australia: Noigroup Publications; 2005.

81. Butler DS, Matheson JE, Boyaci A. *The Sensitive Nervous System.* Adelaide City West, South Australia: Noigroup Publications; 2000.

82. Erbay H. Meralgia paresthetica in differential diagnosis of low-back pain. *Clin J Pain.* 2002;18(2):132-135.

83. Hirabayashi H, Takahashi J, Hashidate H, et al. Characteristics of L3 nerve root radiculopathy. *Surg Neurol.* 2009;72(1):36-40, discussion 40.

84. Tokuhashi Y, Matsuzaki H, Uematsu Y, Oda H. Symptoms of thoracolumbar junction disc herniation. *Spine (Phila Pa 1976).* 2001;26(22):e512-e518.

85. Trummer M, Flaschka G, Unger F, Eustacchio S. Lumbar disc herniation mimicking meralgia paresthetica: case report. *Surg Neurol.* 2000;54(1):80-81.

86. Seror P. Somatosensory evoked potentials for the electrodiagnosis of meralgia paresthetica. *Muscle Nerve.* 2004;29(2):309-312.

87. Seror P. Lateral femoral cutaneous nerve conduction v somatosensory evoked potentials for electrodiagnosis of meralgia paresthetica. *Am J Phys Med Rehabil.* 1999;78(4):313-316.

88. el-Tantawi GA. Reliability of sensory nerve-conduction and somatosensory evoked potentials for diagnosis of meralgia paraesthetica. *Clin Neurophysiol.* 2009;120(7):1346-1351.

89. Chhabra A, Andreisek G, Soldatos T, et al. MR neurography: past, present, and future. *AJR Am J Roentgenol.* 2011;197(3): 583-591.

90. Chhabra A, Del Grande F, Soldatos T, et al. Meralgia paresthetica: 3-Tesla magnetic resonance neurography. *Skeletal Radiol.* 2013;52(6):803-808.

91. Khalil N, Nicotra A, Rakowicz W. Treatment for meralgia paraesthetica. *Cochrane Database Syst Rev.* 2008;(3):CD004159.

92. Khalil N, Nicotra A, Rakowicz W. Treatment for meralgia paraesthetica. *Cochrane Database Syst Rev.* 2012;(12):CD004159.

93. Kadel RE, Godbey WD, Davis BP. Conservative and chiropractic treatment of meralgia paresthetica: review and case report. *J Manipulative Physiol Ther.* 1982;5(2):73-78.

94. Kalichman L, Vered E, Volchek L. Relieving symptoms of meralgia paresthetica using Kinesio taping: a pilot study. *Arch Phys Med Rehabil.* 2010;91(7):1137-1139.

95. Kose O, Ozyurek S. Meralgia paresthetica due to fracture of anterior superior iliac spine in an adolescent. *CJEM.* 2009; 11(6):514.

96. Kotler D. Meralgia paresthetica: case report in policewoman. *JAAPA.* 2000;13(10):39-42, 47.

97. Skaggs CD, Winchester BA, Vianin M, Prather H. A manual therapy and exercise approach to meralgia paresthetica in pregnancy: a case report. *J Chiropr Med.* 2006;5(3):92-96.

98. Houle S. Chiropractic management of chronic idiopathic meralgia paresthetica: a case study. *J Chiropr Med.* 2012;11(1): 36-41.

99. Terrett AG. Meralgia paresthetica: a complication of chiropractic therapy. *J Aust Chiropr Assoc.* 1984;14:29-30.

100. Cao H, Han M, Li X, et al. Clinical research evidence of cupping therapy in China: a systematic literature review. *BMC Complement Altern Med.* 2010;10:70.

101. Cao H, Li X, Liu J. An updated review of the efficacy of cupping therapy. *PLoS One.* 2012;7(2):e31793.

102. Aigner N, Aigner G, Fialka C, Fritz A. Therapy of meralgia paresthetica with acupuncture: two case reports. *Schmerz.* 1997;11(2):113-115. [in German].

103. Wang X-Z, Zhu D-X. Treatment of 43 cases of lateral femoral cutaneous neuritis with pricking and cupping therapy. *J Acupunct Tuina Sci.* 2009;7(6):366-367.

104. Yang XY, Shi GX, Li QQ, et al. Characterization of deqi sensation and acupuncture effect. *Evid Based Complement Alternat Med.* 2013;2013:319734.

105. Moffet HH. How might acupuncture work? A systematic review of physiologic rationales from clinical trials. *BMC Complement Altern Med.* 2006;6:25.

106. Philip CN, Candido KD, Joseph NJ, Crystal GJ. Successful treatment of meralgia paresthetica with pulsed radiofrequency of the lateral femoral cutaneous nerve. *Pain Physician.* 2009; 12(5):881-885.

107. Fowler IM, Tucker AA, Mendez RJ. Treatment of meralgia paresthetica with ultrasound-guided pulsed radiofrequency ablation of the lateral femoral cutaneous nerve. *Pain Pract.* 2012;12(5):394-398.

108. Choi HJ, Choi SK, Kim TS, Lim YJ. Pulsed radiofrequency neuromodulation treatment on the lateral femoral cutaneous nerve for the treatment of meralgia paresthetica. *J Korean Neurosurg Soc.* 2011;50(2):151-153.

109. Hurdle MF, Weingarten TN, Crisostomo RA, et al. Ultrasound-guided blockade of the lateral femoral cutaneous nerve: technical description and review of 10 cases. *Arch Phys Med Rehabil.* 2007;88(10):1362-1364.

110. Tumber PS, Bhatia A, Chan VW. Ultrasound-guided lateral femoral cutaneous nerve block for meralgia paresthetica. *Anesth Analg.* 2008;106(3):1021-1022.

111. de Ruiter GC, Wurzer JA, Kloet A. Decision making in the surgical treatment of meralgia paresthetica: neurolysis versus neurectomy. *Acta Neurochir (Wien).* 2012;154(10): 1765-1772.

112. Ducic I, Dellon AL, Taylor NS. Decompression of the lateral femoral cutaneous nerve in the treatment of meralgia paresthetica. *J Reconstr Microsurg.* 2006;22(2):113-118.

113. Siu TL, Chandran KN. Neurolysis for meralgia paresthetica: an operative series of 45 cases. *Surg Neurol.* 2005;63(1):19-23, discussion 23.

114. Son BC, Kim DR, Kim IS, et al. Neurolysis for meralgia paresthetica. *J Korean Neurosurg Soc.* 2012;51(6):363-366.

115. Emamhadi M. Surgery for meralgia paresthetica: neurolysis versus nerve resection. *Turk Neurosurg.* 2012;22(6):758-762.

116. Tyler TF, Silvers HJ, Gerhardt MB, Nicholas SJ. Groin injuries in sports medicine. *Sports Health.* 2010;2(3):231-236.

117. Iles JD. Adductor injury: a common cause of groin pain often misdiagnosed as hernia. *Can Fam Physician.* 1968;14(11): 58-66.

118. Holmich P. Long-standing groin pain in sportspeople falls into three primary patterns, a "clinical entity" approach: a prospective study of 207 patients. *Br J Sports Med.* 2007;41(4):247-252, discussion 252.

119. Karlsson J, Sward L, Kalebo P, Thomee R. Chronic groin injuries in athletes: recommendations for treatment and rehabilitation. *Sports Med.* 1994;17(2):141-148.

120. Garvey JF, Hazard H. Sports hernia or groin disruption injury? Chronic athletic groin pain: a retrospective study of 100 patients with long-term follow-up. *Hernia.* 2013;18(6): 815-823.

121. Sansone M, Ahlden M, Jonasson P, et al. Can hip impingement be mistaken for tendon pain in the groin? A long-term follow-up of tenotomy for groin pain in athletes. *Knee Surg Sports Traumatol Arthrosc.* 2014;22(4):786-792.

122. Narvani AA, Tsiridis E, Kendall S, et al. A preliminary report on prevalence of acetabular labrum tears in sports patients with groin pain. *Knee Surg Sports Traumatol Arthrosc.* 2003;11(6): 403-408.

123. Bradshaw C, McCrory P, Bell S, Brukner P. Obturator nerve entrapment: a cause of groin pain in athletes. *Am J Sports Med.* 1997;25(3):402-408.

124. Holmich P, Uhrskou P, Ulnits L, et al. Effectiveness of active physical training as treatment for long-standing adductor-related groin pain in athletes: randomised trial. *Lancet.* 1999; 353(9151):439-443.

125. Takizawa M, Suzuki D, Ito H, et al. Why adductor magnus muscle is large: the function based on muscle mor-

phology in cadavers. *Scand J Med Sci Sports*. 2012;24(1):197-203.

126. Thorborg K, Serner A, Petersen J, et al. Hip adduction and abduction strength profiles in elite soccer players: implications for clinical evaluation of hip adductor muscle recovery after injury. *Am J Sports Med*. 2011;39(1):121-126.

127. Caudill P, Nyland J, Smith C, et al. Sports hernias: a systematic literature review. *Br J Sports Med*. 2008;42(12):954-964.

128. Norton-Old KJ, Schache AG, Barker PJ, et al. Anatomical and mechanical relationship between the proximal attachment of adductor longus and the distal rectus sheath. *Clin Anat*. 2013;26(4):522-530.

129. Strauss EJ, Campbell K, Bosco JA. Analysis of the cross-sectional area of the adductor longus tendon: a descriptive anatomic study. *Am J Sports Med*. 2007;35(6):996-999.

130. Davis JA, Stringer MD, Woodley SJ. New insights into the proximal tendons of adductor longus, adductor brevis and gracilis. *Br J Sports Med*. 2012;46(12):871-876.

131. Charnock BL, Lewis CL, Garrett WE Jr, Queen RM. Adductor longus mechanics during the maximal effort soccer kick. *Sports Biomech*. 2009;8(3):223-234.

132. Chang R, Turcotte R, Pearsall D. Hip adductor muscle function in forward skating. *Sports Biomech*. 2009;8(3):212-222.

133. Crow JF, Pearce AJ, Veale JP, et al. Hip adductor muscle strength is reduced preceding and during the onset of groin pain in elite junior Australian football players. *J Sci Med Sport*. 2010;13(2):202-204.

134. Tyler TF, Nicholas SJ, Campbell RJ, McHugh MP. The association of hip strength and flexibility with the incidence of adductor muscle strains in professional ice hockey players. *Am J Sports Med*. 2001;29(2):124-128.

135. Morelli V, Smith V. Groin injuries in athletes. *Am Fam Physician*. 2001;64(8):1405-1414.

136. Renstrom P, Peterson L. Groin injuries in athletes. *Br J Sports Med*. 1980;14(1):30-36.

137. Nicholas SJ, Tyler TF. Adductor muscle strains in sport. *Sports Med*. 2002;32(5):339-344.

138. Holmich P, Thorborg K, Dehlendorff C, et al. Incidence and clinical presentation of groin injuries in sub-elite male soccer. *Br J Sports Med*. 2014;48(16):1245-1250.

139. Hagglund M, Walden M, Ekstrand J. Risk factors for lower extremity muscle injury in professional soccer: the UEFA Injury Study. *Am J Sports Med*. 2013;41(2):327-335.

140. Emery CA, Meeuwisse WH, Powell JW. Groin and abdominal strain injuries in the National Hockey League. *Clin J Sport Med*. 1999;9(3):151-156.

141. Maffey L, Emery C. What are the risk factors for groin strain injury in sport? A systematic review of the literature. *Sports Med*. 2007;37(10):881-894.

142. Grote K, Lincoln TL, Gamble JG. Hip adductor injury in competitive swimmers. *Am J Sports Med*. 2004;32(1):104-108.

143. Franic M, Ivkovic A, Rudic R. Injuries in water polo. *Croat Med J*. 2007;48(3):281-288.

144. Orchard J, James T, Alcott E, et al. Injuries in Australian cricket at first class level 1995/1996 to 2000/2001. *Br J Sports Med*. 2002;36(4):270-274, discussion 275.

145. O'Connor D. Groin injuries in professional rugby league players: a prospective study. *J Sports Sci*. 2004;22(7):629-636.

146. Swan KG Jr, Wolcott M. The athletic hernia: a systematic review. *Clin Orthop Relat Res*. 2007;455:78-87.

147. Sedaghati P, Alizadeh MH, Shirzad E, Ardjmand A. Review of sport-induced groin injuries. *Trauma Mon*. 2013;18(3):107-112.

148. Emery CA, Meeuwisse WH. Risk factors for groin injuries in hockey. *Med Sci Sports Exerc*. 2001;33(9):1423-1433.

149. Hureibi KA, McLatchie GR. Groin pain in athletes. *Scott Med J*. 2010;55(2):8-11.

150. Holmich P, Larsen K, Krogsgaard K, Gluud C. Exercise program for prevention of groin pain in football players: a cluster-randomized trial. *Scand J Med Sci Sports*. 2010;20(6):814-821.

151. Verrall GM, Slavotinek JP, Barnes PG, et al. Hip joint range of motion restriction precedes athletic chronic groin injury. *J Sci Med Sport*. 2007;10(6):463-466.

152. Ibrahim A, Murrell GA, Knapman P. Adductor strain and hip range of movement in male professional soccer players. *J Orthop Surg (Hong Kong)*. 2007;15(1):46-49.

153. Morrissey D, Graham J, Screen H, et al. Coronal plane hip muscle activation in football code athletes with chronic adductor groin strain injury during standing hip flexion. *Man Ther*. 2012;17(2):145-149.

154. Bradley PS, Portas MD. The relationship between preseason range of motion and muscle strain injury in elite soccer players. *J Strength Cond Res*. 2007;21(4):1155-1159.

155. Mens J, Inklaar H, Koes BW, Stam HJ. A new view on adduction-related groin pain. *Clin J Sport Med*. 2006;16(1):15-19.

156. Hrysomallis C. Hip adductors' strength, flexibility, and injury risk. *J Strength Cond Res*. 2009;23(5):1514-1517.

157. Macintyre J, Johnson C, Schroeder EL. Groin pain in athletes. *Curr Sports Med Rep*. 2006;5(6):293-299.

158. Rassner L. Lumbar plexus nerve entrapment syndromes as a cause of groin pain in athletes. *Curr Sports Med Rep*. 2011;10(2):115-120.

159. Paajanen H. "Sports hernia" and osteitis pubis in an athlete. *Duodecim*. 2009;125(3):261-266. [in Finnish].

160. Quah C, Cottam A, Hutchinson J. Surgical management of a completely avulsed adductor longus muscle in a professional equestrian rider. *Case Rep Orthop*. 2014;2014:828314.

161. Dimitrakopoulou A, Schilders EM, Talbot JC, Bismil Q. Acute avulsion of the fibrocartilage origin of the adductor longus in professional soccer players: a report of two cases. *Clin J Sport Med*. 2008;18(2):167-169.

162. Banks DB, MacLennan I, Banks AJ. Adductor longus ruptures in elite sportsmen—pitfalls of surgical repair: a report of two cases. *BMJ Case Rep*. 2013;(Jun 24):2013.

163. Thorborg K, Petersen J, Nielsen MB, Holmich P. Clinical recovery of two hip adductor longus ruptures: a case-report of a soccer player. *BMC Res Notes*. 2013;6:205.

164. Dimitrakopoulou A, Schilders E, Bismil Q, et al. An unusual case of enthesophyte formation following an adductor longus rupture in a high-level athlete. *Knee Surg Sports Traumatol Arthrosc*. 2010;18(5):691-693.

165. Rizio L 3rd, Salvo JP, Schurhoff MR, Uribe JW. Adductor longus rupture in professional football players: acute repair with suture anchors: a report of two cases. *Am J Sports Med*. 2004;32(1):243-245.

166. Schlegel TF, Bushnell BD, Godfrey J, Boublik M. Success of nonoperative management of adductor longus tendon ruptures in National Football League athletes. *Am J Sports Med*. 2009;37(7):1394-1399.

167. Aerts BR, Plaisier PW, Jakma TS. Adductor longus tendon rupture mistaken for incarcerated inguinal hernia. *Injury.* 2014;45(3):639-641.

168. Robertson BA, Barker PJ, Fahrer M, Schache AG. The anatomy of the pubic region revisited: implications for the pathogenesis and clinical management of chronic groin pain in athletes. *Sports Med.* 2009;39(3):225-234.

169. Delahunt E, McEntee BL, Kennelly C, et al. Intrarater reliability of the adductor squeeze test in Gaelic games athletes. *J Athl Train.* 2011;46(3):241-245.

170. Nevin F, Delahunt E. Adductor squeeze test values and hip joint range of motion in Gaelic football athletes with longstanding groin pain. *J Sci Med Sport.* 2014;17(2):155-159.

171. Delahunt E, Kennelly C, McEntee BL, et al. The thigh adductor squeeze test: 45 degrees of hip flexion as the optimal test position for eliciting adductor muscle activity and maximum pressure values. *Man Ther.* 2011;16(5):476-480.

172. Lovell GA, Blanch PD, Barnes CJ. EMG of the hip adductor muscles in six clinical examination tests. *Phys Ther Sport.* 2012;13(3):134-140.

173. Verrall GM, Slavotinek JP, Barnes PG, Fon GT. Description of pain provocation tests used for the diagnosis of sports-related chronic groin pain: relationship of tests to defined clinical (pain and tenderness) and MRI (pubic bone marrow oedema) criteria. *Scand J Med Sci Sports.* 2005;15(1):36-42.

174. Malliaras P, Hogan A, Nawrocki A, et al. Hip flexibility and strength measures: reliability and association with athletic groin pain. *Br J Sports Med.* 2009;43(10):739-744.

175. Branci S, Thorborg K, Nielsen MB. Holmich P. Radiological findings in symphyseal and adductor-related groin pain in athletes: a critical review of the literature. *Br J Sports Med.* 2013;47(10):611-619.

176. Sofka CM, Marx R, Adler RS. Utility of sonography for the diagnosis of adductor avulsion injury ("thigh splints"). *J Ultrasound Med.* 2006;25(7):913-916.

177. Bradley M, Morgan J, Pentlow B, Roe A. The positive predictive value of diagnostic ultrasound for occult herniae. *Ann R Coll Surg Engl.* 2006;88(2):165-167.

178. Grant T, Neuschler E, Hartz W 3rd. Groin pain in women: use of sonography to detect occult hernias. *J Ultrasound Med.* 2011;30(12):1701-1707.

179. Robinson A, Light D, Kasim A, Nice C. A systematic review and meta-analysis of the role of radiology in the diagnosis of occult inguinal hernia. *Surg Endosc.* 2013;27(1):11-18.

180. Branci S, Thorborg K, Bech BH, et al. MRI findings in soccer players with long-standing adductor-related groin pain and asymptomatic controls. *Br J Sports Med.* 2015;49(10):681-691.

181. Zoga AC, Kavanagh EC, Omar IM, et al. Athletic pubalgia and the "sports hernia": MR imaging findings. *Radiology.* 2008;247(3):797-807.

182. Branci S, Thorborg K, Bech BH, et al. The Copenhagen Standardised MRI protocol to assess the pubic symphysis and adductor regions of athletes: outline and intratester and intertester reliability. *Br J Sports Med.* 2015;49(10):692-699.

183. Robinson P, Barron DA, Parsons W, et al. Adductor-related groin pain in athletes: correlation of MR imaging with clinical findings. *Skeletal Radiol.* 2004;33(8):451-457.

184. Schilders E, Talbot JC, Robinson P, et al. Adductor-related groin pain in recreational athletes: role of the adductor enthesis, magnetic resonance imaging, and entheseal pubic cleft injections. *J Bone Joint Surg Am.* 2009;91(10):2455-2460.

185. Silvis ML, Mosher TJ, Smetana BS, et al. High prevalence of pelvic and hip magnetic resonance imaging findings in asymptomatic collegiate and professional hockey players. *Am J Sports Med.* 2011;39(4):715-721.

186. Gallo RA, Silvis ML, Smetana B, et al. Asymptomatic hip/groin pathology identified on magnetic resonance imaging of professional hockey players: outcomes and playing status at 4 years' follow-up. *Arthroscopy.* 2014;30(10):1222-1228.

187. Robinson P, Grainger AJ, Hensor EM, et al. Do MRI and ultrasound of the anterior pelvis correlate with, or predict, young football players' clinical findings? A 4-year prospective study of elite academy soccer players. *Br J Sports Med.* 2015;49(3):176-182.

188. Mei-Dan O, Lopez V, Carmont MR, et al. Adductor tenotomy as a treatment for groin pain in professional soccer players. *Orthopedics.* 2013;36(9):e1189-e1197.

189. Machotka Z, Kumar S, Perraton LG. A systematic review of the literature on the effectiveness of exercise therapy for groin pain in athletes. *Sports Med Arthrosc Rehabil Ther Technol.* 2009;1(1):5.

190. Jansen JA, Mens JM, Backx FJ, et al. Treatment of longstanding groin pain in athletes: a systematic review. *Scand J Med Sci Sports.* 2008;18(3):263-274.

191. Almeida MO, Silva BN, Andriolo RB, et al. Conservative interventions for treating exercise-related musculotendinous, ligamentous and osseous groin pain. *Cochrane Database Syst Rev.* 2013;(6):CD009565.

192. Delmore RJ, Laudner KG, Torry MR. Adductor longus activation during common hip exercises. *J Sport Rehabil.* 2014;23(2):79-87.

193. Jensen J, Holmich P, Bandholm T, et al. Eccentric strengthening effect of hip-adductor training with elastic bands in soccer players: a randomised controlled trial. *Br J Sports Med.* 2014;48(4):332-338.

194. Cheatham SW, Hanney WJ, Kolber MJ, Salamh PA. Adductor-related groin pain in the athlete. *Phys Ther Rev.* 2014;19(5):328-337.

195. Serner A, Jakobsen MD, Andersen LL, et al. EMG evaluation of hip adduction exercises for soccer players: implications for exercise selection in prevention and treatment of groin injuries. *Br J Sports Med.* 2014;48(14):1108-1114.

196. Weir A, Veger SA, Van de Sande HB, et al. A manual therapy technique for chronic adductor-related groin pain in athletes: a case series. *Scand J Med Sci Sports.* 2009;19(5):616-620.

197. Yuill EA, Pajaczkowski JA, Howitt SD. Conservative care of sports hernias within soccer players: a case series. *J Bodyw Mov Ther.* 2012;16(4):540-548.

198. Verrall GM, Slavotinek JP, Fon GT, Barnes PG. Outcome of conservative management of athletic chronic groin injury diagnosed as pubic bone stress injury. *Am J Sports Med.* 2007;35(3):467-474.

199. Chaudhari AM, Jamison ST, McNally MP, et al. Hip adductor activations during run-to-cut manoeuvres in compression shorts: implications for return to sport after groin injury. *J Sports Sci.* 2014;32(14):1333-1340.

200. Miyamoto N, Kawakami Y. Effect of pressure intensity of compression short-tight on fatigue of thigh muscles. *Med Sci Sports Exerc.* 2014;46(11):2168-2174.

201. Lovell DI, Mason DG, Delphinus EM, McLellan CP. Do compression garments enhance the active recovery process after high-intensity running? *J Strength Cond Res.* 2011;25(12):3264-3268.

202. Sear JA, Hoare TK, Scanlan AT, et al. The effects of whole-body compression garments on prolonged high-intensity intermittent exercise. *J Strength Cond Res.* 2010;24(7):1901-1910.

203. Michael JS, Dogramaci SN, Steel KA, Graham KS. What is the effect of compression garments on a balance task in female athletes? *Gait Posture.* 2014;39(2):804-809.

204. Holmich P, Nyvold P, Larsen K. Continued significant effect of physical training as treatment for overuse injury: 8- to 12-year outcome of a randomized clinical trial. *Am J Sports Med.* 2011;39(11):2447-2451.

205. Weir A, Jansen JA, van de Port IG, et al. Manual or exercise therapy for long-standing adductor-related groin pain: a randomised controlled clinical trial. *Man Ther.* 2011;16(2):148-154.

206. Weir A, Jansen J, van Keulen J, et al. Short and mid-term results of a comprehensive treatment program for longstanding adductor-related groin pain in athletes: a case series. *Phys Ther Sport.* 2010;11(3):99-103.

207. Bizzini M, Junge A, Dvorak J. Implementation of the FIFA 11+ football warm up program: how to approach and convince the Football associations to invest in prevention. *Br J Sports Med.* 2013;47(12):803-806.

208. Soligard T, Nilstad A, Steffen K, et al. Compliance with a comprehensive warm-up programme to prevent injuries in youth football. *Br J Sports Med.* 2010;44(11):787-793.

209. Steffen K, Emery CA, Romiti M, et al. High adherence to a neuromuscular injury prevention programme (FIFA 11+) improves functional balance and reduces injury risk in Canadian youth female football players: a cluster randomised trial. *Br J Sports Med.* 2013;47(12):794-802.

210. Grooms DR, Palmer T, Onate JA, et al. Soccer-specific warm-up and lower extremity injury rates in collegiate male soccer players. *J Athl Train.* 2013;48(6):782-789.

211. Owoeye OB, Akinbo SR, Tella BA, Olawale OA. Efficacy of the FIFA 11+ warm-up programme in male youth football: a cluster randomised controlled trial. *J Sports Sci Med.* 2014;13(2):321-328.

212. van Beijsterveldt AM, van de Port IG, Krist MR, et al. Effectiveness of an injury prevention programme for adult male amateur soccer players: a cluster-randomised controlled trial. *Br J Sports Med.* 2012;46(16):1114-1118.

213. Krist MR, van Beijsterveldt AM, Backx FJ, de Wit GA. Preventive exercises reduced injury-related costs among adult male amateur soccer players: a cluster-randomised trial. *J Physiother.* 2013;59(1):15-23.

214. Steffen K, Bakka HM, Myklebust G, Bahr R. Performance aspects of an injury prevention program: a ten-week intervention in adolescent female football players. *Scand J Med Sci Sports.* 2008;18(5):596-604.

215. Tyler TF, Nicholas SJ, Campbell RJ, et al. The effectiveness of a preseason exercise program to prevent adductor muscle strains in professional ice hockey players. *Am J Sports Med.* 2002;30(5):680-683.

216. Messaoudi N, Jans C, Pauli S, et al. Surgical management of sportsman's hernia in professional soccer players. *Orthopedics.* 2012;35(9):e1371-e1375.

217. Robertson IJ, Curran C, McCaffrey N, et al. Adductor tenotomy in the management of groin pain in athletes. *Int J Sports Med.* 2011;32(1):45-48.

218. Gill TJ, Carroll KM, Makani A, et al. Surgical technique for treatment of recalcitrant adductor longus tendinopathy. *Arthrosc Tech.* 2014;3(2):e293-e297.

219. Reference deleted in review.

220. Atkinson HD, Johal P, Falworth MS, et al. Adductor tenotomy: its role in the management of sports-related chronic groin pain. *Arch Orthop Trauma Surg.* 2010;130(8):965-970.

221. Akermark C, Johansson C. Tenotomy of the adductor longus tendon in the treatment of chronic groin pain in athletes. *Am J Sports Med.* 1992;20(6):640-643.

222. Jans C, Messaoudi N, Pauli S, et al. Results of surgical treatment of athletes with sportsman's hernia. *Acta Orthop Belg.* 2012;78(1):35-40.

223. Schilders E, Dimitrakopoulou A, Cooke M, et al. Effectiveness of a selective partial adductor release for chronic adductor-related groin pain in professional athletes. *Am J Sports Med.* 2013;41(3):603-607.

224. Maffulli N, Loppini M, Longo UG, Denaro V. Bilateral mini-invasive adductor tenotomy for the management of chronic unilateral adductor longus tendinopathy in athletes. *Am J Sports Med.* 2012;40(8):1880-1886.

225. Hopp SJ, Culemann U, Kelm J, et al. Osteitis pubis and adductor tendinopathy in athletes: a novel arthroscopic pubic symphysis curettage and adductor reattachment. *Arch Orthop Trauma Surg.* 2013;133(7):1003-1009.

226. Radic R, Annear P. Use of pubic symphysis curettage for treatment-resistant osteitis pubis in athletes. *Am J Sports Med.* 2008;36(1):122-128.

227. Paajanen H, Heikkinen J, Hermunen H, Airo I. Successful treatment of osteitis pubis by using totally extraperitoneal endoscopic technique. *Int J Sports Med.* 2005;26(4):303-306.

228. Williams PR, Thomas DP, Downes EM. Osteitis pubis and instability of the pubic symphysis: when nonoperative measures fail. *Am J Sports Med.* 2000;28(3):350-355.

229. Hechtman KS, Zvijac JE, Popkin CA, et al. A minimally disruptive surgical technique for the treatment of osteitis pubis in athletes. *Sports Health.* 2010;2(3):211-215.

230. Rossidis G, Perry A, Abbas H, et al. Laparoscopic hernia repair with adductor tenotomy for athletic pubalgia: an established procedure for an obscure entity. *Surg Endosc.* 2015;29(2):381-386.

231. Hiti CJ, Stevens KJ, Jamati MK, et al. Athletic osteitis pubis. *Sports Med.* 2011;41(5):361-376.

232. Mandelbaum B, Mora SA. Osteitis pubis. *Oper Tech Sports Med.* 2005;13(1):62-67.

233. Choi H, McCartney M, Best TM. Treatment of osteitis pubis and osteomyelitis of the pubic symphysis in athletes: a systematic review. *Br J Sports Med.* 2011;45(1):57-64.

234. Rodriguez C, Miguel A, Lima H, Heinrichs K. Osteitis pubis syndrome in the professional soccer athlete: a case report. *J Athl Train.* 2001;36(4):437-440.

235. Jarosz BS. Individualized multi-modal management of osteitis pubis in an Australian Rules footballer. *J Chiropr Med.* 2011;10(2):105-110.

236. Beatty T. Osteitis pubis in athletes. *Curr Sports Med Rep.* 2012;11(2):96-98.

237. Khan W, Zoga AC, Meyers WC. Magnetic resonance imaging of athletic pubalgia and the sports hernia: current understanding and practice. *Magn Reson Imaging Clin N Am.* 2013;21(1):97-110.

238. Cunningham PM, Brennan D, O'Connell M, et al. Patterns of bone and soft-tissue injury at the symphysis pubis in soccer players: observations at MRI. *AJR Am J Roentgenol.* 2007;188(3):W291-W296.

239. Larson CM, Sikka RS, Sardelli MC, et al. Increasing alpha angle is predictive of athletic-related "hip" and "groin" pain in collegiate National Football League prospects. *Arthroscopy.* 2013;29(3):405-410.

240. Birmingham PM, Kelly BT, Jacobs R, et al. The effect of dynamic femoroacetabular impingement on pubic symphysis motion: a cadaveric study. *Am J Sports Med.* 2012;40(5): 1113-1118.

241. Sudarshan A. Physical therapy management of osteitis pubis in a 10-year-old cricket fast bowler. *Physiother Theory Pract.* 2013;29(6):476-486.

242. Pham DV, Scott KG. Presentation of osteitis and osteomyelitis pubis as acute abdominal pain. *Perm J.* 2007;11(2): 65-68.

243. Holmich P, Holmich LR, Bjerg AM. Clinical examination of athletes with groin pain: an intraobserver and interobserver reliability study. *Br J Sports Med.* 2004;38(4):446-451.

244. Drew MK, Osmotherly PG, Chiarelli PE. Imaging and clinical tests for the diagnosis of long-standing groin pain in athletes: a systematic review. *Phys Ther Sport.* 2014;15(2): 124-129.

245. Kunduracioglu B, Yilmaz C, Yorubulut M, Kudas S. Magnetic resonance findings of osteitis pubis. *J Magn Reson Imaging.* 2007;25(3):535-539.

246. Besjakov J, von Scheele C, Ekberg O, et al. Grading scale of radiographic findings in the pubic bone and symphysis in athletes. *Acta Radiol.* 2003;44(1):79-83.

247. Lovell G, Galloway H, Hopkins W, Harvey A. Osteitis pubis and assessment of bone marrow edema at the pubic symphysis with MRI in an elite junior male soccer squad. *Clin J Sport Med.* 2006;16(2):117-122.

248. Brennan D, O'Connell MJ, Ryan M, et al. Secondary cleft sign as a marker of injury in athletes with groin pain: MR image appearance and interpretation. *Radiology.* 2005;235(1): 162-167.

249. Balconi G. US in pubalgia. *J Ultrasound.* 2011;14(3): 157-166.

250. Jardi J, Rodas G, Pedret C, et al. Osteitis pubis: can early return to elite competition be contemplated? *Transl Med UniSa.* 2014;10:52-58.

251. Vijayakumar P, Nagarajan M, Ramli A. Multimodal physiotherapeutic management for stage-IV osteitis pubis in a 15-year old soccer athlete: a case report. *J Back Musculoskelet Rehabil.* 2012;25(4):225-230.

252. Grace JN, Sim FH, Shives TC, Coventry MB. Wedge resection of the symphysis pubis for the treatment of osteitis pubis. *J Bone Joint Surg Am.* 1989;71(3):358-364.

253. Grumet RC, Frank RM, Slabaugh MA, et al. Lateral hip pain in an athletic population: differential diagnosis and treatment options. *Sports Health.* 2010;2(3):191-196.

254. Strauss EJ, Nho SJ, Kelly BT. Greater trochanteric pain syndrome. *Sports Med Arthrosc.* 2010;18(2):113-119.

255. Williams BS, Cohen SP. Greater trochanteric pain syndrome: a review of anatomy, diagnosis and treatment. *Anesth Analg.* 2009;108(5):1662-1670.

256. Martin RL, Kelly BT, Leunig M. Reliability of clinical diagnosis in intraarticular hip diseases. *Knee Surg Sports Traumatol Arthrosc.* 2010;18:685-690.

257. Lauder TD. Musculoskeletal disorders that frequently mimic radiculopathy. *Phys Med Rehabil Clin N Am.* 2002;13(3): 469-485.

258. Martin RL, Enseki KR, Draovitch P, et al. Acetabular labral tears of the hip: examination and diagnostic challenges. *J Orthop Sports Phys Ther.* 2006;36(7):503-515.

259. Paluska SA. An overview of hip injuries in running. *Sports Med.* 2005;35(11):991-1014.

260. Bird P, Oakley S, Shnier R, Kirkham B. Prospective evaluation of magnetic resonance imaging and physical examination findings in patients with greater trochanteric pain syndrome. *Arthritis Rheum.* 2001;44(9):2138-2145.

261. Segal NA, Felson DT, Torner JC, et al. Greater trochanteric pain syndrome: epidemiology and associated factors. *Arch Phys Med Rehabil.* 2007;88(8):988-992.

262. Ho GW, Howard TM. Greater trochanteric pain syndrome: more than bursitis and iliotibial tract friction. *Curr Sports Med Rep.* 2012;11(5):232-238.

263. Nielsen RØ, Parner ET, Nohr EA, et al. Excessive progression in weekly running distance and risk of running-related injuries: an association which varies according to type of injury. *J Orthop Sports Phys Ther.* 2014;44(10):739-747.

264. Klauser AS, Martinoli C, Tagliafico A, et al. Greater trochanteric pain syndrome. *Semin Musculoskelet Radiol.* 2013;17(1): 43-48.

265. Lustenberger DP, Ng VY, Best TM, Ellis TJ. Efficacy of treatment of trochanteric bursitis: a systematic review. *Clin J Sport Med.* 2011;21(5):447-453.

266. Lonne JH, Van Kleunen JP. Spontaneous rupture of the gluteus medius and minimus tendons. *Am J Orthop.* 2002;31(10): 579-581.

267. LaBan MM, Weir SK, Taylor RS. "Bald trochanter" spontaneous rupture of the conjoined tendons of the gluteus medius and minimus presenting as a trochanteric bursitis. *Am J Phys Med Rehabil.* 2004;83(10):806-809.

268. Aepli-Schneider N, Treumann T, Müller U, Schmid L. Degenerative rupture of the hip abductors: missed diagnosis with therapy-resistant trochanteric pain of the hips and positive Trendelenburg sign in elderly patients. *Z Rheumatol.* 2012; 71(1):68-74. [in German].

269. Lachiewicz PF. Abductor tendon tears of the hip: evaluation and management. *J Am Acad Orthop Surg.* 2011;19(7): 385-391.

270. Stanton MC, Maloney MD, Dehaven KE, Giordano BD. Acute traumatic tear of gluteus medius and minimus tendons in a patient without antecedent peritrochanteric hip pain. *Geriatr Orthop Surg Rehabil.* 2012;3(2):84-88.

271. Tyler TF, Fukunaga T, Gellert J. Rehabilitation of soft tissue injuries of the hip and pelvis. *Int J Sports Phys Ther.* 2014; 9(6):785-797.

272. Martin RL, Sekiya JK. The interrater reliability of 4 clinical tests used to assess individuals with musculoskeletal hip pain. *J Orthop Sports Phys Ther.* 2008;38(2):71-77.

273. Reiman MP, Goode AP, Hegedus EJ, et al. Diagnostic accuracy of clinical tests of the hip: a systematic review with meta-analysis. *Br J Sports Med.* 2013;47(14):893-902.

274. Lequesne M, Mathieu P, Vuillemin-Bodaghi V, et al. Gluteal tendinopathy in refractory greater trochanter pain syndrome: diagnostic value of two clinical tests. *Arthritis Rheum.* 2008;59(2):241-246.

275. Reese NB, Bandy WD. Use of an inclinometer to measure flexibility of the iliotibial band using the Ober test and the modified Ober test: differences in magnitude and reliability of measurements. *J Orthop Sports Phys Ther.* 2003;33(6): 326-330.

276. Westacott DJ, Minns JI, Foguet P. The diagnostic accuracy of magnetic resonance imaging and ultrasonography in gluteal tendon tears: a systematic review. *Hip Int.* 2011;21(6): 637-645.

277. Chowdhury R, Naaseri S, Lee J, Rajeswaran G. Imaging and management of greater trochanteric pain syndrome. *Postgrad Med J.* 2014;90(1068):576-581.

278. Tibor LM, Sekiya JK. Differential diagnosis of pain around the hip joint. *Arthroscopy.* 2008;24(12):1407-1421.

279. Klauser AS, Martinoli C, Tagliafico A, et al. Greater trochanteric pain syndrome. *Semin Musculoskelet Radiol.* 2013;17(1):43-48.

280. Bewyer DC, Bewyer KJ. Rationale for treatment of hip abductor pain syndrome. *Iowa Orthop J.* 2003;23:57-60.

281. Brinks A, van Rijn RM, Willemsen SP, et al. Corticosteroid injections for greater trochanteric pain syndrome: a randomized controlled trial in primary care. *Ann Fam Med.* 2011;9(3): 225-234.

282. Sayegh F, Potoupnis M, Kapetanos G. Greater trochanter bursitis pain syndrome in females with chronic low back pain and sciatica. *Acta Orthop Belg.* 2004;70(5):423-428.

283. Selkowitz DM, Beneck GJ, Powers CM. Which exercises target the gluteal muscles while minimizing activation of the tensor fascia lata? Electromyographic assessment using fine-wire electrodes. *J Orthop Sports Phys Ther.* 2013;43(2):56-64.

284. Bolgla LA, Uhl TL. Electromyographic analysis of hip rehabilitation exercises in a group of healthy subjects. *J Orthop Sports Phys Ther.* 2005;35(8):487-494.

285. Ebert JR, Bucher TA, Ball SV, Janes GC. A review of surgical repair methods and patient outcomes for gluteal tendon tears. *Hip Int.* 2015;25(1):15-23.

286. Domb BG, Botser I, Giordano BD. Outcomes of endoscopic gluteus medius repair with minimum 2-year follow-up. *Am J Sports Med.* 2013;41(5):988-997.

287. McCormick F, Alpaugh K, Nwachukwu BU, et al. Endoscopic repair of full-thickness abductor tendon tears: surgical technique and outcome at minimum of 1-year follow-up. *Arthroscopy.* 2013;29(12):1941-1947.

288. Van Hofwegen C, Baker CL, Savory CG, Baker CL. Arthroscopic bursectomy for recalcitrant trochanteric bursitis after hip arthroplasty. *J Surg Orthop Adv.* 2013;22(2):143-147.

289. Verrall GM, Esterman A, Hewett TE. Analysis of the three most prevalent injuries in Australian football demonstrates a season to season association between groin/hip/osteitis pubis injuries with ACL knee injuries. *Asian J Sports Med.* 2014;5(3):e23072.

290. DeWitt J, Vidale T. Recurrent hamstring injury: consideration following operative and non-operative management. *Int J Sports Phys Ther.* 2014;9(6):798-812.

291. Verrall GM, Slavotinek J, Barnes P. Diagnostic and prognostic value of clinical findings in 83 athletes with posterior thigh injury: comparison of clinical findings with magnetic resonance imaging documentation of hamstring muscle strain. *Am J Sports Med.* 2003;31(6):969.

292. Prior M, Guerin M, Grimmer K. An evidence-based approach to hamstring strain injury: a systematic review of the literature. *Sports Health.* 2009;1(2):154-164.

293. Petersen J, Hölmich P. Evidence based prevention of hamstring injuries in sport. *Br J Sports Med.* 2005;39(6):319-323.

294. Schmitt B, Tyler T, McHugh M. Hamstring injury rehabilitation and prevention of reinjury using lengthened state eccentric training: a new concept. *Int J Sports Phys Ther.* 2011;7(3): 333-341.

295. Heiderscheit BC, Sherry MA, Silder A, et al. Hamstring strain injuries: recommendations for diagnosis, rehabilitation, and injury prevention. *J Orthop Sports Phys Ther.* 2010;40(2): 67-81.

296. Brooks JH, Fuller CW, Kemp SP, Reddin DB. Incidence, risk, and prevention of hamstring muscle injuries in professional rugby union. *Am J Sports Med.* 2006;34(8):1297-1306.

297. Feeley BT, Kennelly S, Barnes RP, et al. Epidemiology of national football league training camp injuries from 1998-2007. *Am J Sports Med.* 2008;36(8):1597-1603.

298. Askling CM, Tengvar M, Saartok T, Thorstensson A. Proximal hamstring strains of stretching type in different sports: injury situations, clinical and magnetic resonance imaging characteristics, and return to sport. *Am J Sports Med.* 2008;36(9): 1799-1804.

299. Askling C, Saartok T, Thorstensson A. Type of acute hamstring strain affects flexibility, strength, and time to return to pre-injury level. *Br J Sports Med.* 2006;40(1):40-44.

300. Connell DA, Schneider-Kolsky ME, Hoving JL, et al. Longitudinal study comparing sonographic and MRI assessments of acute and healing hamstring injuries. *AJR Am J Roentgenol.* 2004;183(4):975-984.

301. Pedersen IK, Thillemann T, Storm JO. Complete proximal hamstring tendon rupture can be misinterpreted as muscle rupture. *Ugeskr Laeger.* 2012;174(18):1232-1233. [in Danish].

302. Engebretsen AH, Myklebust G, Holme I, et al. Intrinsic risk factors for hamstring injuries among male soccer players: a prospective cohort study. *Am J Sports Med.* 2010;38(6): 1147-1153.

303. Fousekis K, Tsepis E, Poulmedis P, et al. Intrinsic risk factors of non-contact quadriceps and hamstring strains in soccer: a prospective study of 100 professional players. *Br J Sports Med.* 2011;45(9):709-714.

304. Sugiura Y, Saito T, Sakuraba K, et al. Strength deficits identified with concentric action of the hip extensors and eccentric action of the hamstrings predispose to hamstring injury in elite sprinters. *J Orthop Sports Phys Ther.* 2008;38(8):457-464.

305. Lorenz D, Reiman M. The role and implementation of eccentric training in athletic rehabilitation: tendinopathy, hamstring strains, and ACL reconstruction. *Int J Sports Phys Ther.* 2011; 6(1):27-44.

306. Small K, McNaughton LR, Greig M, et al. Soccer fatigue sprinting and hamstring injury risk. *Int J Sports Med.* 2009; 30(8):573-578.

307. Sherry MA, Best TM. A comparison of 2 rehabilitation programs in the treatment of acute hamstring strains. *J Orthop Sports Phys Ther.* 2004;34(3):116-125.

308. Cibulka MT, Rose SJ, Delitto A, Sinacore DR. Hamstring muscle strain treated by mobilizing the sacroiliac joint. *Phys Ther.* 1986;66(8):1220-1223.

309. Worrell TW. Factors associated with hamstring injuries: an approach to treatment and preventative measures. *Sports Med.* 1994;17(5):338-345.

310. Clanton TO, Coupe KJ. Hamstring strains in athletes: diagnosis and treatment. *J Am Acad Orthop Surg.* 1998;6(4):237-248.

311. Kendall FP, McCreary EK, Provance PG. *Muscles: Testing and Function.* Baltimore: Williams & Wilkins; 1993.

312. Cohen S, Bradley J. Acute proximal hamstring rupture. *J Am Acad Orthop Surg.* 2007;15(6):350-355.

313. Kelly BT, Williams RJ, Philippon MJ. Hip arthroscopy: current indications, treatment options, and management issues. *Am J Sports Med.* 2003;31(6):1020-1037.

314. Hitora T, Kawaguchi Y, Mori M, et al. Ischiogluteal bursitis: a report of three cases with MR findings. *Rheumatol Int.* 2008; 29(4):455-458.

315. Nicholas SJ, Tyler TF. Adductor muscle strains in sport. *Sports Med.* 2002;32(5):339-344.

316. Kilcoyne KG, Dickens JF, Keblish D, et al. Outcome of grade I and II hamstring injuries in intercollegiate athletes: a novel rehabilitation protocol. *Sports Health.* 2011;3(6):528-533.

317. Heiser T, Weber J, Sullivan G. Prophylaxis and management of hamstring muscle injuries in intercollegiate football players. *Am J Sports Med.* 1984;12(5):368-370.

318. Brukner P, Nealon A, Morgan C, et al. Recurrent hamstring muscle injury: applying the limited evidence in the professional football setting with a seven-point programme. *Br J Sports Med.* 2014;48(11):929-938.

319. Goode AP, Reiman MP, Harris L, et al. Eccentric training for prevention of hamstring injuries may depend on intervention compliance: a systematic review and meta-analysis. *Br J Sports Med.* 2015;49(6):349-356.

320. Askling C, Karlsson J, Thorstensson A. Hamstring injury occurrence in elite soccer players after preseason strength training with eccentric overload. *Scand J Med Sci Sports.* 2003;13(4): 244-250.

321. Fredericson M, Moore W, Guille M, Beaulieu C. High hamstring tendinopathy in runners: meeting the challenges of diagnosis, treatment, and rehabilitation. *Phys Sportsmed.* 2005; 33(5):32-43.

322. Klingele KE, Sallay PI. Surgical repair of complete proximal hamstring tendon rupture. *Am J Sports Med.* 2002;30(5): 742-747.

323. Domb BG, Linder D, Sharp KG, et al. Endoscopic repair of proximal hamstring avulsion. *Arthrosc Tech.* 2013;2(1): e35-e39.

324. Lefevre N, Bohu Y, Klouche S, Herman S. Surgical technique for repair of acute proximal hamstring tears. *Orthop Traumatol Surg Res.* 2013;99(2):235-240.

325. Sallay PI, Friedman RI, Coogan PG, Garrett WE. Hamstring muscle injuries among water skiers: functional outcome and prevention. *Am J Sports Med.* 1996;24:130-136.

326. Browning KH. Hip and pelvis injuries in runners. *Phys Sportsmed.* 2001;29(1):23-24.

327. DeAngelis NA, Busconi BD. Assessment and differential diagnosis of the painful hip. *Clin Orthop Relat Res.* 2003;406: 11-18.

328. Anderson K, Strickland SM, Warren R. Hip and groin injuries in athletes. *Am J Sports Med.* 2001;29(4):521-533.

329. Adkins SB, Figler RA. Hip pain in athletes. *Am Fam Physician.* 2000;61(7):2109-2118.

330. Johnston CA, Wiley JP, Lindsay DM, Wiseman DA. Iliopsoas bursitis and tendinitis: a review. *Sports Med.* 1998;25(4): 271-284.

331. Blankenaker DG, Tuite MJ. Iliopsoas musculotendinous unit. *Semin Musculoskelet Radiol.* 2008;12(1):13-27.

332. Winston P, Awan R, Cassidy JD, Bleakney RK. Clinical examination and ultrasound of self-reported snapping hip syndrome in elite ballet dancers. *Am J Sports Med.* 2007;35(1): 118-126.

333. Wahl CJ, Warren RF, Adler RS, et al. Internal coxa saltans (snapping hip) as a result of overtraining: a report of 3 cases in professional athletes with a review of causes and the role of ultrasound in early diagnosis and management. *Am J Sports Med.* 2004;32(5):1302-1309.

334. Brunot S, Dubeau S, Laumonier H. Acute inguinal pain associated with iliopectineal bursitis in four professional soccer players. *Diagn Interv Imaging.* 2013;94(1):91-94.

335. Generini S, Matucci-Cerinic M. Iliopsoas bursitis in rheumatoid arthritis. *Clin Exp Rheumatol.* 1993;11(5):549-551.

336. Philippon MJ, Decker MJ, Giphart JE, et al. Rehabilitation exercise progression for the gluteus medius muscle with consideration for iliopsoas tendinitis: an in vivo electromyography study. *Am J Sports Med.* 2011;39(8):1777-1785.

337. Labile C, Swanson D, Garofolo G, Rose DJ. Iliopsoas syndrome in dancers. *Orthop J Sports Med.* 2013;1(3):1-6.

338. Johnston CA, Lindsay DM, Wiley JP. Treatment of iliopsoas syndrome with a hip rotation strengthening program: a retrospective case series. *J Orthop Sports Phys Ther.* 1999;29(4): 218-224.

339. Ingber RS. Iliopsoas myofascial dysfunction: a treatable cause of "failed" low back syndrome. *Arch Phys Med Rehabil.* 1989;70(5):382-386.

340. Irmola T, Heikkilä JT, Orava S, Sarimo J. Total proximal tendon avulsion of the rectus femoris muscle. *Scand J Med Sci Sports.* 2007;17(4):378-382.

341. Bordalo-Rodrigues M, Rosenberg ZS. MR imaging of the proximal rectus femoris musculotendinous unit. *Magn Reson Imaging Clin N Am.* 2005;13:717-725.

342. Ueblacker P, Müller-Wohlfahrt HW, Hinterwimmer S, et al. Suture anchor repair of proximal rectus femoris avulsions in elite football players. *Knee Surg Sports Traumatol Arthrosc.* 2015;23(9):2590-2594.

343. Hughes C, Hasselman CT, Best TM, et al. Incomplete, intrasubstance strain injuries of the rectus femoris muscle. *Am J Sports Med.* 1995;23(4):500-506.

344. Peeler J, Anderson JE. Reliability of the Ely's test for assessing rectus femoris muscle flexibility and joint range of motion. *J Orthop Res.* 2008;26(6):793-799.

345. Gamradt SC, Brophy RH, Barnes R, et al. Nonoperative treatment for proximal avulsion of the rectus femoris in professional American football. *Am J Sports Med.* 2009;37(7):1370-1374.

346. Bass CJ, Connell DA. Sonographic findings of tensor fascia lata tendinopathy: another cause of anterior groin pain. *Skeletal Radiol.* 2002;31(3):143-148.

347. Sahrmann SA. *Diagnosis and Treatment of Movement Impairment Syndromes.* St. Louis: Mosby; 2002.

348. Sutter R, Kalberer F, Binkert CA, et al. Abductor tendon tears are associated with hypertrophy of the tensor fasciae latae muscle. *Skeletal Radiol.* 2013;42(5):627-633.

349. Niemuth PE, Johnson RJ, Myers MJ, Thieman TJ. Hip muscle weakness and overuse injuries in recreational runners. *Clin J Sport Med.* 2005;15(1):14-21.

350. Boyajian-O'Neill LA, McClain RL, Coleman MK, Thomas PP. Diagnosis and management of piriformis syndrome: an osteopathic approach. *J Am Osteopath Assoc.* 2008;108(11):657-664.

351. Cass SP. Piriformis syndrome: a cause of nondiscogenic sciatica. *Curr Sports Med Rep.* 2015;14(1):41-44.

352. Moore KL, Dalley AF, Agur AMR. *Clinically Oriented Anatomy.* 7th ed. Baltimore: Lippincott Williams & Wilkins; 2014.

353. Windisch G, Braun EM, Anderhuber F. Piriformis muscle: clinical anatomy and consideration of the piriformis syndrome. *Surg Radiol Anat.* 2007;29(1):37-45.

354. Pace JB, Nagle D. Piriform syndrome. *West J Med.* 1976;124: 435-439.

355. Papadopoulos EC, Khan SN. Piriformis syndrome and low back pain: a new classification and review of the literature. *Orthop Clin North Am.* 2004;35(1):65-71.

356. Deville WL, van der Windt DA, Dzaferagic A, et al. The test of Lasegue: systematic review of the accuracy in diagnosing herniated discs. *Spine (Phila Pa 1976).* 2000;25(9):1140-1147.

357. Fishman LM, Dombi GW, Michaelsen C, et al. Piriformis syndrome: diagnosis, treatment, and outcome—a 10-year study. *Arch Phys Med Rehabil.* 2002;83(3):295-301.

358. Beatty RA. The piriformis muscle syndrome: a simple diagnostic maneuver. *Neurosurgery.* 1994;34(3):512-514.

359. Kirschner JS, Foye PM, Cole JL. Piriformis syndrome, diagnosis and treatment. *Muscle Nerve.* 2009;40(1):10-18.

360. Chang CW, Shieh SF, Li CM, et al. Measurement of motor nerve conduction velocity of the sciatic nerve in patients with piriformis syndrome: a magnetic stimulation study. *Arch Phys Med Rehabil.* 2006;87(10):1371-1375.

361. Filler AG, Haynes J, Jordan SE, et al. Sciatica of nondisc origin and piriformis syndrome: diagnosis by magnetic resonance neurography and interventional magnetic resonance imaging with outcome study of resulting treatment. *J Neurosurg Spine.* 2005;2(2):99-115.

362. Lewis AM, Layzer R, Engstrom JW, et al. Magnetic resonance neurography in extraspinal sciatica. *Arch Neurol.* 2006;63(10):1469-1472.

363. Hochman MG, Zilberfarb JL. Nerves in a pinch: imaging of nerve compression syndromes. *Radiol Clin North Am.* 2004;42(1):221-245.

364. Pecina HI, Boric I, Smoljanovic T, et al. Surgical evaluation of magnetic resonance imaging findings in piriformis muscle syndrome. *Skeletal Radiol.* 2008;37(11):1019-1023.

365. Fishman LM, Anderson C, Rosner B. Botox and physical therapy in the treatment of piriformis syndrome. *Am J Phys Med Rehabil.* 2002;81(12):936-942.

366. Masala S, Crusco S, Meschini A, et al. Piriformis syndrome: long-term follow-up in patients treated with percutaneous injection of anesthetic and corticosteroid under CT guidance. *Cardiovasc Intervent Radiol.* 2012;35(2):375-382.

367. Yoon SJ, Ho J, Kang HY, et al. Low-dose botulinum toxin type A for the treatment of refractory piriformis syndrome. *Pharmacotherapy.* 2007;27(5):657-665.

368. Al-Al-Shaikh M, Michel F, Parratte B, et al. An MRI evaluation of changes in piriformis muscle morphology induced by botulinum toxin injections in the treatment of piriformis syndrome. *Diagn Interv Imaging.* 2015;96(1):37-43.

369. Tonley JC, Yun SM, Kochevar RJ, et al. Treatment of an individual with piriformis syndrome focusing on hip muscle strengthening and movement reeducation: a case report. *J Orthop Sports Phys Ther.* 2010;40(2):103-111.

370. Benson ER, Schutzer SF. Posttraumatic piriformis syndrome: diagnosis and results of operative treatment. *J Bone Joint Surg Am.* 1999;81(7):941-949.

371. Aboulfetouh I, Saleh A. Neurolysis for secondary sciatic nerve entrapment: evaluation of surgical feasibility and functional outcome. *Acta Neurochir (Wien).* 2014;156(10):1979-1986.

372. Craig A. Entrapment neuropathies of the lower extremity. *PM R.* 2013;5(5 suppl):S31-S40.

373. Moore AE, Stringer MD. Iatrogenic femoral nerve injury: a systematic review. *Surg Radiol Anat.* 2011;33(8):649-658.

374. Antoniadis G, Kretschmer T, Pedro MT, et al. Iatrogenic nerve injuries: prevalence, diagnosis and treatment. *Dtsch Arztebl Int.* 2014;111(16):273-279.

375. Murray IR, Perks FJ, Beggs I, Moran M. Femoral nerve palsy secondary to traumatic iliacus haematoma: a young athlete's injury. *BMJ Case Rep.* 2010;(Oct 22):2010.

376. Roy PC. Electrodiagnostic evaluation of lower extremity neurogenic problems. *Foot Ankle Clin.* 2011;16(2):225-242.

377. Tipton JS. Obturator neuropathy. *Curr Rev Musculoskelet Med.* 2008;1(3–4):234-237.

378. Smoll NR. Variations of the piriformis and sciatic nerve with clinical consequence: a review. *Clin Anat.* 2010;23(1):8-17.

379. Bradshaw C, McCrory P. Obturator nerve entrapment. *Clin J Sport Med.* 1997;7(3):217-219.

380. Binkley JM, Stratford PW, Lott SA, Riddle DL. The Lower Extremity Functional Scale (LEFS): scale development, measurement properties, and clinical application. North American Orthopaedic Rehabilitation Research Network. *Phys Ther.* 1999;79(4):371-383.

4

Femoral Acetabular Impingement and Labral Tears

KEELAN ENSEKI AND DAVE KOHLRIESER

CHAPTER OUTLINE

Injuries to the acetabular labrum and other causes of nonarthritic hip pain have become topics of increased interest in the orthopedic literature. The relatively younger and more active population has received significant attention when the treatment options available for patients with labral injuries are debated. Improved understanding of hip joint function, coupled with advances in diagnostic technology and surgical options, has resulted in increased interest from clinicians.[1] Acetabular labral tears are often associated with other conditions of the joint such as femoral acetabular impingement (FAI) and joint hypermobility. Although lesions of the acetabular labrum have been described in the literature for some time, reporting detailed data for the injury is a more recent occurrence. The true prevalence of acetabular labral tears in the population is unknown and perhaps underreported. The prevalence of labral tears among patients with mechanical hip pain has been estimated to be as high as 88%.[2] In a review of acetabular labral tears, Groh and Herrera[3] estimated prevalence rates between 22% and 55% in patients with groin pain. This chapter places particular emphasis on the group of patients with labral tears that occur secondary to FAI. Pathomechanical factors, common patient-related characteristics, and clinical findings are described. Conservative and surgical treatment is discussed along with considerations for postoperative rehabilitation.

General Information and Anatomic Overview

Acetabular Labrum

The acetabular labrum is a fibrocartilaginous structure that serves to provide stability and optimize load distribution across the joint surfaces.[4] It deepens the concavity of the acetabulum and, when intact, functions with the joint capsule to create a sealing effect at the joint. The labrum has also been suggested to play a protective role in cartilage preservation through decreasing the rate of cartilage consolidation (fluid expression from the matrix) when forces are experienced at the hip joint.[4,5] The controlled rate of consolidation decreases the amount of focal stress experienced at the articular surfaces of the acetabulum, thereby

potentially decreasing the likelihood of chondral lesion development. Acetabular labral tears have been identified as potential sources of hip pain. More recently, lesions of this structure have been suggested to play a role as a precursor to the development of hip osteoarthritis (OA).[6] It has been previously suggested that acetabular labral tears may be an early sign of the changes involved with the development of hip OA.[7] The occurrence of labral tears is suggested to result in focal chondral damage that eventually progresses globally to the development of hip OA. A comprehensive knowledge of the anatomy and biomechanics of the hip and pelvic complex will help clinicians understand the pathomechanical processes associated with acetabular labral tears of the hip joint.

Pathophysiology

The morphologic characteristics of acetabular labral tears have been described in the literature. Lage and associates[8] described four categories of tears (Fig. 4-1): radial flap, radial fibrillated, longitudinal peripheral, and abnormally mobile (partially detached). Radial flap and radial fibrillated

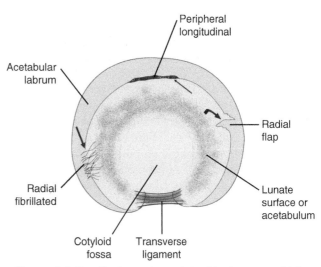

• **Figure 4-1** Classifications of acetabular labral tears: radial flap, radial fibrillated, and peripheral longitudinal. (Adapted from Lage LA, Patel JV, Villar RN. The acetabular labral tear: an arthroscopic classification. *Arthroscopy.* 1996;12:269-272.)

tears both have free ends detached from the acetabulum, with fibrillated tears showing fraying at the detached edge. Longitudinal peripheral tears involve disruption where the labrum meets the acetabulum. Abnormally mobile tears are detached from the acetabulum, thus creating an unstable structure. Radial flap tears are the most commonly observed labral disorders.[8] The most common area for acetabular labral tears to occur is the anterior superior region. This site corresponds to the following: the superior region is subject to the most forces during weight bearing, and the anterior region is thinner and is more likely affected by forces placed on the joint.[1,3] The bony femoral characteristic of cam impingement (described later) also has an established association with anterior superior labral and cartilage lesions.[9] Although the exact relationship between morphologic characteristics of labral tears and prognosis has not been established, the type of tear may influence the choice of procedure (resection versus repair) when a patient undergoes an arthroscopic surgical procedure to address the injury.[10]

The primary risk factors identified for acetabular labral tears are anatomic variants that affect hip joint function and type of physical activity. The association of age with symptomatic labral tears is debatable. Whereas the presence of labral tears does increase with age, the increased presence of hip OA must also be considered when attempting to determine a patient's primary source of pain. Several connective tissue disorders that result in generalized joint hypermobility (Ehlers-Danlos, Down, and Marfan syndromes) are also associated with a higher risk of lesions of the acetabular labrum.

Patient Profile

Because of the nature of injury development, correctly identifying acetabular labral tears as a primary source of symptoms often takes a long time. The condition is often overlooked when the patient is given another diagnosis. The list of differential diagnoses for patients with nonarthritic hip pain is expansive and includes both musculoskeletal and nonmusculoskeletal conditions. Clinicians must carefully consider the patient's history and complete clinical presentation to accurately determine the likelihood of an acetabular labral tear as the primary source of the patient's symptoms.

As previously noted, most persons with symptomatic acetabular labral tears are relatively young and active. Even so, the reported age range for diagnosis of symptomatic labral tears is 8 to 75 years.[3] Labral tears of the hip have been associated with a high proportion of athletes with complaints of hip pain.[11] Athletic activities that have been associated with acetabular labral tears include running, ballet, golf, ice hockey, and soccer.[12]

Persons participating in these activities often maneuver their hips into the extreme limits of the available range of motion (ROM). In the presence of abnormal bony morphology, sport activities that require repetitive end-range positions may elicit intraarticular pain and symptoms, but they may also increase the risk of cartilage and labral injury.[13] For this reason, clinicians should carefully inquire about a

patient's type of activity and correlation with symptoms during clinical evaluation. For clinicians to consider all potential diagnoses that may be applicable in a patient suspected of having a labral disorder, a comprehensive examination of the hip and pelvic complex should be performed. The reader is directed to review Chapter 2 for discussion of the hip examination process. Diagnostic imaging can help confirm the results of clinical examination. The later section on cam impingement discusses the use of imaging to diagnose acetabular labral tears and associated bony abnormalities.

Mechanisms of Injury

Although traumatic injury can occur, the more common mechanisms of injury tend to be the result of anatomic abnormalities that lead to mechanical overloading of the labrum over time. The tendency for damage to occur, when abnormal bony morphology is present, may be increased for those patients who participate in specific activities that increase the mechanical load placed on the hip joint. Heavy labor or athletic activities (as previously listed) may produce these types of forces. These activities are often repetitive. The most commonly described underlying anatomic mechanism of injury in the literature is FAI.[14,15]

Femoral Acetabular Impingement

FAI occurs when premature contact occurs between the proximal femur and the acetabular rim as a result of abnormal morphologic variations of the hip joint. Anatomic variants associated with FAI involve bony abnormalities of the femoral head and acetabulum. FAI tends to occur with specific movements of the hip joint. These movements typically involve flexion, internal rotation, or adduction. FAI is of particular concern in the younger, relatively active population.[12] FAI may lead to acetabular labral tears and subsequent chondral damage in some patients.[16] Although the specific etiology of FAI is not well understood, classification of the bony abnormalities related to FAI has been well described in the literature. The most common descriptions of FAI mechanisms include cam (femoral head and neck), pincer (acetabular), or mixed (cam and pincer) variations of impingement. Figure 4-2 illustrates the observed variations of FAI. The pathoanatomic features, common imaging findings, and distinguishing pathologic characteristics associated with FAI are discussed here.

Cam Impingement

Cam impingement is the result of excessive bone in the region of the femoral head and neck junction. The processes responsible for this abnormality are not well understood. Investigators have suggested that cam deformities may result from processes or events that potentially disturb development of the bone such as slipped capital femoral epiphysis.[17] When someone participates in repetitive activity requiring end ROMs (particularly flexion, internal rotation, or adduction), the femur makes premature contact

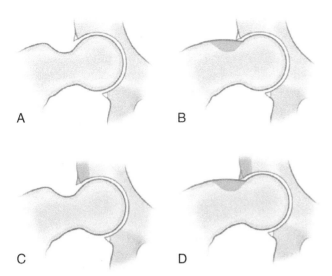

A

B

C

D

• **Figure 4-2** Mechanisms of Femoral Acetabular Impingement. **A,** Normal clearance of the hip. **B,** Cam type. **C,** Pincer type. **D,** Mixed type. (Modified from Lavigne M, Parvizi J, Beck M, et al. Anterior femoroacetabular impingement: part I. Techniques of joint preserving surgery. *Clin Orthop Relat Res.* 2004;418:61-66.)

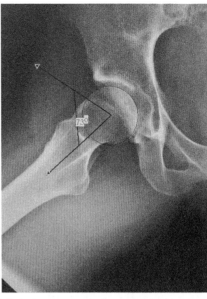

• **Figure 4-3** Alpha Angle. A reference line is the drawn from the center of the femoral head through the femoral neck. A second line is drawn from the center of the femoral head to the location where bone exists outside the drawn circular border. The angle formed between the two lines is the alpha angle. An alpha angle of 73 degrees is associated with cam femoral acetabular impingement.

into the acetabular rim and labral tissue.[11] An example of a sport-specific activity requiring this ROM is a soccer kick. With repetitive exposure to these forces, the labrum often fails at the bony interface where it attaches into the acetabulum, and a tear results. As time passes, the labral tears may progress to chondral damage on the articulating surfaces of the femur or acetabulum. Cam deformities have been commonly associated with labral and chondral damage in the anterior superior region of the hip joint.[9] Currently, a small body of evidence suggests that cam FAI is more prevalent in younger to middle-aged male patients.[18,19] Investigators have suggested that participation in high-impact activity at a young age may contribute to the development of the CAM deformity in this population.[13]

Plain radiographic imaging is routinely used when attempting to confirm FAI as an anatomic factor that may play a role in a patient's symptomatic presentation. Plain radiographs may also identify the presence of degenerative joint changes, which may be a differential diagnosis or prognostic factor in patients with FAI or tears of the acetabular labrum.[20] Radiographs can help clinicians determine the specific impingement mechanism (cam, pincer, or mixed) and the magnitude of variation from normal values. Cam impingement can be identified by specific findings on plain radiographic imaging. These findings indicate an increased diameter of the femoral neck or excessive bony formation in the region of the femoral head-neck junction that results in a decreased head-neck offset.[21]

The alpha angle is useful in measuring femoral head-neck offset and examining sphericity of the femoral head. The alpha angle can be measured from examining anteroposterior (AP), cross-table lateral, or modified Dunn views.[20,22] The alpha angle is measured by creating a circle around the peripheral borders of the femoral head. A reference line is then drawn from the center of the femoral head through the femoral neck. A second line is drawn from the center of the femoral head to the location where bone exists outside the circular border. The angle formed between the two lines is the alpha angle. The reported values for normal alpha angles vary, with the upper limits ranging from 50 to 60 degrees.[22,23] Barton and colleagues[24] determined the alpha angle to be 91% sensitive and 88% specific for identification of cam FAI when using a Dunn view. Figure 4-3 demonstrates an alpha angle value associated with cam impingement. Although not a technical measurement, the appearance of cam impingement on an AP radiograph is often identified as a "pistol grip deformity." The nonspherical head blends with the femoral neck to give the appearance of a pistol handle.

Currently, magnetic resonance arthrography (MRA) is the most common imaging modality used to identify acetabular labral tears and chondral damage.[25] When FAI of the hip joint is identified, clinicians may wish to determine whether an acetabular labral tear has developed secondary to the condition. MRA imaging is the modality of choice in confirming acetabular labral tears. A gadolinium-based contrast agent is introduced into the joint by injection before imaging is performed. This approach has been suggested to allow better intraarticular visualization and more detailed imagery of the articular surfaces when compared with standard magnetic resonance imaging (MRI). Enseki and associates[12] reviewed a number of studies that examined the sensitivity and specificity of MRA in identifying labral tears. The studies reviewed reported values of sensitivity ranging from 71% to 100%[26-29] and specificity ranging from 44% to 100%,[27,29] when compared with arthroscopic visualization as the gold standard.

Although not routinely applied in examination of patients with suspected FAI or acetabular labral tears, other imaging options may be useful in determining the potential role of other pathologic conditions in the presentation of hip pain. Additional imaging options include MRI, computed tomography (CT), diagnostic ultrasound, and bone scan. CT technology provides the ability to create three-dimensional imaging of the hip that provides further information on joint architecture.[12] This modality may prove useful in presurgical planning for complicated cases because it allows the surgeon to visualize the size and location of all possible impingement sources. This modality does not provide information on the acetabular labrum. The inclusion of three-dimensional CT imaging allows the surgeon to define more clearly the amount of bone to remove in each location; this is more difficult to determine during arthroscopic techniques. The use of an arthroscopic surgical approach allows only limited or intermittent visualization of the bony contour during the procedure. The high level of radiation exposure with CT imaging typically limits the application to complicated cases.[30]

Pincer Impingement

Pincer impingement is an innominate bone abnormality that is characterized by excessive coverage of the acetabulum over the femoral head. Several variations of increased acetabular overhang that may create pincer impingement have been described. The presence of an excessively deep acetabular fossa creates a condition of general overcoverage (coxa profunda). Coxa profunda has been debated as an underlying mechanism for pincer FAI, with no definitive agreement on the presence or strength of the relationship.[31,32] Another condition that results in general overcoverage of the femoral head is acetabular protrusio (protrusio acetabuli, acetabular protrusion). Acetabular protrusio occurs when the femoral head is abnormally located toward the midline of the body secondary to medial displacement of the acetabular wall. In comparison with coxa profunda and acetabular protrusion, a retroverted acetabulum may result in focal anterior overcoverage of the femoral head. Coxa profunda, acetabular protrusion, and acetabular retroversion may occur in combination with each other. The osseous characteristics associated with pincer impingement have been reported to be more prevalent in female patients.[33] The relationship of pincer FAI and chondral damage has not been as strongly established when compared with the relationship of cam FAI and cartilage injuries.[34]

Plain radiograph imaging is useful for identifying osseous abnormalities associated with pincer FAI. Measurements that can be used to identify the presence of general acetabular overcoverage include the lateral center edge angle (LCEA) and the Tönnis angle (also reported at the acetabular index). The LCEA and the Tönnis angle are measured on AP radiographs of the pelvis with the hip positioned in 20 degrees of hip internal rotation.[20] The LCEA and Tönnis angle are

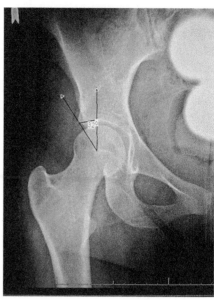

• **Figure 4-4** Lateral Center Edge Angle (LCEA). The LCEA is measured on an anteroposterior radiograph by drawing a vertical line down through the center of the femoral head and a second line from the center of the femoral head to the edge of the acetabulum. An LCEA of 33 degrees is considered normal.

radiographic indices that are routinely used to examine characteristics of the acetabular roof and the amount of coverage provided by the femoral head.[20] The LCEA is a measurement of the amount of coverage afforded to the femoral head by the acetabulum. This angle is measured on an AP radiograph by drawing a vertical line down through the center of the femoral head and a second line from the center of the femoral head to the edge of the acetabulum (Fig. 4-4).[20] Normal LCEA values vary by reference, but typically they are listed between 25 and 40 degrees. A measurement greater than 40 degrees is considered excessive and is associated with coxa profunda. In a study of 55 patients undergoing surgical treatment for FAI, Kutty and colleagues[35] found 81% sensitivity and 100% specificity values for using the 40-degree threshold to determine acetabular overcoverage and pincer FAI. The ratio of the femoral head not covered by the acetabulum is termed the Tönnis angle.[36] This measurement is used to assess the acetabular roof in the coronal plane.[20] A normal Tönnis angle is between 0 and 10 degrees. A Tönnis angle less than 0 degrees is associated with pincer FAI.[37] The literature evaluating the reliability of the Tönnis angle when used to diagnose FAI is scant.

Focal anterior superior overcoverage associated with acetabular retroversion can be identified on plain radiographs by the presence of a crossover sign.[38] The crossover sign is assessed using an AP radiograph. The position of the anterior and posterior walls is evaluated. If the acetabulum is positioned normally, the line formed by the anterior wall remains medial to the line formed by the posterior wall. When the acetabulum is in a retroverted position, the lines representing the anterior and posterior walls cross to

TABLE 4-1	Radiograph Findings Associated With Femoral Acetabular Impingement			
FAI Variation:	**Pistol Grip Deformity**	**Alpha Angle**	**Lateral Center Edge Angle**	**Crossover Sign**
Cam	Present	>50-60 degrees	Normal	Normal
Pincer	Normal	Normal	>40 degrees (coxa profunda)	Present (acetabular retroversion)
Mixed	Present	Present	Variable	Variable

FAI, Femoral acetabular impingement.

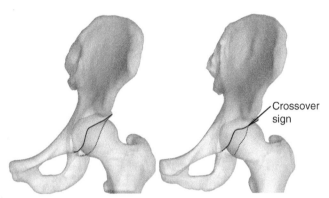

Crossover sign

• **Figure 4-5** Normal acetabular position (*right*) compared with a retroverted position (*left*) as indicated by a crossover sign. (From Henak CR, Carruth ED, Anderson AE, et al. Finite element predictions of cartilage contact mechanics in hips with retroverted acetabula. *Osteoarthritis Cartilage.* 2013;21(10):1522-1529.)

form an "X" pattern. Figure 4-5 displays normal acetabular position and retroversion as indicated by a crossover sign. The validity and reliability of the crossover sign in diagnosing pincer FAI have not been agreed on in the literature. In a study of 43 pelvis samples from cadavers, Jamali and associates[39] found the crossover sign to be 96% sensitive and 95% specific in determining pincer FAI. Conversely, Zaltz and colleagues[40] found that 19 of 38 subjects identified with a crossover sign on plain radiographs did not have overcoverage of the acetabulum when examined with CT scanning.

As with the case of cam FAI, other modalities such as MRI, CT, diagnostic ultrasound, and bone scan may be used on selected occasions. The applications of such modalities follow the same logic as with cam FAI cases. These imaging methods are reserved for when atypical information is required or for presurgical planning for difficult cases.

Mixed Impingement

Although FAI is commonly described as resulting from a cam or pincer deformity, most patients diagnosed with FAI have a combination of both forms of morphology. This is referred to as mixed pincer and cam impingement.[41] Beck and associates[9] reported that 86% of patients with FAI

present with a combination of both forms of impingement, with only 14% presenting with pure cam or pincer impingement. The literature examining the reliability of specific radiographic measurements and mixed-type FAI is minimal.

It is important for clinicians to remember that symptomatic FAI is the product of both anatomic variations and patient-specific activity patterns. Patients with FAI characteristics who do not participate in activities requiring significant ROM in specific planes or who do not participate in repetitive activity may not become symptomatic.[42] Although radiographic evidence of FAI is a useful tool in diagnosis and treatment, other sources of pain in the hip region must be considered and appropriately included or eliminated through the process of structured, thorough clinical evaluation of the patient. Table 4-1 summarizes the radiograph findings associated with FAI.

Joint Hypermobility and Instability

Joint hypermobility of the hip has been described as a risk factor for musculoskeletal pain, especially at regions that tend to be exposed to higher mechanical forces (anterior capsule and labrum).[43] Generalized capsular hyperlaxity and focal hypermobility have been associated with the development of acetabular labral tears.[43,44] Global ligamentous hyperlaxity associated with connective tissue disorders, such as Ehlers-Danlos disease, Down syndrome, and Marfan syndrome, has also been described as a significant risk factor for the development of acetabular labral tears.[45] The Beighton score has been described as a method of identifying joint global hyperlaxity in patients (see Chapter 2).

Focal hypermobility of the hip joint most commonly manifests as anterior capsular hyperlaxity associated with repetitive and forceful activities that place the hip joint at end-range hip external rotation or extension, thus possibly compromising the integrity of the capsular tissue in this region, as well as creating attenuation of the iliofemoral ligament.[12] If the iliofemoral ligament's ability to restrict excessive motion is compromised, the labrum may be exposed to increased stress that raises the risk of structural failure and injury.[46] Athletes such as dancers and gymnasts who participate in activities requiring repetitive and forceful hip and pelvic rotation have been noted to develop focal anterior laxity.[43,47] This topic is further discussed in Chapter 8.

Several bony abnormalities occurring at the hip joint may contribute to instability or hypermobility. Insufficient coverage of the femoral head by the acetabulum or excessive inclination of the acetabulum has been described as potentially affecting the stability of the hip joint. Various imaging studies may be used in determining the possible contribution of osseous anatomy to symptoms in patients with hip pain secondary to joint hypermobility.

Plain film radiographs are commonly implemented early during the evaluation process for patients with hip pain, to aid in the differential diagnosis and identify the presence of pathologic bony anatomy features associated with instability of the joint. The previously described LCEA and Tönnis angle measurements are useful in identifying the insufficient coverage of the femoral head that is often associated with hip joint dysplasia. Hips with LCEA measurements less than 25 degrees are considered to be dysplastic.[26] Hips with a Tönnis angle greater than 10 degrees are considered to be at risk for structural instability.[26,36] Patients with acquired focal hypermobility of the hip joint may have no associated bony abnormalities, and therefore plain radiographic imaging findings may be normal for these patients.

Cartilage Lesions of the Hip Joint

The degree and specific pattern of cartilage damage associated with FAI or hypermobility and acetabular labral tears may be of clinical interest, particularly when considering the prognosis of patients with these disorders. Beck and colleagues[9] studied 302 hips to determine whether specific anatomic variations affected the pattern of labral damage and cartilage degeneration. These investigators noted distinct differences in cartilage wear patterns when comparing the conditions of cam and pincer impingement. They observed that cam impingement was associated with focal anterior superior chondral damage that occurred as a result of separation of the cartilage from the labrum in a shearing manner. In contrast, pincer impingement was associated with more circumferential cartilage damage around the acetabulum. These investigators concluded that with pincer impingement, the labrum is crushed between the femoral neck and the acetabular rim, often leading to ossification of the labrum. Isolated cam or pincer FAI was not commonly observed in isolation. The most common presentation was a mixed type of both entities. These variations of acetabular labrum lesions were suggested to result in different patterns of cartilage damage.

Summary

The acetabular labrum plays a significant role in normal hip function. Injury to the acetabular labrum has been associated with pain and dysfunction. Numerous factors may lead to the development of labral compromise. Variations in bony anatomy may lead to FAI or joint instability. Labral

tears have been associated with chondral damage. Cam and pincer FAI create distinct patterns of cartilage lesions. Identifying acetabular labral tears and associated conditions can be a challenging process. Successful diagnosis depends on an understanding of hip joint anatomy and structured clinical examination, and it may be assisted with the use of imaging modalities.

Differential Diagnosis of Related Conditions

The clinical evaluation of patients with suspected nonarthritic hip and groin pain is challenging because of numerous competing differential diagnoses that often produce overlapping symptom presentations.[45,48] Although a common clinical priority is differentiating among the various causes (musculoskeletal and nonmusculoskeletal) of hip pain, clinicians should consider the coexistence of multiple conditions in conjunction with a intraarticular disorder that may require specific intervention considerations to maximize the patient's rehabilitation potential. Several conditions examined in the literature may produce similar symptoms or complicate the presentation of patients with acetabular labral tears. Conditions that occur adjacent to the hip joint may refer pain or other symptoms to this region. Lumbar radiculopathy, pelvic floor dysfunction, and peripheral nerve entrapment should be considered or ruled out during the process of evaluating a patient with the presentation of localized hip joint involvement and other suspicious symptoms. The reader is encouraged to review Chapter 2.

The association of FAI with the clinical syndrome of athletic pubalgia has been described in the literature. Athletic pubalgia or sports hernia is an overuse syndrome that has been observed to be more prevalent in patients with FAI. Controversy remains regarding the specific anatomic structure responsible for pain and symptoms experienced in this population. However, it is generally accepted that the spectrum of athletic pubalgia injuries are the result of compromise of the musculature and or fascial attachments to the anterior pubis that leads to weakening of the abdominal or posterior inguinal wall.[49] Hammoud and associates[50] examined 38 consecutive professional athletes for an association of FAI and athletic pubalgia in a retrospective case series. These investigators found that 32% of the athletes who underwent arthroscopy to address FAI had undergone surgical procedures to address athletic pubalgia in the past. Additionally, 39% of patients reported relief of athletic pubalgia symptoms with surgical procedures to address FAI alone.

FAI has been associated with decreased hip and pelvic ROM.[51,52] The limited ROM associated with FAI may contribute to soft tissue injuries of the hip resulting from the increased strain experienced by these structures during repetitive physical activities.[50] Investigators have suggested that decreased hip ROM predisposes athletes to injury secondary to the resulting compensatory pelvic motion or trunk hyperextension during sport-specific movements.[53,54] Birmingham and colleagues[55] examined the effects of simulated cam FAI on pubic symphysis movement in cadaver hips. Transverse plane ROM was measured at the pubic symphysis. The investigators noted a significant increase in internal rotation motion at the pubic symphysis in the cam FAI group. The clinical diagnosis of athletic pubalgia is a process of exclusion. The reader is encouraged to review Chapter 5.

An emerging body of literature has identified extraarticular causes of hip impingement that are associated with patients who have poor outcomes after intraarticular surgical procedures. The types of extraarticular causes of impingement may include central iliopsoas impingement, subspine impingement, and ischiofemoral impingement. Central iliopsoas impingement is a source of anterior hip pain and has been linked to acetabular labral tears. This type of impingement causes a distinct pattern of anterior labral damage that does not extend into the anterosuperior portion of the labrum (e.g., 1- to 2-o'clock position). The damage often occurs directly adjacent to the iliopsoas tendon at the 2- to 3-o'clock position of the anterior labrum, is often confirmed via MRA, and is often treated with a surgical release of the tendon.[55a] It has been postulated that the impingement may be caused by one of two mechanisms: (1) a repetitive traction injury by the iliopsoas tendon that is scarred on adherence to the capsule-labrum complex of the hip or (2) a tight or inflamed iliopsoas tendon that causes impingement during hip extension.[56] Subspine impingement is caused by a prominent anterior inferior iliac spine (AIIS) abnormally contacting the distal femoral neck during hip flexion.[57] This may be caused by excessive muscular activity of the rectus femoris during repetitive knee flexion with hip extension, resulting in an avulsion injury of the AIIS. This repetitive traction injury is common in running sports and in sports such as soccer that involve rapid high-energy kicking.[57] Upon healing, this often results in an enlarged bony protrusion at the AIIS that abnormally abuts the femoral neck during movements into hip flexion.[56] Subspine impingement has been related to CAM-type FAI and may be corrected surgically.[56] Ischiofemoral impingement is characterized by a narrowed space between the ischial tuberosity and the lesser trochanter, resulting in repetitive pinching of the quadratus femoris muscle.[57-57b] The impingement has been reported to be mainly congenital but may also be acquired from a hip fracture or superior medial migration of the hip joint as seen with OA.[56] Other forms of atypical hip impingement include greater trochanteric/pelvic impingement, abnormal femoral antetorsion, abnormal pelvic and acetabular tilt, and extreme hip motions.[56-57]

The presence of radicular symptoms originating from lumbar or sacral regions may make the evaluation and treatment of patients with FAI and acetabular labral tears more difficult. Referred pain from the lower lumbar or sacral nerve roots typically causes symptoms in the gluteal region or posterior thigh. Fortunately, the referral patterns extend distal to the gluteal and posterior thigh as well, thus enabling the clinician to recognize the radicular presentation. Upper lumbar nerve roots may produce anterior thigh and groin pain and should be assessed through appropriate neurologic screening tests during the clinical examination.[58] A complete discussion of nerve root patterns may be found in Chapter 10. Pudendal neuropathy is typically produced from compression and may manifest as groin pain and parasthesia.[58] Pudendal neurapraxia has been reported in patients undergoing hip arthroscopy.[58a] Postoperative pudendal neurapraxia is typically a transient event.[10] Obturator nerve entrapment may also produce exertional groin pain and adductor muscle weakness. Obturator nerve entrapment has been associated with significant adductor muscular development in athletes. Bradshaw and associates[58b] conducted a case series investigation that described 32 cases of athletes presenting with exercise-induced medial thigh pain secondary to fascial entrapment of the obturator nerve. Lateral femoral cutaneous nerve involvement (meralgia paresthetica) is generally not challenging to differentiate from a mechanical hip disorder. Symptoms are sensory related (anterior and lateral thigh), with no motor changes. The surgical procedure during hip arthroscopy or hip replacement by the anterior approach may contribute to the development of this condition. In a review of the literature, Cheatham and colleagues[59] discussed other orthopedic surgical procedures involving the hip, spine, or pelvis as potential causes of iatrogenic meralgia paresthetica. When evaluating patients who present with nonmechanical signs or symptoms or vague clinical examination results, neurologic influences should be considered. This rationale should be employed in both conservative treatment and postoperative settings.

Clinical Examination

A detailed and structured approach to clinical examination is imperative in implicating acetabular labral tears and associated conditions as the primary cause of a patient's symptoms occurring in the hip region. The reader is directed to Chapter 2 for a comprehensive description of this approach. An outline describing the approach for clinical evaluation of patients from the labral tear and FAI population, as described in this section, is contained in Box 4-1.

Demographics and Patient Interview

Basic demographic information helps clinicians determine whether a patient falls into the typical age range for acetabular labral tear and FAI. As previously mentioned, these conditions typically occur in the younger population. In relatively older individuals, OA of the hip may become a more likely primary diagnosis. Persons older than 50 years of age with hip pain of gradual onset have a higher likelihood of hip OA.[60]

Although traumatic injury is a possible cause of acetabular labral tears, most often the onset is gradual, and the tears

• BOX 4-1 **Clinical Examination Approach for Patients With Suspected Acetabular Labral Tears or Associated Conditions**

History (Through Self-Report Questionnaire and Interview)

- Demographics: age, gender, living situation, and so forth
- Onset
  - Traumatic
  - Gradual
- Symptom description or chief complaint
  - Pain
  - Stiffness
  - Paresthesia
  - Burning or shooting
  - Locking or catching
  - Weakness
  - Subjective feeling of instability
- Symptom location
- Anterior or groin*
- Medial thigh or adductor region
  - Lateral thigh or greater trochanter region*
  - Buttock or gluteal region
- Functional limitations
  - Activities of daily living
  - Labor- or sport-specific
- Prior injury
  - Hip or other lower extremity joints
    - Nature of previous injury and description of symptoms
    - Previous treatment and reported effectiveness
  - Previous low back injury
  - Previous surgical procedure
- Childhood disorders
  - Legg-Calvé-Perthes disease
  - Slipped capital epiphysis
  - Congenital dysplasia
- Other significant past medical history

Physical Examination: Observation and Inspection

- Static observation
  - Lower extremity alignment
    - Knee (valgus, varus, patellar position), foot position
    - Lumbar spine (increased or decreased lordosis)
    - Indicators of leg-length discrepancy

- Pelvic landmarks: palpate ASIS, PSIS, iliac crests
- Muscle atrophy
- Gait observation

Selective Tissue Tension Testing

- Range of motion testing
  - Active
  - Passive
  - Resisted
    - General muscle groups of hip and pelvis
    - Specific muscles

Palpation of Anatomic Landmarks

- Anterior region: ASIS, femoral triangle and contents
- Lateral region: greater trochanter, bursae and proximal iliotibial band region, gluteus medius muscle belly
- Posterior region: PSIS, ischial tuberosity, sciatic nerve

Flexibility

- Thomas test/modified Thomas test
- Ober test
- Hamstring length
- Adductor group

Clinical Tests

- FABER test
- Impingement test (FADIR)
- Log roll test (anterior laxity)
- Resisted straight leg raise test
- Scour test
- Craig test (femoral anteversion)

Accessory Motion and Joint Mobility Testing

- Joint distraction assessment

Determination of Leg-Length Discrepancy

- Weight bearing
- Non–weight bearing

ASIS, Anterior inferior iliac spine; *FABER,* flexion abduction external rotation; *FADIR,* flexion adduction internal rotation; *PSIS,* posterior inferior iliac spine.
*Presence of "C-sign"?

---

result from an associated underlying condition (FAI or hypermobility).[12] When injury is traumatic, it is often associated with a mechanism of sudden twisting or pivoting.[45] Hyperflexion or forced squatting positions have also been associated with labral injury.[61] Persons who participate in activities that require repetitive movements into positions of end-range extension, flexion, or internal rotation that potentially create impingement or excessive stress on the passive stabilizers of the hip joint may be at higher risk to develop acetabular labral tears. Specific sporting activities that have been associated with the development of acetabular labral tears include golf, soccer, ice hockey, running, and dancing.[62,63]

The patient's description of symptoms may be beneficial when attempting to determine whether an acetabular tear is the primary cause of a patient's hip pain. Pain is the most common complaint and may be described as sharp or aching.[37] The primary location of pain is typically the groin region, but pain may also occur in the lateral thigh region.[46,64] The presence of deep pain in a distribution that the patient can demonstrate by cupping the hand above the greater trochanter is often reported as the "C-sign" (Fig. 4-6), indicative of potential intraarticular pain.[65] This should not be confused with superficial palpable pain that is often noted with tensor fasciae latae tendinitis, proximal iliotibial band (ITB) irritation, or trochanteric bursitis. Mechanical symptoms such as clicking, popping, or catching may be noted with acetabular tears.[29,66] However, extraarticular conditions such as a snapping iliopsoas tendon or ITB may also cause audible symptoms[67] (see Chapter 3).

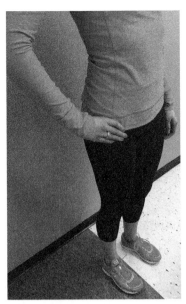

• **Figure 4-6** C-Sign of the Hip. The hand is cupped around the anterolateral region of the thigh.

Symptoms that occur in atypical locations or are described with a quality different from pain should cue the clinician to consider alternate or significant concurrent conditions. The complaint of stiffness, particularly when occurring in the morning, is often associated with hip OA.[60] Reports of paresthesia, burning, or radiating pain may indicate peripheral nerve involvement or involvement of the lumbosacral spine complex (e.g., meralgia paresthetica). Pain may also occur at the tendinous insertions of the pelvis (anterior superior iliac spine, posterior superior iliac spine, ischial tuberosity). Gluteal region pain may indicate lumbar or sacral spine involvement. Pain in adjacent regions, such as the knee and lumbopelvic areas, should be noted because these areas may be involved as part of the cause or result of underlying injury mechanisms.[68]

Physical Examination

Basic principles of structured musculoskeletal examination should be followed when evaluating a patient with symptoms that are expected to originate from involvement of the acetabular labrum and associated hip disorders.[45] Assessment of lower extremity alignment, posture, gait, active range of motion (AROM) and passive range of motion (PROM), flexibility, strength, and joint mobility helps the clinician determine the contribution of various structures in proximity to the hip joint.

Posture Assessment

Static and postural observation may yield findings that predispose a patient with FAI to become symptomatic. An exaggerated valgus position of the knee may predispose the hip to move into excessive adduction and internal rotation with weight-bearing activities. This motion may contribute to the symptomatic presentation of patients with FAI.[69]

Austin and associates[69] described controlling excessive hip adduction and internal rotation as an effective method to decrease symptoms of a patient with FAI. Pelvic position in the sagittal plane and the associated lumbar spine position should be noted. Of particular concern are exaggerated anterior pelvic tilt and concurrent increased lumbar lordosis. Ross and colleagues[70] found that dynamic anterior pelvic tilt results in an earlier occurrence of FAI through movement of the hip in flexion and internal rotation. If this postural tendency is noted, further investigation to determine the underlying causes and whether they are treatable is warranted.

Gait Observation

Although no specific gait pattern is associated with FAI or acetabular labral tears, gait examination can be used to determine the effect of impairments on function.[20] If gait deviations are noted, further examination should be performed to determine responsible impairments. Lewis and Sahrmann[71] observed that patients who ambulate with anterior hip pain often tend to ambulate with a swayback posture (posterior displacement of upper torso and anterior displacement of the pelvis) and symptomatically improve when posture is corrected to a more normal position. These investigators examined 15 healthy persons walking with 3 postural variations (normal, swayback, and forward flexed). Those persons walking with a swayback posture demonstrated higher peak hip extension angles, hip flexor moments, and hip flexion angular impulse when compared with subjects walking with a normal posture.[71] Tendencies of the pelvis to drop excessively into adduction or internal rotation in stance phase should be recognized. As previously mentioned, this pattern of movement has been associated with symptomatic FAI.[69] Decreased peak angles of adduction, extension, and internal rotation have been reported in patients with symptomatic FAI.[72] The clinician should note any abnormalities with gait such as an abductor-deficient pattern, asymmetrical step lengths, or excessive foot internal or external rotation during limb advancement.[73] Additionally, the occurrence of abnormal or excessive movements at the lumbopelvic complex to compensate for insufficient or painful hip motion should be noted.

Functional Testing

In addition to gait, the clinician should observe the patient during performance of basic functional movements and assess the presence of pain or compensatory movement patterns. The use of total body functional movement assessment is recommended to assist in the identification of regional impairments local to and distal to the symptomatic region that may be contributing to symptoms.[74] An example of one such tool is the Selective Functional Movement Assessment. Whether a formal functional movement assessment tool is used or not, important information can be gained from assessing movements such as gait, sit to stands or squats, and step-downs. These basic movement patterns can be assessed in any clinic setting with minimal

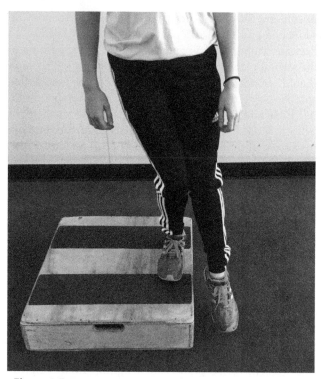

• **Figure 4-7** The patient demonstrates valgus collapse (excessive hip adduction and internal rotation) during a "step-down" maneuver, indicating weak hip abductors and external rotators.

equipment and can provide additional information to the basic orthopedic examination. Sit to stand and squatting are basic activities of daily living (ADLs) repeated often throughout the day. This movement pattern should be assessed to identify any pain provocation or deviations, because a typical sit to stand transfer requires approximately 105 degrees of hip flexion.[75] Figure 4-7 demonstrates weakness of the hip abductors and external rotators resulting in valgus collapse of the lower extremity during a "step-down" maneuver.

Range-of-Motion Testing

Selective tissue tension testing should be used to differentiate deficits in PROM, AROM, and muscle strength. When assessing PROM, the quality of end feel should be examined to determine any observed limitations that are caused by insufficient muscle length, capsular restriction, or bony block or derangement. A marked loss of internal rotation (<15 degrees), particularly in the relatively older population, may indicate the presence of degenerative changes within the hip joint.[76] When AROM values are markedly less than PROM values, a strength deficit should be suspected. The results of selective tissue tension testing may be particularly useful in guiding treatment.

Strength Assessment

Strength assessment in all planes of motion should be included in the standard examination of any patient whose

symptoms may be secondary to an acetabular labral tear or associated condition of the hip joint. Although evaluation in all planes of movement should be performed, clinicians should note that specific patterns of weakness have been described in patients with nonarthritic pain.[77,78] Harris-Hayes and associates[77] compared hip muscle strength differences in 35 younger adults (18 to 40 years old) with chronic hip joint pain against 35 asymptomatic matched controls. The controls were matched by sex, age within 5 years, body mass index, and limb side. Diagnoses of the test group included cam FAI, pincer FAI, structural instability, and hip pain without notable radiographic findings for bony abnormalities. The investigators found that when compared with controls, the patients with chronic hip pain did exhibit weakness of the hip abductor and external rotator muscles groups. Furthermore, a trend of weakness of the uninvolved hip for the group with chronic hip pain was also identified. Casartelli and colleagues[79] found that patients ($n = 15$) with symptomatic FAI produced less peak hip flexor torque when compared with healthy controls ($n = 15$). This finding was consistent in both isometric and isokinetic conditions. However, when analyzing electromyography (EMG) data, the investigators found that fatigability of the hip flexor muscle groups was not more pronounced when compared with controls. Weakness of hip adductors in patients with FAI has also been described.[78]

Lumbopelvic strength should also be considered during the evaluation process of patients with suspected acetabular labral tears. Although many differences exist in functional anatomy and pathologic process, an analogy can be made to the well-established concept of proximal stabilization that is often employed when evaluating patients with suspected pathologic conditions of the shoulder joint complex. Much like the scapular complex, the lumbopelvic complex must maintain appropriate stabilization to provide a solid foundation for use of the peripheral joints. The lower abdominal muscles may be of particular interest because of their role in controlling dynamic anterior pelvic tilt. As previously mentioned, the presence of dynamic anterior pelvic tilt has been correlated with FAI occurring earlier in the motions of flexion and internal rotation.[70] Deficient lumbopelvic control may contribute to the development of lumbopelvic instability and sacroiliac joint disorders, which are commonly observed in conjunction with FAI and labral tears.

Muscle Length Assessment

A flexibility assessment of the hip and pelvic musculature should be performed to identify any muscle length impairments that may be contributing to abnormal movement patterns that increase the risk of symptoms in patients with labral tears of the hip. A differential diagnosis to consider when evaluating patients suspected of having intraarticular hip dysfunctions is the involvement of hip and pelvic musculotendinous structures.[12,45] The iliopsoas muscle complex should be of particular interest. Damage to the labrum caused by excessive iliopsoas friction and even cases of iliopsoas impingement have been described in the literature.[80] Internal coxa saltans (snapping hip) may be caused by snapping of the iliopsoas tendon across the anterior femoral head or joint capsule.[81] The Thomas test can be used to evaluate flexibility of the iliopsoas complex and ITB complex.[20] Lateral hip pain is often associated with trochanteric bursitis or proximal ITB inflammation. The Ober test can also be used to evaluate flexibility of the ITB complex.[20]

Joint Mobility Testing

Joint mobility testing may be useful in determining whether capsular mobility deficits are present in patients with acetabular labral tears. This determination may be particularly useful in patients with symptoms related to FAI. As discussed, FAI may be part of the degenerative process eventually leading to OA of the hip joint.[6,82] The benefits of joint mobilization have been reported in patients with hip OA.[83] Decreased joint mobility or pain relief with accessory motion testing is often considered an indication for the use of joint mobilization techniques. Because of the variable but relatively small amount of translational movement that occurs at the hip joint,[84] joint mobility may best be assessed through long-axis distraction. Given that current clinical practice guidelines recommend manual therapy as a potential intervention option for patients with nonarthritic hip pain, joint mobility testing should be considered as part of clinicians' examination methodology.[12]

Clinical Tests

Certain clinical tests have been described as useful in diagnosing acetabular tears or the underlying conditions associated with tears. Clinicians should have an understanding of which clinical tests are supported by the evidence in patients with nonarthritic hip pain. If a patient is younger, is involved in cutting or pivoting sports, and is found to have positive findings on a cluster of the following tests, the clinician should suspect the presence of an acetabular labral tear or an intraarticular disorder.[45]

Flexion Abduction External Rotation Test

The flexion abduction external rotation (FABER), or Patrick test, is intended to indicate the irritability of the hip joint in relation to passive movement (Fig. 4-8). The test can also serve as a general indicator of hip joint mobility. The FABER test may elicit pain in various regions (anterior, lateral, and posterior), and it may symptomatically implicate structures other than the hip joint, such as the sacroiliac joint when the test causes symptoms in the sacroiliac joint region.

Procedure

The patient assumes the supine position. The heel of the patient's test extremity is placed above the opposite knee, thus allowing that hip to be in a flexed, abducted, and externally rotated position. The pelvis is stabilized at the anterior superior iliac spine of the contralateral side. Instruct

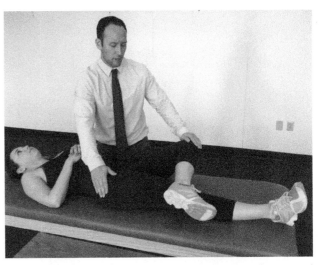

• **Figure 4-8** The patient is placed in the flexion abduction external rotation (FABER) test position. Groin pain is associated with a potential hip joint disorder.

the patient to indicate whether symptoms are provoked by the assumed position. General mobility can be estimated by measuring the distance from the lateral knee of the test leg to the treatment surface. If tolerated, overpressure can be placed at the medial surface of the knee toward the treatment surface. This additional pressure may elicit symptoms when passive stabilizers of the joint are loaded in this end-range position.

Interpretation

Pain (groin, lateral hip region, buttock) that resembles the patient's primary symptoms is considered a positive finding, although identification of a specific pain generator with this test is difficult. The location of symptoms produced during this test must be considered when attempting to differentiate between hip joint involvement (typically groin pain) and sacroiliac joint dysfunction (often buttock pain).[65] Differences in general hip mobility between the involved and noninvolved extremity should also be noted.

The studies examining diagnostic accuracy of the FABER test are inconsistent in regard to condition specificity, study methods, and overall quality.[20,85] The FABER test has a reported sensitivity range of 57% to 100% and a specificity range of 25% to 100% when used to identify intraarticular disorders.[85,86] Martin and Sekiya[87] reported a positive likelihood ratio of 0.73 (95% confidence interval [CI]: 0.41, 0.77) and a negative likelihood ration of 2.2 (95% CI: 0.8, 6).

Flexion Adduction Internal Rotation Test

The flexion adduction internal rotation (FADIR) test is intended to identify symptomatic anterior impingement occurring at the hip joint (Fig. 4-9). The patient is placed in a position associated with anterior hip joint impingement, and symptom reproduction is monitored. It is suggested that patients with acetabular labral tears secondary to FAI often report pain with this test.

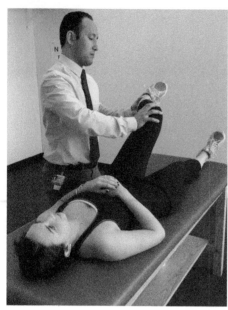

• **Figure 4-9** The patient is placed in the flexion adduction internal rotation (FADIR) test position. Complaints of groin pain are associated with symptomatic femoral acetabular impingement.

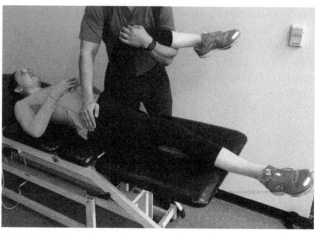

• **Figure 4-10** Internal Rotation and Over Pressure (IROP) Test. The patient is placed in 90 degrees of flexion and end-range internal rotation. A posteriorly directed force is placed through the femur. Reproduction of pain (typically in the groin) indicates an intraarticular hip disorder.

Procedure

The patient assumes the supine position. The symptomatic hip and knee are passively flexed to 90 degrees. The hip is then passively internally rotated and horizontally adducted to the end ROM. Instruct the patient to note provocation of symptoms during performance of the test.

Interpretation

Pain (typically in the groin region) that reproduces the patient's primary symptoms is considered a positive finding. Clinicians should exert caution when interpreting pain that occurs in areas other than the groin region. Tension or pressure placed across soft tissues (muscle, tendons, bursae) may elicit pain in other areas around the hip region.

When attempting to identify acetabular labral tears or other symptomatic intraarticular disorders, the FADIR test has a reported sensitivity range of 75% to 100%, and specificity range of 10% to 100%.[11,87,88] In a systematic review, Reiman and associates[88] reported a negative likelihood ratio range from 0.04 to 2.2 and a positive likelihood ratio range from 0.86 to 2.4.

Internal Rotation Over Pressure Test

The internal rotation over pressure (IROP) test is intended to identify symptomatic hip joint disorders (Fig. 4-10). The patient is placed in a position associated with anterior hip joint impingement; anterior-to-posterior pressure is then applied through the femur, and symptom reproduction is monitored. It is suggested that patients with acetabular labral tears and other intraarticular disorders often report pain with this test.

Procedure

The patient assumes the supine position. The test hip and knee are passively flexed to 90 degrees. The hip is then passively internally rotated to the end ROM. Posterior pressure is then applied through the axis of the femur. The patient is instructed to note provocation of symptoms during performance of the test.

Interpretation

Pain (typically in the groin region) that resembles the patient's primary symptoms is considered a positive finding.[86] Clinicians should exert caution when interpreting pain that occurs in areas other than the groin region. Tension or pressure placed across soft tissues (muscle, tendons, bursae) may elicit pain in other areas around the hip region.

A small body literature has examined the IROP test. Maslowski and colleagues[86] found sensitivity and specificity to be 0.91 (95% CI: 0.68, 0.99) and 0.18 (95% CI: 0.05, 0.40), respectively. Additionally, these investigators calculated a negative predictive value of 0.17 (95% CI: 0.04, 0.40) and positive predictive value of 0.88 (95% CI: 0.67, 0.98).[86]

Log Roll Test

The log roll test is intended to identify anterior capsular-ligamentous hyperlaxity of the hip joint (Fig. 4-11).[12] Additionally, this test has been described as a method of assessing symptoms of intraarticular disorders.[65]

Procedure

The patient assumes the supine position. The examiner grasps the patient's thighs, and the hips are moved through passive internal and external rotation. After the maneuver

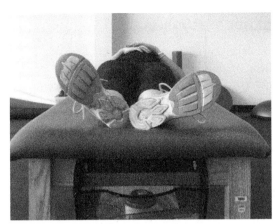

• **Figure 4-11** Positive Log Roll Test Result. After the hips are passively moved through internal and external rotation, the left foot is rotated further outward. This may indicate anterior laxity of the left hip joint.

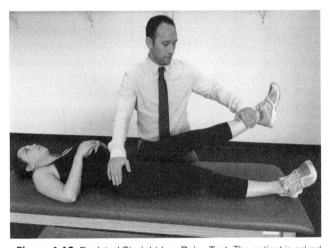

• **Figure 4-12** Resisted Straight Leg Raise Test. The patient is asked to perform a straight leg raise maneuver against resistance. Reproduction of groin pain may indicate irritability of the anterior hip capsule, acetabular labrum, or iliopsoas complex.

is performed several times, the hips are allowed to rest. The resting positions of the involved and noninvolved extremities are compared.

Interpretation
A notable increase of external rotation ROM in the involved hip is considered positive for hyperlaxity of the anterior capsular-ligamentous joint structures. Additionally, motion-induced pain in the groin or anterior lateral region of the thigh may indicate an associated intraarticular disorder of the hip joint. No diagnostic validity has been reported for the log roll test.[89]

Resisted Straight Leg Raise Test
The resisted straight leg raise test is intended to identify potential irritability of the anterior joint capsule or acetabular labrum (Fig. 4-12).[20] Isometric contraction of the iliopsoas muscle is thought to place tension through the tendon across these structures.

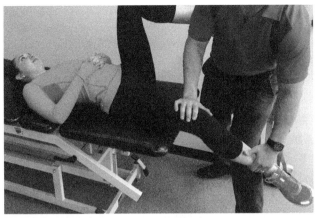

• **Figure 4-13** Posterior Rim Impingement Test. The patient is supine with the legs hanging freely. Both knees are drawn toward the chest, and the leg not being tested is stabilized by the patient. The clinician lowers the test hip into extension. Then the hip is passively abducted and externally rotated. Reproduction of posterior symptoms may indicate posterior hip impingement.

Procedure
The patient assumes the supine position. The test hip is actively flexed (knee remains extended) to approximately 30 degrees. The patient is instructed to maintain this movement as the examiner applies force into extension. The patient is instructed to note if groin pain is provoked by the test procedure.

Interpretation
The reproduction of groin pain when an extension force is applied to the patient's hip may indicate irritability of the anterior hip capsule, acetabular labrum, or iliopsoas complex.[86] Maslowski and associates[86] found a sensitivity of 0.59 (95% CI: 0.34, 0.82) and specificity of 0.32 (95% CI: 0.14, 0.55). They calculated a negative likelihood ratio of 1.28 and a positive likelihood ratio of 0.87.

Posterior Rim Impingement Test
The posterior rim impingement test is used to assess the congruence of the posterolateral aspect of the femoral neck and the posterior acetabular rim clinically (Fig. 4-13).[75]

Procedure
This test is performed by positioning the patient supine at the foot of the examination table and allowing the legs to hang freely at the hip. Instruct the patient to draw both knees up toward chest. While the patient holds the lower extremity not being examined in this flexed position, the clinician lowers the patient's opposite leg off of the table into a position of extension. From this position, the hip is abducted and externally rotated in an attempt to reproduce the patient's symptoms.[75]

Interpretation
Reproduction of the patient's posterior hip pain when the leg is taken through this arc of motion may indicate

posterior impingement between the posterior acetabular rim and the posterior aspect of the femoral head and neck. It has also been reported that if anterior pain is recreated in the position, it may indicate the presence of hip instability.[1,75] Data to evaluate the clinometric properties of this test are scant.

Clustering of Clinical Tests

A limited but growing body of research has examined the use of clinical tests in patients with nonarthritic hip pain. More recent studies have often focused on the use of clinical tests and the population of patients with FAI. Martin and Sekiya[87] conducted a study that examined the interrater reliability of the FABER test, FADIR test, log roll test, and greater trochanter palpation in patients with a mean age of 42 years (range, 18 to 76 years; SD, 15.4). These investigators found moderate to substantial agreement for all four tests. Acceptable reliability (moderate or greater as defined by a kappa coefficient >0.40) was found for the FABER test, log roll test, and tenderness with greater trochanter palpation. Kappa coefficients with 95% CIs were 0.63 (95% CI: 0.43 to 0.83) for the FABER test, 0.58 (95% CI: 0.29 to 0.87) for the FADIR test; 0.61 (95% CI: 0.41 to 0.81) for the log roll test, and 0.66 (95% CI: 0.48 to 0.84) for tenderness to palpation at the greater trochanter. All four tests demonstrated low bias index values (0.06 to 0.08). Higher bias index values can inflate the kappa coefficient. However, because of a high prevalence index (0.76) for FAI, the FADIR test was not considered reliable. A high prevalence index is correlated with an increased likelihood that the test result is positive by chance agreement.

Maslowski and colleagues[86] examined pain provocation maneuvers before and after diagnostic intraarticular injection to determine the validity of the tests in the diagnosis of intraarticular hip disorders. If pain decreased greater than or equal to 80% after the injection, the symptom was considered to originate from within the hip joint. They found the most sensitive tests to be the FABER test, with a sensitivity of 0.82 (95% CI: 0.57 to 0.96), and the IROP test, with a sensitivity of 0.91 (95% CI: 0.68 to 0.99). The IROP test is performed similarly to the FADIR test, with added posterior overpressure. None of the tests showed high specificity (e.g., most had many false-positive results), with the resisted straight leg raise showing the highest value of 0.32 (95% CI: 0.14 to 0.55). The tests with the highest positive predictive value were the IROP and FABER tests, with respective values of 0.47 (95% CI: 0.29 to 0.64) and 0.46 (95% CI: 0.28 to 0.65). The IROP demonstrated the highest negative predictive value of 0.71 (95% CI: 0.25 to 0.98). These tests seem to have the ability to identify pathologic processes when present; however, they also tend to be associated with a high false-positive rate. Thus, a complete examination offers the best clinical utility, with special tests reserved as a means of confirmation. The results of this study justify the use of these tests for purposes of screening, as opposed to confirming specific disorders.

Diagnostic Injection

The use of an image-guided injection consisting of a local anesthetic or steroid compound for diagnostic purposes is common practice when a labral tear or a disorder such as FAI is suspected.[20] A therapeutic effect may be derived from this procedure as well. The patient is instructed to rate the pain and record activities that provoke symptoms. After the injection is administered into the hip joint, the patient is asked again to rate the pain and attempt activities that were previously noted as symptomatic. A decrease of symptoms following the injection helps to confirm that the patient's symptoms originate from an intraarticular source. The commonly observed pattern of intraarticular involvement is a decrease of pain, followed by an eventual return of symptoms. The timeframe for pain relief from the local anesthetic when the hip joint is the source of symptoms is often between 3 and 4 hours.[90,91] Kivlan and associates[91] found that coexisting extraarticular disease did not affect the pain relief response derived from the injection when cartilage damage was present. These investigators reviewed 72 consecutive subjects undergoing hip arthroscopy and performed 3 analyses of covariance based on subdivisions of type of impingement, labral disease severity, and type of chondral disorder. The results indicated that there was no significant main effect on percentage of symptom relief of injection from the type of impingement or from the severity of labral disease. The type of chondral lesion was found to have a significant main effect on the percentage of symptom relief from injection ($P < 0.05$). The results indicated that patients with mild chondral disease of the acetabulum and those with acetabular delamination had significantly greater relief when compared with patients lacking chondral disorders.[91]

Early Intervention and Symptom Prevention for Femoral Acetabular Impingement

In rare cases in which a patient is known to have the anatomic features consistent with FAI (radiographic or clinical evidence) but is asymptomatic with ADLs or other physical activity, measures may be taken in an attempt to prevent the development of symptoms. As is the case with symptomatic FAI, advice and education regarding activity modification are indicated for patients with asymptomatic FAI. The education provided should be tailored to address the specific functional demands, impairments identified, and the pathologic characteristics of the patient.[12] It is recommended that a patient should avoid activities that place the hip joint in impingement positions that may eventually create pain or other associated symptoms. Specifically, movements that require end-range hip flexion, internal rotation, and adduction should be avoided or modified in patients with FAI to avoid potential mechanical force that could be placed on the acetabular labrum.[12,92] Patients with FAI should be educated to avoid deep squatting exercises.

Lamontagne and colleagues[51] found that patients with cam FAI demonstrated a significant decrease in maximal squat depth when compared with normal subjects.

Assessment of basic ADLs such as sitting, sit to stand transfers, ambulation, sleeping position, and stair negotiation should be performed for patients with known FAI anatomic characteristics. These positions and activities should be evaluated to determine whether the patient is able to perform these tasks without creating a predisposition to developing pain or symptoms.[12] If the alignment or movement pattern employed during these tasks is likely to contribute to pain or symptoms, instruction on activity modification should be provided as part of the preventive approach.[93]

In addition to ADLs, work-related or fitness and athletic activities should be evaluated and modified as necessary to limit movements that may become painful and increase the shear forces experienced at the hip joint. Ergonomic assessment and modification of a patient's work environment, such as raising office chair height to keep the hips flexed less than 90 degrees, may decrease the potential for creating joint irritation and pain in the presence of FAI. A comparable example of a fitness-related activity modification for this population would be to elevate the seat height on a stationary cycle to limit excessive hip flexion.[12] Recommendations may be made for these patients to avoid or appropriately modify any sport-specific movements that require repetitive or forceful end-range positions of the hip joint.

Rehabilitation Considerations for Nonsurgical Management of Symptomatic Femoral Acetabular Impingement

The initial management of symptomatic FAI should include a period of conservative management. A trial of conservative treatment spanning approximately 8 to 12 weeks has been suggested before surgical intervention is considered.[1,3,12] Conservative management often includes physical therapy intervention and antiinflammatory medications, and it may also include image-guided intraarticular injections.[12,94]

Patient Education

Similar to preventive management, education plays a significant role in the treatment of symptomatic FAI. The emphasis of conservative management should initially be placed on patient education and activity modification to decrease inflammation and pain resulting from excessive mechanical forces associated with the FAI condition. Postural education emphasizing the avoidance of excessive pelvic tilt and posterior placement of the torso in relation to the pelvis (swayback posture) may help minimize forces placed on the acetabular labrum and other anterior joint structures.[71,93] Patients should be advised to avoid performance of excessive or repetitive movement into deep hip flexion or internal rotation.[12] Active patients may have

to modify their exercise programs to achieve these modifications. Ergonomic recommendations such as adjusting a patient's office chair height may also be useful.

Treatment of the Acute Presentation

The goals of physical therapy during the acute phase of symptoms include alleviation of pain and gradual restoration of joint ROM and mobility. It is recommended that patients avoid any aggravating activities, especially those involving repetitive end-range movements, and take nonsteroidal antiinflammatory medications (as recommended or appropriately prescribed) during the acute phase.[20] Interventions included during this period consist of low-grade joint mobilization techniques and PROM. To improve ROM, the patient is encouraged to begin stationary cycling with minimal resistance with the seat set high enough to avoid painful hip flexion.[20] If available, it is recommended that an upright stationary bicycle be used rather than a recumbent bicycle, to limit the amount of hip flexion sufficiently during this early period of rehabilitation. The resistance level can gradually be progressed as tolerated by the patient. Theoretically, the inclusion of cold modalities or electrical stimulation for pain alleviation may be of some benefit during the initial stages of injury management.

Impairment-Based Interventions

As the acute presentation of inflammation and pain decreases, interventions should be progressed to include non–pain-provoking flexibility and strengthening exercises. The goal at this point in the rehabilitation process is to correct muscular imbalances or asymmetries throughout the lower extremities or lumbopelvic region.[95] A thorough evaluation should be completed to develop an individualized rehabilitation program to address any identified clinical impairments.

Muscle Flexibility Exercises

Stretching exercises should be prescribed with caution and only after muscle length testing and ROM end-feel assessment have been completed. Stretching exercises commonly target the piriformis, iliopsoas, quadriceps, and ITB.[20] The patient should be educated to avoid stretching at an excessive intensity or forcing the joint into an ROM that recreates intraarticular pain.

Hip Muscle Strengthening

Muscular strengthening exercises should be recommended to address strength deficits and imbalances throughout the involved lower extremity as indicated by clinical examination. The clinician should assess the patient's movement strategies and include additional strengthening exercises for weakness in regions or at joints away from the hip such as at the knee or ankle that may be contributing to abnormal movement patterns. Strength deficits of the contralateral limb should be addressed as well. Progressive

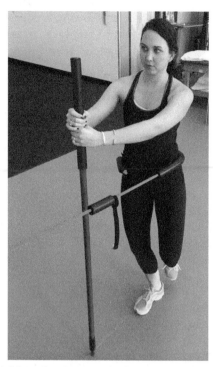

• **Figure 4-14** Weight-Bearing Hip External Rotation. The patient uses her external rotators to move the pelvis on the fixed femur while using her abductors to maintain frontal plane stability of the pelvis.

resistance exercises should initially be performed in hip mid-ROM positions that do not produce joint pain or other symptoms consistent with FAI. Strengthening exercises should be progressed as tolerated by the patient and should emphasize strengthening into all planes of movement. The strengthening program should specifically target the hip abductors, external rotators,[77] and core musculature.[20] These muscle groups play a crucial role in maintaining a level pelvis and preventing valgus collapse throughout the lower extremity during activities that involve maintaining a single leg stance position.[69,96] Additionally, exercises biasing the gluteus maximus should be included because the upper fibers of this muscle have been reported to assist in hip abduction. Weakness can therefore contribute to excessive adduction of the lower extremity.[69] Figure 4-14 demonstrates weight-bearing external rotation (pelvis moving on the fixed lower extremity) against resistance while maintaining frontal plane stability with the hip abductors.

Lumbopelvic Stabilization

Core muscle and lumbopelvic stabilization exercises should be considered as standard components in the conservative management of patients with symptomatic FAI. Poor lumbopelvic control in the sagittal plane, which can lead to excessive anterior pelvic tilt during functional movements, promotes a position of impingement at the hip and thus may produce inflammation and continued pain.[70] Core muscle retraining and stabilization exercises should be initiated at an intensity appropriate to the patient's strength and neuromuscular control level. Exercises should gradually be

progressed to more demanding exercises and positions only once correct completion of each task is demonstrated. These exercises should be initiated in a non–weight-bearing supine position and progressed to include more functional upright postures. It is recommended that stabilization exercises be performed in intermediate postures such as quadruped and half-kneeling before having patients in more functional upright positions. This enables the clinician to identify more easily any asymmetries or compensatory strategies used by the patient to complete exercises in standing or sport-specific postures.[54] As previously mentioned, the gluteus maximus contributes to dynamic control of the pelvis and lower extremity by limiting adduction of the lower extremity. Developing adequate strength throughout this muscle group is also important because of its role in controlling hip or trunk position in the sagittal plane and in force transfer from the lower extremities to the trunk.[97]

Neuromuscular Control Exercises

In addition to developing adequate strength throughout these aforementioned muscle groups, neuromuscular reeducation strategies may be useful in the conservative management of FAI. As previously stated, weakness of the hip abductors or external rotators can lead to abnormal movement patterns and excessive motion throughout the involved lower extremity. Decreased dynamic pelvic control and the related excessive motion in the frontal and transverse planes have been implicated as factors associated with the presence of pain symptoms in patients diagnosed with FAI.[69]

Joint Mobilization

A trial of manual therapy including joint mobilization may be beneficial for patients with symptomatic FAI. Indications for the use of joint mobilization techniques include the presence of hip pain and decreased PROM, coupled with a capsular end feel at end ROM.[12] Initially, techniques may include low-grade mobilization application in midrange positions that emphasize joint distraction techniques to achieve pain modulation (Fig. 4-15). In the absence of a bony end feel, joint mobilization can be progressed to include graded techniques at higher intensities closer to the end range of available motion. Caution should be applied when applying joint mobilization techniques in positions of end-range flexion or internal rotation to patients with FAI. As previously discussed, some patients with FAI may be progressing to the development of hip OA.[82] Current clinical practice guidelines recommend the use of manual therapy for patients with FAI and hip OA.[12,60]

Surgical Options for Femoral Acetabular Impingement and Acetabular Labral Tears

The advancement of surgical options for the younger, more active population with nonarthritic hip pain has been a rapidly growing interest in the fields of orthopedic and sports medicine. Improved understanding of hip joint

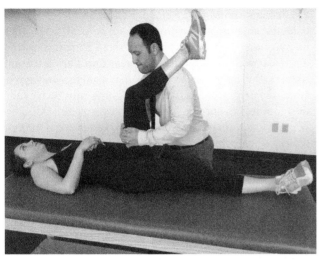

• **Figure 4-15** Lateral Distraction of the Hip Joint Performed at 90 Degrees of Hip Flexion.

function, better diagnostic methods, and less invasive means of surgical intervention have led to a rapidly growing number of patients undergoing procedures to address hip disorders.[1,10,48,98] Injuries to the acetabular labrum and associated conditions may be surgically addressed. Such conditions include acetabular labral tears, FAI, focal joint laxity, focal chondral lesions, torn ligamentum teres, and loose body removal.[1,20] Arthroscopy has been the most common surgical method used to address nonarthritic hip pain. Montgomery and associates[99] reported a 365% increase of hip arthroscopy procedures in the United States. This indicated an increased incidence rate of 1.2 cases per 10,000 in 2004 to 5.58 cases per 10,000 in 2009. A 600% increase of the procedure performed by surgeons who recently passed their certification examination series between 2006 and 2010 was reported.[98] Most procedures were performed on patients between 20 and 39 years of age, with no observed differences between female and male patients.[99] The initial focus of hip arthroscopy was to address acetabular labral lesions, with débridement being the most common procedure performed. However, with improved understanding of the disease spectrum and development of surgical techniques, the procedure has evolved to include addressing FAI or joint hyperlaxity as underlying causes of labral injury. Although not routinely used, open and mini-open procedures have been described and successfully used for FAI.[16,100]

The body of evidence supporting the efficacy of hip arthroscopy in addressing acetabular labral tears and associated conditions is relatively young but growing. Most recent studies tend to focus on surgery to address symptomatic FAI. Kemp and colleagues[101] conducted a systematic review investigating the outcomes after hip arthroscopy. Although these investigators found reports of significant pain relief and functional improvement up to 10 years after the surgical procedures, this trend could be confirmed only for up to 28 months in patients specifically undergoing osteoplasty (removal of excessive bone) to address FAI, secondary to limited follow-up time. Larson and Giveans[102] reported

significant improvement in outcomes measures in 75% of patients undergoing arthroscopy to address FAI at a minimum of 1-year follow-up. Age has been identified as a factor affecting patient-related outcomes after hip arthroscopy. Wilkin and associates[103] studied 41 hip arthroscopy patients who were older than 45 years of age. The investigators found that patients older than 45 years of age did not tend to show significant clinical improvement and experienced a higher reoperation rate (including conversion to total hip arthroplasty and resurfacing procedures) after undergoing arthroscopy for acetabular labral tear débridement. Often concurrent with age, the presence of arthritic changes within the hip joint has been associated with negative outcomes after hip arthroscopy.[104] Philippon and colleagues[105] reported that a preoperative joint space of 2 mm or less significantly increased the chance of an additional total hip arthroplasty procedure in patients undergoing hip arthroscopy. Ayeni and associates[106] conducted a systematic review examining the arthroscopic management of labral tears in patients with FAI. These investigators found that better clinical outcomes were reported for patients undergoing labral repair versus those undergoing débridement procedures.

A commonly stated goal of hip arthroscopy procedures is to decelerate the progression to hip OA and related total hip arthroplasty procedures. Bedi and colleagues[6] reported an increase of circulating biomarkers related to cartilage degradation and inflammation in athletes with FAI. Beck and associates[9] confirmed an increased risk of cartilage damage with the presence of FAI. However, beyond basic science studies and the aforementioned evidence supporting positive outcomes after hip arthroscopy, no definitive evidence supports the theory that arthroscopic hip procedures decrease the rate of hip OA progression.

Identifying Surgical Candidates

Identifying ideal surgical candidates for hip arthroscopy shares the same challenges as evaluating patients with nonarthritic pain in the hip region. Recognizing the primary source of a patient's symptoms is crucial in ensuring effective surgical treatment. Although guidelines to determining surgical candidates vary, common criteria often involve a combination of the patient's history and subjective reports, appropriate clinical examination findings, significant imaging results, and failure of conservative care. The criteria listed are discussed previously in this chapter. Diagnostic injection is often used to confirm that the patient's symptoms are intraarticular. If the patient sufficiently meets the diagnostic criteria for an intraarticular hip disorder and conservative care has failed, he or she may be considered an ideal surgical candidate.

Arthroscopic Procedures of the Hip Joint

Burman[107] first described hip arthroscopy for diagnostic purposes in 1931. Suzuki and colleagues[108] described a tear of the acetabular labrum in 1986. The earliest described and most commonly performed arthroscopic procedures for the hip joint were resection procedures for a torn acetabular labrum.[1,10] Formal arthroscopic approaches for this purposes were described in 1988 by Glick[109] (the lateral position) and in 1994 by Byrd[110] (the supine position). Early in the procedure's development, isolated resection of a labral tear was relatively common.[10,48] As the understanding of the etiology and underlying conditions related to the development of labral tears progressed, procedures evolved to include measures specifically directed to address these conditions (most commonly FAI).

Currently, hip arthroscopy is performed with the patient in either the supine or the lateral position.[10,109,110] The hip is placed under traction to allow adequate access to the intraarticular space; 8 to 10 mm of distraction is required to perform most procedures.[10] This typically requires 25 to 50 pounds of force.[10] If inadequate traction is provided, iatrogenic cartilage damage may occur as instrumentation is navigated in the joint space. Excessive traction may result in injury (often transient) of neurovascular structures around the proximal hip and perineum area.[10,111] Specialized flexible scope instrumentation is used to gain access to the joint through up to three portals: anterior, anterolateral, and posterolateral.[10,112] A capsulotomy is often performed to allow improved visualization of structures.

Although no consensus exists on repair of the capsule when a capsulotomy is performed, Frank and associates[113] reviewed 64 consecutive cases of arthroscopy to address FAI. Patients underwent either partial or complete repair after capsulotomy was performed as part of the arthroscopic procedure. The investigators found that patients undergoing complete capsular repair reported significantly better scores on the Hip Outcome Score (HOS) sport-specific subscale and had no incidences of revision (compared with 4 revision procedures for the partial repair group).[113]

Acetabular Labrum Resection and Repair Procedures

Typically, resection procedures have been most often performed on degenerative or fibrillated tears of the acetabular labrum.[1] The procedure can be compared to partial meniscectomy procedures of the knee, in which an attempt is made to débride and remove unstable tissue that is potentially affecting joint function, back to a stable base. When tissue is salvageable, labral resection has given way to labral repair procedures to maximize tissue preservation and optimize joint function.[114]

Procedures involving the repair of acetabular labral lesions have become more popular in recent times. Acute, longitudinal, or peripheral tears are most often amendable to surgical repair procedures.[115] The specific method of repair depends on the nature of injury. In cases in which the labrum is detached from the acetabular wall, bioabsorbable anchors may be used to fixate the torn portion back to the bony origin. Midsubstance tears can be repaired using bioabsorbable sutures.[112] Ayeni and colleagues[106] performed

a systematic review that yielded 6 studies for a total of 490 patients undergoing arthroscopy to address FAI. These investigators specifically compared those patients undergoing repair with those undergoing resection during the procedure. The investigators found that patients undergoing labral repair procedures reported significantly better function on region-specific outcome instruments (Modified Harris Hip, Non-arthritic Hip, HOS, and Merle d'Aubigne scores) when compared with patients undergoing débridement. Domb and associates[116] compared outcomes of patients undergoing labral reconstruction versus labral resection. At a minimum of 2 years of follow-up, these investigators found, among patients with irreparable labral tears, that the reconstruction group ($n = 11$) scored better than the resection group ($n = 22$) on the Non-arthritic Hip Score and the HOS ADL subscale.[116]

Procedures to Address Femoral Acetabular Impingement

Arthroscopic surgery to address symptomatic FAI has been rapidly increasing in popularity. As previously mentioned, open and mini-open procedures to address FAI have been performed with relatively successful outcomes. Matsuda and colleagues[117] reported equivalent clinical outcomes when comparing the open, mini-open, and arthroscopic intervention to address FAI. However, arthroscopic intervention was associated with a reduced occurrence of significant complications. Femoral osteoplasty is performed to address cam FAI. The procedure involves removing excessive bone in the femoral head-neck junction region and attempting to reshape the femoral head to the ideal spherical shape.[118] In the case of pincer FAI, a rim trimming or acetabuloplasty procedure is performed. The acetabular rim is resected in an attempt to resemble the normal structure and provide sufficient but not excessive coverage of the femoral head.[119] The intention of both femoral osteoplasty and acetabular rim trimming is to provide sufficient joint ROM to avoid articular damage that may be caused over time by FAI.

Another surgical procedure for the management of FAI is performed through open hip dislocation. This procedure allows for complete visualization of the femoral head and acetabulum.[120] The procedure involves a greater trochanteric osteotomy and anterior capsulotomy. After the capsulotomy has been performed, the femoral head can be dislocated anteriorly, providing a 360-degree view of the femoral head and acetabulum.[120,121] The sites of impingement are then identified, and excess bone is removed from femoral head and neck or the acetabular rim. Any intraarticular disorder such as cartilage damage or labral disorder is identified and addressed.[120,121] The open surgical dislocation procedure allows good visualization of the joint and treatment of all pathologic processes present. However, it is a substantial operation with some disadvantages when compared with the arthroscopic approach, including greater soft tissue trauma, greater blood loss, longer recovery time as a result of osteotomy, and disruption of the ligamentum teres.[120] The minimally invasive arthroscopic technique does not require extensive hospitalization and allows for quicker rehabilitation and recovery.[120]

Capsular Modification Procedures

Patients who present with hyperlaxity and capsular redundancy of the hip may be candidates for capsular modification to restore tension properties to the capsular structures. Procedures such as thermal modification and capsular plication have received limited attention in the literature, which consists primarily of case series.[43] Plication of the iliofemoral ligament with a bioabsorbable suture has been used in the treatment of focal anterior instability of the hip joint.[1] Caution must be used during the rehabilitation process, to protect capsuloligamentous tissue affected by thermal modification or plication procedures. In the common example of plication of the iliofemoral ligament to address anterior instability, external rotation would be limited for at least 4 weeks in the early stage of recovery.[10] Although the general consensus is that arthroscopy has no role in the treatment of hip dysplasia, some investigators have debated a limited use for the technique in patients with borderline dysplasia.[122] Surgical options for severe hip dysplasia include more invasive procedures such as periacetabular osteotomy (PAO) procedures.[123]

Microfracture Procedures

Microfracture procedures may be used to address focal chondral lesions during arthroscopic surgery of the hip joint. McCarthy and associates[7] observed that more than 73% of patients with a labral tear or fraying had chondral damage. Arthroscopic microfracture procedures have been suggested as effective for medium-sized, full-thickness articular lesions of the femoral head and acetabulum.[1] A surgical awl is used to create microfracture lesions in the subchondral bone to bring bone marrow and better blood supply to the articular surface.[10] Over time, the released material forms a clot that eventually develops into fibrocartilage. Fibrocartilage does not have the structural resilience of the native hyaline cartilage that lines the articular surfaces. Therefore, concerns exist regarding the durability of tissue after microfracture procedures. Philippon and colleagues[124] examined nine patients undergoing revision hip arthroscopy who underwent microfracture of the acetabulum during their primary arthroscopic surgical procedure. During the revision procedure, the investigators directly measured the percentage of fill in chondral defects and found that eight of nine patients demonstrated 95% to 100% coverage of isolated acetabular chondral defects.

McDonald and associates[125] examined the return to play rate and level for elite male athletes undergoing hip arthroscopy with and without microfracture procedures. These investigators found no statistically significant difference between the microfracture ($n = 39$) and nonmicrofracture ($n = 81$, total of 94 hips when counting bilateral cases) groups. Seventy-seven percent of athletes in the microfracture group compared with 84% in the group without microfracture returned to play, with an average of 3 years of follow-up. Further investigation of microfracture techniques may allow routine use of the procedure for patients with focal cartilage lesions of the hip joint.

Tendon Release Procedures

Patients with recurrent extraarticular snapping hip syndrome (coxa saltans) or chronic tendon irritation that does not respond to conservative treatment may be candidates for arthroscopic tendon release and lengthening procedures. The two most frequently released tendon structures are the iliopsoas and the ITB, with iliopsoas release being the more common of the two procedures.[1] Arthroscopic release procedures are very often performed in conjunction with surgical procedures to address acetabular labral disorders; however, these procedures can be performed in isolation as well. Cascio and colleagues[80] described labral injuries caused by iliopsoas impingement. They described a method of arthroscopic psoas release combined with labral repair. A significant improvement in patient-reported outcomes was noted. Generally positive outcomes have been reported for isolated arthroscopic iliopsoas release procedures.[126] Arthroscopic ITB release for external snapping hip syndrome has been reported as effective, matching the outcomes of open procedures described for the same condition.[127]

Complications Associated With Hip Arthroscopic Surgery

Hip arthroscopy has been described as a relatively safe surgical procedure with complication rates reported between 1.3% and 1.6% worldwide.[10] Although the occurrence is low, complications have been reported. Similar to other orthopedic surgical procedures such as arthroscopic knee procedures, complications including deep venous thrombosis, infection, neurovascular injury, and excessive loss of blood are all possible.[112,128] There are reports of complications specific to arthroscopic procedures at the hip. Such complications include, but are not limited to, surgical traction-related injuries to the neurovascular structures, fluid extravasation, avascular necrosis, cartilage damage or injury, excessive or inadequate resection of underlying osseous disorders, development of heterotrophic ossification, and the formation of intraarticular adhesions.[128,129] Of these complications of hip arthroscopic procedures, traction-related injuries are the most commonly reported. Typically, these injuries consist of neurapraxias (loss of nerve transmission) of the pudendal or sciatic nerves and are believed to be associated with the total amount of time in which the lower extremity is placed under traction during the operation.[128] In most reported cases, neurapraxias after hip arthroscopy resolve with time and require no further interventions.[130] Although extremely rare, femoral neck fractures after arthroscopic surgery to address FAI and anterior hip dislocations following arthroscopy to address capsular laxity have been reported.[131,132]

Clinicians involved in the postoperative care of patients after surgical procedures should familiarize themselves with potential complications and the clinical presentation of patients experiencing these issues. Concerning observations include excessive or uncontrollable pain not related to movement, incision regions that are bleeding excessively or that appear inflamed, change in organ function, and unexplainable change of mental status. It is imperative that clinicians recognize an abnormal clinical presentation or atypical postoperative progression and communicate these findings to the surgical team immediately. Prompt communication or referral is important in helping to ensure that serious conditions are avoided or minimized and the rehabilitation progression is not delayed.[48]

Postoperative Rehabilitation Following Hip Arthroscopy

As is the case with hip arthroscopy, the development of corresponding postoperative rehabilitation protocols for such procedures is an ongoing process.[48] Despite numerous descriptions of postoperative care in the literature, the evidence to support current programs is relatively weak.[133,134] Cheatham and associates[133] conducted a systematic review to evaluate current evidence on postoperative rehabilitation following hip arthroscopy procedures. These investigators found the highest quality of literature to be case reports, which are descriptive, with no studies comparing different approaches of postoperative rehabilitation. Although the program structure and number of rehabilitation stages vary by author, overlap in the underlying principles for existing protocols is substantial. In the following sections, rehabilitation for postoperative care of hip arthroscopy patients is described based on the available published recommendations and taking into account variations of tissue healing characteristics and patient population demands. When applicable, objective criteria are emphasized. Box 4-2 describes a general four-phase postoperative rehabilitation program for hip arthroscopy. Finally, the need for development of postoperative rehabilitation protocols based on clinical milestones is discussed. In the clinical setting, clinicians often encounter patients who have undergone surgical procedures to address multiple issues. In such cases, rehabilitation must be based on the most conservative approach for each performed procedure. For example, a patient undergoing a combined osteoplasty and capsular modification procedure will have to follow rehabilitation guidelines that are more conservative for weight bearing and ROM progression when compared with a patient undergoing isolated labral tear débridement.

Immediate Postoperative Care

The goal of immediate postoperative rehabilitation is to achieve a solid foundation on which the later stages of rehabilitation will be developed. This stage lasts approximately 2 weeks. An attempt is made to control excessive inflammation and optimize the healing environment. Although no specific evidence of modalities effectiveness on the postarthroscopy hip exists, ice and other physical agents may be used, based on theoretical reasoning. Various structures affected by the surgical procedure must be protected to allow healing during this time of vulnerability. Clinicians must consider the typical healing properties and timeframes of the tissues involved and plan rehabilitation activities accordingly.

Patient Education

Clinicians should review postoperative goals, precautions, and guidelines for activity progression with the patient. Patient education regarding proper posture and joint positioning is provided. Many postoperative protocols suggest that the patient spend a predetermined amount of time in the prone position to prevent development of hip flexor or anterior capsule tightness. The patient should also be instructed to monitor for unexpected changes in status that may indicate a postoperative complication.

Postoperative Bracing

A postoperative brace may be prescribed to limit excessive ROM for variable time periods after the procedure (Fig. 4-16).[10] The brace is set on the surgeon's discretion and may vary by procedure. However, the most common allowance for ROM is between 0 and 80 degrees of flexion in the sagittal plane. It does not allow abduction and has no effect on motion in the transverse plane. An immobilizer system may be issued to prevent excessive external rotation of the hip while the patient is sleeping.[10,20,135]

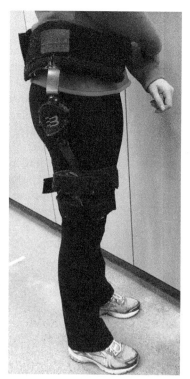

• **Figure 4-16** Postoperative Hip Brace.

Phase I: Immediate Postoperative Phase of Rehabilitation Program (1 to 2 Weeks)

Goals
- Decrease postoperative pain, inflammation, and swelling.
- Protect soft tissue repair.
- Prevent postoperative stiffness and adhesions.
- Restore basic muscle activation patterns.
- Normalize gait pattern with assistive device.

Precautions
- Avoid excessive weight bearing on the involved lower extremity.
- Avoid supine straight leg raise exercises.
- Limit symptom provocation during rehabilitation.
- Emphasize compliance with ice and antiinflammatory medications.

Range of Motion (Avoid Symptom Provocation)
- Circumduction at resting position, progress amount of flexion per tolerance
- Supine IR and ER passive ROM in resting position
- Supine log rolling with emphasis on internal rotation
- Progress to prone IR and ER passive ROM
- Stationary bike (one half to full revolution with elevated seat height, no resistance)

Flexibility
- Opposite knee to chest
- Prone positioning (progress duration per tolerance)
- Prone knee flexion

Edema Control and Muscle Activation
- Gluteal and quadriceps setting exercises (supine then prone)
- Ankle pumps
- Short arc quads
- Transverse abdominis contractions
- Prone terminal knee extension
- Pain-free isometric strengthening in all planes except hip flexion

Criteria to Progress to Next Phase
- Minimal to no pain at rest (<3/10)
- Neutral, pain free hip extension ROM
- Adequate gluteal, quadriceps, transverse abdominis muscle activation
- No increased pain with prone positioning

Phase II: Early Postoperative Phase of Rehabilitation Program (2 to 4 Weeks)

Goals
- Decrease postoperative pain and inflammation.
- Restore pain-free ROM necessary for ambulation and ADLs.
- Improve muscular strength and endurance for ambulation and ADLs.

Precautions
- ER limited to 20 degrees if capsular closure was performed
- ER and extension limited if capsulectomy was performed
- Avoidance of hyperextension and ER >20 degrees if labral repair was performed
- Avoidance of premature weaning from assistive device for ambulation

Range of Motion
- Continued circumduction ROM
- Continued stationary bicycle
- Progressed duration of prone positioning
- Quadruped heel sits for pain-free progression of flexion ROM

Flexibility
- Prone quadriceps stretch
- Prone prop positioning
- Progression to lunge position hip flexor stretch at week 3 or 4

Muscle Activation and Strengthening
- Initiation of pain-free isometric hip flexion at week 3
- Pain-free isotonic strengthening in all planes except hip flexion
- Recommended interventions:
  - Prone hip extension over pillows (avoid hyperextension)
  - Assisted progressing to active supine hip abduction
  - Bridges
  - Knee extension
  - Quadruped hip extension
  - Standing TKE
  - Partially loaded active external rotation
  - Standing hip abduction with IR
  - Bilateral leg press (<90 degrees of hip flexion, limited resistance)
  - Sit to stands from elevated height and mini-squats
  - Single leg stance balance

Criteria to Progress to Next Phase
- No reactive pain with exercise; no persistent pain after exercise
- Patient verbalizes <3/10 pain with rehabilitation and daily activities
- No complaints of anterior hip pain
- Demonstration of 10 seconds of single leg stance without deviations or pain
- Ability to ambulate with no deviations and without use of an assistive device. (Patient must verbalize pain-free community ambulation without an assistive device.)

Phase III: Intermediate Postoperative Phase of Rehabilitation Program (5 to 12 Weeks)

Goals
- Maintain adequate flexibility and full passive and active ROM.
- Restore adequate muscular strength, neuromuscular control, and endurance for progression of instrumental ADLs.
- Progress activity level without intraarticular or extraarticular irritation.
- Improve ROM and flexibility to allow for progression toward sport-specific movements.

Precautions
- Any symptom provocation should alter or slow down progression of interventions.

Range of Motion and Flexibility
- Continued ROM from previous phases
- Progressed stationary bicycle duration and added resistance
- Active pain-free FABER ROM
- Progression to end-range stretching in all planes at end of phase. (Avoid symptom provocation.)

Flexibility
- Initiation of standard lower extremity flexibility and stretching program

Strengthening
- Continuation of previous progressive gluteal and quadriceps strengthening exercises
- Progression allowed if exercises are pain free
- Recommended interventions:
  - Progression from bilateral to unilateral leg press
  - Step-ups and step-downs emphasizing lumbopelvic stabilization

Continued

• BOX 4-2 **Four-Phase General Hip Arthroscopy Postoperative Rehabilitation Protocol—cont'd**

- Side planks and prone planks
- Side-lying hip abduction without compensations
- Bridging progressions
- Single leg stance external rotation
- Side stepping with band resistance
- Single leg dead lifts
- Single leg mini-squats
- Progressed single leg balance and proprioceptive exercises

Conditioning
- Core muscle strengthening progressed to include multiplane exercises
- Cardiovascular conditioning to include elliptical, stair stepper, bicycle with resistance

Criteria to Progress to Next Phase
- Pain-free hip ROM that is symmetric to uninvolved lower extremity
- Demonstrated ability to ambulate for 10 minutes at patient's preferred speed without deviations
- Demonstrated ability to complete repeated lateral and forward step-downs from short step height without loss of pelvic or lower extremity control
- Completion of 30 correct repetitions of prone hip extension from 0 to 20 degrees without demonstrating abnormal muscle firing patterns or compensations
- Completion of 20 repetitions of active hip flexion from position of hip extension to 90 degrees of hip flexion without pain or pinching while in single leg stance on the uninvolved limb

Phase IV: Late Phase of Postoperative Rehabilitation Program (13 to 24 Weeks)
Goals
- Demonstrate an ability to return to sport or work activities safely at the preinjury level.
- Progress muscular strength, endurance, and power to meet the requirements of sport.

Precautions
- Caution should be taken not to progress or return to sport prematurely.
- Any symptom provocation should delay or alter progression.

Range of Motion and Flexibility
- Sport-specific end-range stretching in all planes. (Avoid symptom provocation.)

Strengthening
- Multiplanar weight-bearing sport-specific exercises
- Recommended interventions:
  - Split stance cable chops and lifts
  - Multidirectional lunges
- Inclusion of lower extremity plyometric exercises as appropriate to sport
- Example exercises:
  - Bilateral hopping progressions
  - Unilateral hopping progressions
  - Box jumps

Conditioning
- Initiation of return to jogging progression
- Initiation of agility training
- Example interventions:
  - Ladder drills
  - Forward and backward shuttle run
  - Lateral shuffle and shuttle run

Example Return-to-Sport Criteria
- Hip Outcome Score sport subscale score of ≥78
- Demonstrated ability to perform all sport-specific activities without kinetic collapse or complaints of decreased confidence or symptoms
- Demonstrated >90% limb symmetry index with all single leg hopping tests
- Vail Hip Sport Test score of 20/20

ADLs, Activities of daily living; *ER,* external rotation; *FABER,* flexion abduction external rotation; *IR,* internal rotation; *ROM,* range of motion; *TKE,* terminal knee extension.

Protected Weight Bearing

To protect healing tissues and limit inflammation, it is typically recommended that patients use bilateral axial crutches to allow for a period of partial weight bearing in the early phases of recovery. This time period of protected weight bearing can vary depending on the surgical procedure performed and is discussed in more detail. It is recommended that the use of crutches is continued until the patient can demonstrate a normalized gait pattern without the use of an assistive device even if this persists beyond the recommended timeframes.[48,136] Progressing to full weight-bearing gait with compensatory patterns may lead to setbacks in recovery caused by excessive intraarticular or extraarticular irritation or inflammation.[48]

Early Range of Motion

Early, protected ROM, including application of gentle circumduction passive motion, is emphasized to avoid excessive joint stiffness and development of intraarticular adhesions.[129] Intraarticular adhesions are recognized complications encountered during postoperative rehabilitation and have been noted as factors in revision procedures.[129,137,138] The stationary bicycle is used early in the rehabilitation process to emphasize regaining joint ROM in the sagittal plane.[10] Caution should be taken to adjust the stationary bicycle seat to a sufficient height that allows the patient to move the bicycle through appropriate motion without significant pain in the lower extremity. Limiting hip flexion to no more than 90 degrees while pedaling is typically recommended for the stationary bicycle.

Therapeutic Exercise

Another goal of early rehabilitation is to reestablish neuromuscular control of the hip and pelvic musculature. Non–weight-bearing exercises emphasizing gentle lower extremity AROM or isometric strengthening are typically prescribed.

TABLE 4-2   Rehabilitation Concerns Following Specific Hip Arthroscopy Procedures

Procedure	Weight Bearing	Range of Motion	Strength
Labral resection	PWB up to 2 weeks	As tolerated	Dictated by any weight bearing and ROM precautions
Labral repair	PWB 2-4 weeks	Variable	Dictated by any weight bearing and ROM precautions
Osteoplasty	PWB 4-6 weeks	As tolerated; do not force impingement position	Dictated by any weight bearing and ROM precautions
Microfracture	PWB 4-8 weeks *Occasional NWB	Variable	Dictated by any weight bearing and ROM precautions
Capsular modification	Variable	Limit ER and extension for anterior modification Limit IR and flexion for posterior modification	Dictated by any weight bearing and ROM precautions
Tendon release	PWB up to 2 weeks	As tolerated	Iliopsoas release: hold supine straight leg raise for 4 weeks ITB: hold side-lying straight leg raise for 3-4 weeks

ER, External rotation; IR, internal rotation; ITB, iliotibial band; NWB, non–weight bearing; PWB, partial weight bearing (typically 30 pounds, foot flat); ROM, range of motion.
*For combined procedures, the most conservative guideline of each performed procedure should be selected from each category.

Examples of exercises initially prescribed following hip arthroscopy include ankle AROM exercises, pelvic tilt activities, and isometric strength exercises (quadriceps, hamstring, and gluteal muscles). The use of exercises involving contraction of the hip flexors is delayed to avoid irritation of the iliopsoas tendon and bursae.[48]

Postoperative Concerns for Specific Procedures

Acetabular Labral Resection

Rehabilitation guidelines for arthroscopic surgical procedures to address acetabular labral tears vary according to the invasiveness of the procedure performed and the location of damage, as well as whether other procedures were performed to address underlying conditions related to the individual patient's presentation (Table 4-2).[10,20,48,136] The approach to rehabilitation following isolated resection of a labral tear is relatively unrestrictive. The primary concern is to keep joint and associated soft tissue inflammation at a reasonable level to ensure an optimal healing environment. Patients are typically allowed to bear weight partially immediately and are often fully weight bearing within 2 weeks.[10] Early ROM is encouraged, and progression toward full motion is typically dictated by the patient's tolerance. The progression of strength activities is limited primarily by the patient's tolerance and any restrictions of ROM or weight bearing. Although the postoperative guidelines for patients undergoing labral resection allow for a somewhat expeditious recovery, clinicians must recognize signs of an overly aggressive approach.[20,48,136] Persistent or increasing pain, a

regression of function, or an increase in mechanical symptoms warrants reevaluation and modification of the plan of care.

Acetabular Labral Repair

The invasive nature of labral repair procedures in comparison with labral resection procedures typically necessitates more restrictive postoperative guidelines. ROM restrictions may apply and depend on the location, size, and method of repair. An attempt is made to avoid placing excessive stress on the area of repair. Compared with resection procedures, more restrictive weight-bearing precautions are often assigned to patients undergoing labral repair. Partial weight bearing (often 30 pounds, foot flat) is typically recommended for up to 4 weeks postoperatively.[134] Specific concerns exist when the repair is performed on the anterior superior (weight-bearing) region of the labrum. Strengthening exercises are progressed as allowed by the ROM and weight-bearing status.

Procedures to Address Femoral Acetabular Impingement (Osteoplasty or Acetabuloplasty)

Femoral osteoplasty or acetabuloplasty or rim trimming may be performed to remove the excessive bone associated with cam and pincer FAI. The initial concern specific to these procedures is to protect the integrity of the remaining bone, in particular the femoral neck following osteoplasty to address cam FAI.[75] Prolonged partial weight bearing (often 30 pounds, foot flat) is typically prescribed for 4 to 6 weeks.[20,135] Although rare, stress fracture of the femoral neck has been described after hip arthroscopic osteoplasty to address cam FAI.[131] ROM precautions vary for procedures to address FAI, but they often are very similar to the recommendations for labral resection and repair procedures.[135] If a substantial capsulectomy was performed during the surgical procedure, the patient may have specific ROM precautions. In such cases, typically, external rotation and extension are limited, with no consensus on the specific amount in the literature. Caution should be applied with joint movement into end-range flexion, internal rotation, and horizontal addiction (common impingement positions) because this may approximate bone exposed during the procedure. This approximation may create groin pain or a "pinching" sensation. Early in rehabilitation, strength exercises that significantly stress the femoral neck should be approached with caution. Clinicians should progress resisted single leg exercises and jumping exercises slowly to allow careful monitoring of the patient's response to such activities.

Capsular Modification Procedures

Capsular plication and thermal modification procedures to address capsular laxity of the hip joint have been described in the literature.[1,43] The primary postoperative concerns for patients undergoing such procedures are preservation and protection of the newly established tension characteristics of the capsuloligamentous structures of the hip. To achieve these goals, a prolonged period of limited ROM is required postoperatively. The specific limitations vary depending on the area of the capsule that was stabilized. The most commonly performed procedures address attenuation of the anterior capsule or iliofemoral ligament. Anterior stabilization procedures necessitate prolonged limitation of external rotation and extension of the hip.[10,20,48,139] In the more rare case of posterior capsule stabilization, flexion and internal rotation are limited.[10,20,48,139] The specific ROM limitations for each procedure vary in the literature.[20] ROM limitations for arthroscopic procedures of the hip joint typically last at least 4 weeks.[10,20]

Microfracture Procedures

When microfracture procedures are performed to address focal chondral lesions, clinicians must prioritize providing protection by minimizing the shear forces experienced at the exposed joint surfaces. The rehabilitation precautions used for microfracture procedures of the hip are modified from guidelines used for patients undergoing microfracture of the knee joint.[10] Weight-bearing precautions are modified to provide the optimal environment for formation of fibrocartilage. Patients are typically partially weight bearing for 4 to 8 weeks.[134,139] In rare cases, patients may be assigned non–weight-bearing status. However, non–weight-bearing status of the hip joint may produce the unwanted effects of increased anterior hip forces and overactivity of the hip flexors.[93,136] Clinicians should also use additional caution when considering applying joint mobilization techniques to this group of patients. Distraction-based techniques allow safe mobilization of the joint capsule if the physical examination yields results suggesting hypomobility. Joint distraction techniques minimize shearing secondary to the force being applied perpendicular to the articular surfaces. Direction-specific mobilization techniques may place unwanted shear forces across the articular surfaces.

Tendon Release Procedures

Arthroscopic tendon release for the iliopsoas or ITB tissues creates requires specific considerations when initiating strength activities. Premature or excessive stress across these structures during the rehabilitation program may result in prolonged or increased inflammation. Hip flexor tendinopathy has been recognized as a disorder with an increased risk during the rehabilitation process.[48,135,136] To decrease the likelihood of excessive inflammation of these structures, activities that excessively load the hip flexors (supine straight leg raises) and ITB (side-lying leg raises) are not performed for approximately 4 weeks after tissue release procedures are performed.[10,135] Additionally, caution should be taken when performing soft tissue mobilization to these areas.

Common Rehabilitation Complications Following Hip Arthroscopy

To reduce the risk of complications or delayed recovery, it is important that an individualized and structured rehabilitation program be developed and followed. Several postoperative complications that directly affect or are the result of rehabilitation activities have been described. Regardless of the surgical procedure performed, intraarticular adhesions have been reported as a cause of postoperative pain and failure following hip arthroscopic surgical procedures of the hip joint.[129,137,138] Cited risk factors for intraarticular adhesion development include age younger than 30 years, a modified Harris Hip Score lower than 50, no microfracture procedure performed, and a postoperative rehabilitation program without passive joint circumduction activities.[129] Recognition of these risk factors allows clinicians to identify patients who may be at an elevated risk for adhesion development and ensure that their rehabilitation program emphasizes early ROM, including joint circumduction activities.[48]

With the exception of complications inherent to the surgical procedure, many problems during recovery may be preventable by appropriate implementation of the rehabilitation program. Complications during rehabilitation are frequently caused by an overly aggressive approach in which the intensity or volume of exercise is progressed prematurely, thus resulting in overloading of the extraarticular or intraarticular structures of the hip that, in turn, leads to increased inflammation and pain.[48] Many of these issues in recovery occur during the transitional periods between phases and stages of the rehabilitation protocol.[75,136] These transitional periods involve greater loading of the joint (increased weight bearing) or increased demands on the musculature (increasing exercise volume and intensity). Tendinopathy of the hip flexor muscles, bursitis, joint effusion, muscular imbalances, low back pain, and sacroiliac joint pain are common rehabilitation complications.[135,136]

Caution should be taken when a patient is weaning off crutches postoperatively because this is a transitional period with a higher risk for the development of complications. A patient should continue to use the appropriate assistive device until he or she can ambulate without deviations. Allowing patients to ambulate with faulty gait pattern characteristics can lead to intraarticular or extraarticular irritation. Hip joint effusion contributes to gluteal muscle inhibition.[140] To recognize and prevent unexpected increases of pain and decreased gluteal strength, clinicians should use objective measures (strength, ROM, gait quality), as opposed to basing protocol progression decisions solely on time elapsed after the operation.

The highly active population, particularly those patients involved in organized sports, is already predisposed to joint overloading by the aspiration to return to sport or activity as quickly as possible.[75] This aspiration can lead clinicians and patients to progress through the recovery and rehabilitation phases too rapidly. As the patient progresses, the clinician should base progression decisions on the patient's ability to demonstrate mastery of all interventions at the current level with the appropriate ROM, dynamic control, and proprioception.[48,135]

Functional and Activity Progression Considerations for Patients With Acetabular Labral Tears and Femoral Acetabular Impingement (Nonoperative and Postoperative)

With a paucity of research examining specific rehabilitation protocols (nonoperative and postoperative) for treatment of acetabular labral tears and associated conditions such as FAI, a substantially smaller proportion of the available evidence evaluates functional progression and return-to-sport issues in this population. This facet of rehabilitation is particularly important because these patients are typically active and often athletic. Clinicians should attempt to assess a patient's readiness to return to higher-level physical activity and provide treatment strategies that meet the demands of these patients.

An emphasis should be placed on developing appropriate neuromuscular control to participate in more strenuous activities. Dynamic stabilization and perturbation activities can help active patients prepare for the demands of stabilizing the hip and pelvic complex when they experience external forces that occur in random directions and of variable magnitude during athletic endeavors (Fig. 4-17).[12] Although applicable to all patient categories mentioned to this point, stabilization activities may be particularly useful for the hypermobile population. Static balance activities should be progressed to include variable surfaces and performance of multiple tasks (using upper and lower

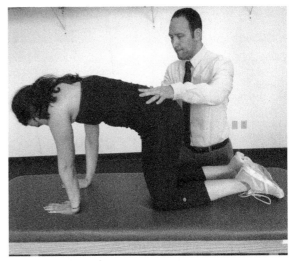

• **Figure 4-17** Perturbation Training. The patient assumes the quadruped position and then must maintain the position as the therapist applies randomly directed forces of various magnitudes to challenge the stability of the pelvis.

extremities). If the patient participates in a specific sport, these activities should be progressed to represent the demands of that sport. Clinicians should remember to ensure that the patient has achieved the ability to execute the current rehabilitation task properly before advancing the level of activity. Inappropriate progression, before a patient has achieved the necessary prerequisite skill set, may result in unwanted compensation strategies, as well as excessive loading of the joint.[136]

Functional testing and return-to-play criteria for patients with acetabular labral tears and FAI are minimally described in the literature. No specific descriptions of functional testing protocols exist for patients with nonoperative nonarthritic hip pain. Currently, clinicians must use the few validated tests that are condition specific in combination with functional tests and measures validated for active patients with other lower extremity injuries. Tranovich and colleagues[20] described return-to-play criteria for patients undergoing hip arthroscopy that were modified from a postoperative anterior cruciate ligament reconstruction rehabilitation program. Criteria for progression include tolerance to all prescribed exercises for strength, agility, running, and plyometric activities. Once these activities are tolerated at 100% effort and the surgeon clears the patient, the patient must then pass a specific return-to-play test (Box 4-3). The return-to-play test consists of 12 functional tasks or tests that involve various combinations of squatting, jumping, landing, pivoting, cutting, and multidirectional movement. Many of the tasks are graded based on the performance of the surgical leg compared with the nonsurgical leg (either time or distance). A patient must score 90% or higher on the surgical leg (compared with the nonsurgical leg) to pass the test. Two functional tests are timed. Specific criteria are given to determine the threshold to achieve a passing time for the tests.

- Complete a 10- to 20-minute dynamic warm-up (stationary bicycle, elliptical, treadmill jogging, flexibility and stretching routine).
- Practice each exercise/test at 25%, 50%, 75%, and 100% effort.
- Complete two to three measured trials of each exercise or test.
- Included exercises and tests:
  1. 10 repetitions maximum single leg squat
  2. Triple broad jump, landing last on one foot
  3. Single leg diagonal cross over jump
  4. Single leg forward jump
  5. Single leg lateral jump
  6. Single leg medial jump
  7. Single leg rotating jump
  8. Single leg vertical jump
  9. Single leg triple jump
  10. Timed 10-m single leg hop
  11. 10-yard lower extremity functional test (includes sprint and back pedal, shuffle, carioca, sprint; recommended times: male patients, 18 to 22 seconds; female patients, 20 to 24 seconds)
  12. 10-yard proagility drill

Another return-to-sport clearance test is the Vail Hip Sport Test. This objective test allows clinicians to give an individual a score out of 20 possible points (optimal) based on their performance of 4 sport-cord–resisted multiplanar exercises. The 4 exercises are single leg squat completed for 3 minutes, lateral bounding for 100 seconds, diagonal bounding completed for 100 seconds, and forward lunge onto raised step for 2 minutes. Currently, the test has not been shown to be reliable. The test is reported to be clinically valuable because it provides a controlled method for the clinician to assess muscle strength, endurance, and dynamic control during multiplanar tasks.[75]

As clinicians continue to focus on refining the return-to-play and functional progression criteria for patients with acetabular labral tears and FAI, tests that will be included in such protocols must be validated. In addition to physical performance measures, a need exists to determine threshold scores for validated patient-reported outcome (PRO) measurements that can be included in return-to-play or functional progression criteria.

Patient-Reported Outcome Measurements for Patients With Labral Tears and Femoral Acetabular Impingement

Advances in recognition of pathologic conditions of the hip joint and related treatment options created a need for outcome measurements that captured the needs and characteristics of the population of patients experiencing such injuries. Until recently, most PRO tools for patients with

hip injuries were designed to reflect the characteristics of patients with hip OA or hip fractures or surgical procedures related to these conditions (total hip arthroplasty or open reduction and internal fixation).[12,48] Some PROs were developed for use in patients with postoperative and non-operative nonarthritic hip pain.[141,142] A selection of these PROs is discussed in this section. Currently, no single PRO is considered superior for use in patients with symptomatic FAI.[143]

Hip Outcome Score

The HOS is a 36-item (17 ADL items, 9 sport items) PRO designed to assess performance in patients with nonarthritic hip pain.[144] Items are scored from 0 to 4. A score of 0 represents being "unable to do," whereas a score of 4 represents "no difficulty." The total score is calculated for each subscale (ADL and sport) and is then divided by the total number of points possible (60 for ADLs, 36 for sport, if all questions are answered) and multiplied by 100 to derive a percentage score. A higher score indicates a higher reported level of function. The HOS has demonstrated high test-retest reliability, construct validity, and content reliability when assessed for patients undergoing hip arthroscopy.[144] The minimal clinically important difference (MCID) for the HOS is 9 points for the ADL subscale and 6 points for the sport subscale.[144] The HOS has shown excellent responsiveness for patients 7 months after hip arthroscopy.[144]

Thirty-Three-Item International Hip Outcome Tool

The 33-item International Hip Outcome Tool (IHOT-33) was developed as part of a multicenter, multidisciplinary effort examining more than 400 patients (16 to 60 years of age) with hip pain.[145] The IHOT-33 PRO covers several domains: symptoms and functional limitations; sports and recreational physical activities; job-related concerns; and social, emotional, or lifestyle concerns. Items are rated using a visual analog scale (0 to 100), with 100 being the best possible score for each item. Face and content validity for the IHOT-33 have been established for patients with nonarthritic hip pain. The MCID after hip arthroscopy has been reported to be 6 points. Test-retest reliability was reported as moderate to good (intraclass correlation coefficient of 0.78).[145]

Copenhagen Hip and Groin Outcome Score

The Copenhagen Hip and Groin Outcome Score (HAGOS) was developed with the intention of assessing characteristics of young to middle-aged, physically active patients with hip pain.[146] The HAGOS contains 6 subscales: pain, other symptoms, physical function in daily living, function in sports and recreation, participation in physical activities, and hip-related quality of life. Each question has 5 options, and they are scored from 0 to 4, taking the past week into consideration. The score for each category is normalized, with an optimal score of 100 (no symptoms). The HAGOS has shown substantial test-retest reliability across all subscales, with intraclass correlation coefficient values ranging from 0.82 to 0.91. Construct validity and responsiveness of the HAGOS have been confirmed.[147] Changes greater than 5.2 points are considered detectable for any of the subscales.[143]

Summary

Acetabular labral tears of the hip joint continue to be a debated topic in the orthopedic and sports medicine community. The options available for diagnosis and treatment of nonarthritic hip pain have expanded at a substantial rate since 2000. FAI is the most studied and debated etiologic mechanism for the development of acetabular labral tears. However, clinicians should be aware of the numerous differential diagnoses, particularly capsular instability, that must be considered when evaluating a patient with nonarthritic hip pain. Being relatively early in the process of understanding the progression and consequences of FAI, clinicians may still be on the learning curve in regard to establishing standardized treatment recommendations for this population of patients. To assess and treat patients with acetabular labral tears secondary to FAI or other underlying conditions effectively, clinicians must employ a structured approach to examination, understand the pathomechanical process of the involved injury mechanisms, and use intervention techniques based on the best evidence available.

Case Studies

Examples of acetabular impingement and labral tear are provided in Case Studies 4-1 and 4-2.

CASE STUDY 4-1

Nonoperative Treatment of Symptomatic Femoral Acetabular Impingement

Patient History

A 31-year-old man presented to an outpatient physical therapy clinic with a complaint of right groin pain. The patient was self-referred in a state that allows direct access to physical therapy treatment. He noted a 4-week history of groin pain associated with his increased participation in road cycling. The patient cycles regularly on variable inclined and declined surfaces in a rural setting for at least 25 miles, four times per week. The pain was most noticeable when he was positioned in a low stance with hips flexed deeply (aero position) while descending hills and when he was sitting at his work desk for several hours the day after intense training. Pain levels reached 5 out of 10 during cycling activity and 4 out of 10 when sitting at the desk. Occasional crepitus did randomly occur and at times was associated with residual groin pain. Once the patient became symptomatic, pain typically persisted for the remainder of the day. Ambulation and activities of daily living (ADLs) were minimally affected, with the exception of sitting longer than 2 hours and deep squatting activities. He also noted minor stiffness when awakening the day after cycling intensely. He was not taking any medications at the time of evaluation.

The patient reported a history of undergoing a lumbar fusion procedure 3 years ago at the region of L2 to L3. He participated in a full regimen of postoperative physical therapy and returning to all ADLs and fitness activities. Otherwise, he did not note any significant medical history.

Other than participation in cycling approximately 5 months per year, the patient led a relatively sedentary lifestyle. He worked as a computer analyst and did not participate in any other regular fitness activities. He lived in a two-story home with his wife and two young children.

Systems Review

Observation yielded a 31-year-old, 6-foot 1-inch, 225-pound man (mesomorph) in minimal distress. His standing posture showed a relative anterior tilt of the pelvis in static standing. He was unremarkable for any other deviations of the spine or lower extremities. The patient's gait pattern was symmetrical, and velocity was within normal limits.

Tests and Measures

A Hip Outcome Score (HOS) was issued to assess the patient's functional limitations associated with his current hip pain. The HOS was chosen for ease of administration, level of support in the literature, and inclusion of a sport subscale. The patient reported a score of 79% on the ADL subscale and 61% on the sport subscale (100% optimal).

Because the patient presented in a direct access situation and had a history of lumbar spine involvement, a lower-quarter screening examination was performed. Assessment of myotomes, dermatomes, and reflexes was completed. Additionally, active range of motion (ROM) of the lumbar spine, assessment of pelvic landmark position, and tests to evaluate potential sacroiliac joint involvement were implemented. Results of all lower-quarter screening tests and measures were negative.

Next, physical examination specific to the hip region was completed. Passive ROM was symmetrical and within normal limits for both hips. The patient did note that groin pain and the feeling of stiffness were increased both when the hip was placed at end-range extension and when it was placed at end-range internal rotation with the hip flexed to 90 degrees. He demonstrated weakness on the involved side, with abduction and external rotation of the right hip measuring 4/5.

Continued

Nonoperative Treatment of Symptomatic Femoral Acetabular Impingement—cont'd

The patient also demonstrated difficulty maintaining a posterior pelvic tilt while lowering the legs from 90 degrees of hip flexion to the table (leg lowering test for lower abdominal strength). Groin pain (2 out of 10) was noted with manual muscle testing for abduction. Flexibility tests showed tightness for the hamstrings, piriformis, and iliopsoas on the left side. Results of the flexion abduction external rotation (FABER) test were negative. Groin pain (4 out of 10) was increased when the flexion adduction internal rotation (FADIR) tests were performed on the involved side. Additionally, with long-axis distraction of the left hip, baseline pain decreased (0 out of 10), and decreased joint mobility was noted when compared with the uninvolved side when assessed with long-axis distraction.

Evaluation, Diagnosis, and Prognosis

Based on the patient's history, observation, and physical examination, it was determined that the likelihood was high that the patient's pain and dysfunction were caused by femoral acetabular impingement (FAI). The patient demonstrated strength, flexibility, and joint mobility deficits that have been suggested to occur with this patient population. Additionally, the activity of cycling consists of repetitive flexion of the hip, a mechanism correlated with symptomatic FAI.

Intervention

An intervention plan to address the patient's impairments was initiated. Additionally, measures to minimize the progression of potential degenerative changes were recommended. Manual and self-stretch activities were used to address the lack of flexibility for the psoas and piriformis and the hamstring tightness observed during the physical examination. Long-axis and lateral distraction of the hip joint was performed each session to address lack of capsular mobility around the hip joint. Progressive strength activities were prescribed, with a progression from non–weight-bearing to weight-bearing exercises as tolerated. Strengthening activities were performed in ranges that would not engage the joint in positions of impingement. To avoid impingement during strengthening exercises, the patient was instructed to avoid flexion beyond 90 degrees and hip internal rotation past neutral when the hip was in a flexed position. Activities to enhance lumbopelvic control were prescribed.

Activity modification and patient education were provided in an attempt to decrease joint irritability and encourage preservation of joint integrity. The patient agreed to cycle three times per week with the seat elevated to a height that eliminated any pain or pinching. Additionally, he raised the height and reclined the back of his desk chair at work. The patient was treated for 3 weeks, for a total of six visits.

After 3 weeks, the patient's strength and muscle flexibility were symmetrical. All results of tests for joint involvement were now negative except the FADIR test, which still produced groin pain. Although passive ROM remained normal, the patient continued to note stiffness at the end range of hip extension. Decreased mobility was still present with long-axis distraction. The patient could now cycle three times per week. Groin pain was still reported if the patient attempted to increase frequency or total miles of cycling. Manual therapy was modified to include joint distraction at 100 degrees of hip flexion. The patient performed the home program and followed the recommended activity modification for 2 weeks, with a formal follow-up appointment in physical therapy scheduled at that time.

After the 3-week reevaluation, it was recommended the patient arrange a consultation for professionally fitting his bicycle. The fitting was performed by a physical therapist who also had extensive training in bicycle fitting evaluation. After evaluation, the patient's cycle parameters were adjusted to decrease his overall amount of hip flexion while on the bicycle.

Reexamination

After 2 weeks of independently performing the home program and modified activity (including riding on the adjusted bicycle), the patient reported to the clinic for formal reevaluation. At this time, the patient reported no pain with cycling, no pain with ADLs, and minor soreness when sitting in very low chairs or couches for prolonged periods of time. Physical examination found no deficits in ROM, strength, flexibility, or joint mobility. The FADIR test was still painful, when significant overpressure was applied. The patient completed an additional HOS questionnaire. He scored 95% on the ADL subscale and 88% on the sport subscale. Both scores represent significant improvements from his baseline assessment.

Discharge From Physical Therapy

Following formal reexamination, the patient was discharged. He was reporting minimal pain and showed significant improvement on the HOS outcome tool. The patient was to continue performing his home program independently to maintain optimal strength and flexibility. Modifications of the patient's cycling activities were suggested to minimize symptoms consistent with FAI. It was suggested that he avoid consecutive days of cycling if possible, basically training every other day. The patient included 1 day of swimming per week to allow cardiovascular training with less repetitive hip movement isolated in the sagittal plane.

The patient elected to consult an orthopedic surgeon to evaluate the hip joint for purposes of confirmation of clinical presentation. Plain radiographs of the hip and pelvis were obtained. FAI of the cam type (excessive bone at the femoral head-neck junction) was identified. Additionally, minor degenerative changes in the anterior superior portion of the joint were noted. No further intervention was recommended because the patient was reporting minimal symptoms at that time.

CASE STUDY 4-2

Rehabilitation After Hip Arthroscopy With Labral Repair and Osteoplasty

Patient History

A 20-year-old male patient presented to an outpatient physical therapy clinic with complaints of postoperative pain and soreness after undergoing hip arthroscopy 4 days earlier. The patient reported gradually worsening groin and hip pain for 3 months preoperatively. He denied a specific mechanism of injury, but he initially felt minor groin pain after playing in a recreational basketball game. The pain and discomfort began to limit sport participation and eventually escalated to point where he was unable to sit through class or perform basic activities of daily living (ADLs) without intensification of symptoms. He reported decreased confidence in using his lower extremities and an occasional catching sensation when negotiating stairs. Nonsteroidal antiinflammatory medications were used, with only short-term relief of symptoms. After 3 weeks of consistent pain with ADLs, the patient consulted his primary care physician, who ordered plain radiographic imaging and referred him for magnetic resonance arthrography and consultation with a specialist.

The patient was diagnosed with femoral acetabular impingement (FAI) resulting from cam-type morphology with the presence of an acetabular labral tear in the anterior superior portion of the joint. The patient was referred to physical therapy to attempt 4 to 6 weeks of conservative management before proceeding with surgical intervention.

Preoperative Physical Therapy

The focus of this case study is to describe the postoperative course of rehabilitation. The specific details of the preoperative physical therapy treatments are not described in detail. The emphasis of the preoperative physical therapy visit was placed on patient education and activity modification to decrease intraarticular irritation and pain. ADLs and recreational activities were modified to avoid end-range positions or positions that recreated the patient's pain and symptoms. Low-intensity active and passive range-of-motion (ROM) exercises were included to optimize functional ROM. Gluteal and core muscle strengthening exercises were included in non–pain-provoking positions to improve dynamic control and muscular endurance during functional activities to limit intraarticular irritation and pain. After 4 weeks, the patient continued to have groin pain that limited any progression toward his previous level of activities. The patient elected to proceed with surgical intervention.

Postoperative Physical Therapy

The postoperative protocol used for this patient is listed in Box 4-2. The patient presented for the first postoperative visit 4 days following arthroscopic surgery with one caregiver present. He rated his pain at 5 out of 10 on a verbal 11-point pain scale. The patient scored a 22 on the Hip Outcome Score (HOS) ADL subscale. He was demonstrating correct use of bilateral axial crutches and weight bearing as tolerated on the right lower extremity with ambulation. On questioning, he was compliant with frequent use of ice modalities and the initial home exercise program consisting of gluteal setting, quadriceps setting, and ankle plantar and dorsiflexion active ROM exercises provided by the surgical center. The patient's incisions were clean and dry, without excessive erythema or drainage. Distal sensation and pulses were intact and symmetrical to contralateral lower extremity. Baseline

measurements of bilateral hip ROM were assessed in the supine position. Left hip measurements were flexion to 65 degrees, extension to –5 degrees (5 degrees less than the contralateral side), abduction to 25 degrees, external rotation to 20 degrees, and internal rotation to 15 degrees. Right hip measurements were flexion to 110 degrees, abduction to 35 degrees, extension to at least neutral, external rotation to 35 degrees, and internal rotation to 30 degrees. Strength testing of left hip was deferred at this time because of the patient's postoperative status.

The first treatment session focused on patient education specific to the postoperative protocol, activity modification, pain-free ROM, and neuromuscular reeducation and activation exercises. Circumduction ROM exercises were performed with the hip in resting position to reduce the risk of postoperative adhesions and improve joint ROM. The patient's caregiver was educated on technique and importance of continued performance as part of the initial home exercise program. Pain-free passive ROM was performed in the directions of internal rotation, external rotation, and abduction. External rotation ROM was limited to 20 degrees because of labral repair precautions. The patient was then instructed on the performance of gluteal setting, transverse abdominis activation, quadriceps setting, and short arc knee extension exercises. Pain-free isometric exercises targeting hip abductor and adductor muscles were also included. The patient was positioned prone for several minutes to emphasize neutral hip position and prevent anterior soft tissue tightness. Ice was applied to the patient's hip after completion of treatment to limit or reduce any reactive pain or swelling of superficial tissues.

A plan of care was established, with the frequency of physical therapy visits being once per week. This was determined to be sufficient during the early postoperative period because of the patient's ability to demonstrate independence with exercises and the availability of a caregiver to perform passive ROM and circumduction at home. The goals of the early postoperative rehabilitation period were to reduce postoperative inflammation and pain, to improve ROM to allow normalization of the patient's gait pattern, and to improve gluteal muscle strength and muscular endurance, thus allowing for ambulation without assistive devices.

At the second and third physical therapy sessions, interventions were progressed to improve ROM and develop strength sufficient to produce a normalized gait pattern. An upright stationary bicycle with an elevated seat height and minimal resistance was used to promote self-guided pain-free ROM. Internal and external rotation passive ROM was performed in the prone position emphasizing neutral hip extension. Care was taken to limit hip extension beyond neutral or external rotation beyond 20 degrees. Hip flexion ROM was performed by having the patient complete quadruped rocking exercises from the quadruped position. To reduce anterior soft tissue tightness, the patient was instructed in prone knee bends and prone terminal knee extension exercises. Strengthening exercises were progressed from isometric exercises to include active ROM or isotonic strength activities. Some additional activities added at this time were prone hip extension over pillows to avoid hyperextension, bridges, and partial weight-bearing hip external rotation with use of a stool. The home exercise program was updated to

Continued

Rehabilitation After Hip Arthroscopy With Labral Repair and Osteoplasty—cont'd

include all strengthening exercises completed during the visit once correct technique was demonstrated.

At the following visit, the patient continued to demonstrate hip drop when ambulating without crutches. The patient was instructed to continue using crutches until strength improved. At this time, the ROM and flexibility exercises were progressed to include hip extension beyond neutral and external rotation beyond 20 degrees. Anterior soft tissue or hip flexor stretching was progressed to include stretches performed in a lunge or Thomas test position. Pain-free passive and active ROM exercises were initiated in a position of flexion abduction and external rotation. Strengthening exercises continued to emphasize gluteal and lower extremity strengthening in pain-free midrange positions. Full weight-bearing unilateral strengthening exercises were not yet included in the patient's program because he had not yet returned to pain-free community ambulation. At this time, the frequency of physical therapy was increased from once per week to twice per week to ensure monitored progression of strength and dynamic pelvic control.

At the next follow-up visit, the patient was 5 weeks postoperative and now demonstrated the ability to ambulate without an assistive device and demonstrated no gait deviations. At this time, instructions to wean from crutches for community ambulation were provided. The goals of this intermediate phase of rehabilitation were to increase ROM and strength further, thereby allowing the patient to return to ADLs, and to address any acquired muscular imbalances present throughout the lower extremities and lumbopelvic region. A flexibility and stretching program was developed emphasizing the iliopsoas, quadriceps, and adductor muscle groups. General lower extremity strengthening exercises were progressed as tolerated by the patient. Gluteal strengthening exercises were progressed based on the patient's ability to demonstrate proper technique and not use compensatory strategies. Examples of gluteal muscle strengthening exercises included in this phase include single leg bridges, single leg step-up and step-down exercises, and lateral stepping with band resistance. The patient was provided a home exercise program, which included use of strengthening equipment at his recreation center, with an emphasis on general lower body strengthening. Education was provided, instructing the patient to avoid any positions that created groin or hip pain. He was also instructed to initiate exercise at higher repetition ranges and then, once comfortable with the movement pattern of a specific exercise, increase weight to level where he was reaching fatigue between 8 and 12 repetitions.

After 12 weeks and total of 17 physical therapy visits, the patient could be progressed to the next phase of the rehabilitation program, which included initiation of a return-to-running program. The criteria to progress from this phase were 0 out of 10 verbal pain rating with ADLs, an HOS ADL subscale score of 89% or higher, no pain or compensation with 10 minutes of continuous ambulation, and the ability to perform repetitive lateral and forward single leg step-downs without kinetic collapse into a valgus position. The patient's ROM measurements were flexion to 115 degrees, extension to 15 degrees, abduction to 35 degrees, internal rotation to 35 degrees, and external rotation to 35 degrees. He rated his pain as 0 out of 10 with low-level activities and scored 91% on the

HOS ADL subscale. He demonstrated the ability to perform repetitive single leg mini-squats and well as repetitive lateral and forward step-downs without loss of lumbopelvic control or valgus collapse throughout the lower extremity. At this point, the rehabilitation program was modified to include progressive strengthening exercises that used movement patterns similar to those required by recreational and sport activities. The frequency of formal physical therapy visits was decreased to once every 10 to 14 days.

Return-to-Sport Progression

At 16 weeks postoperatively, the patient had progressed through the return to running progression with minimal soreness and was tolerating 20 minutes of continuous jogging. The rehabilitation program was progressed to include higher-level sport-specific movements including sprinting, cutting, and pivoting maneuvers. Before inclusion of these activities, the patient demonstrated appropriate lumbopelvic and lower extremity control during multidirectional step-down tasks and low-intensity plyometric exercises. These exercises were introduced at a 50% to 75% effort level and progressed toward 100% intensity over several weeks. As the patient began to tolerate predetermined cutting and pivoting maneuvers, agility and change in direction drills to verbal commands were included. The patient was also encouraged to begin specific conditioning activities with the team as well as individual skill development drills specific to his sport of choice. In this case, drills included ball handling drills, short-range jump shots, and layups.

At the time of the twenty-third physical therapy session (25 weeks after the surgical procedure), the patient was without complaints of pain or soreness when performing agility and sport-specific conditioning activities. To determine readiness for return to sport, the patient completed a battery of tests during this session to identify objectively any impairments or risk factors for potential injury or reinjury. The patient completed the HOS and scored 97% on the ADL subscale and a 76% on the sport subscale. Single leg hop testing included single hop for distance, triple hop for distance, triple crossover hop for distance, and timed 6-m hop. The patient demonstrated greater than 90% limb symmetry index with all hopping tests.

Discharge From Physical Therapy

The examination findings were communicated to the referring surgeon, and the recommendation was to return the patient to previous sport activities gradually. The patient was instructed to begin with half-court scrimmages of short duration and gradually increase duration and intensity of play. Once he felt conditioned enough and was tolerating all half-court play without concerns, he could progress to full-court scrimmages of shorter duration. He was provided a general recommendation of resting 24 hours if any soreness resulted from playing and not to return to participation until soreness resolved. The patient was encouraged to follow up with the surgeon or physical therapist if soreness persisted more than 5 to 7 days. The patient did not experience any hindrances during return-to-sport progression and did not require any further physical therapy care.

References

1. Kelly BT, Williams RJ 3rd, Philippon MJ. Hip arthroscopy: current indications, treatment options, and management issues. *Am J Sports Med*. 2003;31(6):1020-1037.

2. Fitzgerald RH Jr. Acetabular labrum tears: diagnosis and treatment. *Clin Orthop Relat Res*. 1995;311:60-68.

3. Groh MM, Herrera J. A comprehensive review of hip labral tears. *Curr Rev Musculoskelet Med*. 2009;2(2):105-117.

4. Ferguson SJ, Bryant JT, Ganz R, Ito K. An in vitro investigation of the acetabular labral seal in hip joint mechanics. *J Biomech*. 2003;36(2):171-178.

5. Ferguson SJ, Bryant JT, Ganz R, Ito K. The influence of the acetabular labrum on hip joint cartilage consolidation: a poroelastic finite element model. *J Biomech*. 2000;33(8):953-960.

6. Bedi A, Lynch EB, Sibilsky Enselman ER, et al. Elevation in circulating biomarkers of cartilage damage and inflammation in athletes with femoroacetabular impingement. *Am J Sports Med*. 2013;41(11):2585-2590.

7. McCarthy JC, Noble PC, Schuck MR, et al. The Otto E. Aufranc Award: the role of labral lesions to development of early degenerative hip disease. *Clin Orthop Relat Res*. 2001;393:25-37.

8. Lage LA, Patel JV, Villar RN. The acetabular labral tear: an arthroscopic classification. *Arthroscopy*. 1996;12(3):269-272.

9. Beck M, Kalhor M, Leunig M, Ganz R. Hip morphology influences the pattern of damage to the acetabular cartilage: femoroacetabular impingement as a cause of early osteoarthritis of the hip. *J Bone Joint Surg Br*. 2005;87(7):1012-1018.

10. Enseki KR, Martin RL, Draovitch P, et al. The hip joint: arthroscopic procedures and postoperative rehabilitation. *J Orthop Sports Phys Ther*. 2006;36(7):516-525.

11. Narvani AA, Tsiridis E, Kendall S, et al. A preliminary report on prevalence of acetabular labrum tears in sports patients with groin pain. *Arthroscopy*. 2003;11(6):403-408.

12. Enseki KR, Harris-Hayes M, White DM, et al. Nonarthritic hip joint pain. *J Orthop Sports Phys Ther*. 2014;44(6):A1-A32.

13. Agricola R, Bessems JH, Ginai AZ, et al. The development of cam-type deformity in adolescent and young male soccer players. *Am J Sports Med*. 2012;40(5):1099-1106.

14. Peelle MW, Della Rocca GJ, Maloney WJ, et al. Acetabular and femoral radiographic abnormalities associated with labral tears. *Clin Orthop Relat Res*. 2005;441:327-333.

15. Wenger DE, Kendell KR, Miner MR, Trousdale RT. Acetabular labral tears rarely occur in the absence of bony abnormalities. *Clin Orthop Relat Res*. 2004;426:145-150.

16. Parvizi J, Leunig M, Ganz R. Femoroacetabular impingement. *J Am Acad Orthop Surg*. 2007;15(9):561-570.

17. Leunig M, Casillas MM, Hamlet M, et al. Slipped capital femoral epiphysis: early mechanical damage to the acetabular cartilage by a prominent femoral metaphysis. *Acta Orthop Scand*. 2000;71(4):370-375.

18. Hack K, Di Primio G, Rakhra K, Beaule PE. Prevalence of cam-type femoroacetabular impingement morphology in asymptomatic volunteers. *J Bone Joint Surg Am*. 2010;92(14):2436-2444.

19. Gosvig KK, Jacobsen S, Sonne-Holm S, Gebuhr P. The prevalence of cam-type deformity of the hip joint: a survey of 4151 subjects of the Copenhagen Osteoarthritis Study. *Acta Radiol*. 2008;49(4):436-441.

20. Tranovich MJ, Salzler MJ, Enseki KR, Wright VJ. A review of femoroacetabular impingement and hip arthroscopy in the athlete. *Phys Sportsmed*. 2014;42(1):75-87.

21. Notzli HP, Wyss TF, Stoecklin CH, et al. The contour of the femoral head-neck junction as a predictor for the risk of anterior impingement. *J Bone Joint Surg Br*. 2002;84-B(4):556-560.

22. Tannast M, Siebenrock KA, Anderson SE. Femoroacetabular impingement: radiographic diagnosis—what the radiologist should know. *AJR Am J Roentgenol*. 2007;188(6):1540-1552.

23. Pollard TC, Villar RN, Norton MR, et al. Femoroacetabular impingement and classification of the cam deformity: the reference interval in normal hips. *Acta Orthop*. 2010;81(1):134-141.

24. Barton C, Salineros MJ, Rakhra KS, Beaulé PE. Validity of the alpha angle measurement on plain radiographs in the evaluation of cam-type femoroacetabular impingement. *Clin Orthop Relat Res*. 2011;469(2):464-469.

25. Zaragoza E, Lattanzio PJ, Beaule PE. Magnetic resonance imaging with gadolinium arthrography to assess acetabular cartilage delamination. *Hip Int*. 2009;19(1):18-23.

26. Burnett RS, Rocca GJD, Prather H, et al. Clinical presentation of patients with tears of the acetabular labrum. *J Bone Joint Surg Am*. 2006;88(7):1448-1457.

27. Czerny C, Hofmann S, Neuhold A, et al. Lesions of the acetabular labrum: accuracy of MR imaging and MR arthrography in detection and staging. *Radiology*. 1996;200(1):225-230.

28. Freedman BA, Potter BK, Dinauer PA, et al. Prognostic value of magnetic resonance arthrography for Czerny stage II and III acetabular labral tears. *Arthroscopy*. 2006;22(7):742-747.

29. Keeney JA, Peelle MW, Jackson J, et al. Magnetic resonance arthrography versus arthroscopy in the evaluation of articular hip pathology. *Clin Orthop Relat Res*. 2004;429:163-169.

30. Tannast M, Kubiak-Langer M, Langlotz F, et al. Noninvasive three-dimensional assessment of femoroacetabular impingement. *J Orthop Res*. 2007;25(1):122-131.

31. Nepple JJ, Lehmann CL, Ross JR, Schoenecker PL. JC. C. Coxa profunda is not a useful radiographic parameter for diagnosing pincer-type femoroacetabular impingement. *J Bone Joint Surg Am*. 2013;95(5):412-423.

32. Anderson LA, Kapron AL, Aoki SK, Peters CL. Coxa profunda: is the deep acetabulum overcovered? *Clin Orthop Relat Res*. 2012;470(12):3375-3382.

33. Gosvig KK, Jacobsen S, Sonne-Holm S, et al. Prevalence of malformations of the hip joint and their relationship to sex, groin pain, and risk of osteoarthritis: a population-based survey. *J Bone Joint Surg Am*. 2010;92(5):1162-1169.

34. Anderson LA, Peters C, Park BB, et al. Acetabular cartilage delamination in femoroacetabular impingement: risk factors and magnetic resonance imaging diagnosis. *J Bone Joint Surg Am*. 2009;91(2):305-313.

35. Kutty S, Schneider P, Faris P, et al. Reliability and predictability of the centre-edge angle in the assessment of pincer femoroacetabular impingement. *Int Orthop*. 2012;36(3):505-510.

36. Tonnis D. *Congenital dysplasia and Dislocation of the Hip in Children and Adults*. Berlin, Germany: Springer; 1987.

37. Clohisy JC, Knaus ER, Hunt DM, et al. Clinical presentation of patients with symptomatic anterior hip impingement. *Clin Orthop Relat Res*. 2009;467(3):638-644.

38. Bellaiche L, Lequesne M, Gedouin JE, et al. Imaging data in a prospective series of adult hip pain in under-50 year-olds. *Orthop Traumatol Surg Res*. 2010;96(8 suppl):S44-S52.

39. Jamali AA, Mladenov K, Meyer DC, et al. Anteroposterior pelvic radiographs to assess acetabular retroversion: high validity of the "cross-over-sign. *J Orthop Res*. 2007;25(6):758-765.

40. Zaltz I, Kelly BT, Hetsroni I, Bedi A. The crossover sign over-estimates acetabular retroversion. *Clin Orthop Relat Res.* 2013;471(8):2463-2470.

41. Hong SJ, Shon WY, Lee CY, et al. Imaging findings of femoroacetabular impingement syndrome: focusing on mixed-type impingement. *Clin Imaging.* 2010;34(2):116-120.

42. Register B, Pennock AT, Ho CP, et al. Prevalence of abnormal hip findings in asymptomatic participants: a prospective, blinded study. *Am J Sports Med.* 2012;40(12):2720-2724.

43. Philippon MJ. The role of arthroscopic thermal capsulorrhaphy in the hip. *Clin Sports Med.* 2001;4:817-829.

44. Boykin RE, Anz AW, Bushnell BD, et al. Hip instability. *J Am Acad Orthop Surg.* 2011;19(6):340-349.

45. Martin RL, Enseki KR, Draovitch P, et al. Acetabular labral tears of the hip: examination and diagnostic challenges. *J Orthop Sports Phys Ther.* 2006;36(7):503-515.

46. Philippon MJ, Maxwell RB, Johnston TL, et al. Clinical presentation of femoroacetabular impingement. *Knee Surg Sports Traumatol Arthrosc.* 2007;15(8):1041-1047.

47. Epstein DM, Rose DJ, Philippon MJ. Arthroscopic management of recurrent low-energy anterior hip dislocation in a dancer: a case report and review of literature. *Am J Sports Med.* 2010;38(6):1250-1254.

48. Enseki K, Kohlrieser D. Rehabilitation following hip arthroscopy: an evolving process. *Int J Sports Phys Ther.* 2014;9(6):765-773.

49. Kachingwe A, Grech S. Proposed algorithm for the management of athletes with athletic pubalgia: a coordination of the core and extremities of athletes. *N Am J Sports Phys Ther.* 2009;4(2):70-82.

50. Hammoud S, Bedi A, Magennis E, et al. High incidence of athletic pubalgia symptoms in professional athletes with symptomatic femoroacetabular impingement. *Arthroscopy.* 2012;28(10):1388-1395.

51. Lamontagne M, Kennedy MJ, Beaulé PE. The effect of cam FAI on hip and pelvic motion during maximum squat. *Clin Orthop Relat Res.* 2009;467(3):645-650.

52. Brisson N, Lamontagne M, Kennedy MJ, Beaulé PE. The effects of cam femoroacetabular impingement corrective surgery on lower-extremity gait biomechanics. *Gait Posture.* 2013;37:258-263.

53. Verrall G, Slavotinek J, Barnes P, et al. Spriggins AJ. Hip joint range of motion restriction precedes athletic chronic groin injury. *J Sci Med Sport.* 2007;10(6):463-466.

54. Becker LC, Kohlrieser DA. Conservative management of sports hernia in a professional golfer: a case report. *Int J Sports Phys Ther.* 2014;9(6):851-860.

55. Birmingham PM, Kelly BT, Jacobs R, et al. The effect of dynamic femoroacetabular impingement on pubic symphysis motion: a cadaveric study. *Am J Sports Med.* 2012;40(5):1113-1118.

55a. Domb BG, Shindle MK, McArthur B, et al. Iliopsoas impingement: a newly identified cause of labral pathology in the hip. *HSS J.* 2011;7(2):145-150.

56. Sutter R, Pfirrmann CWA. Atypical hip impingement. *AJR Am J Roentgenol.* 2013;201(3):W437-W442.

57. de Sa D, Cargnelli S, Catapano M, et al. Femoroacetabular impingement in skeletally immature patients: a systematic review examining indications, outcomes, and complications of open and arthroscopic treatment. *Arthroscopy.* 2015;31(2):373-384.

57a. Lee S, Kim I, Lee SM, Lee J. Ischiofemoral impingement syndrome. *Ann Rehabil Med.* 2013;37(1):143-146.

57b. Stafford GH, Villar RN. Ischiofemoral impingement. *J Bone Joint Surg Br.* 2011;93(10):1300-1302.

58. Anderson K, Strickland SM, Warren RF. Hip and groin injuries in athletes. *Am J Sports Med.* 2001;29(4):521-533.

58a. Papavasiliou AV, Bardakos NV. Complications of arthroscopic surgery of the hip. *Bone Joint Res.* 2012;1(7):131-144.

58b. Bradshaw C, McCrory P, Bell S, Brukner P. Obturator nerve entrapment: a cause of groin pain in athletes. *Am J Sports Med.* 1997;25(3):402-408.

59. Cheatham SW, Kolber MJ, Salamh PA. Meralgia paresthetica: a review of the literature. *Int J Sports Phys Ther.* 2013;8(6):883-893.

60. Cibulka MT, White DM, Woehrle J, et al. Hip pain and mobility deficits—hip osteoarthritis: clinical practice guidelines linked to the international classification of functioning, disability, and health from the orthopaedic section of the American Physical Therapy Association. *J Orthop Sports Phys Ther.* 2009;39(4):A1-A25.

61. Mason JB. Acetabular labral tears in the athlete. *Clin Sports Med.* 2001;4:779-790.

62. Guanche CA, Sikka RS. Acetabular labral tears with underlying chondromalacia: a possible association with high-level running. *Arthroscopy.* 2005;21(5):580-585.

63. Stull JD, Philippon MJ, LaPrade RF. "At-risk" positioning and hip biomechanics of the Peewee ice hockey sprint start. *Am J Sports Med.* 2011;39(suppl):29S-35S.

64. Martin RL, Kelly BT, Leunig M, et al. Reliability of clinical diagnosis in intraarticular hip diseases. *Knee Surg Sports Traumatol Arthrosc.* 2010;18(5):685-690.

65. Domb BG, Brooks AG, Byrd JW. Clinical examination of the hip joint in athletes. *J Sport Rehabil.* 2009;18(1):3-23.

66. McCarthy JC, Busconi B. The role of hip arthroscopy in the diagnosis and treatment of hip disease. *Orthopedics.* 1995;18(8):753-756.

67. Lewis CL. Extra-articular snapping hip: a literature review. *Sports Health.* 2010;2(3):186-190.

68. Sueki DG, Cleland JA, Wainner RS. A regional interdependence model of musculoskeletal dysfunction: research, mechanisms, and clinical implications. *J Man Manip Ther.* 2013;21(2):90-102.

69. Austin AB, Souza RB, Meyer JL, Powers CM. Identification of abnormal hip motion associated with acetabular labral pathology. *J Orthop Sports Phys Ther.* 2008;38(9):558-565.

70. Ross JR, Nepple JJ, Philippon MJ, et al. Effect of changes in pelvic tilt on range of motion to impingement and radiographic parameters of acetabular morphological characteristics. *Am J Sports Med.* 2014;42(10):2402-2409.

71. Lewis CL, Sahrmann SA. Effect of posture on hip angles and moments during gait. *Man Ther.* 2015;20(1):176-182.

72. Hunt MA, Guenther JR, Gilbart MK. Kinematic and kinetic differences during walking in patients with and without symptomatic femoroacetabular impingement. *Clin Biomech (Bristol, Avon).* 2013;28(5):519-523.

73. Poultsides LA, Bedi A, Kelly BT. An algorithmic approach to mechanical hip pain. *HSS J.* 2012;8(3):213-224.

74. Wainner RS, Whitman JM, Cleland JA, Flynn TW. Regional interdependence: a musculoskeletal examination model whose time has come. *J Orthop Sports Phys Ther.* 2007;37(11):658-660.

75. Wahoff M, Dischiavi S, Hodge J, Pharez JD. Rehabilitation after labral repair and femoroacetabular decompression: criteria-based progression through the return to sport phase. *Int J Sports Phys Ther.* 2014;9(6):813-826.

76. Altman R, Alarcon G, Appelrouth D, et al. The American College of Rheumatology criteria for the classification and reporting of osteoarthritis of the hip. *Arthritis Rheum.* 1991; 34(5):505-514.

77. Harris-Hayes M, Mueller MJ, Sahrmann SA, et al. Persons with chronic hip joint pain exhibit reduced muscle strength. *J Orthop Sports Phys Ther.* 2014;44(11):890-898.

78. Casartelli NC, Maffiuletti NA, Item-Glatthorn JF, et al. Hip muscle weakness in patients with symptomatic femoroacetabular impingement. *Osteoarthritis Cartilage.*2011;19(7): 816-821.

79. Casartelli NC, Leunig M, Item-Glatthorn JF, et al. Hip flexor muscle fatigue in patients with symptomatic femoroacetabular impingement. *Int Orthop.* 2012;36(5):967-973.

80. Cascio BM, King D, Yen YM. Psoas impingement causing labrum tear: a series from three tertiary hip arthroscopy centers. *J la State Med Soc.* 2013;165(2):88-93.

81. Allen WC, Cope R. Coxa saltans: the snapping hip revisited. *J Am Acad Orthop Surg.* 1995;3(5):303-308.

82. Sierra RJ, Trousdale RT, Ganz R, Leunig M. Hip disease in the young, active patient: evaluation and nonarthroplasty surgical options. *J Am Acad Orthop Surg.* 2008;16(12):689-703.

83. Hoeksma HL, Dekker J, Ronday HK, et al. Comparison of manual therapy and exercise therapy in osteoarthritis of the hip: a randomized clinical trial. *Arthritis Rheum.* 2004;51(5): 722-729.

84. Harding L, Barbe M, Shepard K, et al. Posterior-anterior glide of the femoral head in the acetabulum: a cadaver study. *J Orthop Sports Phys Ther.* 2003;33(3):118-125.

85. Tijssen M, van Cingel R, Willemsen L, de Visser E. Diagnostics of femoroacetabular impingement and labral pathology of the hip: a systematic review of the accuracy and validity of physical tests. *Arthroscopy.* 2012;28(6):860-871.

86. Maslowski E, Sullivan W, Forster HJ, et al. The diagnostic validity of hip provocation maneuvers to detect intra-articular hip pathology. *PM R.* 2010;2(3):174-181.

87. Martin R, Sekiya J. The interrater reliability of 4 clinical tests used to assess individuals with musculoskeletal hip pain. *J Orthop Sports Phys Ther.* 2008;38(2):71-77.

88. Reiman MP, Goode AP, Cook CE, et al. Diagnostic accuracy of clinical tests for the diagnosis of hip femoroacetabular impingement/labral tear: a systematic review with meta-analysis. *Br J Sports Med.* 2015;49(12):811.

89. Reiman MP, Thorborg K. Clincal examination and physical assessment of hip joint–related pain in athletes. *Int J Sports Phys Ther.* 2014;9(6):737-755.

90. Byrd JW, Jones KS. Diagnostic accuracy of clinical assessment, magnetic resonance imaging, magnetic resonance arthrography, and intra-articular injection in hip arthroscopy patients. *Am J Sports Med.* 2004;32(7):1668-1674.

91. Kivlan BR, Martin RL, Sekiya JK. Response to diagnostic injection in patients with femoroacetabular impingement, labral tears, chondral lesions, and extra-articular pathology. *Arthroscopy.* 2011;27(5):619-627.

92. Safran MR, Giordano G, Lindsey DP, et al. Strains across the acetabular labrum during hip motion: a cadaveric model. *Am J Sports Med.* 2011;39(suppl):92S-102S.

93. Lewis CL, Sahrmann SA. Acetabular labral tears. *Phys Ther.* 2006;86(1):110-121.

94. Smith J, Hurdle MF. Accuracy of sonographically guided intra-articular injections in the native adult hip. *J Ultrasound Med.* 2009;28:329-335.

95. Yazbek PM, Ovanessian V, Martin RL, Fukuda TY. Nonsurgical treatment of acetabular labrum tears: a case series. *J Orthop Sports Phys Ther.* 2011;41(5):346-353.

96. Leetun DT, Ireland ML, Willson JD, et al. Core stability measures as risk factors for lower extremity injury in athletes. *Med Sci Sports Exerc.* 2004;36(6):926-934.

97. Willson JD, Dougherty CP, Ireland ML, Davis IM. Core stability and its relationship to lower extremity function and injury. *J Am Acad Orthop Surg.* 2005;13(5):316-325.

98. Bozic KJ, Chan V, Valone FH 3rd, et al. Trends in hip arthroscopy utilization in the United States. *J Arthroplasty.* 2013;28(8 suppl):140-143.

99. Montgomery SR, Ngo SS, Hobson T, et al. Trends and demographics in hip arthroscopy in the United States. *Arthroscopy.* 2013;29(4):661-665.

100. Cohen SB, Huang R, Ciccotti MG, et al. Treatment of femoroacetabular impingement in athletes using a mini-direct anterior approach. *Am J Sports Med.* 2012;40(7):1620-1627.

101. Kemp JL, Collins NJ, Makdissi M, et al. Hip arthroscopy for intra-articular pathology: a systematic review of outcomes with and without femoral osteoplasty. *Br J Sports Med.* 2012;46(9): 632-643.

102. Larson CM, Giveans MR. Arthroscopic management of femoroacetabular impingement: early outcomes measures. *Arthroscopy.* 2008;24(5):540-546.

103. Wilkin G, March G, Beaule PE. Arthroscopic acetabular labral debridement in patients forty-five years of age or older has minimal benefit for pain and function. *J Bone Joint Surg Am.* 2014;96(2):113-118.

104. McCormick F, Nwachukwu BU, Alpaugh K, Martin SD. Predictors of hip arthroscopy outcomes for labral tears at minimum 2-year follow-up: the influence of age and arthritis. *Arthroscopy.* 2012;28(10):1359-1364.

105. Philippon MJ, Briggs KK, Carlisle JC, Patterson DC. Joint space predicts THA after hip arthroscopy in patients 50 years and older. *Clin Orthop Relat Res.* 2013;471(8):2492-2496.

106. Ayeni OR, Adamich J, Farrokhyar F, et al. Surgical management of labral tears during femoroacetabular impingement surgery: a systematic review. *Knee Surg Sports Traumatol Arthrosc.* 2014;22(4):756-762.

107. Burman M. Arthroscopy or the direct visualization of joints. *J Bone Joint Surg.* 1931;4:669-695.

108. Suzuki S, Awaya G, Okada Y, et al. Arthroscopic diagnosis of ruptured acetabular labrum. *Acta Orthop Scand.* 1986;57(6): 513-515.

109. Glick JM. Hip arthroscopy using the lateral approach. *Instr Course Lect.* 1988;37:223-231.

110. Byrd JW. Hip arthroscopy utilizing the supine position. *Arthroscopy.* 1994;10(3):275-280.

111. Clarke MT, Arora A, Villar RN. Hip arthroscopy: complications in 1054 cases. *Clin Orthop Relat Res.* 2003;406:84-88.

112. Kelly BT, Weiland DE, Schenker ML, Philippon MJ. Arthroscopic labral repair in the hip: Surgical technique and review of the literature. *Arthroscopy.* 2005;21:1496-1504.

113. Frank RM, Lee S, Bush-Joseph CA, et al. Improved outcomes after hip arthroscopic surgery in patients undergoing T-capsulotomy with complete repair versus partial repair for femoroacetabular impingement: a comparative matched-pair analysis. *Am J Sports Med.* 2014;42(11):2634-2642.

114. Pennock AT, Philippon MJ, Briggs KK. Acetabular labral preservation: surgical techniques, indications, and early outcomes. *Oper Tech Orthop.* 2010;20(4):217-222.

115. Garrison JC, Osler MT, Singleton SB. Rehabilitation after arthroscopy of an acetabular labral tear. *N Am J Sports Phys Ther*. 2007;2(4):241-250.

116. Domb BG, El Bitar YF, Stake CE, et al. Arthroscopic labral reconstruction is superior to segmental resection for irreparable labral tears in the hip: a matched-pair controlled study with minimum 2-year follow-up. *Am J Sports Med*. 2014;42(1): 122-130.

117. Matsuda DK, Carlisle JC, Arthurs SC, et al. Comparative systematic review of the open dislocation, mini-open, and arthroscopic surgeries for femoroacetabular impingement. *Arthroscopy*. 2011;27(2):252-269.

118. Ejnisman L, Philippon MJ. Lertwanich P. Femoroacetabular impingement: the femoral side. *Clin Sports Med*. 2011;30(2): 369-377.

119. Colvin AC, Koehler SM, Bird J. Can the change in center-edge angle during pincer trimming be reliably predicted? *Clin Orthop Relat Res*. 2011;469(4):1071-1074.

120. Domb BG, Stake CE, Botser B, Jackson TJ. Surgical dislocation of the hip versus arthroscopic treatment of femoroacetabular impingement: a prospective matched-pair study with average 2-year follow-up. *Arthroscopy*. 2013;29(9):1506-1513.

121. Ganz R, Gill TJ, Gautier E, et al. Surgical dislocation of the adult hip a technique with full access to the femoral head and acetabulum without the risk of avascular necrosis. *J Bone Joint Surg Br*. 2001;83(8):1119-1124.

122. Domb BG, Stake CE, Lindner D, et al. Arthroscopic capsular plication and labral preservation in borderline hip dysplasia: two-year clinical outcomes of a surgical approach to a challenging problem. *Am J Sports Med*. 2013;41(11):2591-2598.

123. Hartig-Andreasen C, Soballe K, Troelsen A. The role of the acetabular labrum in hip dysplasia: a literature overview. *Acta Orthop*. 2013;84(1):60-64.

124. Philippon MJ, Schenker ML, Briggs KK, Maxwell RB. Can microfracture produce repair tissue in acetabular chondral defects? *Arthroscopy*. 2008;24(1):46-50.

125. McDonald JE, Herzog MM, Philippon MJ. Return to play after hip arthroscopy with microfracture in elite athletes. *Arthroscopy*. 2013;29(2):330-335.

126. Ilizaliturri VM Jr, Buganza-Tepole M, Olivos-Meza A, et al. Central compartment release versus lesser trochanter release of the iliopsoas tendon for the treatment of internal snapping hip: a comparative study. *Arthroscopy*. 2014;30(7):790-795.

127. Ilizaliturri VM, Martinez-Escalante FA, Chaidez PA, Camacho-Galindo J. Endoscopic iliotibial band release for external snapping hip syndrome. *Arthroscopy*. 2006;22(5):505-510.

128. Mather R III, Reddy A, Nho S. Complications of hip arthroscopy. In: *Operative Hip Arthroscopy*. New York, NY: Springer; 2013:403-409.

129. Willimon S, Briggs K, Philippon MJ. Intra-articular adhesions following hip arthroscopy: a risk factor analysis. *Knee Surg Sports Traumatol Arthrosc*. 2014;22(4):822-825.

130. Beck M, Leunig M, Parvizi J. Anterior femoroacetabular impingement: part II. Midterm results of surgical treatment. *Clin Orthop Relat Res*. 2004;418:67-73.

131. Ayeni OR, Bedi A, Lorich DG, Kelly BT. Femoral neck fracture after arthroscopic management of femoroacetabular impingement: a case report. *J Bone Joint Surg Am*. 2011;93(9):e47.

132. Ranawat AS, McClincy M, Sekiya JK. Anterior dislocation of the hip after arthroscopy in a patient with capsular laxity of the hip: a case report. *J Bone Joint Surg Am*. 2009;91(1): 192-197.

133. Cheatham SW, Enseki KR, Kolber MJ. Post-operative rehabilitation after hip arthroscopy: a search for the evidence. *J Sport Rehabil*. 2014;[Epub ahead of print].

134. Spencer-Gardner L, Eischen JJ, Levy BA, et al. A comprehensive five-phase rehabilitation programme after hip arthroscopy for femoroacetabular impingement. *Knee Surg Sports Traumatol Arthrosc*. 2014;22(4):848-859.

135. Enseki KR, Martin R, Kelly BT. Rehabilitation after arthroscopic decompression for femoroacetabular impingement. *Clin Sports Med*. 2010;29(2):247-255, viii.

136. Malloy P, Malloy M. Draovitch P. Guidelines and pitfalls for the rehabilitation following hip arthroscopy. *Curr Rev Musculoskelet Med*. 2013;6(3):235-241.

137. Aprato A, Jayasekera N, Villar RN. Revision hip arthroscopic surgery: outcome at three years. *Knee Surg Sports Traumatol Arthrosc*. 2014;22(4):932-937.

138. Bogunovic L, Gottlieb M, Pashos G, et al. Why do hip arthroscopy procedures fail? *Clin Orthop Relat Res*. 2013;471(8): 2523-2529.

139. Edelstein J, Ranawat A, Enseki KR, et al. Post-operative guidelines following hip arthroscopy. *Curr Rev Musculoskelet Med*. 2012;5(1):15-23.

140. Freeman S, Mascia A, McGill S. Arthrogenic neuromusculature inhibition: a foundational investigation of existence in the hip joint. *Clin Biomech (Bristol, Avon)*. 2013;28(2):171-177.

141. Hinman RS, Dobson F, Takla A, et al. Which is the most useful patient-reported outcome in femoroacetabular impingement? Test-retest reliability of six questionnaires. *Br J Sports Med*. 2014;48(6):458-463.

142. Kivlan BR, Martin R. Outcome instruments for the hip: a guide to implementation. *Orthop Phys Ther Practice*. 2013;25(3): 162-169.

143. Harris-Hayes M, McDonough CM, Leunig M, et al. Clinical outcomes assessment in clinical trials to assess treatment of femoroacetabular impingement: use of patient-reported outcome measures. *J Am Acad Orthop Surg*. 2013;21(suppl 1): S39-S46.

144. Martin RL, Philippon MJ. Evidence of reliability and responsiveness for the hip outcome score. *Arthroscopy*. 2008;24(6): 676-682.

145. Mohtadi NG, Griffin DR, Pedersen ME, et al. Multicenter Arthroscopy of the Hip Outcomes Research Network. The development and validation of a self-administered quality-of-life outcome measure for young, active patients with symptomatic hip disease: the International Hip Outcome Tool (iHOT-33). *Arthroscopy*. 2012;28(5):595-605.

146. Thorborg K, Hölmich P, Christensen R, et al. The Copenhagen Hip and Groin Outcome Score (HAGOS): development and validation according to the COSMIN checklist. *Br J Sports Med*. 2011;45(6):478-491.

147. Thorborg K, Roos EM, Bartels EM, et al. Validity, reliability and responsiveness of patient-reported outcome questionnaires when assessing hip and groin disability: a systematic review. *Br J Sports Med*. 2010;44(16):1186-1196.

5

Musculoskeletal Sources of Abdominal and Groin Pain: Athletic Pubalgia, Hernias, and Abdominal Strains

AIMIE F. KACHINGWE

CHAPTER OUTLINE

Investigators have estimated that 5% to 18 % of athletes present to their physicians with activity-restrictive groin or lower abdominal pain.[1-3] Groin pain is particularly common in sports requiring athletes to perform repetitive kicking, twisting, or turning at high speeds including soccer, football, basketball, track and field, tennis, and hockey.[3-10] Despite the prevalence of groin pain, the literature is filled with puzzling and often contradictory information on the etiology, presentation, diagnosis, and treatment of groin pain in athletes.[10] Diagnosing groin pain is often complicated by confounding symptoms and concomitant injuries that make diagnostic differentiation challenging.[1,4-6,11-13] This chapter focuses on three of the most common dysfunctions leading to lower abdominal or groin pain: abdominal strains, inguinal hernias, and sports hernias or athletic pubalgia.

Abdominal Strains

Abdominal strains can involve the rectus abdominis, internal and external oblique, and transversus abdominis muscles. "Side strains" implicate the oblique muscles—most typically the internal oblique, but external oblique strains have also been documented.[14] It is purported that muscle strains typically occur in muscles (e.g., the hamstrings) crossing two joints, with a high percentage of type II fibers, and active during volitional eccentric muscle activity.[15] Muscles such as the rectus abdominis that are nonarticular and multilaminated are often found to be injured during eccentric contractions during highly specific and volitional sports movements such as serving in tennis, bowling in cricket, spiking in volleyball, smashing in tennis, or batting, and pitching in baseball.[15]

Anatomy of the Abdominal Muscles

Four primary muscles constitute the abdominal wall: the rectus abdominis, the internal and external obliques, and the transversus abdominis. The rectus abdominis consists of two vertically oriented components, with each muscle having two tendinous origins—the larger lateral head originates from the upper border of the pubic crest, and a medial head arises from the anterior pubic symphysis (Fig. 5-1). The rectus abdominis medial head blends with fibers from the contralateral rectus and with the ligaments covering the anterior pubic symphysis.[16] The rectus inserts superiorly onto the cartilages of the fifth, sixth, and seventh ribs and the xiphoid process (Fig. 5-2). The two vertical muscles are separated by the linea alba and are reinforced by three transverse fibrous bands, called tendinous intersections, that run horizontally and blend with the anterior rectus sheath to give the muscle its "six-pack" appearance.[16-20]

The rectus abdominis is enclosed in a sheath formed by the aponeurosis of the internal and external obliques and transversus abdominis. The posterior sheath ends at a point midway between the umbilicus and pubic symphysis at the linea semicircularis or arcuate line (Fig. 5-3). Superior to

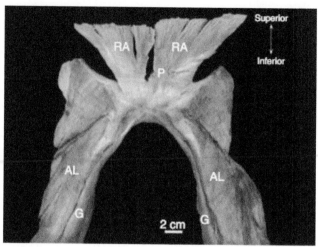

• **Figure 5-1** Anterior view of the pubic symphysis showing the tendinous origins of the rectus abdominis (RA)—the larger lateral head originating from the upper border of the pubic crest and the smaller medial head originating from the anterior pubic symphysis. Note how the medial head blends with its contralateral counterpart to reinforce the anterior pubic symphysis. The pyramidalis (P) also originates from the anterior pubis and anterior pubic ligament. *AL*, Adductor longus; *G*, gracilis. (From Becker I, Woodley SJ, Stringer MD. The adult human pubic symphysis: a systematic review. *J Anat.* 2010;217: 475-487.)

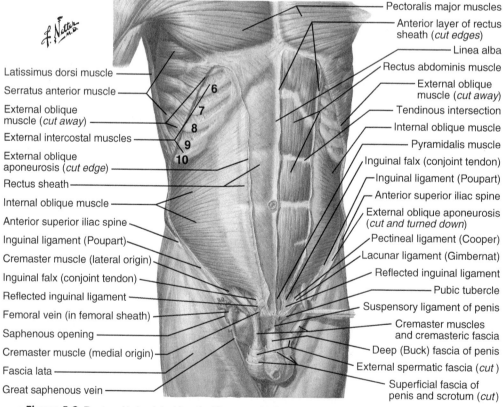

• **Figure 5-2** Rectus Abdominis Muscle. The pyramidalis is a small triangular muscle anterior to the rectus abdominis and enclosed in the same rectus sheath. Note how it diminishes in size as it runs superiorly—eventually blending into the linea alba midway between the umbilicus and pubis. The cremaster muscle originates from the inguinal ligament. Its fibers are continuous with the internal oblique and sometimes the transversus. (Netter illustration from www.netterimages.com. © Elsevier Inc. All rights reserved.)

the arcuate line, the internal oblique aponeurosis divides at the lateral margin of the rectus into two lamellae: one passing anterior to the rectus and blending with the aponeurosis of the external obliques to become the anterior rectus sheath and the other passing posterior to the rectus and blending with the aponeurosis of the transversus abdominis (known as the inguinal falx or the conjoint tendon) to form the posterior sheath (Fig. 5-4, *A*).[17] Inferior to the arcuate line, the aponeurosis of all three muscles passes anterior to the rectus (Fig. 5-4, *B*), and thus the

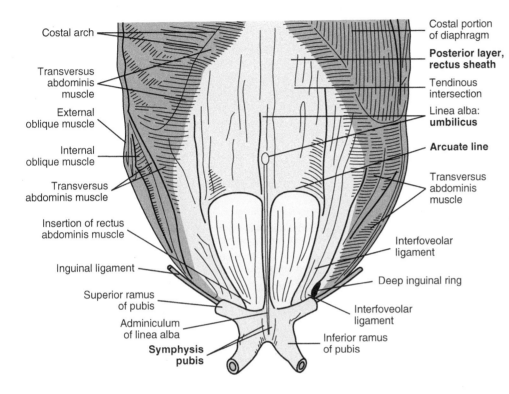

• **Figure 5-3** Internal view of the anterior abdominal wall provides an excellent view of the posterior sheath of rectus abdominis. Note that the posterior sheath ends at the arcuate line midway between the umbilicus and pubic symphysis. (Redrawn from Clemente CD. *Anatomy: A Regional Atlas of the Human Body.* 3rd ed. Baltimore: Urban & Schwarzenberg; 1987.)

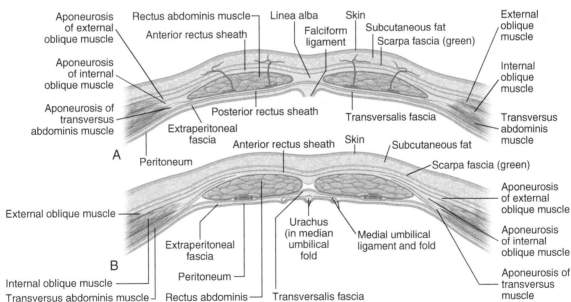

• **Figure 5-4 A,** Superior to the arcuate line, the aponeurosis of the internal oblique muscle splits—the anterior portion joints the aponeurosis of the external oblique to become the anterior layer of the rectus sheath, whereas the posterior portion joins the aponeurosis of the transversus abdominis to become the posterior layer of the rectus sheath. The anterior and posterior layers of the rectus sheath join medially at the linea alba. **B,** Inferior to the arcuate line, the aponeurosis of the internal oblique does not split, but it continues anterior to the rectus abdominis to join both the aponeurosis of the external oblique and transversus abdominis to become the anterior layer of the rectus sheath. Thus, the posterior wall of the rectus abdominis muscle lies directly on the transversalis fascia. (From Song DH, Neligan PC. *Plastic Surgery.* Vol 4: *Trunk and Lower Extremity.* 3rd ed. London: Saunders; 2013.)

posterior border of the recti is separated from the peritoneum only by the transversalis fascia.[17] The drawing by Netter[20] of the internal view of the anterior abdominal wall shows how, when the transversalis fascia is cut, the posterior aspect of the rectus abdominis is directly exposed inferior to the arcuate line (Fig. 5-5). At the medial border of the rectus, the anterior and posterior rectus sheaths merge again at the linea alba.[17]

The obliquus externus abdominis, more commonly referred to as the external oblique, is the largest and most superficial of the abdominal muscles; its muscular portion occupies the anterior lateral abdomen, and its aponeurosis occupies the anterior abdominal wall (Fig. 5-6).[17] It originates with eight fleshy digitations from the external surfaces and inferior borders of ribs 5 to 12, as well as the adjacent serratus anterior and latissimus dorsi muscles. Fibers from the lower ribs pass inferiorly in a nearly vertical fashion to insert onto the anterior half of the outer lip of the iliac crest, whereas fibers from the middle and upper fibers are directed inferior and medial to become an aponeurosis.[17] The external oblique aponeurosis blends with the contralateral aponeurosis, covering the entire anterior abdomen. Superiorly,

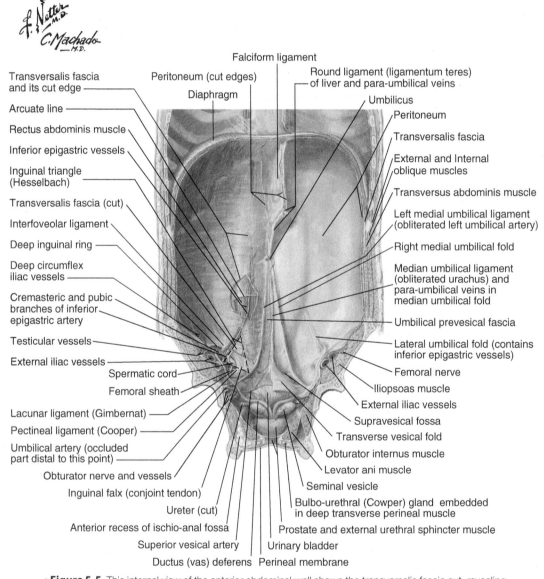

• **Figure 5-5** This internal view of the anterior abdominal wall shows the transversalis fascia cut, revealing the arcuate line. Superior to the arcuate line is the posterior sheath of the rectus abdominis. Inferior to the arcuate line, the rectus abdominis muscle directly contacts the transversalis fascia. Note the orifice in the transversalis fascia for the deep inguinal ring, which is bounded medially by the inferior epigastric vessels. Located medial to the deep inguinal ring, the Hesselbach triangle is bounded laterally by the inferior epigastric vessels, medially by the lateral border of the rectus abdominis, and inferiorly by the inguinal ligament. (Netter illustration from www.netterimages.com. © Elsevier Inc. All rights reserved.)

the fibers of the external oblique muscle communicate with the pectoralis major. In the middle, its fibers interlace with the contralateral obliques to form the linea alba. The inferior fibers attach to the pubic tubercle and pectineal line (Fig. 5-7).[17]

Acting bilaterally, the external oblique muscle flexes the trunk and posteriorly tilts the pelvis (Fig. 5-8). When it acts unilaterally, or if one side is stiffer than the other, lateral flexion and contralateral rotation of the trunk result.[21-26]

The inguinal (Poupart) ligament is the portion of the external oblique aponeurosis extending between the anterior superior iliac spine (ASIS) and the pubic tubercle, and it is a thick band that folds inward (Fig. 5-9).[17] The lacunar (Gimbernat) ligament (see Fig. 5-9) is a distal portion of the external oblique aponeurosis that is reflected from its pubic tubercle attachment to connect to the pectineal line. The lacunar ligament is approximately 1.25 cm long—larger in males than in females—and it has an almost horizontal orientation in an erect posture. The lacunar ligament is triangular, with its apex at the pubic tubercle, its posterior margin attaching to the pectineal line, and its anterior margin attaching to the inguinal ligament. The lacunar ligament forms the medial boundary of the femoral ring (discussed later in this chapter).[17]

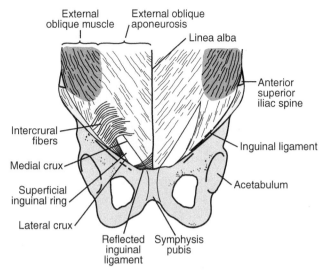

• **Figure 5-7** The inferior fibers of the external oblique aponeurosis attach on the pubic tubercle and pectineal line. A few fibers from the external oblique pass posterior to the medial crux to form the reflected inguinal ligament. The superficial inguinal ring is a slitlike opening in the distal aponeurosis of the external oblique muscle. (Redrawn from Clemente CD. *Anatomy: A Regional Atlas of the Human Body*. 3rd ed. Baltimore: Urban & Schwarzenberg; 1987.)

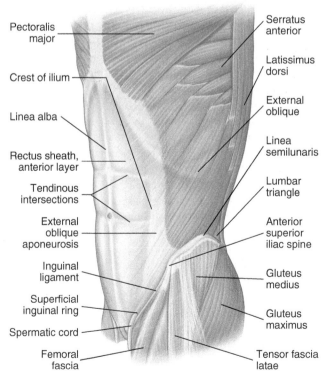

• **Figure 5-6** External Oblique Muscle. (From Standring S, ed. *Gray's Anatomy: The Anatomical Basis of Clinical Practice*. 41st ed. London: Churchill Livingstone; 2016.)

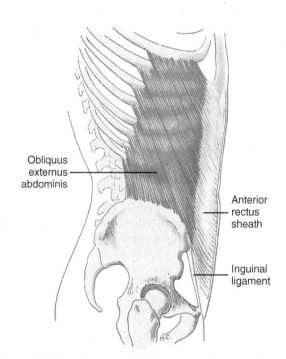

• **Figure 5-8** Attachments of the External Oblique Muscle. Acting bilaterally, the external oblique flexes the trunk and posteriorly tilts the pelvis. Unilateral contraction, or one side is stiffer than the other, would lead to lateral flexion and contralateral rotation of the trunk. (Modified from Luttgens K, Hamilton N: *Kinesiology: Scientific Basis of Human Motion*. 9th ed. Madison, Wis.: Brown and Benchmark; 1997.)

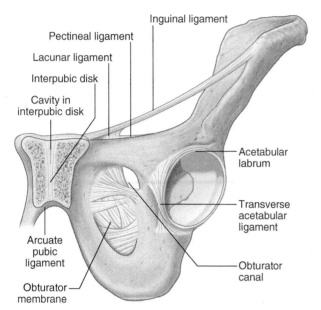

• **Figure 5-9** The inguinal ligament is the portion of the external oblique aponeurosis the folds inward, extending between the anterior superior iliac spine and the pubic tubercle. The lacunar ligament is a distal portion of the external oblique aponeurosis. It is triangular, with its apex attaching at the pubic tubercle, the posterior margin attaching to the pectineal line, and the anterior margin attaching to the inguinal ligament. The pectineal (Cooper) ligament extends laterally from the base of the lacunar ligament to attach along the pectineal line. (From Standring S, ed. *Gray's Anatomy: The Anatomical Basis of Clinical Practice.* 41st ed. London: Churchill Livingstone; 2016.)

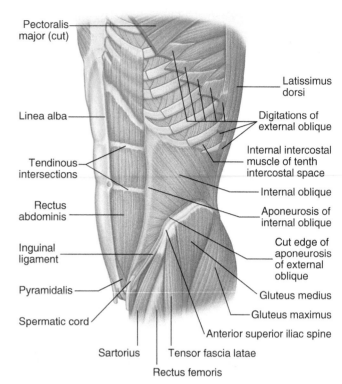

• **Figure 5-10** Internal Oblique Muscle. (From Standring S, ed. *Gray's Anatomy: The Anatomical Basis of Clinical Practice.* 41st ed. London: Churchill Livingstone; 2016.)

The pectineal (Cooper) ligament is another fibrous extension from the lacunar ligament (see Fig. 5-9) that extends laterally from the base of the lacunar ligament to attach along the pectineal line. The pectineal ligament helps to reinforce the pectineal fascia, as well as the linea alba.[17]

From its pectineal line attachment, a few fibers from the external oblique aponeurosis pass superiorly and medially, behind the medial crus of the subcutaneous inguinal ring, to form a thin triangular fibrous band called the reflected inguinal ligament (triangular fascia) (see Fig. 5-7).[17] The reflected inguinal ligament blends with the lacunar ligament and the medial inferior crus of the subcutaneous inguinal ring to help reinforce the subcutaneous inguinal ring. The reflected inguinal ligament also blends with the contralateral reflected inguinal ligament to reinforce the distal linea alba,[17] and it is discussed later in this chapter.

The obliquus internus abdominis muscle, also known as the internal oblique, is deep to the external oblique and forms the second abdominal layer (Fig. 5-10). Its fibers originate from the lateral half of the inguinal ligament, from the anterior two thirds of the middle lip of the iliac crest, and from the posterior lamella of the lumbodorsal fascia.[17] The portion of the internal oblique that originates most posteriorly passes almost vertically and superiorly to insert onto the cartilages of the tenth, eleventh, and twelfth ribs

to become continuous with the internal intercostal muscle. Internal oblique fibers originating from the middle third of the iliac crest run obliquely superiorly and medially. They culminate in an aponeurosis that divides at the lateral border of the rectus to become the anterior and posterior lamellae that envelop the rectus. Internal oblique fibers originating from the anterior third of the iliac crest run horizontally, become tendinous, and pass in front to the rectus abdominis to insert into the linea alba.[17] The internal oblique fibers originating from the inguinal ligament arch inferiorly and medially across the spermatic cord in the male and the round ligament in the female. These fibers become tendinous, join with the transversus abdominis to form the inguinal aponeurotic falx (conjoint tendon), and insert onto the pubic crest and medial aspect of the pectineal line behind the lacunar ligament immediately behind the subcutaneous inguinal ring (Figs. 5-11 and 5-12).[17]

Acting bilaterally, the internal oblique flexes the trunk and posteriorly tilts the pelvis (Fig. 5-13). However, unilateral contraction or stiffness leads to lateral flexion and ipsilateral trunk rotation.[21-26]

The internal and external oblique muscles are effective axial rotators of the trunk, with the external oblique being a contralateral rotator and the internal oblique an ipsilateral rotator. During active axial rotation in one direction,

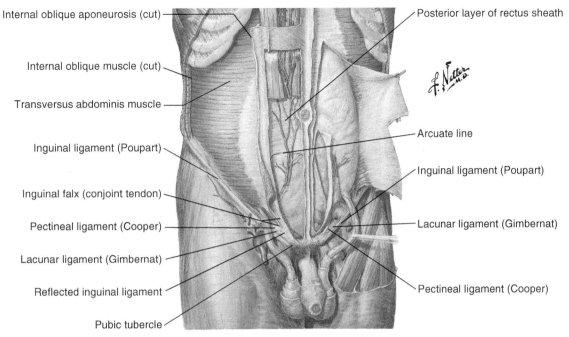

Internal oblique aponeurosis (cut)

Internal oblique muscle (cut)

Transversus abdominis muscle

Inguinal ligament (Poupart)

Inguinal falx (conjoint tendon)

Pectineal ligament (Cooper)

Lacunar ligament (Gimbernat)

Reflected inguinal ligament

Pubic tubercle

Posterior layer of rectus sheath

Arcuate line

Inguinal ligament (Poupart)

Lacunar ligament (Gimbernat)

Pectineal ligament (Cooper)

• **Figure 5-11** The internal oblique fibers originating from the inguinal ligament join with the transversus abdominis to form the inguinal falx or conjoint tendon. It inserts onto the pubic crest and medial pectineal line posterior to the lacunar ligament. (Netter illustration from www.netterimages.com. © Elsevier Inc. All rights reserved.)

the external oblique on the contralateral side works synergistically with the internal oblique on the ipsilateral side to produce a diagonal line of force through the muscles' midline through their attachment on the linea alba.[21,25,27-29]

The deepest abdominal layer is the transversus abdominis, named accordingly because of the nearly horizontal orientation of its fibers (Fig. 5-14). It arises from the lateral third of the inguinal ligament, the anterior three fourths of the inner lip of the iliac crest, the inner surfaces of the cartilages of ribs 6 to 12, fibers from the diaphragm, and the lumbodorsal fascia. The lower fibers curve inferiorly and medially to converge with the internal oblique to form the conjoint tendon and insert onto the crest of the pubis and pectineal line (see Figs. 5-11 and 5-12). The rest of the muscle inserts into the linea alba—the upper three fourths passes behind the rectus to blend with the posterior lamella of the internal oblique aponeurosis, and the lower one fourth passes anterior to the rectus.[17]

The nearly horizontal orientation of the transversus abdominis makes it ideal for compressing the abdomen and stabilizing the lumbopelvic region through its attachments on the thoracolumbar fascia, where it works to limit intersegmental lumbar spine motion.[22,30,31] Studies have found that the transversus abdominis contracts milliseconds before the lower extremity musculature before foot strike during running and before upper extremity elevation or throwing motions.[32] Several fine-wire electromyography (EMG) studies have found bilateral activation of the transversus

abdominis during axial rotation, and thus this muscle appears to function more as a stabilizer for the obliques than as a torque generator by stabilizing the ribs, linea alba, and thoracolumbar fascia.[25,33,34]

A few additional muscles are present in the abdominal region. The pyramidalis is a small triangular muscle located in the inferior abdomen anterior to the rectus abdominis and enclosed in the same sheath (see Fig. 5-2). It originates at the anterior pubis and anterior pubic ligament (see Fig. 5-1), and it passes superiorly, where it diminishes in size and eventually inserts into the linea alba midway between the umbilicus and the pubis (see Fig. 5-2). The pyramidalis functions to tense the linea alba.[17]

The cremaster is a thin muscle consisting of fasciculi originating from the middle of the inguinal ligament, where its fibers are continuous with the internal oblique and sometimes the transversus (see Fig. 5-2).[17] It passes along the lateral aspect of the spermatic cord and descends with it through the subcutaneous inguinal ring to form a series of loops that unite to form the cremasteric fascia covering the spermatic cord and testis (Fig. 5-15). The fibers then ascend along the medial side of the spermatic cord to insert on to the pubic tubercle and crest and onto the front of the sheath of the rectus abdominis.[17]

Incidence

Although athletic communities anecdotally purport that abdominal injuries are fairly common, few epidemiologic

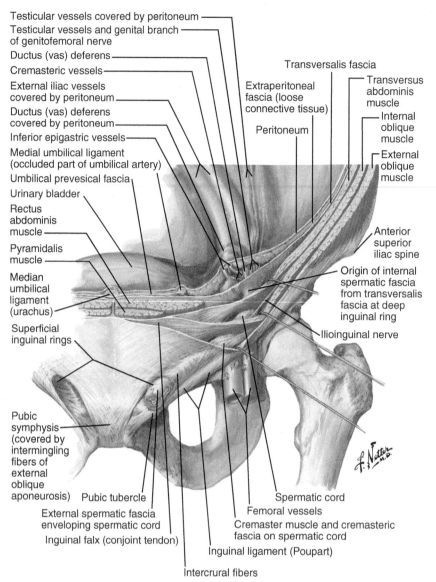

Testicular vessels covered by peritoneum
Testicular vessels and genital branch of genitofemoral nerve
Ductus (vas) deferens
Cremasteric vessels
External iliac vessels covered by peritoneum
Ductus (vas) deferens covered by peritoneum
Inferior epigastric vessels
Medial umbilical ligament (occluded part of umbilical artery)
Umbilical prevesical fascia
Urinary bladder
Rectus abdominis muscle
Pyramidalis muscle
Median umbilical ligament (urachus)
Superficial inguinal rings
Pubic symphysis (covered by intermingling fibers of external oblique aponeurosis)
Pubic tubercle
External spermatic fascia enveloping spermatic cord
Inguinal falx (conjoint tendon)
Intercrural fibers
Inguinal ligament (Poupart)
Cremaster muscle and cremasteric fascia on spermatic cord
Femoral vessels
Spermatic cord
Ilioinguinal nerve
Origin of internal spermatic fascia from transversalis fascia at deep inguinal ring
Anterior superior iliac spine
External oblique muscle
Internal oblique muscle
Transversus abdominis muscle
Transversalis fascia
Peritoneum
Extraperitoneal fascia (loose connective tissue)

• **Figure 5-12** The aponeurosis of the transversus abdominis joins the aponeurosis of the internal oblique to form the inguinal falx, or conjoint tendon. Note the deep inguinal ring. Note the internal spermatic fascia, a continuation of the transversalis fascia that envelops the spermatic cord. (Netter illustration from www.netterimages.com. © Elsevier Inc. All rights reserved.)

studies support their incidence.[19,22,35] Abdominal injuries have been documented primarily through published case studies in throwing and racquet sports including baseball, tennis, handball, and cricket, as well as in soccer.[14,18,19,36-39]

A 19-year retrospective review of the Major League Baseball disabled list[35] reported that abdominal muscle strains constituted 5% of all baseball injuries, with 92% of these injuries specially classified as internal or external oblique or intercostal strains, 1% classified as rectus abdominis strains, and 7% classified as general "abdominal muscle strains." In addition, 44% of abdominal strains occurred in pitchers and 56% in position players, and although an upward trend of more abdominal strains within this 20-year period was noted, the injury rate remained fairly constant in the past decade.[35] A prospective study of English professional soccer

teams[40] reported that torso injuries constituted 7% of all injuries, and a study of youth soccer players found that abdominal injuries constituted 1% of all injuries.[41]

Presentation of Abdominal Strain

Internal oblique abdominal strains, also referred to as side strains, typically manifest with sudden, sharp onset of anterolateral pain along the anterolateral inferior border of one or more of ribs 9 to 12, with localized tenderness and pain on muscular contraction or passive stretching that may arise during deep inspiration.[36,37,39] The pain typically manifests after or during throwing, swinging, or twisting movements, and it often results in forced withdrawal from athletic competition.[14,36,37,39,42,43] The injury site and pain

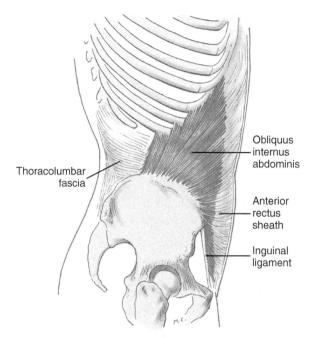

• **Figure 5-13** Attachments of the Internal Oblique Muscle. Acting bilaterally, the internal oblique flexes the trunk and posteriorly tilts the pelvis. Unilateral contraction, or if one side is stiffer than the other, would lead to lateral flexion and ipsilateral trunk rotation. (Modified from Luttgens K, Hamilton N. *Kinesiology: Scientific Basis of Human Motion.* 9th ed. Madison, Wis.: Brown and Benchmark; 1997.)

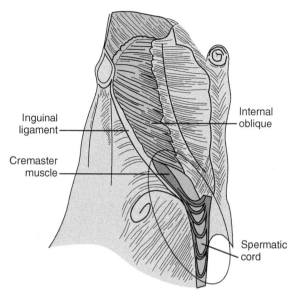

• **Figure 5-15** The cremaster muscle passes lateral to the spermatic cord and descends through the superficial inguinal ring. It forms a series of loops that cover the spermatic cord and testis. (Redrawn from Gray H. *Anatomy of the Human Body.* Philadelphia: Lea & Febiger, 1918; Bartleby.com, 2000. www.bartleby.com/107/. [October 28, 2015].)

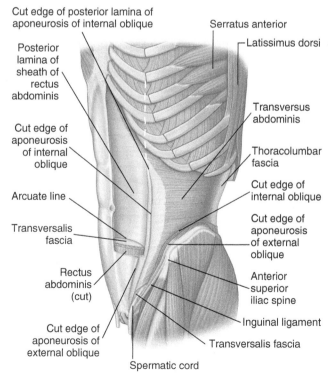

• **Figure 5-14** Transversus Abdominis Muscle. (From Standring S, ed. *Gray's Anatomy: The Anatomical Basis of Clinical Practice.* 41st ed. London: Churchill Livingstone; 2016.)

are typically on the contralateral side of the dominant arm,[18,19,35,36] and the pain often appears when the athlete is asked to perform resisted ipsilateral side flexion to the painful side when starting from either contralateral side flexion or neutral.[36] Only one case of an external oblique strain in a professional soccer player has been documented, and the injury manifested in a manner very similar to that of the internal oblique strain as discussed.[14]

Strains of the internal oblique often involve the anterolateral fibers where the muscle inserts into the eleventh rib.[36,39,44,45] These muscle fibers are primarily responsible for lateral trunk flexion, and the tearing is thought to occur during the late cocking and early acceleration stages of throwing, when the nondominant arm is torqued backward from a hyperextended position to allow the dominant arm to follow through and release the ball.[37] EMG studies have found that muscle activity in the contralateral obliques and transversus abdominis increases 75% to 100% during the acceleration phase of throwing, ball release, and follow-through.[46]

Rectus abdominis strains typically manifest with anterior abdominal wall pain below the umbilicus.[18,19,22] Edema may be present, along with point tenderness distal to the umbilicus and muscle guarding. Passive trunk flexion often relieves or decreases acute pain, whereas active contraction with resisted trunk or hip flexion or passive trunk extension exacerbates symptoms.[22,47] Abdominal pain that is constant or increased with isometric abdominal contraction is termed the Carnett sign and is used in the differential diagnosis to distinguish abdominal muscular disorders from intraabdominal injury.[48] Thomson and Francis[48] reported that a positive Carnett sign corresponded to normal laparotomy findings, thus ruling out intraabdominal disorders, in 23 of 24 emergency department admissions of patients with acute abdominal pain. Abdominal wall injuries caused by direct trauma may result in muscular hematoma and complaints of abdominal pain accompanied by nausea and vomiting. Rectus sheath hematomas often manifest with a bluish discoloration in the periumbilical region, known as the Cullen sign, approximately 72 hours after the injury.[22,47]

Imaging

Although abdominal strains can be diagnosed by clinical sign and symptom presentation, imaging can help determine the exact site, status, and severity of the injury.[39] Increased use of magnetic resonance imaging (MRI) has led to specific documentation of abdominal injuries, especially in professional athletes.[18,35] MRI can be used to identify the anatomic site of injury accurately, as well as to rule out additional lesions such as osteochondral injuries.[37]

Diagnostic ultrasound examination is typically easily accessible and less costly than MRI, and it appears to be a sensitive and valuable tool for detecting abdominal strains.[18,39,45] A case series report using ultrasound to diagnose rectus sheath hematomas found sensitivities ranging from 100% to 30%.[49] This wide variation of false-negative results from 0% to 70% suggests that the examination depends on the operator's expertise. A positive ultrasound result is characterized by disruption of the normal echogenic fibrillar pattern or muscle fibril disruption, edema, and hemorrhage 10 to 28 mm below the umbilicus.[18,19,45]

Etiology

Abdominal wall injuries can occur as a result of direct trauma,[22,47] during an abrupt movement of the torso such as during throwing, spiking, or serving, or they can be caused by repetitive trunk rotation in sports such as golf or racquet sports.[22] The most common mechanism of injury is sporting activity in which trunk rotation is critical for generating power. The abdominal muscles are integral for transferring forces from the lower extremities to the upper extremity during throwing or racquet sports, and they work eccentrically to decelerate the trunk.[35,37,45,46,50-53] EMG analysis of professional baseball players documented that batting and pitching activities require the abdominal muscles not only to function to stabilize the trunk, but also to create axial torque.[46,53] These high-demand, volitional movements require an intricate balance of muscle concentric and eccentric activity. Thus, any asymmetry of muscular strength or length can significantly affect other muscles, and injuries are often the result of excessive, unbalanced eccentric muscle contraction. Investigators have suggested that after a muscular strain, the muscle is weaker and thus at increased risk for further injury compared with normal muscle.[15] Evidence does suggest that recurrence of abdominal muscle strain is common.[36]

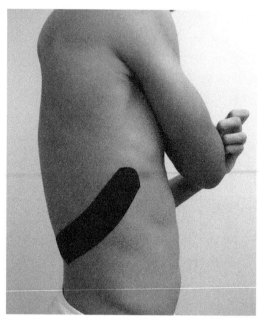

• **Figure 5-16** Kinesiotaping technique for an internal oblique strain at its attachment to the eleventh rib. The patient is placed in a pain-free position of contralateral sidebending and slight contralateral rotation and extension to lengthen the muscle. To inhibit the painful aspect of the muscle, the tape is started just proximal to its insertion at approximately the tenth rib. It is applied with a peel-and-stick technique, maintaining the built-in tension of the tape, running inferiorly and slightly posterior, ending on the lumbodorsal fascia.

Treatment

Treatment of abdominal muscle strains can be divided into phases according to injury presentation. During the acute inflammatory phase (typically from injury to 72 hours), rehabilitation often includes rest, ice, electrotherapy, and antiinflammatory medication.[19,36] Patients may also obtain relief with either a compression support device or taping (Fig. 5-16). Athletes are progressed according to symptom presentation, with special attention paid to the absence of pain reported with activities. After approximately day 4, athletes can start gentle isometric abdominal contraction as long as no pain is reported with muscular activity, and modalities such as electrotherapy and ice are continued. When no signs of edema or inflammation are noted, soft tissue massage can be incorporated, especially in areas surrounding the focal injury site.

When pain with active contraction and daily activities is no longer present, patients can begin gentle concentric strengthening exercises, light stretching, and conditioning, with the focus on correcting any muscular strength and length imbalances. Exercises are gradually progressed to include eccentric exercises, core strengthening, and plyometric exercise, with the focus on returning to sport-related activities as the patient tolerates.[19,36] Reported recovery time to return to sport has been 1 to 70 days in cricket bowlers,[36] 4 to 6 weeks for elite tennis players,[18,37] and 27 to 33 days for professional baseball pitchers.[39]

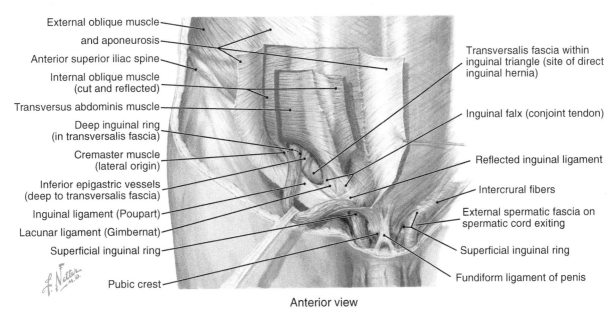

Anterior view

• **Figure 5-17** The inguinal canal is bounded anterior by the external oblique aponeurosis and posteriorly by the transversalis fascia, with medial reinforcement from the conjoint tendon and reflected inguinal ligament. The inguinal floor is formed by the inguinal and lacunar ligaments, and its roof is formed by arching fibers of the internal oblique and transversus abdominis muscles. The deep inguinal ring is located at the proximal end of the inguinal canal. (Netter illustration from www.netterimages.com © Elsevier Inc. All rights reserved.)

In professional sports, athletes are often given an ultrasound-guided corticosteroid injection at the injured site.[36,39] Stevens and colleagues[39] reported that corticosteroid injections enabled professional baseball pitchers to return to pitching at full speed in a mean of 21 days and return to able status in a mean of 30.7 days, compared with the typical recovery time of 6 to 10 weeks,[44] with no reinjury reported in long-term follow up. Corticosteroid injections for the treatment of muscular injuries are controversial because of concerns about incomplete healing, rupture, and risk of infection.[39] However, in rat studies, a single dose of dexamethasone given to an acutely strained muscle facilitated recovery of contractile tension without adverse effects.[54] A retrospective review of corticosteroid injections for severe hamstring injuries in professional football players found no adverse side effects, decreased time before return to play, and lessened game and practice time missed.[55] Also becoming increasingly more common in professional sports is platelet-rich plasma (PRP) injections of a growth factor that is thought to stimulate and enhance tissue healing.[56,57] Despite anecdotal evidence and increased popularity, evidence is lacking that PRP injections hasten healing.[14,58] Athletes are often withheld from participating in their sport until they are able to perform the skills necessary for the sport with appropriate intensity.[22]

Abdominal Wall Hernias

Anatomy of the Inguinal Canal

The inguinal canal is an oblique canal measuring approximately 4 cm long that runs parallel and a little superior to the inguinal ligament (Fig. 5-17). Throughout its length, the inguinal canal is bounded anteriorly by the aponeurosis of the external oblique, with a small contribution from the internal oblique in its lateral third. The transversalis fascia forms the posterior wall of the inguinal canal, with medial reinforcement by the conjoint tendon and reflected inguinal ligament. The floor is formed by the superior surface of both the inguinal and lacunar ligaments, and the roof is formed by the arching fibers of the internal oblique and transversus abdominis muscles. The sides of the inguinal canal are reinforced by intercrural (medial and lateral crura) fibers (Fig. 5-18).[17]

The inguinal canal has two openings: a superficial (external) inguinal ring and a deep (internal) inguinal ring. The superficial (external) ring is a slitlike opening in the distal aponeurosis of the external oblique muscle just superior and lateral to the pubic crest (see Fig. 5-7). The ring is somewhat triangular, measuring approximately 2.5 cm. It is bound inferiorly by the pubic crest, on either side by margins of the external oblique aponeurosis named the medial and lateral crus, and superiorly by a series of curved intercrural fibers. The strong inferior crus forms the floor of the ring and consists of the inferior portion of the inguinal ligament that inserts onto the pubic tubercle and on which the spermatic cord or round ligament rests. The superior crus attaches to the front of the pubic symphysis and interfaces with the contralateral superior crus.[17]

At the proximal end of the inguinal canal is the deep (internal) inguinal ring, also known as the abdominal inguinal ring (see Fig. 5-17). It is located midway between the ASIS and the pubic symphysis, approximately 1.25 cm above the inguinal ligament (see Fig. 5-12). It is bordered

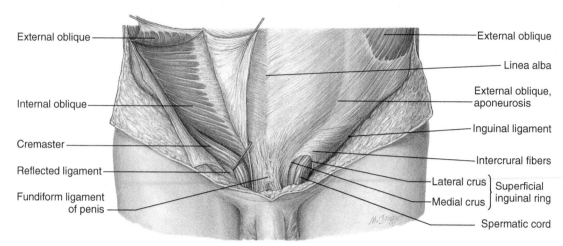

• **Figure 5-18** The intercrural fibers span the distance between the medial and lateral crus of the external oblique aponeurosis, thus helping to reinforce the inguinal canal. (From Putz R, Pabst R, eds. *Sobotta Atlas of Human Anatomy.* 14th ed. Munich: Urban & Fischer, an imprint of Elsevier GmbH; 2006.)

superiorly and laterally by the transversus abdominis and inferiorly and medially by the inferior epigastric vessels.[17] The deep inguinal ring is an opening in the transversalis fascia for the passage of the spermatic cord and ilioinguinal nerve in males and the round ligament of the uterus and ilioinguinal nerve in females.[59,60] Netter's[20] internal view of the anterior abdominal wall shows the orifice in the transversalis fascia (see Fig. 5-5). The deep inguinal ring is much larger in male than in female anatomy, and in males the fascial opening continues as a thin membrane, called the internal spermatic fascia, that envelops the spermatic cord and testis (see Fig. 5-12).[17]

Another important anatomic area of the abdominal wall is the inguinal triangle, also known as the Hesselbach triangle (see Fig. 5-5). The Hesselbach triangle is bounded laterally and superiorly by the inferior epigastric vessels, medially by the lateral border of the rectus abdominis, and inferiorly by the inguinal ligament, and it is located medial to the deep inguinal ring.[17]

The femoral artery exits inferior to the inguinal ligament midway between the ASIS and the pubic symphysis (Fig. 5-19). The first 4-cm segment of the femoral artery is enclosed together with the femoral vein within the fibrous femoral sheath (see Fig. 5-19), a continuation of the abdominal transversalis fascia downward and posterior to the inguinal ligament. The femoral vessels are surrounded anteriorly by this femoral sheath and posteriorly by the iliac fascia. The femoral sheath is shaped like a short tunnel that becomes narrow and fuses approximately 5 cm below the inguinal ligament and is reinforced anteriorly by a fibrous band called the deep crural arch (Fig. 5-20). The femoral sheath is compartmentalized vertically to contain the femoral artery laterally and the femoral vein in the middle, whereas the medial compartment is termed the femoral canal. The conical femoral canal measures approximately 1.25 cm and is bounded anteriorly by the inguinal ligament, posteriorly by the pectineus muscle, medially by the

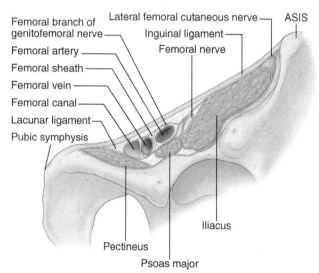

• **Figure 5-19** The femoral artery and vein are enclosed together within the fibrous femoral sheath. *ASIS,* Anterior superior iliac spine. (From Standring S, ed. *Gray's Anatomy: The Anatomical Basis of Clinical Practice.* 40th ed. London: Churchill Livingstone; 2008.)

lacunar ligament, and laterally by the femoral vein's fibrous sheath.[17]

Types and Incidence of Abdominal Hernias

The diagnosis of abdominal wall hernia is made in 1.7% of the population and in 4% of persons older than 45 years of age.[61] Inguinal hernias account for 75% of all abdominal wall hernias, whereas the other 25% are noninguinal, including umbilical, epigastric, incisional, and femoral hernias.[61,62]

Although the exact incidence and prevalence of inguinal hernias are unknown, the incidence of inguinal hernia repair is 27% in men and 3% in women.[63-66] The two classes of inguinal hernias are direct and indirect. Both types of

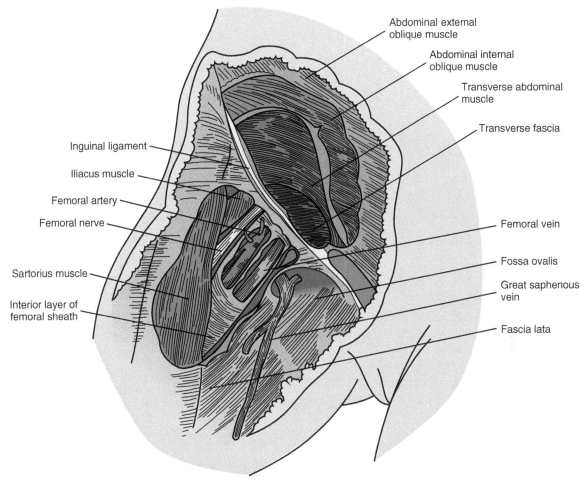

• **Figure 5-20** The femoral sheath is shaped like a short tunnel that fuses 5 cm inferior to the inguinal ligament. This "tunnel" is compartmentalized vertically to contain the femoral artery laterally, femoral vein centrally, and femoral canal medially. (Redrawn from Gray H. *Anatomy of the Human Body*. Philadelphia: Lea & Febiger, 1918; Bartleby.com, 2000. www.bartleby.com/107/. [October 28, 2015].)

hernia protrude through the inguinal canal and exit through or near the superficial inguinal ring, but the point of entry into the inguinal canal differs.[60,66] At its point of entry, direct hernias protrude within the Hesselbach triangle, medial to the epigastric vessels, whereas indirect hernias protrude through the deep inguinal ring, lateral to the epigastric vessels (Fig. 5-21).[17,60,63] In males, 50% of inguinal hernias are indirect, and 40% are direct. In females, 70% of inguinal hernias are indirect, 10% are direct hernias, and 20% are femoral hernias.[64,66,67]

An indirect inguinal hernia occurs when a sac containing peritoneum contents protrudes through the deep inguinal ring. An indirect inguinal hernia is also known as a congenital hernia because the cause is embryonic failure of the processus vaginalis to close. This type of inguinal hernia is more prevalent and is typically diagnosed in younger patients; most patients younger than 25 years of age who present with a hernia have an indirect hernia.[63]

Boys and men are more likely to develop an indirect inguinal hernia than are girls and women because the testicles and blood vessels pass through the inguinal canal before birth, thus making the deep ring less likely to close

completely and making the ring larger.[63] The incidence of indirect hernias is increased in persons with a close family history of the condition.[63,66,68-70] Although an indirect inguinal hernia is often congenital, it may also result from an increase in intraabdominal pressure during strenuous activities such as lifting or straining during sports or with a medical condition leading to increased pressure on the region such as a chronic cough, chronic constipation, excess weight, or pregnancy.[63,66,70-72] Smoking is also a risk factor.[66,73,74] In male patients, indirect hernias are always covered by internal spermatic fascia, so if an inguinal hernia is located within the male scrotum, it is an indirect hernia.[17]

The protruding abdominal sac of an indirect inguinal hernia may become pinched during exercise and straining, thereby causing pain. If the abdominal sac becomes pinched and the blood supply to the hernia is compromised, the hernia become "incarcerated" or "strangulated."[60,63] The incidence of incarceration or strangulation is estimated to be 0.3% to 3% per year, depending on the definition.[66,75-78] Strangulation occurs 10 times more often in indirect inguinal hernias than in direct hernias because of a comparably

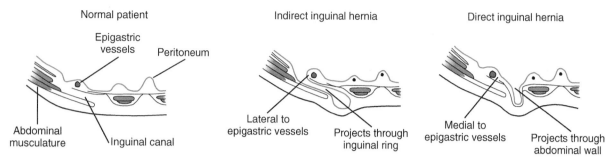

Normal patient   Indirect inguinal hernia   Direct inguinal hernia

Epigastric vessels   Peritoneum   Lateral to epigastric vessels   Projects through inguinal ring   Medial to epigastric vessels   Projects through abdominal wall

Abdominal musculature   Inguinal canal

• **Figure 5-21** Regional Anatomy of the Inguinal Canal. Both types of hernia exit at the superficial inguinal ring; however, their point of entry differs. An indirect inguinal hernia protrudes through the deep inguinal ring, lateral to the epigastric vessels, and exits as an elliptical swelling. A direct inguinal hernia protrudes within the Hesselbach triangle, medial to the epigastric vessels, and protrudes directly forward as a more symmetrical circular swelling. (Redrawn from O'Rahilly R, Müller F, Carpenter S, et al: *Basic Human Anatomy: A Regional Study of Human Structure* [online version/Dartmouth Geisel Medical School, Hanover, NY]. Copyright © O'Rahilly 2008.)

smaller orifice.[66,79-81] Hernia incarceration or strangulation can lead to intestinal obstruction, resulting in potential ischemia, gangrene, and even death, and thus requires emergency surgery. Emergency surgical treatment of a strangulated inguinal hernia has a higher associated mortality than elective surgical treatment of inguinal hernia (>5% versus <0.5%).[82,83]

Direct inguinal hernias occur when retroperitoneal fat herniates through the transversalis fascia secondary to weakness or tearing of the transversalis fascia within the Hesselbach triangle. This tearing may result from increased intraabdominal pressure during strenuous activities such as lifting or straining or in sport. Thus, direct inguinal hernias are acquired and are more common in 40- to 50-year old persons.[60,63,66]

Femoral hernias occur when peritoneum protrudes into the femoral sheath or canal posterior and inferior to the inguinal ligament as a result of weakness of the transversalis fascia.[62] Femoral hernias are extremely rare, accounting for only 3% of all hernias and found primarily in women.[66,67] Femoral hernias account for one fifth to one third of all groin hernias in women, but only 2% in men,[67,84] and 50% of men with a femoral hernia have a concomitant direct inguinal hernia, compared with only 3% of women.[85] It is speculated that femoral hernia is more common in women compared with men because of its association with pregnancy and childbirth.[86] In addition, a prospective fresh-cadaver study of women who had undergone femoral hernia repair[87] found that the distances between the pubic tubercle and the medial margin of the femoral vein and between the inguinal and Cooper ligaments were much larger in these subjects compared with subjects who did not undergo repair. This finding suggests that the wider bone structure in women may lead to stretching of the fascia, with eventual weakening the fascia and predisposition to femoral hernia.

Diagnosing a femoral hernia is challenging because the hernia is often asymptomatic until strangulation or incarceration occurs.[62] The typical presentation of a femoral hernia comprises "achy" abdominal pain, signs of intestinal obstruction,[84] and a small nonreducible palpable bulge below the inguinal ligament lateral and inferior to the pubic tubercle.[67,88] Given the challenge of diagnosis using clinical signs and symptoms, imaging is often necessary, including ultrasound, MRI, and computed tomography (CT). Although all imaging techniques have high accuracy in diagnosing a femoral hernia,[62] ultrasound is most typically used because of its high accuracy (up to 100% sensitivity and specificity),[89] wide availability, low cost, and reduced exposure to radiation.[62]

Because femoral hernias are more likely to become incarcerated or strangulated as a result of their narrow orifice, and because they have a 10-fold risk of mortality, immediate surgical repair is advised.[62,67,88,90] Repairs typically consist of closure with nonabsorbable sutures that may be reinforced using the pectineal (Cooper) ligament.[84] The recurrence rate after femoral hernia repair is only 2%.[85] Postoperative return to activities is similar to that after inguinal hernias (discussed later), including limiting strain to the area for 2 to 3 weeks and gradual return to activities that avoid symptom reproduction.[62,91]

Umbilical hernias manifest near the naval in an area naturally weakened by the vessels of the umbilical cord.[17] These hernias often appear in infants soon after birth, and 95% resolve spontaneously by age 3 to 4 years.[92] Umbilical hernias can also manifest in adults in response to excessive pressure from being overweight or from coughing or pregnancy,[62,93] and in the athletic population, they can manifest from increased abdominal pressure in activities such as powerlifting.[94] Umbilical hernias are typically asymptomatic, and they appear as a nonpainful palpable bulge at the umbilicus in adults.[95] Although they rarely become incarcerated, umbilical hernias in adults and unresolved hernias in infants are often treated surgically to prevent worsening and possible incarceration. Umbilical hernias have a high success rate when treated operatively; treatment involves defect closure and suture placement or a mesh prosthesis.[96] Postoperative guidelines are similar to those for femoral hernias and inguinal hernias, as subsequently discussed.

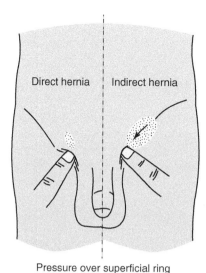

• **Figure 5-22** Site of palpation for indirect and direct inguinal hernias at the superior aspect of the scrotum.

Presentation of Inguinal Hernias

Clinical examination typically suffices in the diagnosis of an inguinal hernia because diagnosing an inguinal hernia by means of a physical examination has a sensitivity of 75% to 92% and a specificity of 93%.[97,98] Indirect and direct inguinal hernias result in a palpable bulge with increased abdominal pressure in the groin at the top of, or within, the scrotum (Fig. 5-22). This small bulge is elicited during examination by palpating the inguinal canal and asking the patient to cough while standing. The hernia is reducible if it appears intermittently, such as during standing or straining, and can be manually pushed back into the abdominal cavity with minimal pressure or when the patient lies supine, in contrast to an irreducible hernia, which remains outside the abdominal cavity permanently even with pressure.[60,63] A direct hernia protrudes directly forward and appears as a symmetrical, circular swelling, whereas an indirect hernia has a more oblique route and thus appears as a more elliptical swelling. However, differentiating between direct and indirect inguinal hernias clinically by using anatomic landmarks is unreliable and is necessary only to rule out a femoral hernia because treatment is identical for both direct and indirect inguinal hernias.[79-81]

Pain from an inguinal hernia, if present, is typically described as a deep, aching pain in the inguinal or scrotal region.[63] However, approximately one third of patients electing to undergo surgical hernia repair have no pain and little to no limitation of daily activities.[60,77] A study of 323 patients undergoing inguinal hernia repair found that, before the operation, at rest 27% had no pain, 54% had "mild pain" (<10 on a 1- to 100-point scale), and 1.5% had severe pain (>50 out of 100), and during movement 16% had no pain, 42% had mild pain, and 10% had severe pain. In addition, no association was observed between pain intensity and location type of hernia.[99]

Imaging

If a patient has obscure or vague pain, or has intermittent swelling not palpable during examination, a diagnostic investigation is recommended.[66] Ultrasonography is a useful noninvasive adjunct to the physical examination; its specificity of 81% to 100% and sensitivity of 33% to 100% compared with surgical exploration in the diagnosis of an inguinal hernia suggests that the accuracy of this technique depends on the examiner's experience.[97,100-103] MRI has a sensitivity of 95% and a specificity of 96% and is also useful in diagnosing inflammation, tumors, and other musculotendinous dysfunctions.[66,104] A CT scan has a limited place in the diagnosis of an inguinal hernia even though its sensitivity is 83% and its specificity is 67% to 83%.[66] Herniography is a radiographic diagnostic technique using fluoroscopy-guided injection of a contrast medium into the peritoneal cavity.[105,106] Herniography is highly reliable for detecting inguinal hernias[104-107]; moreover, it has a reported sensitivity of 100% and a specificity of 98% to 100%.[107] In the diagnosis of hernias, herniography has been found to be superior to MRI, possibly because of the difficulty of having the patient perform a Valsalva maneuver (forced expiration against a closed glottis) while statically supine.[104] However, herniography has limited use in the United States as a result of potential complications including accidental bowel puncture, despite a reported 1% incidence of complications,[106,108] given that less invasive techniques with nearly equal accuracy are available. All things considered, the typical diagnostic investigative course of action is to first perform an ultrasound examination; if findings are negative, then perform an MRI with a Valsalva maneuver, and if MRI results are negative, perform herniography.[66]

Treatment

Minimally symptomatic direct and indirect inguinal hernias are typically initially treated with "watchful waiting" to assess whether they become more symptomatic.[66] Given that historically most diagnosed inguinal hernias are operated on, the natural course of an untreated inguinal hernia is rarely documented.[66] Studies have found similar outcomes between men with minimally symptomatic inguinal hernias that were surgically repaired compared with men who were treated with watchful waiting.[75,109] This finding suggests that watchful waiting is a reasonable option for men with minimally symptomatic inguinal hernias, and if the hernia becomes more painful or the pain interferes with normal activities, than repair is suggested.[75,109] The primary rationale for watchful waiting as the first course of treatment is to avoid potential postoperative pain syndrome, or inguinodynia—pain or discomfort lasting longer than 3 months after the surgical procedure—a somewhat common complaint after surgical repair of inguinal hernias. Studies report that 3% to 6% of patients undergoing hernia repair have severe pain, and 30% have mild pain, 1 year after inguinal hernia repair.[82,110,111] Thus, investigators have suggested that patients with moderate to severe pain undergo surgical repair, whereas patients with no pain should undergo a trial of watching waiting because the repair may make their pain worse.[99]

Evidence-based guidelines suggest that all men who are older than 30 years of age and who have a symptomatic inguinal hernia should be operated on to reduce symptoms and prevent complications such as incarceration or strangulation.[66] Inguinal hernia repair is one of the most frequently performed surgical procedures in the United States, with an estimated 600,000 operations performed annually.[112,113] Surgery can be laparoscopic/endoscopic or open. A review of the literature reveals that, compared with open repair, laparoscopic procedures result in longer operation times but less severe postoperative pain, fewer complications, and a quicker return to normal activities.[114,115] Surgical procedures include the following: herniotomy, in which the hernia sac is removed without any repair; herniorrhaphy, which is repair without any reinforcement; and hernioplasty, which consists of herniotomy combined with reinforcement using the patient's own tissue (autogenous) or a heterogeneous material such as mesh.[116] The procedure used is selected based on the surgeon's preference and the hernia presentation. The mesh is typically a synthetic nonabsorbable polypropylene flat mesh.[66] Laparoscopic hernioplasty using mesh repair results in fewer recurrences than techniques not using mesh and also reduces the incidence of chronic inguinodynia.[117-119] Either the open or endoscopic mesh repair is a recommended option for treating a unilateral inguinal hernia because both procedures have similar outcomes, provided the surgeon is experienced in that procedure.[118,120] Endoscopic techniques are technically more demanding and thus are more dependent on the surgeon's experience.[91,121]

The Lichtenstein technique is the best evaluated and most popular of the open mesh techniques. It has been associated with low morbidity, can be performed as a same-day surgical procedure using local anesthesia, and has low recurrence rates (≤4%) in long-term studies.[122,123] Although endoscopic mesh techniques require a longer operation time than the open mesh procedure, they result in a lower incidence of wound infection and hematoma formation, have a faster recovery time and thus earlier return to normal activities, and have a reduced incidence of chronic inguinodynia compared with the open mesh techniques.[117,124] Endoscopic mesh repair is chosen for treating inguinal hernias in women because they have a higher risk of hernia recurrence following an open repair[125,126] and a greater risk of presenting with a concomitant femoral hernia, thus suggesting that endoscopic mesh repair should be used to cover both inguinal and femoral hernias simultaneously.[66]

If a nonmesh procedure is selected, the Shouldice technique, a modern version of the original Bassini procedure, has been found to be the most effective.[127] The Shouldice technique involves repairing the posterior wall of the inguinal canal and the internal ring by suturing several layers with a continuous nonsoluble monofilament suture; it has considerably better outcomes than other nonmesh techniques and results in a lower recurrence rate (15% versus 33%).[128]

Postsurgical Considerations and Rehabilitation

Inguinal hernia repair can be easily performed as a same-day surgical procedure, regardless of the technique used.[66] Typical postoperative recovery for an anterior open approach without mesh is 6 weeks.[129] Research reveals that patients recover 4 days earlier on average after an open mesh procedure than after a conventional nonmesh open repair, and they recover 7 days earlier on average following an endoscopic mesh operation than after an open mesh technique.[117-120,124,130-135]

Following inguinal hernia repair, patients were historically informed to resume activities as their symptoms allowed but to avoid heavy weight lifting for 2 to 3 weeks.[66] This limitation of heavy physical lifting was based primarily on expert opinion and low-level evidence suggesting that physical strain leads to an increase in intraabdominal pressure that subsequently causes inguinal hernias and thus possible reinjury.[66,136,137] This opinion led to ambiguous guidelines to avoid "heavy weight lifting" for 2 to 3 weeks without specifying the threshold of heavy lifting.[66,136,137] Current research suggests that after an initial 3-week period of reduced protected activity to allow wound healing, no difference in hernia recurrence is noted among groups informed to resume all occupational and recreational activities without restrictions, those informed to return to activity but reduce strain for an additional 2 to 3 weeks, and those remaining inactive for 3 months.[138-140] Thus, no evidence exists of a relationship between an increase in intraabdominal pressure with activities and hernia recurrence.[136,137] Mesh reconstruction of an inguinal hernia that is placed through an open or laparoscopic procedure has full loading strength immediately after wound closure that is not endangered by physical activity of any type, including heavy lifting.[136] Therefore, physical activity of any type, including heavy lifting, does not endanger the repair. The only limiting factor for resumption of activity after herniotomy is not recurrence risk, but pain.[82,136,141-143] Because laparoscopic hernia repair is associated with less postoperative pain,[120,144,145] laparoscopic repair facilitates earlier resumption of work and daily activity.[66,145] Thus, current evidence suggests that patients be allowed to return to their regular activities, regardless of the physical strain involved, immediately after healing of the skin wound if analgesics are administered.[136] Because most inguinal hernias are treated surgically, guidelines governing conservative rehabilitation are few or absent.

Sports Hernia or Athletic Pubalgia

Another dysfunction manifesting as groin pain is a "sports hernia." A sports hernia is defined as weakness of the posterior inguinal wall or muscular and fascial injury to structures attaching to the anterior pubis without a clinically recognizable hernia that manifests as severe lower abdominal, pubic, or groin pain with exertion.[3,7,10,146,147] The term athletic pubalgia may be more appropriate than sports hernia when referring to this injury, given that no actual palpable hernia is present.[3,6-8,10,13,146-152] All things considered, the origin of athletic pubalgia is more of a syndrome than a specific injury.[150,152]

Anatomy

The anatomy of the lower abdominal and groin region is very complex. As discussed earlier in the section on inguinal hernia, the pubic region has many muscular, aponeurosis, and fascial attachments. Any adverse stresses to these structures, such as a volitional eccentric contraction or repetitive stresses, can adversely affect these distal pubic attachments.

The rectus abdominis has two direct tendinous origins on the pubis: laterally on the pubic crest and medially on the anterior pubic symphysis (see Fig. 5-1). Fibers from this medial head blend with fibers from the contralateral medial rectus head and anterior pubic symphysis ligaments to reinforce the anterior pubis and distal linea alba. The anterior rectus abdominis and its anterior sheath are also reinforced by the pyramidalis, which helps stabilize and tension the linea alba.[17]

The anterior rectus sheath contains fibers from the aponeurosis of the external and internal obliques, as well as the transversus abdominis (see Fig. 5-12). In addition, fibers from the internal oblique merge with the transversus abdominis to become the conjoint tendon and insert onto the pubic crest and medial aspect of the pectoral line behind the lacunar ligament.[17]

Fibers from the inferior aspect of external oblique have direct attachments to the pubic tubercle and pectineal line. In addition, there are various aponeurosis and facial attachments: the inguinal ligament attaches distally on the pubic tubercle, the lacunar ligament reflects from the pubic tubercle attachment to connect to the pectineal line, and the pectineal ligament attaches to the pectineal line to help reinforce the pectineal fascia and anterior pubis (see Fig. 5-2). The reflected inguinal ligament also reinforces the distal linea alba.[17]

The rectus abdominis and adductor longus share a common aponeurosis attachment at the anterior inferior aspect of the pubic body, 1 to 2 cm from the symphyseal midline.[153,154] In Figure 5-23, a photograph from a cadaveric specimen shows the common attachment of the right rectus abdominis and adductor longus tendons. A sagittal MRI scan (Fig. 5-24) also shows the aponeurosis of the rectus abdominis and the adductor longus where the aponeurosis is seen as a dark band of fibers extending along the anterior inferior aspect of the pubic body, 1 to 2 cm from the symphyseal midline.[154] In addition, fibrous continuity is present between the aponeurosis of the anterior distal rectus sheath and the contralateral adductor longus[154] (Fig. 5-25). Thus, any abnormal forces placed on the rectus abdominis or the

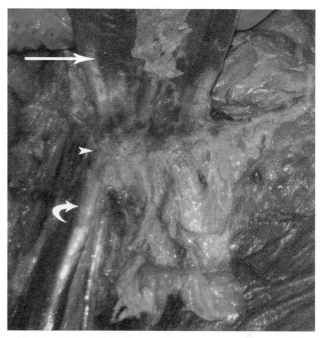

• **Figure 5-23** Photograph of a cadaver specimen revealing the common attachment *(straight arrow)* of the right rectus abdominis *(arrowheads)* and adductor longus *(curved arrow)* tendon. (From Omar IM, Zoga AC, Kavanagh EC, et al. Athletic pubalgia and "sports hernia": optimal MR imaging technique and findings. *RadioGraphics.* 2008;28:1415-1438.)

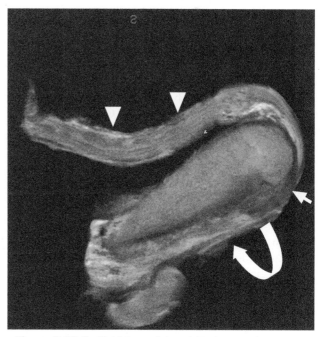

• **Figure 5-24** Sagittal intermediate-weighted magnetic resonance imaging revealing the common aponeurosis *(straight arrow)* between the rectus abdominis *(arrowheads)* and adductor longus *(curved arrow)*. The aponeurosis appears as a dark band of fibers extending along the anterior-inferior aspect of the pubic body, 1 to 2 cm from the symphyseal midline. (From Omar IM, Zoga AC, Kavanagh EC, et al. Athletic pubalgia and "sports hernia": optimal MR imaging technique and findings. *RadioGraphics.* 2008;28:1415-1438.)

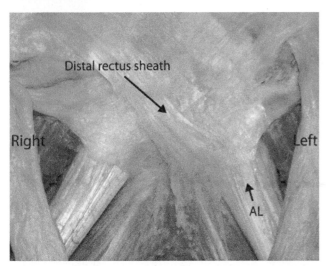

• **Figure 5-25** Photograph of a cadaver specimen revealing a dominant extension of the right anterior rectus sheath crossing superficial to the left. On both sides, the fibrous continuity between the contralateral adductor longus (AL) is evident. (From Norton-Old KJ, Schache AG, Barker PJ, et al. Anatomical and mechanical relationship between the proximal attachment of the adductor longus and the distal rectus sheath. *Clin Anat.* 2013; 26:522-530.)

adductor longus can have a direct effect on the other. See Chapter 3 for more information on adductor longus disorders.

Incidence

Athletic pubalgia is becoming a more widely diagnosed condition affecting primarily athletes. Media coverage of high-profile athletes diagnosed with, and treated for, the condition has heightened awareness of the condition. These athletes include the following: National Football League members Donovan McNabb, Tom Brady, and Adrian Peterson; National Hockey League members Clayton Stoner, the late Rick Rypien, and Brad Larsen; Major League Baseball players Torii Hunter and Chris Duncan; professional soccer's Benjamin Benditson; and collegiate basketball players J.T. Thompson and Jodie Meeks.[10,155-157] The question remains whether athletic pubalgia is becoming more prevalent or whether the diagnosis is simply a new term for an old diagnosis.[1,5,146,158,159] The increasing incidence of this condition as reported by the media may, in part, be explained by heightened awareness and interest in the athletic arena.[155]

Athletic pubalgia is found in high-performance recreational, high school, and professional athletes. The incidence is highest in sports involving running, kicking, cutting, explosive turns, and changing direction, as well as activities requiring an athlete to push hard against resistance such as linemen in football or hockey.[160] The most common sports in the United States in which the incidence of athletic pubalgia is highest include soccer, ice hockey, and American football, but the disorder has also been reported in rugby, cricket, martial arts, basketball, baseball, tennis, swimming, and long-distance running.[7,146,155,160-164]

Athletic pubalgia has the highest reported incidence in male athletes.[*] Some investigators speculate that the lower incidence in female athletes may be explained by the relatively lower level of female participation in high-intensity sports compared with male athletes,[7] a hypothesis discredited by the increasing number of women training and competing at high levels in similar sports. A more plausible explanation of the lower incidence of athletic pubalgia in female athletes takes into account the anatomic differences between the male and female pelvis.[7,154,167-169] The female pelvis has been observed to have larger, more robust distal rectus abdominis attachments and convergence of aponeurosis fibers from both sides crossing the midline along the anteroinferior pubic symphysis, an anatomic finding not seen in most male patients.[154] In addition, the shape of the female pelvis changes muscle alignment and contraction, which may, in turn, affect the dynamic neuromuscular control of the hip and pelvis during sporting activities such as kicking.[170] Finally, the female pelvis is wider and has a larger subpubic angle that may aid in the transference of forces away from the pubic region to the rest of the innominate bones or the lower extremities.[154,171] These anatomic and biomechanical differences in the female pelvis may distribute muscular forces more effectively and help stabilize the pubic region, thus protecting the female pelvis from repetitive stress injuries such as athletic pubalgia.[7,154,168,169]

Presentation of Athletic Pubalgia

The physical examination starts with a detailed subjective history consisting of the following: background information of the present injury; past medical history; the nature, behavior, location, and duration of symptoms; relieving and aggravating factors; earlier episodes; accounts of sport and daily activities; use of over-the-counter and prescription medications; and the presence of any symptoms suggestive of systemic disease.[172] Patients with athletic pubalgia present with complaints of "deep" groin or lower abdominal pain with exertion or sports-related activities including kicking, sprinting, sidestepping, cutting, or transitioning from supine to sitting.[†] Although mild discomfort at rest is acceptable to make this diagnosis, pain with exertion is a hallmark.[12,150,173,175] Patients report that the pain is "deeper," "more intense," and "more proximal" than a typical groin strain.[‡]

Symptoms typically start after approximately 5 minutes of exertion, and once symptoms have started, the athlete can often play through the pain to finish a game, but usually at less than 100% capacity.[174] Symptoms are typically relieved after 6 to 24 hours of rest, only to return on resumption of the activity or sport.[§] After a game, the

---

*References 3, 5, 9, 146, 147, 155, 159, 165, and 166.
†References 6, 7, 10, 12, 13, 146, 147, 155, 156, 161-163, 166, 169, 173, and 174.
‡References 6, 7, 146, 148, 166, 169, 174, and 176.
§References 3, 7, 10, 12, 146, 148, 156, and 166.

athletes often have discomfort and complaints of "throbbing" in the lower groin and "stiffness" in the morning that typically resolves after 1 to 2 days of rest, only to increase again with the sport activity.[169,174]

Symptoms are typically unilateral, although some patients report bilateral pain or symptoms that started unilaterally and progressed to bilaterally.[‖] The onset of athletic pubalgia symptoms is often insidious; however, most patients can retrospectively recall a specific traumatic event after the groin symptoms are already present.[¶]

Approximately 20% to 40% of patients report pain with sneezing and coughing.[#] Symptoms may radiate into the perineum, inner thigh, or scrotum, and approximately 10% to 30% of male patients report testicular pain.[**]

The physical examination consists of a postural assessment, functional assessment, measurement of thoracolumbar and hip active range of motion,[179] joint accessory motion testing of the hip and lumbar spine,[180] manual muscle testing and length testing of the musculature attaching to the pelvis, neurologic assessment, palpation of muscular and bony structures, and applicable special tests of the sacroiliac, hip, and lumbar region. It is imperative that the clinician conducts a thorough physical examination to treat the objective signs and symptoms accordingly.

Hip disorders can be excluded based on negative findings after performing the flexion abduction external rotation (FADER) and flexion adduction internal rotation (FADIR) tests and the hip scouring test (see Chapter 2 for discussion of test performance). Lumbosacral disorders should be ruled out as well (see Chapter 11 for a discussion of lumbosacral differential diagnosis). Although a sacroiliac joint (SIJ) dysfunction may not be the primary cause, it may be involved in an inflammatory process, especially if the patient has underlying pelvic instability. Thus, the clinician should include pelvic compression and distraction tests. These tests have been shown to have fairly good reliability and high levels of diagnostic validity for diagnosing SIJ dysfunction.[181-184] Positive findings in two of four SIJ special tests of the Laslett cluster[182] (thigh thrust, ASIS distraction, ASIS compression, and sacral thrust) have a sensitivity of 88, a specificity of 78, a positive likelihood ratio of 4.00, and a negative likelihood ratio of 0.16, suggesting that the evidence strongly supports the use of this cluster. Palpation of bony landmarks can be used to assess static pelvic position; however, this manual assessment has been found to have poor interrater and intrarater reliability.[184,185]

Impairments of muscle length and strength can adversely influence pelvic alignment and thus force attenuation of the pelvic musculature. Muscle length tests should include the Thomas test for hip flexor muscle length, the Ober test for iliotibial band and tensor fasciae latae length, and the straight leg raise test for hamstring length. Strength testing

of the pelvis and hips should include the iliopsoas, hamstrings, quadriceps, gluteus maximus, and gluteus medius. Assessment of hip active range of motion and hip joint accessory motion is also invaluable.

The two most important muscle resistance tests that may help confirm the diagnosis of athletic pubalgia are resisted hip adduction and resisted abdominal curl-up.[174] Referred pain along the adductor longus tendons during resisted hip adduction is a common complaint with athletic pubalgia, with 35% of patients reporting referred pain along the adductor longus tendon with resisted adduction.[7,146,148,173,186,187] A common test for adductor-related groin pain is the adductor squeeze test.[188,189] Delahunt and associates[188] found the highest adductor EMG activity with the legs positioned in 45 degrees of hip flexion, whereas Lovell and colleagues[190] found similar EMG and force values at 0 and 45 degrees of flexion; these findings suggest that the test be conducted in both hip flexion positions. Verrall and associates[191] found that the test had a sensitivity of 55%, a specificity of 95%, a positive predictive value of 93%, and a negative predictive value of 34% compared with MRI. Refer to Chapter 3 for a more detailed description of this test.

Next, the examiner should test resisted abdominal curl-up in two positions. The examiner tests resisted abdominal curl-up, first with the patient's legs flexed and then with the legs extended (lengthening the rectus abdominis), to look for reproduction of symptoms near the pubic ramus.

The physical examination should conclude with palpation of the abdomen, inguinal area, testes, pubic symphysis, SIJ, and lumbar spine. A common finding with athletic pubalgia is point tenderness over the superior lateral pubis.[††] The practitioner should also palpate 2 to 3 cm of the inguinal floor laterally and slightly superior to the pubic tubercle while the patient performs the Valsalva maneuver.[6,10,155,156,173] In a patient with athletic pubalgia, this gentle pressure replicates his or her unilateral discomfort, or the examiner will not feel the fascia tighten, a finding suggesting tearing or inguinal ring dilation.[3,148,155,156] Also during this part of the physical examination, it is important that the practitioner ensure that no palpable hernia is present.

In a retrospective review of six collegiate athletes with athletic pubalgia, Kachingwe and Grech[174] identified five hallmark signs and symptoms (Box 5-1). The diagnosis of athletic pubalgia relies heavily on the patient's subjective history and physical examination. The differential diagnosis of athletic pubalgia is often one of exclusion by ruling out other pathologic conditions, such as the lack of a palpable inguinal hernia, and verifying the presence of the five hallmark signs and symptoms.[3,10,146,156,174] Determining the exact cause of an athlete's groin pain may be elusive secondary to the lengthy differential diagnostic possibilities, the high degree of symptom overlap among different groin

‖References 3, 7, 8, 143-148, 156, 166, 169, and 174.
¶References 6, 10, 12, 146, 156, 166, 174.
#References 6, 8, 13, 146, 148, 149, 155, and 156.
**References 2, 7, 8, 13, 146, 148, 156, 166, 169, 174, 177, and 178.

††References 8, 146, 147, 155, 158, 166, 173, 187, and 192.

disorders, and the possibility that multiple dysfunctions may coexist in one patient.[166]

Differential Diagnosis

Various diagnoses must be ruled out when considering the diagnosis of athletic pubalgia. Genitourinary disorders should be excluded. Although female athletes may present with signs and symptoms suggestive of athletic pubalgia, surgical exploration and diagnostic testing often find gynecologic causes of their symptoms, including endometriosis and ovarian cysts.[3,7,146,147] Thus, if a female patient complains of lower abdominal pain that is cyclic and accompanies menstruation, endometriosis must be ruled out (see Chapter 9). Patients with a confirmed diagnosis of athletic

pubalgia may also have concomitant genitourinary disease. A study of 12 patients with a preoperative diagnosis of athletic pubalgia who underwent surgical treatment revealed that 50% had either lymphoma of the spermatic cord or nonspecific attenuation of the inguinal floor (42%), whereas only 8% had a tear of the rectus abdominis insertion.[146] Surgical exploration studies have also reported that a few patients have a minor direct or indirect inguinal hernia in combination with the posterior wall deficiency.[7,152,159,166,193-195]

In male patients, reports of upper scrotum pain may be secondary to inflammation or entrapment of the ilioinguinal nerve.[169,196] The ilioinguinal nerve originates from the ventral ramus of L1, passes between the external and internal oblique abdominal muscles, and continues through the inguinal canal to innervate the skin of the scrotum in men and the labia majora in women, the mons pubis, and the adjacent medial aspect of the thigh; this nerve also has distributions to the internal oblique and transversus abdominis (Fig. 5-26).[17] The ilioinguinal nerve can be injured with a direct hernia or repair leading to further weakening of the internal oblique or transversus abdominis and thus the conjoint tendon.[169,196] Other peripheral nerves that, if entrapped, can lead to groin pain include the obturator, femoral, iliohypogastric, pudendal, genitofemoral, and lateral femoral cutaneous nerve.[12,154,197] Please refer to Chapter 1 for a more detailed description of the pelvic neuroanatomy. A thorough neurologic screening may reveal whether the groin pain is being referred from the SIJ, sciatic nerve, or lumbar

---

• BOX 5-1   Five Hallmark Signs and Symptoms of Athletic Pubalgia

1. Deep groin or lower abdominal pain
2. Pain exacerbated by sport-specific activities (e.g., kicking, sprinting, cutting) and temporarily relieved with rest
3. Palpable tenderness over the superior-lateral pubis 2 to 3 cm superior-lateral to the pubic tubercle near the rectus abdominis insertion or its lateral edge or at the conjoined tendon-rectus interface
4. Pain with resisted hip adduction
5. Pain with resisted curl-up

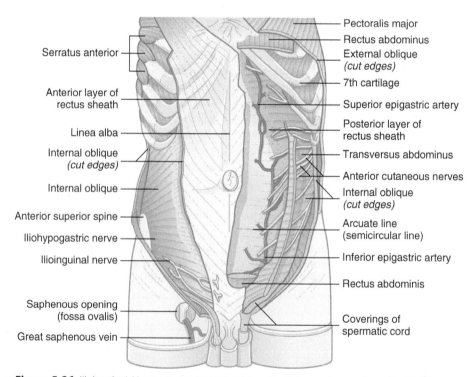

• **Figure 5-26** Ilioinguinal Nerve. In the inguinal region, the ilioinguinal nerve branch of L1 becomes superficial in the region of the superficial inguinal ring. It can be injured or compressed by an inguinal hernia or repair. (From Wei F, Mardini S. *Flaps and Reconstructive Surgery.* London: Saunders; 2009.)

nerve root or whether peripheral nerve entrapment is present.[154]

Various hip-associated causes of groin pain must be ruled out when diagnosing athletic pubalgia, including acetabular labral tear, femoral acetabular impingement, osteoarthritis, snapping hip syndrome, bursitis, iliopsoas tendinitis, avascular necrosis, and iliotibial band syndrome.[154] Please refer to Chapter 2 for an overview of diagnosis and treatment of hip disorders.

Groin pain has many pubic symphyseal causes, including adductor tendinopathy, iliopsoas tendinopathy, osteitis pubis, and rectus abdominis and adductor longus aponeurosis injury.[154,155,169,176,186,198] Osteitis pubis, or pubic symphysis stress injury, was found in 19% of 100 athletes presenting with chronic groin pain.[169,198] Its cause is believed to be pubic instability resulting from chronic repetitive shear or distraction from unbalanced tensile stresses across the pubic symphysis thus leading to an inflammatory response.[169,198] Radiographs show subchondral sclerosis, symphyseal irregularity, and bone resorption,[154,169] and MRI scans show marrow edema and bone erosion.[199,200] Symptom presentation is often insidious in onset, with pain centered over the pubis that may refer to the suprapubic region, adductor origin, and lower abdominals.[4,198] Pain manifests during kicking, running, jumping, and twisting, with tenderness to palpation over the pubic symphysis or pubic tubercle.[4,176,198] Treatment of osteitis pubis includes rest, activity modification including limited high-impact weight-wearing activities and resisted adduction, stabilization with an external support, and addressing any length-strength muscular imbalances.[4,198] The finding that osteitis pubis responds favorably to nonsteroidal antiinflammatory medications and corticosteroid injections suggests that the concomitant tenoperiosteal injury may be the source of pain because bone does not respond well to corticosteroids.[169] Osteitis pubis may take up to 12 months to heal, especially in the presence of underlying instability.[176,201-203]

Iliopsoas tendinopathy may manifest with pain during resisted or active hip flexion, passive hip extension, and tenderness to palpation lateral to the femoral artery within the femoral triangle.[176] MRI is accurate with high sensitivity and specificity for confirming this diagnosis.[204] Treatment includes rest, nonsteroidal antiinflammatory medications, gentle abdominal bracing not using the hip flexors, and addressing any muscle length-strength imbalances. Specific muscle strengthening or stretching of the iliopsoas should not be started until pain resolves and only if indicated.[154,176]

Adductor longus tendinopathy manifests either at the tendon's insertion on the pubic bone or at its convergence with the conjoint tendon and pubic aponeurotic plate.[169] Adductor longus tendinopathy is a common concomitant finding with other diagnoses including athletic pubalgia, conjoint tendinopathy, rectus abdominis tendinopathy, and osteitis pubis. Isolated adductor longus tendinopathy was found in only 3% of athletes with chronic groin pain.[169] Adductor longus tendinopathy manifests with pain in the proximal thigh, tenderness over the proximal adductor longus tendon, and pain reproduction with resisted hip adduction, passive abduction, and occasionally hip extension.[154,176] Strain to the adductor longus aponeurosis is evidenced on MRI.[154] Treatment of adductor longus tendinopathy includes rest, antiinflammatory medications, gentle lumbopelvic stabilization exercises, and addressing any muscle length-strength imbalances. If conservative treatment is not successful, an adductor release can be performed surgically. Please refer to Chapter 3 for an overview of diagnosis and treatment of adductor tendinopathy.

Confounding the athletic pubalgia diagnostic dilemma is the issue that patients often have concomitant injuries manifesting with very similar subjective complaints and objective findings. Multiple coexisting dysfunctions have been reported in 27% to 95% of athletes presenting with chronic groin pain.[‡‡] An example is osteitis pubis (see Chapter 3), whose presentation makes it difficult to distinguish from adductor strain and athletic pubalgia, and it was found to coexist in 19% of patients with athletic pubalgia.[§§] Patients with documented osteitis pubis treated with the typical athletic pubalgia mesh technique were able to return to competition even though their MRI documented the osteitis pubalgia remained.[12,148] Multiple studies have also documented concomitant adductor longus tendinopathy in patients with athletic pubalgia.[‖‖] Often, surgical findings reveal that athletic pubalgia, adductor longus tendinopathy, and osteitis pubic are all present in athletes with groin pain.[169,207]

Diagnostic Testing

The role of diagnostic imaging, including radiographs, ultrasound, MRI, CT scans, and bone scans, in diagnosing athletic pubalgia is being debated.[155] Dynamic assessment of the inguinal region with real-time ultrasound is currently advocated for the diagnosis of athletic pubalgia.[173,187] The accuracy of ultrasound is examiner dependent, but if the examiner is experienced, ultrasound examination can detect conjoint tendon dysfunction in a noninvasive manner without exposure to radiation.[173] Diagnostic ultrasound is used to establish posterior inguinal wall deficiency by placing the probe over the medial aspect of the inguinal region and asking the patient to "strain," such as by performing a half sit-up.[173] The test result is positive if the patient has an abnormal bulge, or increase in cross-sectional area, in the posterior inguinal wall, in contrast to the degree of canal closure exhibited under load in a normal inguinal canal.[158,186,208] This abnormal ultrasound finding must be correlated with symptoms, including palpable tenderness, for the diagnosis to be made because an asymptomatic bulge of the posterior inguinal canal has been found in 16% to 20% of athletes.[187,209] Although diagnostic ultrasound has

---

‡‡References 4, 8, 159, 169, 178, 205, and 206.
§§References 5, 9, 10, 13, 148, 165, 166, and 207.
‖‖References 157, 162, 165, 169, 173, 186, 198, and 206.

minimal associated cost and risk yet fair sensitivity, its specificity is low.[§]

Studies reported that MRI has approximately a 10% sensitivity in diagnosing athletic pubalgia,[147,156,165,212] a finding suggesting a limited utility for diagnosing this condition. MRI is useful for detecting muscle injury.[##] Zoga and associates,[200] in a retrospective study comparing MRI with surgery, reported a 68% sensitivity and a 100% specificity for rectus abdominis disorders and an 86% sensitivity and an 89% specificity for adductor disorders. More recent studies reported that MRI can be useful in detecting hyperintensity of the superficial inguinal ring and conjoint tendon associated with athletic pubalgia if the examiner is knowledgeable on reading the images.[10,165,198,200,208] Omar and colleagues[154] reported a common surgical finding of injury along the lateral border of the rectus abdominis, just proximal to its pubic attachment or at the origin of the adductor longus. Studies have documented that only a few patients with athletic pubalgia present with a tear of the rectus abdominis muscle on MRI.[7,12,146,148,165] Nonspecific MRI findings, including osteitis pubis, inflammation, attenuation of the abdominal wall myofascial layers, and small pelvic avulsion fractures, are typical with these patients[7,9,12,165] Omar and associates[154] developed a standardized MRI protocol to enhance the role of this imaging technique as a tool to diagnose athletic pubalgia accurately. Plain radiographs can detect pubic asymmetry, leg-length discrepancy, osteitis pubis, hip joint disorders, fractures, and avulsion fractures.[155,156,169,173,198]

Other investigative procedures that are medically invasive include laparoscopy and herniography. Although herniography can be of value in diagnosing athletic pubalgia, it is inappropriately invasive and controversial, and thus its use is minimal in the United States.[6,10,150,165,194,213] Laparoscopy, an endoscopic examination of the abdominal or pelvic cavity involving topical anesthesia and a small incision through the abdominal or pelvic cavity, can be used to diagnose and surgically repair athletic pubalgia.[10,147,176,193] This procedure has reported high success in diagnosing athletic pubalgia, and in addition to its diagnostic value, the endoscope can be used to repair the posterior wall deficiency in the same session.[147]

Etiology

Various schools of thought exist regarding the etiology of athletic pubalgia. The first hypothesis is that the condition is a muscular injury or disruption of any of the muscular, aponeurosis, or fascial insertions onto the anterior superior pubis and pubic symphysis.[152,214]

An additional hypothesis of the etiology of athletic pubalgia is weakness of the transversalis fascia over the posterior wall of the inguinal canal, a condition very similar to direct inguinal hernia but without peritoneal protrusion through the transversalis fascia. Operative findings report that many patients have an injury of the conjoined tendon or transversalis fascia that leads to weakening of the posterior inguinal wall[***] or multiple sites of defect in these structures (Fig. 5-27).[†††]

Multiple surgical studies of patients with athletic pubalgia have reported a high incidence of muscular and fascial injury to the aforementioned attachments onto the anterior pubis, in addition to weakening of the posterior inguinal floor.[7,195,216] The posterior wall of the inguinal canal is

---

[§]References 10, 147, 150, 166, 186, 187, 210, and 211.
[##]References 3, 8, 13, 147, 150, 155, 156, 166, 169, 173, 193, 200, and 212.

[***]References 3, 7, 148, 166, 187, 193, and 215.
[†††]References 7, 8, 10, 148, 152, 156, 165, and 166.

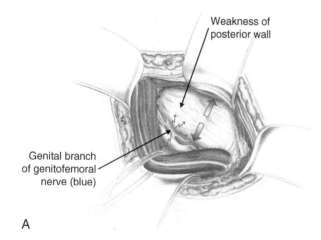

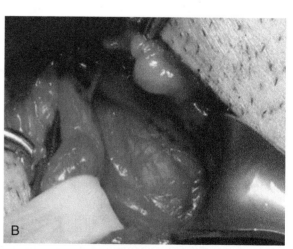

Weakness of posterior wall

Genital branch of genitofemoral nerve (blue)

A

B

• **Figure 5-27** Intraoperative drawing (**A**) and photograph (**B**) showing a localized bulge of the posterior wall causing compression of the genital branch of the genitofemoral nerve. (**A** and **B,** Copyright Dr. U. Muschaweck. **B,** From Minnich JM, Hanks JB, Muschaweck U, et al. Diagnosis and treatment highlighting a minimal repair surgical technique. *Am J Sports Med.* 2011;39:1341-1349.)

covered by transversalis fascia that may bulge on the medial aspect of the Hesselbach triangle, or tearing of the rectus abdominis, conjoined tendon, or the interface between the two may occur.[158,217] This localized "bulge" may compress on the genital branch of the genitofemoral nerve,[92] but again the bulge is not palpable. Although the posterior wall of the inguinal floor may tear during one strenuous effort, often it may weaken as a result of repetitive stresses, thereby resulting in a small bulge that is not considered a true "hernia" because it has not quite broken through the tissue. Therefore, current evidence suggests that the etiology of athletic pubalgia is a combination of (1) a large tear or multiple microtears involving muscular and fascial attachments onto the anterior pubis, (2) hernia-like symptoms related to the proximity of the tears to the medial margin of the superficial inguinal ring, and (3) myofascial lesion or lesions extending through the superficial ring and leading to weakness of the inguinal canal posterior wall.[154,158] The source of reported pain may not be the bulge from the posterior inguinal canal but rather the conjoint tendon disorder.[173]

The muscular or fascial attachments onto the anterior pubis are subjected to repetitive microtrauma from chronic shearing forces across the pubic symphysis, especially with repetitive hip adduction or abduction and hip flexion or extension.[7,148,156,165,218] During these motions, the pubic symphysis functions as a pivot point into which both the rectus abdominis and adductor longus insert, thereby potentially leading to a muscular "tug of war," and thus force transfer between the lumbopelvic and femoroacetabular joints.[218] Excessive lumbar or hip hyperextension forces further increase the stress on the pubic symphysis and lead to progressive microstress to the fascial attachments onto the pubic symphysis.[7,9,149,150]

The rectus abdominis and adductor longus blend together to form a common anatomic unit called an aponeurosis, and they share a common aponeurosis attachment at the anterior inferior aspect of the pubic body, 1 to 2 cm from the symphyseal midline (see Fig. 5-24).[154,198] Given the common aponeurosis, the rectus abdominis and adductor longus are relative antagonists during hip extension and rotation because the rectus abdominis elevates the pubic region, whereas the adductor longus places an anterior inferior force vector on the pubis.[154] Injury to one tendon predisposes a person to injury of the opposing tendon by disrupting the normal biomechanics and influencing the shear forces across the pubis.[198,200,206] Because the common aponeurosis of the rectus abdominis and adductor longus tendons is located along the anterior aspect of the pubic symphysis, movements such as hip extension may lead to eventual avulsion of the tendon and tearing in the aponeurosis.[154]

A cadaveric study by Norton-Old and colleagues[153] found that the adductor longus communicated with the contralateral distal rectus sheath, pubic symphysis, ilioinguinal ligament, anterior capsule, and contralateral adductor longus tendon. The researchers also used a strain gauge and found that simulated mechanical load across one of the adductor longus tendons had varying, yet significant, effects on the strain measured at the ipsilateral and contralateral rectus sheath. Studies using cadaveric dissection documented that rectus abdominis tendon tears can affect pelvic alignment and adductor anatomy.[7,12] When the rectus abdominis tendon is severed or weak in comparison with strong adductors, the pelvis will tilt anteriorly, thus leading to increased pressure directly over the adductor compartment and making it more vulnerable to bony projections on the superior edge of the inferior pubic ramus.[7,12]

Abnormal mechanical load and force attenuation on the anterior pelvis may be heightened by lower leg misalignment, excessive anterior pelvic tilt from poor abdominal and lumbar stability, poor posture, or muscular strength or length imbalances.[‡‡‡] As an example, a person with hip flexor muscle shortness or relative stiffness, limited mobility of the anterior hip capsule, and limited passive hip extension may lack active hip extension range and thus may compensate with excessive lumbar spine extension that leads to increased force attenuation on the anterior pelvis. Many athletes with athletic pubalgia describe a hyperextension injury in which the biomechanical pivot point during the offending motion is the anterior pelvis or pubic symphysis.[7,149] These imbalances of muscular forces, in time, result in chronic damage to the pubic symphysis, as well as to the tendons and fascia, either in isolation or combination.[206] This may explain why the cause of groin pain is often not due to a single injury, but rather the coexistence of two or more disorders.[13] Predisposition to repetitive pubic bone trauma may be heightened by poor blood supply to the pubic bone.[2] The pubic symphysis receives blood supply through the subchondral bone,[219] and damage to subchondral bone is related to cartilage degeneration elsewhere in the body.[220]

Sport-specific activities involving repetitive unilateral extremity dominant jumping, side-to-side motion, and kicking may eventually lead to significant unilateral differences in muscle strength and length that result in pelvic imbalance and strain to the pubic symphysis.[146,166,193,212]

Treatment

Only one prospective, randomized clinical trial has compared the outcomes of conservative treatment with surgical repair for treating athletes with athletic pubalgia.[221] Ekstrand and Ringborg[221] divided 66 soccer players with athletic pubalgia that was confirmed with herniography or nerve block into 1 of 4 groups: a control group, a nonsteroidal antiinflammatory medication and physical therapy group, an individual physical training group, or an open surgical repair group. At the 6-month follow-up, the only group with statistically significant improvement in their symptoms and ability to return to sport was the surgical group, a

---

‡‡‡References 8, 10, 13, 149, 150, 155, 165, and 198.

finding suggesting that conservative treatment is not as effective as surgery for treating this condition.[221] Conservative treatment of athletic pubalgia remains controversial, stemming in part from the limited evidence on the efficacy of conventional rehabilitation compared with surgical outcomes. Evidence supporting the effectiveness of physical therapy rehabilitation in the treatment of this condition is scarce, and early studies report mixed outcomes.[1,8,13,174,222]

Most physicians agree that a trial of physical therapy rehabilitation should be the first option in treating an athlete with suspected athletic pubalgia and negative findings on physical examination. What remains controversial is the length of time constituting a "trial," and the answer depends on the nature of the injury, the level of performance expected of the athlete, and the length of time before the athlete is expected to return to a preinjury level

of play.[174] A published flow chart[174] suggests a decision-making process for determining the course of rehabilitation or surgical treatment when presented with an athlete with athletic pubalgia (Fig. 5-28). If the athlete is presenting with the five hallmark signs and symptoms of athletic pubalgia and heard or felt a lower abdominal "tear" during the activity, then the athlete should consider undergoing a surgical examination and subsequent repair if she or he is off season and not expected to return to sport within 4 months. If the athlete is scheduled to return to sport within 4 months, a 3- to 4-week trial of rehabilitation is advocated, with rehabilitation continued if sufficient improvement is made at the end of the trial period to allow return to sport within required time frame. If the athlete did not hear or feel tearing, a lengthier trial of rehabilitation (6 weeks) is advocated. Athletes presenting with the characteristic signs and

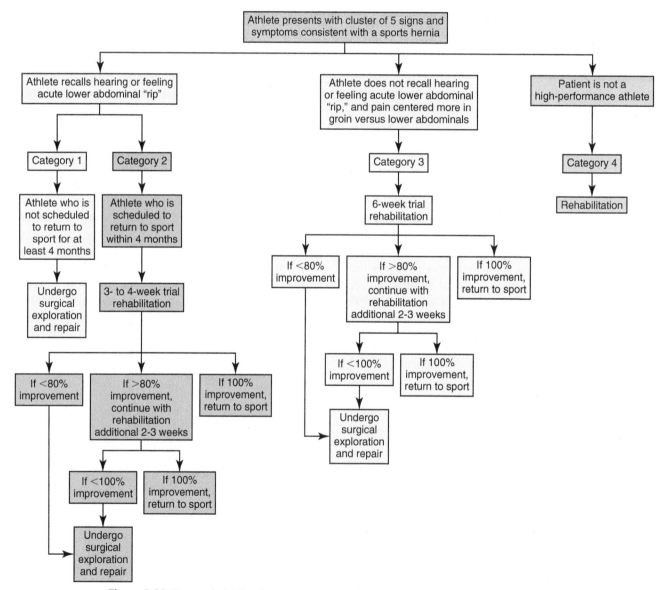

• **Figure 5-28** *Proposed algorithm for the management of an athlete with a suspected athletic pubalgia.* (From Kachingwe AF, Grech S. Proposed algorithm for the management of athletes with athletic pubalgia (sports *hernia*). *J Orthop Sports Phys Ther.* 2008;38:768-781.)

symptoms of athletic pubalgia undergo similar rehabilitation to address common objective findings, whether the definitive diagnosis has been given or not, and the course of rehabilitation versus surgical treatment is followed according to their outcomes. The flow chart[174] serves as a template to guide rehabilitation because outcomes may be variable, as a result of many factors such as the patient's motivation, level of pain tolerance, level of function, demands of the sport, demands of position played within his or her sport, and timing of injury relative to the patient's competitive season.

Little published guidance on the conservative course of treatment of athletic pubalgia is available. Physical therapy should emphasize lumbopelvic stability and restoration of pelvic symmetry through stretching the shortened musculature and strengthening the weak muscles that may have initially contributed to the injury.[146]

Soft tissue mobilization techniques can focus on any stiff posterior, superior, and lateral pelvic musculature and fascia, including the gluteus maximus, gluteus medius, tensor fasciae latae and iliotibial band, latissimus dorsi, erector spinae, and quadratus lumborum. Myofascial techniques may be incorporated to address significant myofascial restrictions of the lumbar spine and pelvis. The physical therapist should avoid myofascial techniques to the anterior abdominals, adductor insertion sites, or inguinal musculature because stresses to these areas may further compromise vulnerable tissue.

Joint mobilizations can be used to address any hypomobility of the pelvis or hips. Pelvic mobilizations may include posterior ilium rotational mobilization in patients with an anterior rotation positional fault and subsequent hypomobility of posterior rotation or anterior ilium rotational mobilization in patients with a posterior rotation positional fault and subsequent hypomobility of anterior pelvic rotation. In patients with innominate asymmetry, pelvic anterior and posterior rotations can be followed by the high-velocity, low-amplitude grade V SIJ gapping technique (Fig. 5-29). The grade V SIJ gapping technique has

been shown to be effective at decreasing pain associated with SIJ dysfunction.[223,224]

Hip mobilizations may include hip anterior or posterior glides to address hip passive accessory motion hypomobility that results in a decrease in active range of motion (Fig. 5-30). Any lumbar segmental hypomobility can be addressed with central or unilateral posterior-to-anterior mobilizations.

Neuromuscular reeducation and stretching techniques can be used to assist in maintaining muscle length and/or strength impairments. Passive stretching to hip musculature can be performed to address muscles that are short or stiff.[174]

Performing exercise is an integral component of rehabilitation because it addresses any strength impairments that may have contributed to the diagnosis of athletic pubalgia. Rehabilitation should include dynamic stretching of the iliopsoas, quadriceps, hamstrings, hip internal and external rotators, and adductors if these structures are found to be short or stiff. Strengthening should focus on lumbopelvic stabilization during the initial 6 weeks after injury. Research documents that the transversus abdominis and the internal and external obliques and rectus abdominis are activated to promote the generation of spinal stiffness before initiation of upper extremity movement.[225-227] It can be assumed that facilitating the motor control of the lumbar stabilization musculature would be of upmost importance in athletes, especially those whose sport involves volitional motions of the arms. Once the athlete is able to perform basic lumbopelvic stabilization exercises while maintaining a neutral spine without pain, exercises can be progressed to include strengthening of specific pelvic muscles as indicated.

Various lumbopelvic stabilization programs serve as excellent platforms for initiating stabilization, including the Sahrmann program[228] and the Watkins-Randall trunk stabilization program.[229] Athletes are started with isometric exercise, and once they establish proper technique without pain at one level of the program, they are advanced through the various levels of increasing difficulty.

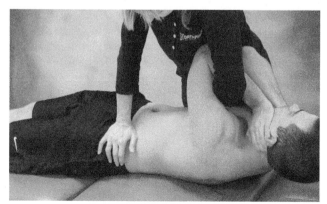

• **Figure 5-29** Performing a small-amplitude, high-velocity thrust sacroiliac joint (SIJ) iliac gapping technique to address pelvic asymmetry or SIJ-related pain.

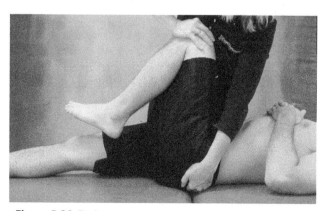

• **Figure 5-30** Performing a posterior glide hip mobilization to address right hip joint hypomobility.

Beginning at 3 to 6 weeks following the onset of symptoms or after the surgical procedure, and after establishing a certain mastery of lumbar isometric stabilization, the patient may begin sport-specific rehabilitation exercises. Multiplane joint motion emphasizing eccentric muscle contractions in a weight-bearing position is the foundation of the sport-specific exercises. The exercises closely replicate the motions taking place within his or her sport, and therefore the exercises may be varied depending on the demands of patient's sport and the level of function the patient demonstrates.

The choice of sport-specific exercises must be determined in an educated manner based on a full understanding of function as it relates to the demands of the patient's sport and position within the sport. Consideration of the pathologic features, the stage of healing, and the current functional ability of the patient must also be taken into account. Constant and consistent evaluation is needed to determine the threshold limitations of successful function and have the patient perform rehabilitation within those limitations. Patients should be progressed based on the level of functional recovery, demonstration of proper technique, and resolution of pain. It is important to evaluate and rehabilitate a patient in a manner that is consistent with the demands of the sport because it will be easier to determine readiness for return to play.

Physicians typically allow the athletes to return to play once they have no pain with sport-specific activities, including sprinting and cutting and can complete an abdominal curl-up and bilateral straight leg raise with resisted hip adduction without symptoms.[169] In one case series,[174] athletes were allowed to return to full participation within their sport once they were able to demonstrate an 80% to 100% functional level. These athletes attended an average of 7.2 sessions (range, 3 to 15); the patients who underwent surgical treatment had a mean of 6.7 sessions, and those who did not had a mean of 7.7 sessions.[174]

Surgical Intervention

If conservative intervention fails in the treatment of athletic pubalgia, surgical intervention is the next course of action.[6,149,187] Although some clinicians believe that surgery should be the last resort, others believe that it is the only way truly to correct the condition because the injury will become symptomatic again as soon as the patient returns to his or her sporting activity.[3,156] Surgical intervention may also be the immediate option if the patient has an acute onset with recollection of pubic musculature "tearing or ripping" and if the patient is a collegiate or professional athlete in whom a lengthy trial of rehabilitation may be impossible.[4,12,174]

The traditional surgical repair of athletic pubalgia involves an open procedure in which the inferior edge of the rectus abdominis muscle, the conjoined tendon, or the transversalis fascia is reattached to the pubis and inguinal ligaments with concomitant repair of the posterior wall of the inguinal canal, often reinforced with polypropylene

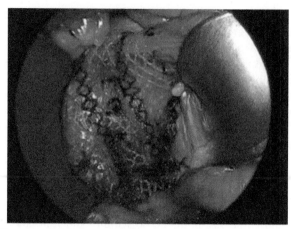

• **Figure 5-31** Intraoperative photograph showing an open procedure with mesh repair of a disrupted posterior inguinal floor. (From Minnich JM, Hanks JB, Muschaweck U, et al. Diagnosis and treatment highlighting a minimal repair surgical technique. *Am J Sports Med*. 2011; 39:1341-1349.)

mesh (Fig. 5-31).[6,7,149,150,156] If the patient has preoperative involvement of the adductor longus tendon, the surgeon may opt to perform a concurrent adductor tenotomy, typically fractional lengthening.[§§§]

An increasingly common surgical procedure is a laparoscopic procedure consisting of preperitoneal insertion of polypropylene mesh to cover and reinforce all potential hernia defects in the posterior abdominal wall.[6,10,146-148,166] The polypropylene mesh is fixed with some type of glue or tacks. Advantages of the endoscopic repair include less postoperative pain, smaller incisions, faster recovery rate, and the ability to perform diagnostic laparoscopy before the repair.[3,10,147,166,176]

Postsurgical Considerations and Rehabilitation

Early outcome studies using laparoscopic repair revealed high success rates to return to preinjury level of play within a relatively short time period.[6,12,146-148,177] Regardless of the operative approach for repair of athletic pubalgia, surgeons report good to excellent outcomes and quick return to previous level of activity.[3,166] Diaco and colleagues[148] and Meyers and associates[7] reported that 88% to 97% of athletes returned to their preinjury level of play within 3 months after the operation, Ahumada and associates[146] reported that 100% of athletes returned to this level within 4 months, and Kumar and colleagues[231] and van Veen and associates[166] reported that 88% to 93% of athletes returned to their preinjury level of play within 6 months postoperatively. Surgical outcomes for nonathletes have not been as favorable; suggested reasons include presurgical omission of exertion pain and adductor symptoms and the confounding issue of workers' compensation claims.[7,156]

---

§§§References 4, 6, 7, 146, 149, 152, 156, 166, 215, and 230.

If surgical treatment is elected, the typical postsurgical goal is for the athlete to return to play within 6 to 8 weeks.[146,166] If the athlete has a chronic condition or if multiple injuries were involved with the diagnosis of athletic pubalgia, the athlete may need as much as 6 months of rehabilitation before returning to play.[146] Immediately after the operation, the patient should rest for 3 to 4 weeks, particularly avoiding heavy lifting and sudden movement,[146] to allow incisional healing before starting rehabilitation. Physical therapy is initiated anywhere from 1 to 4 weeks postoperatively.[146]

Case Study

An example of right groin and lower abdominal pain is given in Case Study 5-1.

CASE STUDY 5-1

Right Groin and Lower Abdominal Pain

The patient is a 21-year-old collegiate basketball player with a physician's diagnosis of right hip flexor and adductor strain who presented with a 2-week history of insidious-onset right groin and lower abdominal pain. He reports that the pain has been increasing in intensity over the past 2 weeks and occasionally radiates into his testicles. The pain is rated at 7 to 8 out of 10 on a visual analog scale with any basketball-related activities and is described as "deep and achy." He has no pain at rest. He also complains of left groin and lower abdominal pain rated at 2 out of 10 and that comes on only after the onset of right groin pain. He reports that he did "pull" his left groin 1 year ago playing basketball; the condition remained during the season, but he rested over the summer and it resolved. As for aggravating factors, he is unable to participate in basketball practice because of pain, and he has 8 out of 10 pain with running and 7 out of 10 pain when transferring from supine to long sitting. He reports no pain with ejaculation. Easing factors are rest and ice. He is taking 500 mg of nonsteroidal antiinflammatory medications twice a day, and the medication does ease his symptoms somewhat. His past medical history is unremarkable except for his left groin injury 1 year ago. He is a right-handed shooter and jumps primarily from his left leg. Diagnostic tests: Radiographs were negative. Oswestry Disability Questionnaire: 20%.

Case Study Objective Tests and Measures, Physical Therapist Diagnosis, and Physical Therapy Intervention

Observation and symmetry	Left iliac crest and PSIS higher, left ASIS lower than right Hypertrophied lumbar paraspinal musculature		
Active Range of Motion	**Hip**	**Right (Degrees)**	**Left (Degrees)**
	Flexion	110	112
	Extension	8	5
	External rotation		
	Sitting	28	**15**
	Prone	30	**10**
	Internal rotation		
	Sitting	**19**	29
	Prone	**22**	30
	Abduction	40	**25 (produced pain in bilateral lower abdomen)**
	Adduction	30	40
Manual Muscle Testing		**Right**	**Left**
	Iliopsoas	3+ (produced pain in anterior hip and right abdomen)	3+ (produced pain in left abdomen; tested stronger [4−] with posterior pelvic tilt but still painful)
	Gluteus maximus	4	4− (produced pain in left abdomen that decreased when tested with more hip flexion)
	Posterior gluteus medius	4−	3+
	Hamstrings	4+	4
	Adductors	3+ (produced pain in right abdomen)	3+ (produced pain in left abdomen)
	Hip external rotation	4	3+
	Hip internal rotation	3+ (produce slight pain anterior hip and abdomen)	4

Continued

CASE STUDY 5-1

Right Groin and Lower Abdominal Pain—cont'd

Tenderness to palpation	Moderate tenderness to right > left iliopsoas tendon
	Moderate tenderness to distal rectus abdominis right > left at pubic insertion
	No tenderness over adductor longus tendon
Muscle length	Positive Thomas test for iliopsoas shortness and stiffness left > right (Fig. 5-32).
	Positive hamstring 90/90 and SLR for hamstring stiffness right > left
	Positive Ober test for ITB and TFL shortness and stiffness left > right
Special tests	Positive Gillet standing march test on left
	Positive forward bending test on left
	Negative ASIS compression and distraction tests
	Negative Craig test (12 degrees of internal rotation) bilaterally
	Pain with resisted hip adduction supine at:
	0 degrees of abduction (produced 3/10 left > right groin pain)
	45 degrees of abduction (produced 3/10 bilateral lower abdominal pain)
	Pain with resisted sit-ups
Passive accessory motion	Right hip posterior glide 2/6 hypomobility (see Fig. 5-31)
	Left ilium posterior rotation 2/6 hypomobility
Physical therapist diagnosis	Acute on chronic right > left rectus abdominis strain with signs and symptoms consistent with athletic pubalgia; right iliopsoas tendinopathy from:
	Left anterior pelvic tilt
	Left hip iliopsoas and TFL and ITB too short and stiff in relation to external obliques
	External obliques, internal obliques, and transversus abdominis not stiff enough
	Left > right posterior gluteus medius too long and weak
	Left ilium anterior rotation positional fault with hypomobility of ilium posterior rotation
	Right posterior pelvic tilt with hip anterior glide syndrome
	Right external rotators too short and stiff
	Hypomobility of right hip posterior glide
	Shortness of right > left hamstrings
	Dominance of hamstring over gluteus maximus
PT intervention and outcome	6 sessions of rehabilitation (twice/week for 3 weeks)
	PT consisting of therapeutic exercises to correct imbalances of muscles crossing the pubis:
	Strengthening of weak muscles (Figs. 5-33 and 5-34)
	Lengthening of shortened muscles (soft tissue mobilization, stretching)
	Lumbosacral stabilization exercises
	Joint mobilizations to correct hypomobility
	Modalities
	Instruction of a home exercise program and activity modification
	Patient then returned to playing basketball with minimal "soreness" during practice. Played at 100% for 1 month; then symptoms returned that forced him to quit during game; unable to return. Underwent endoscopic surgical procedure with bilateral mesh placement 6 weeks later. Returned for two sessions of PT 6 weeks postoperatively; then self-discharged because of full return of sport-specific activities without symptoms.

ASIS, Anterior superior iliac spine; *ITB,* iliotibial band; *PT,* physical therapy; *PSIS,* posterior superior iliac spine; *SLR,* straight leg raise; *TFL,* tensor fasciae latae.
A grade of 2 (on a scale from 0 to 6) indicates a slight restriction of movement that is treated with mobilization and stretching.

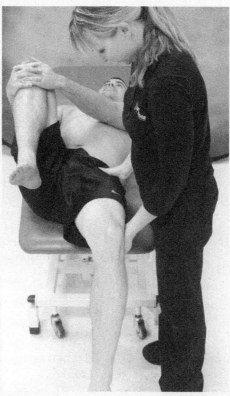

• **Figure 5-32** The Thomas test assesses the muscle length or stiffness of the iliopsoas, the tensor fasciae latae (TFL) and iliotibial band (ITB), and the rectus femoris. In this photograph, the therapist is stabilizing the anterior superior iliac spine to assess muscle length. The TFL and ITB, the iliopsoas, and the rectus femoris may all be short as the hip is in flexion and abduction.

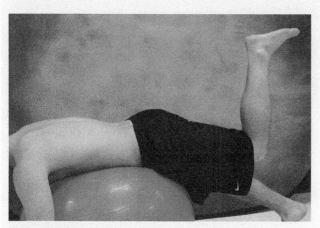

• **Figure 5-33** Strengthening the hip extensors by having the patient performing hip extension from a prone position over the Swiss ball.

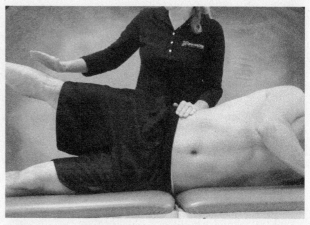

• **Figure 5-34** Strengthening the gluteus medius by having the patient perform hip abduction in a side-lying position. The patient should be cued to maintain slight hip extension and external rotation to avoid focus on the tensor fasciae latae and iliotibial band.

References

1. Syme G, Wilson J, Mackenzie K, Macleod D. Groin pain in athletes. *Lancet*. 1999;353:1444.

2. Holmich P. Adductor-related groin pain in athletes. *Sports Med Arthrosc Rev*. 1997;5:285-291.

3. Moeller JL. Sportsman's hernia. *Curr Sports Med Rep*. 2007; 6:111-114.

4. Anderson K, Strickland SM, Warren R. Hip and groin injuries in athletes. *Am J Sports Med*. 2001;29:521-533.

5. Holmich P. Long-standing groin pain in sportspeople falls into three primary patterns, a "clinical entity" approach: a prospective study of 207 patients. *Br J Sports Med*. 2007;41:247-252, discussion 252.

6. Lynch SA, Renstrom PA. Groin injuries in sport: treatment strategies. *Sports Med*. 1999;28:137-144.

7. Meyers WC, Foley DP, Garrett WE, et al. Management of severe lower abdominal or inguinal pain in high-performance athletes. *Am J Sports Med*. 2000;28:2-8.

8. LeBlanc KE, LeBlanc KA. Groin pain in athletes. *Hernia*. 2003;7:68-71.

9. Daigeler A, Belyaev O, Pennekamp WH. MRI findings do not correlate with outcome in athletes with chronic groin pain. *J Sports Sci*. 2007;6:71-76.

10. Swan KG, Wolcott M. The athletic hernia: a systematic review. *Clin Orthop Relat Res*. 2006;455:78-87.

11. Holmich P, Holmich JR, Bjerg AM. Clinical examination of athletes with groin pain: an intraobserver and interobserver reliability study. *Br J Sports Med*. 2004;38:446-451.

12. Meyers WC, Lanfranco A, Castellanos A. Surgical management of chronic lower abdominal and groin pain in high-performance athletes. *Curr Sports Med Rep*. 2002;1:301-305.

13. Morelli V, Smith V. Groin injuries in athletes. *Am Fam Physician*. 2001;64:1405-1414.

14. Dauty M, Menu P, Dubois C. Uncommon external abdominal oblique muscle strain in a professional soccer player: a case report. *BMC Res Notes*. 2014;7:684-687.

15. Garrett WE. Muscle strain injuries. *Am J Sports Med*. 1996;24: 2-8.

16. Sinnatamby CS, ed. *Last's Anatomy*. 10th ed. Edinburgh: Churchill Livingstone; 1999.

17. Gray H. *Anatomy of the Human Body*. 20th ed. Philadelphia: Lea & Febiger; 1918.

18. Connell D, Ali K, Javid M, et al. Sonography and MRI of rectus abdomens muscle strain in elite tennis players. *AJR Am J Roentgenol*. 2006;187:1457-1461.

19. Balius R, Pedret C, Pacheco L, et al. Rectus abdominis muscle injuries in elite handball players: management and rehabilitation. *J Sports Med*. 2011;2:69-73.

20. Netter FH. *Atlas of Human Anatomy*. 5th ed. Philadelphia: Saunders; 2010.

21. Andersson EA, Grundstrom H, Thorstensson A. Diverging intramuscular activity patterns in back and abdominal muscles during trunk rotation. *Spine (Phila Pa 1976)*. 2002;27:E152-E160.

22. Johnson R. Abdominal wall injuries: rectus abdominis strains, oblique strains, rectus sheath hematoma. *Curr Sports Med Rep*. 2006;5:99-103.

23. Kumar S, Narayan Y, Zedka M. An electromyographic study of unresisted trunk rotation with normal velocity among healthy subjects. *Spine (Phila Pa 1976)*. 1996;21:1500-1512.

24. McGill SM. Electromyographic activity of the abdominal and low back musculature during the generation of isometric and dynamic axial trunk torque: implications for lumbar mechanics. *J Orthop Res*. 1991;9:91-103.

25. Neumann DA. *Kinesiology of the Musculoskeletal System: Foundations for Rehabilitation*. 2nd ed. St. Louis: Mosby; 2010.

26. Ng J, Parnianpour M, Richardson CA, Kippers V. Functional roles of abdominal and back muscles during isometric axial rotation of the trunk. *J Orthop Res*. 2001;19:463-471.

27. Arjmand N, Shirazi-Adl A, Parnianpour M. Trunk biomechanics during maximum isometric axial torque exertions in upright standing. *Clin Biomech (Bristol, Avon)*. 2008;23:969-978.

28. Hoek van Dijke GA, Snijders CJ, Stoeckart R, Stam HJ. A biomechanical model on muscle forces in the transfer of spinal load to the pelvis and legs. *J Biomech*. 1999;32: 927-933.

29. Urquhart DM, Hodges PW, Story IH. Postural activity of the abdominal muscles varies between regions of these muscles and between body positions. *Gait Posture*. 2005;22:295-301.

30. Barker PJ, Briggs CA, Bogeski G. Tensile transmission across lumbar fasciae in unembalmed cadavers: effects of tension to various muscular attachments. *Spine (Phila Pa 1976)*. 2004; 29:129-138.

31. Tesh KM, Dunn JS, Evans JH. The abdominal muscles and vertebral stability. *Spine (Phila Pa 1976)*. 1987;12:501-508.

32. Hodges PW, Richardson CA. Altered trunk muscle recruitment in people with low back pain with upper limb movement at different speeds. *Arch Phys Med Rehabil*. 1999;80:1005-1012.

33. Cresswell AG, Grundstrom H, Thorstensson A. Observations on intraabdominal pressure and patterns of abdominal intramuscular activity in man. *Acta Physiol Scand*. 1992;144:409-418.

34. Urquhart DM, Hodges PW. Differential activity of regions of transversus abdominis during trunk rotation. *Eur Spine J*. 2005;14:393-400.

35. Conte SA, Thompson MM, Marks MA, Dines JS. Abdominal muscle strains in professional baseball. *Am J Sports Med*. 2012; 40:650-656.

36. Humphries D, Jamison M. Clinical and magnetic resonance imaging features of cricket bowler's side strain. *Br J Sports Med*. 2004;38:E21.

37. Maquirriain J, Ghisi JP. Uncommon abdominal muscle injury in a tennis player: internal oblique strain. *Br J Sports Med*. 2006;40:462-463.

38. Maquirriain J, Ghisi JP, Mazzucco J. Abdominal muscles strain injuries in the tennis player: treatment and prevention. *Med Sci Tennis*. 2002;3:14-15.

39. Stevens KJ, Crain JM, Akizuki KH, Beaulieu CF. Imaging and ultrasound-guided steroid injection of internal oblique muscle strains in baseball pitchers. *Am J Sports Med*. 2010;38: 581-585.

40. Hawkins RD, Fuller CW. A prospective epidemiological study of injuries in four English professional football clubs. *Br J Sports Med*. 1999;33:196-203.

41. Price RJ, Hawkins RD, Hulse MA, Hodson A. The Football Association medical research programme: an audit of injuries in academy youth football. *Br J Sports Med*. 2004;38:466-471.

42. Lehman RC. Thoracoabdominal musculoskeletal injuries in racquet sports. *Clin Sports Med*. 1988;7:267-276.

43. O'Neal ML, McCown K, Poulis GC. Complex strain injury involving an intercostal hematoma in a professional baseball player. *Clin J Sport Med.* 2008;18:372-373.

44. Connell DA, Jhamb A, James T. Side strains: a tear of internal oblique musculature. *AJR Am J Roentgenol.* 2003;181:1511-1517.

45. Obaid H, Nealon A, Connell D. Sonographic appearance of side strain injury. *AJR Am J Roentgenol.* 2008;191:264-267.

46. Watkins RG, Dennis S, Dillin WH. Dynamic EMG analysis of torque transfer in professional baseball pitchers. *Spine (Phila Pa 1976).* 1989;14:404-408.

47. Chang CJ, Graves DW. Athletic injuries of the thorax and abdomen. In: Mellion M, Walsh WM, Madden C, eds. *Team Physician's Handbook.* 3rd ed. Philadelphia: Hanley and Belfus; 2002:441-459.

48. Thomson H, Francis D. Abdominal-wall tenderness: a useful sign in the acute abdomen. *Lancet.* 1977;2:1053-1054.

49. Thia EWH, Low JJH, Wee HY. Rectus sheath haematoma mimicking an ovarian mass. *Int J Gynaecol Obstet.* 2003;2:1.

50. Bartlett RM. The biomechanics of the discus throw: a review. *J Sports Sci.* 1992;10:467-510.

51. Chow JW, Shim JH, Lim YT. Lower trunk muscle activity during the tennis serve. *J Sci Med Sport.* 2003;6:512-518.

52. Pink M, Perry J, Jobe FW. Electromyographic analysis of the trunk in golfers. *Am J Sports Med.* 1993;21:385-388.

53. Shaffer B, Jobe FW, Pink M, Perry J. Baseball batting. An electromyographic study. *Clin Orthop Relat Res.* 1993;292:285-293.

54. Hakim M, Hage W, Lovering RM, et al. Dexamethasone and recovery of contractile tension after a muscle injury. *Clin Orthop Relat Res.* 2005;439:235-242.

55. Levine WN, Bergfeld JA, Tessendorf W, Moorman CT. Intra-muscular corticosteroid injection for hamstring injuries: a 13-year experience in the National Football League. *Am J Sports Med.* 2000;28:297-300.

56. Mishra A, Pavelko T. Treatment of chronic elbow tendinosis with buffered platelet-rich plasma. *Am J Sports Med.* 2006;34:1774-1778.

57. Sanchez M, Anitua E, Orive G, et al. Platelet-rich therapies in the treatment of orthopaedic sport injuries. *Sports Med.* 2009;39:345-354.

58. Nguyen RT, Borg-Stein J, McInnis K. Application of platelet-rich plasma in musculoskeletal and sports medicine: an evidence-based approach. *PM R.* 2011;3:226-250.

59. Friemert B, Faoual J, Holldobler G, et al. A prospective randomized study on inguinal hernia repair according to the Shouldice technique: benefits of local anesthesia. *Chirurg.* 2000;71:52-57. [in German].

60. Jenkins JT, O'Dwyer PJ. Inguinal hernias. *BMJ.* 2008;336:269-272.

61. Kingsnorth A, LeBlanc K. Hernias: inguinal and incisional. *Lancet.* 2003;362:1561-1571.

62. Cabry RJ, Thorell E, Heck K, et al. Understanding noninguinal abdominal hernias in the athlete. *Curr Sports Med Rep.* 2014;13:86-93.

63. Purkayastha S, Chow A, Athanasiou T, et al. Inguinal hernia. *BMJ Clin Evid.* 2008;7:1-146.

64. Primatesta P, Goldacre MJ. Inguinal hernia repair: incidence of elective and emergency surgery, readmission and mortality. *Int J Epidemiol.* 1996;25:835-839.

65. Rutkow IM. Epidemiologic, economic, and sociologic aspects of hernia surgery in the United States in the 1990s. *Surg Clin North Am.* 1998;78:941-951.

66. Simons MP, Aufenacker T, May-Nielsen M, et al. European Hernia Society guidelines on the treatment of inguinal hernia in adult patients. *Hernia.* 2009;13:343-403.

67. Kark AE, Kurzer M. Groin hernias in women. *Hernia.* 2008;12:267-270.

68. Klinge U, Zheng H, Si ZY, et al. Altered collagen synthesis in fascia transversals of patients with inguinal hernia. *Hernia.* 1999;4:181-187.

69. Lau H, Fang C, Yuen WK, Patil NG. Risk factors for inguinal hernia in adult males: a case-control study. *Surgery.* 2007;141:262-266.

70. Liem MS, van der Graaf Y, Zwart RC, et al. Risk factors for inguinal hernia in women: a case-control study. The Coala trial group. *Am J Epidomiol.* 1997;146:721-726.

71. Carbonell JF, Sanchez JL, Peris RT, et al. Risk factors associated with inguinal hernias: a case control study. *Eur J Surg.* 1993;159:481-486.

72. Flich J, Alfonso JL, Delgado F, et al. Inguinal hernia and certain risk factors. *Eur J Epidemiol.* 1992;8:277-282.

73. Pleumeekers HJ, De Gruijl A, Hofman A, et al. Prevalence of aortic aneurysm in men with a history of inguinal hernia repair. *Br J Surg.* 1999;86:1155-1158.

74. Sorensen LT, Friis E, Jorgensen T, et al. Smoking is a risk factor for recurrence of groin hernia. *World J Surg.* 2002;26:397-400.

75. Fitzgibbons RJ, Giobbie-Hurder A, Gibbs JO, et al. Watchful waiting vs repair of inguinal hernia in minimally symptomatic men. *JAMA.* 2006;295:285-292.

76. Gallegos NC, Dawson J, Jarvis M, Hobsley M. Risk of strangulation in groin hernias. *Br J Surg.* 1991;78:1171-1173.

77. Hair A, Duffy K, McLean J, et al. What effect does the duration of an inguinal hernia have on patient symptoms? *J Am Coll Surg.* 2001;193:125-129.

78. Rai S, Chandra SS, Smile SR. A study of the risk of strangulation and obstruction in groin hernias. *Aust N Z J Surg.* 1998;68:650-654.

79. Kark A, Kurzer M, Waters KJ. Accuracy of clinical diagnosis of direct and indirect inguinal hernia. *Br J Surg.* 1994;81:1081-1082.

80. McIntosh A, Hutchinson A, Roberts A, Withers H. Evidence-based management of groin hernia in primary care: a systematic review. *Fam Pract.* 2000;17:442-447.

81. Ralphs DN, Brain AJ, Grundy DJ, Hobsley M. How accurately can direct and indirect inguinal hernias be distinguished? *Br Med J.* 1980;280:1039-1040.

82. Bay-Nielsen M, Kehlet H, Strand L, et al. Quality assessment of 26,304 herniorrhaphies in Denmark: a prospective nation-wide study. *Lancet.* 2001;358:1124-1128.

83. Nilsson H, Stylianidis G, Haaparanki M, et al. Mortality after groin hernia surgery. *Ann Surg.* 2007;245:656-660.

84. Deveney KE. Hernias and other lesions of the abdominal wall. In: Doherty GM, ed. *Current Surgical Diagnosis and Treatment.* New York: McGraw-Hill; 2010.

85. Malangoni MA, Rosen MJ. Hernias. In: Townsend CM, Beauchamp RD, Evers BM, Mattox KL, eds. *Sabiston Textbook of Surgery.* 19th ed. Philadelphia: Saunders; 2012.

86. Temiz A, Akcora B, Temiz M, Canbolant E. A rare and frequently unrecognized pathology in children: femoral hernia. *Hernia.* 2008;12:553-556.

87. Kovachev LS. The femoral hernia: some necessary additions. *Int J Clin Med*. 2014;5:752-765.

88. Whalen HR, Kidd GA, O'Dwyer PJ. Femoral hernias. *BMJ*. 2011;343.

89. Snyder CL. Current management of umbilical abnormalities and related anomalies. *Semin Pediatr Surg*. 2007;16:41-49.

90. Dahlstrand U, Wollert S, Nordin P, et al. Emergency femoral hernia repair. *Ann Surg*. 2009;249:672-676.

91. Buhck H, Untied M, Bechstein WO. Evidence-based assessment of the period of physical inactivity required after inguinal herniotomy. *Langenbecks Arch Surg*. 2012;397:1209-1214.

92. Muschaweck U. Umbilical and epigastric hernia repair. *Surg Clin North Am*. 2003;83:1207-1221.

93. Jackson OJ, Moglen LH. Umbilical hernia: a retrospective study. *Calif Med*. 1970;113:8-11.

94. Dickerman RD, Smith A, Stevens QE. Umbilical and bilateral inguinal hernias in a veteran powerlifter: is it a pressure overload syndrome? *Clin J Sport Med*. 2004;14:95-96.

95. Salameh JR. Primary and unusual abdominal wall hernias. *Surg Clin North Am*. 2008;88:45-60.

96. LeBlanc KA. Incisional, epigastric and umbilical hernias. In: Cameron JL, Cameron AM, eds. *Current Surgical Therapy*. 10th ed. Philadelphia: Saunders; 2011:497-501.

97. Kraft BM, Kolb H, Kuckuk B, et al. Diagnosis and classification of inguinal hernias. *Surg Endosc*. 2003;17:2021-2024.

98. van den Berg JC, de Valois JC, Go PM, Rosenbusch G. Radiological anatomy of the groin region. *Eur Radiol*. 2000;10:661-670.

99. Page B, Paterson C, Young D, O'Dwyer PJ. Pain from primary inguinal hernia and the effect of repair on pain. *Br J Surg*. 2002;89:1315-1318.

100. Alam A, Nice C, Uberoi R. The accuracy of ultrasound in the diagnosis of clinically occult groin hernias in adults. *Eur Radiol*. 2005;15:2457-2461.

101. Bradley M, Morgan D, Pentlow B, Roe A. The groin hernia: an ultrasound diagnosis? *Ann R Coll Surg Engl*. 2003;85:178-180.

102. Lilly MC, Arregui ME. Ultrasound of the inguinal floor for evaluation of hernias. *Surg Endosc*. 2002;16:659-662.

103. Robinson P, Hensor E, Lansdown MJ, et al. Inguino-femoral hernia: accuracy of sonography in patients with indeterminate clinical features. *AJR Am J Roentgenol*. 2006;187:1168-1178.

104. Leander P, Ekberg O, Sjoberg S, Kesek P. MR imaging following herniography in patients with unclear groin pain. *Eur Radiol*. 2000;10:1691-1696.

105. Garner JP, Patel S, Glaves J, Ravi K. Is herniography useful? *Hernia*. 2006;10:66-69.

106. Heise CP, Sproat IA, Starling JR. Peritoneography (herniography) for detecting occult inguinal hernia in patients with inguinodynia. *Ann Surg*. 2002;235:140-144.

107. Calder F, Evans R, Neilson D, Hurley P. Value of herniography in the management of occult hernia and chronic groin pain in adults. *Br J Surg*. 2000;87:824-825.

108. Toms AP, Dixon AK, Murphy JM. Illustrated review of new imaging techniques in the diagnosis of abdominal wall hernias. *Br J Surg*. 1999;86:1243-1249.

109. O'Dwyer PJ, Chung L. Watchful waiting was as safe as surgical repair for minimally symptomatic inguinal hernias. *Evid Based Med*. 2006;11:73.

110. Callesen T, Bech K, Kehlet H. Prospective study of chronic pain after groin hernia repair. *Br J Surg*. 1999;86:1528-1531.

111. MRC Laparoscopic Groin Hernia Trial Group. Laparoscopic versus open repair of groin hernia: a randomized comparison. *Lancet*. 1999;354:185-190.

112. Holzheimer RG. First results of Lichtenstein hernia repair with Ultrapro-mesh as cost saving procedure: quality control combined with a modified quality of life questionnaire (SF-36) in a series of ambulatory operated patients. *Eur J Med Res*. 2004;9:323-327.

113. Holzheimer RG. Inguinal hernia: classification, diagnosis and treatment: classic, traumatic and sportman's hernia. *Eur J Med Res*. 2005;10:121-134.

114. EU Hernia Trialist Collaboration. Laparoscopic compared with open methods of groin hernia repair: systematic review of randomized controlled trials. *Br J Surg*. 2000;37:860-867.

115. Memon MA, Cooper NJ, Memon B, et al. Meta-analysis of randomized clinical trials comparing open and laparoscopic inguinal hernia repair. *Br J Surg*. 2003;90:1479-1482.

116. *Stedman's Medical Dictionary*. 28th ed. Baltimore: Lippincott Williams & Wilkins; 2005.

117. Bittner R, Sauerland S, Schmedt CG. Comparison of endoscopic techniques vs Shouldice and other open non mesh techniques for inguinal hernia repair: a meta-analysis of randomized controlled trials. *Surg Endosc*. 2005;19:605-615.

118. McCormack K, Wake B, Perez J, et al. Laparoscopic surgery for inguinal hernia repair: systematic review of effectiveness and economic evaluation. *Health Technol Assess*. 2005;9:1-203, iii-iv.

119. Scott NW, McCormack K, Graham P, et al. Open mesh versus non-mesh for repair of femoral and inguinal hernia. *Cochrane Database Syst Rev*. 2002;(4):CD002197.

120. Schmedt CG, Sauerland S, Bittner R. Comparison of endoscopic procedures vs Lichtenstein and other open mesh techniques for inguinal hernia repair: a meta-analysis of randomized controlled trials. *Surg Endosc*. 2005;19:188-199.

121. Reuben B, Neumayer L. Surgical management of inguinal hernia. *Adv Surg*. 2006;40:299-317.

122. Amid PK, Shulman AG, Lichtenstein IL. Open "tension-free" repair of inguinal hernias: the Lichtenstein technique. *Eur J Surg*. 1996;162:447-453.

123. Lichtenstein IL, Shulman AG, Amid PK, Montllor MM. The tension-free hernioplasty. *Am J Surg*. 1989;157:188-193.

124. McCormack K, Scott NW, Go PM, et al. Laparoscopic techniques versus open techniques for inguinal hernia repair. *Cochrane Database Syst Rev*. 2003;(1):CD001785.

125. Bay-Nielsen M, Kehlet H. Inguinal herniorrhapy in women. *Hernia*. 2006;10:30-33.

126. Koch A, Edwards A, Haapaniemi S, et al. Prospective evaluation of 6895 groin hernia repairs in women. *Br J Surg*. 2005;92:1553-1558.

127. Simons MP, Kleijnen J, van Geldere D, et al. Role of the Shouldice technique in inguinal hernia repair: a systematic review of controlled trials and a meta-analysis. *Br J Surg*. 1996;83:734-738.

128. Beets GL, Oosterhuis KJ, Go PM, et al. Long-term followup (12-15 years) of a randomized controlled trial comparing Bassini-Stetten, Shouldice, and high ligation with narrowing of the internal ring for primary inguinal hernia repair. *J Am Coll Surg*. 1997;185:352-357.

129. Salcedo-Wasicek MC, Thirlby RC. Postoperative core after inguinal herniorrhapy: a case-controlled comparison of patients receiving workers' compensation vs patients with commercial insurance. *Arch Surg*. 1995;130:29-32.

130. Bringman S, Ramel S, Heikkinen TJ, et al. Tension-free inguinal hernia repair: TEP versus mesh-plug versus Lichtenstein. A prospective randomized controlled trial. *Ann Surg*. 2003;237: 142-147.

131. Chung RS, Rowland DY. Meta-analyses of randomized controlled trials of laparoscopic vs conventional inguinal hernia repairs. *Surg Endosc*. 1999;13:689-694.

132. Grant AM. Laparoscopic versus open groin hernia repair: meta-analysis of randomized trials based on individual patient data. *Hernia*. 2002;6:2-10.

133. Heikkinen TJ, Haukipuro K, Huikko A. A cost and outcome comparison between laparoscopic and Lichtenstein hernia operations in a day-case unit: a randomized prospective study. *Surg Endosc*. 1998;12:1199-1203.

134. Kuhry E, van Veen RN, Langeveld HR, et al. Open or endoscopic total extraperitoneal inguinal hernia repair? A systematic review. *Surg Endosc*. 2007;21:161-166.

135. Lau H, Patil NG, Yuen WK. Day-case endoscopic totally extra peritoneal inguinal hernioplasty versus open Lichtenstein hernioplasty for unilateral primary inguinal hernia in males: a randomized trial. *Surg Endosc*. 2006;20:76-81.

136. Buhck H, Untied M, Bechstein WO. Evidence-based assessment of the period of physical inactivity required after inguinal herniotomy. *Langenbecks Arch Surg*. 2012;397:1209-1214.

137. Hendry PO, Paterson-Brown S, de Beaux A. Work related aspects of inguinal hernia: a literature review. *Surgeon*. 2008;6: 361-365.

138. Bourke JB, Taylor M. The clinical and economic effects of early return to work after elective inguinal hernia repair. *Br J Surg*. 1978;65:728-731.

139. Bourke JB, Lear PA, Taylor M. Effect of early return to work after elective repair of inguinal hernia: clinical and financial consequences at one year and three years. *Lancet*. 1981;2: 623-625.

140. Taylor EW, Dewar EP. Early return to work after repair of a unilateral inguinal hernia. *Br J Surg*. 1983;70:599-600.

141. Callesen T, Bech K, Nielsen R, et al. Pain after groin hernia repair. *Br J Surg*. 1998;85:1412-1414.

142. Callesen T. Inguinal hernia repair: anaesthesia, pain and convalescence. *Dan Med Bull*. 2003;50:203-218.

143. Gillion JF, Fagniez PL. Chronic pain and cutaneous sensory changes after inguinal hernia repair: comparison between open and laparoscopic techniques. *Hernia*. 1999;3:75-80.

144. Aasvang EK, Gmaehle E, Hansen JB, et al. Predictive risk factors for persistent postherniotomy pain. *Anesthesiology*. 2010;112:957-969.

145. Bittner R, Arregui ME, Bisgaard T, et al. Guidelines for laparoscopic (TAPP) and endoscopic (TEP) treatment of inguinal hernia. *Surg Endosc*. 2011;25:2773-2843.

146. Ahumada LA, Ashruf S, Espinosa-de-los-Monteros A. Athletic pubalgia: definition and surgical treatment. *Ann Plast Surg*. 2005;55:393-396.

147. Kluin J, den Hoed PT, van Linschoten R, et al. Endoscopic evaluation and treatment of groin pain in the athlete. *Am J Sports Med*. 2004;32:944-949.

148. Diaco JF, Diaco DS, Lockhart L. Sports hernia. *Oper Tech Sports Med*. 2005;13:68-70.

149. Larson CM, Lohnes JH. Surgical management of athletic pubalgia. *Oper Tech Sports Med*. 2002;10:228-232.

150. Nelson EN, Kassarjian A, Palmer WE. MR imaging of sports-related groin pain. *Magn Reson Imaging Clin N Am*. 2005;13: 727-742.

151. Seidenberg PH, Childress MA. Managing hip tendon and nerve injuries in athletes: an understanding of both the hip and neighboring areas helps the diagnosis. *J Musculo Med*. 2005;22: 337-343.

152. Taylor DC, Meyers WC, Moylan JA, et al. Abdominal musculature abnormalities as a cause of groin pain in athletes. *Am J Sports Med*. 1991;19:239-242.

153. Norton-Old KJ, Schache AG, Barker PJ, et al. Anatomical and mechanical relationship between the proximal attachment of adductor longus and the distal rectus sheath. *Clin Anat*. 2013;26:522-530.

154. Omar IM, Zoga AC, Kavanagh EC, et al. Athletic pubalgia and "sports hernia": optimal MR imaging technique and findings. *Radiographics*. 2008;28:1415-1438.

155. Caudill P, Nyland J, Smith C, et al. Sports hernias: a systematic literature review. *Br J Sports Med*. 2008;42:954-964.

156. Joesting DR. Diagnosis and treatment of sportsman's hernia. *Curr Sports Med Rep*. 2002;1:121-124.

157. Meyers WC, Yoo E, Devon ON, et al. Understanding "sports hernia" (athletic pubalgia): the anatomic and pathophysiologic basis for abdominal and groin pain in athletes. *Oper Tech Sports Med*. 2012;20:33-45.

158. Litwin DE, Sneider EB, McEnaney PM. Athletic pubalgia (sports hernia). *Clin Sports Med*. 2011;30:417-434.

159. Lovell G. The diagnosis of chronic groin pain in athletes: a review of 189 cases. *Aust J Sci Med Sport*. 1995;27:76-79.

160. Brown RA, Mascia A, Kinnear DG, et al. An 18-year review of sports groin injuries in the elite hockey player: clinical presentation, new diagnostic imaging, treatment, and results. *Clin J Sport Med*. 2008;18:221-226.

161. O'Connor D. Groin injuries in professional rugby players: a prospective study. *J Sports Sci*. 2004;22:629-636.

162. Orchard J, James T, Alcott E, et al. Injuries in Australian cricket at first class level 1995/1996 to 2000/2001. *Br J Sports Med*. 2002;36:270-274.

163. Robertson BA, Barker PJ, Fahrer M, Schache AG. The anatomy of the pubic region revisited: implications for the pathogenesis and clinical management of chronic groin pain in athletes. *Sports Med*. 2009;39:225-234.

164. Werner J, Hagglund M, Walden M, Ekstrand J. U.E.F.A. injury report: a prospective report of hip and groin injuries in professional football over seven consecutive seasons. *Br J Sports Med*. 2009;43:1036-1040.

165. Albers SL, Spritzer CE, Garrett WE, Meyers WC. MR findings in athletes with pubalgia. *Skeletal Radiol*. 2001;30:270-277.

166. van Veen RN, de Baat P, Heijboer MP. Successful endoscopic treatment of chronic groin pain in athletes. *Surg Endosc*. 2007; 21:189-193.

167. Diesen DL, Pappas TN. Sports hernias. *Adv Surg*. 2007;41: 177-187.

168. Garvey JF. Sports hernia: controversies and skepticism. *Aspetar Sports Med*. 2012;1:67-69.

169. Garvey JF, Hazard H. Sports hernia or groin disruption injury? Chronic athletic groin pain: a retrospective study of 100 patients with long-term follow-up. *Hernia*. 2014;18:815-823.

170. Brophy RH, Backus S, Kraszewski AP, et al. Difference between sexes in lower extremity alignment and muscle activation during soccer kick. *J Bone Joint Surg Am*. 2010;92:2050-2058.

171. Sanborn CF, Jankowski CM. Physiological considerations for women in sports. *Clin Sports Med*. 1994;13:315-327.

172. Boissonnault WG. *Primary Care for the Physical Therapist: Examination and Triage*. 2nd ed. St. Louis: Saunders; 2010.

173. Garvey JF, Read JW, Turner A. Sportsman hernia: what can we do? *Hernia*. 2010;14:17-25.

174. Kachingwe AF, Grech S. Proposed algorithm for the management of athletes with athletic pubalgia (sports hernia): a case series. *J Orthop Sports Phys Ther*. 2008;38:768-781.

175. Biedert RM, Warnke K, Meyer S. Symphysis syndrome in athletes: surgical treatment for chronic lower abdominal, groin and adductor pain in athletes. *Clin J Sport Med*. 2003;13:278-284.

176. Nam A, Brody F. Management and therapy for sports hernia. *J Am Coll Surg*. 2008;206:154-164.

177. Hackney RG. The sports hernia: a cause of chronic groin pain. *Br J Sports Med*. 1993;27:58-62.

178. Morelli V, Espinosa L. Groin injuries and groin pain in athletes. Part 2. *Prim Care Clin Office Pract*. 2005;32:185-200.

179. Norkin CC, White DJ. *Measurement of Joint Motion: A Guide to Goniometry*. 4th ed. Philadelphia: F.A. Davis; 2009.

180. Gonnella C, Paris SV, Kutner M. Reliability in evaluating passive intervertebral motion. *Phys Ther*. 1982;62:436-444.

181. Freburger JK, Riddle DL. Using published evidence to guide the examination of the sacroiliac joint region. *Phys Ther*. 2001;81:1135-1143.

182. Laslett M, Aprill CN, McDonald B, Young SB. Diagnosis of sacroiliac joint pain: validity of individual provocation tests and composites of tests. *Man Ther*. 2005;10:207-218.

183. Laslett M, Williams M. The reliability of selected pain provocation tests for sacroiliac joint pathology. *Spine (Phila Pa 1976)*. 1994;19:1243-1249.

184. Potter NA, Rothstein JM. Intertester reliability for selected clinical tests of the sacroiliac joint. *Phys Ther*. 1985;11:1661-1675.

185. O'Haire C, Gibbons P. Inter-examiner and intra-examiner agreement for assessing sacroiliac anatomical landmarks using palpation and observation: a pilot study. *Man Ther*. 2000;5:13-20.

186. Drew MK, Osmotherly PG, Chiarelli PE. Imaging and clinical tests for the diagnosis of long-standing groin pain in athletes: a systematic review. *Phys Ther Sport*. 2014;15:124-129.

187. Orchard JW, Read JW, Neophyton J, Garlick D. Groin pain associated with ultrasound finding of inguinal canal posterior wall deficiency in Australian rules footballers. *Br J Sport Med*. 1998;32:134-139.

188. Delahunt E, McEntee BL, Kennelly C, et al. Intrarater reliability of the adductor squeeze test in gaelic games athletes. *J Athl Train*. 2011;46:241-245.

189. Nevin F, Delahunt E. Adductor squeeze test values and hip joint range of motion in Gaelic football athletes with long-standing groin pain. *Med Sci Sports Sci*. 2014;17:155-159.

190. Lovell GA, Blanch PD, Barnes CJ. EMG of the hip adductor muscles in six clinical examination tests. *Phys Ther Sport*. 2012;13:134-140.

191. Verrall GM, Slavotinek JP, Barnes PG, Fon GT. Description of pain provocation tests used for the diagnosis of sports-related chronic groin pain: relationship of tests to defined clinical (pain and tenderness) and MRI (pubic bone marrow edema) criteria. *Scand J Med Sci Sports*. 2005;15:36-42.

192. Larson CM. Sports hernia/athletic pubalgia: evaluation and management. *Sports Health*. 2014;6:139-144.

193. Edelman DS, Selesnick H. "Sports" hernia: treatment with biologic mesh. *Surg Endosc*. 2006;20:971-973.

194. Kesek P, Ekberg O, Westlin N. Herniographic findings in athletes with unclear groin pain. *Acta Radiol*. 2002;43:603-608.

195. Polglase AL, Frydman GM, Framer KC. Inguinal surgery for debilitating chronic groin pain in athletes. *Med J Aust*. 1991;155:674-677.

196. Gilmore J. Groin pain in the soccer athlete: fact, fiction and treatment. *Clin Sports Med*. 1998;17:787-793.

197. Akita K, Niga S, Yamato Y, et al. Anatomic basis of chronic groin pain with special reference to sports hernia. *Surg Radiol Anat*. 1999;21:1-5.

198. McSweeney SE, Naraghi A, Salonen D, et al. Hip and groin pain in the professional athlete. *Can Assoc Radiol J*. 2012;63:87-99.

199. Kavanagh EC, Koulouris G, Ford S. MR imaging of groin pain in the athlete. *Sermin Musculoskelet Radiol*. 2006;10:197-207.

200. Zoga AC, Kavanagh EC, Omar IM, et al. Athletic pubalgia and the "sports hernia": MR imaging findings. *Radiology*. 2008;247:797-807.

201. Haider NR, Syed RA, Dermady D. Osteitis pubis: an important pain generator in women with lower pelvis or abdominal pain: a case report and literature review. *Pain Physician*. 2005;8:145-147.

202. Holt MA, Keen JS, Graf BK, Helwig DC. Treatment of osteitis pubis in athletes: results of corticosteroid injections. *Am J Sports Med*. 1995;23:601-605.

203. O'Connell MJ, Powell T, McCaffrey NM, et al. Symphyseal cleft injection in the diagnosis and treatment of osteitis pubis in athletes. *AJR Am J Roentgenol*. 2002;179:955-959.

204. Shin AY, Morin WD, Gorman JD. The superiority of magnetic resonance imaging in differentiating the cause of hip pain in endurance athletes. *Am J Sports Med*. 1996;24:168-176.

205. Ekberg O, Persson NH, Abrahamsson PA, et al. Longstanding groin pain in athletes and multidisciplinary approach. *Sports Med*. 1988;6:56-61.

206. Robinson P, Barron DA, Parsons W, et al. Adductor-related groin pain in athletes: correlation of MR imaging with clinical findings. *Skeletal Radiol*. 2004;33:451-457.

207. Mens J, Inklaar H, Koes BW. A new view on adduction-related groin pain. *Clin J Sport Med*. 2006;16:15-19.

208. Koulouris G. Imaging review of groin pain in elite athletes: an anatomic approach to imaging findings. *AJR Am J Roentgenol*. 2008;191:962-972.

209. Gullmo A. Herniography: the diagnosis of hernia in the groin and incompetence of the pouch of Douglas and pelvic floor. *Acta Radiol Suppl*. 1980;361:1-76.

210. Fon LJ, Spence RA. Sportsman's hernia. *Br J Surg*. 2000;87:545-552.

211. Hagan I. Sonography reveals causes of acute or chronic groin pain: real-time patient contact allows practitioners to localize discomfort, characterize pathology, and perform essential maneuvers. *Diagn Imaging*. 2007;29:33-39.

212. Lacroix VJ, Kinnear DG, Mulder DS. Lower abdominal pain syndrome in National Hockey League players: a report of 11 cases. *Clin J Sport Med*. 1998;8:5-9.

213. Smedberg SG, Broome AE, Gulimo A, Roos H. Herniography in athletes with groin pain. *Am J Surg*. 1985;149:378-382.

214. Gilmore O. Gilmore's groin: ten years experience of groin disruption—a previously unsolved problem in sportsmen. *Sports Med Soft Tissue Trauma*. 1991;3:12-14.

215. Malycha P, Lovell G. Inguinal surgery in athletes with chronic groin pain: "sportsman's" hernia. *Aust NZ J Surg.* 1992;62:123-125.

216. Muschaweck U, Berger LM. Sportsmen's groin–diagnostic approach and treatment with the minimal repair technique: a single-center uncontrolled clinical review. *Sports Health.* 2010;2:216-221.

217. Minnich JM, Hanks JB, Muschaweck U, et al. Diagnosis and treatment highlighting a minimal repair surgical technique. *Am J Sports Med.* 2011;39(6):1341-1349.

218. Meyers WC, Greenleaf R, Saad A. Anatomic basis for evaluation of abdominal and groin pain in athletes. *Oper Tech Sports Med.* 2005;13:55-61.

219. da Rocha RC, Chopard RP. Nutrition pathways to the pubic symphysis pubis. *J Anat.* 2004;204:209-215.

220. Goldring MB, Goldring SR. Articular cartilage and subchondral bone in the pathogenesis of osteoarthritis. *Ann NY Acad Sci.* 2010;119:230-237.

221. Ekstrand J, Ringborg S. Surgery versus conservative treatment in soccer players with chronic groin pain: a prospective randomized study in soccer players. *Eur J Sports Traum Relat Res.* 2001;23:141-145.

222. Unverzagt CA, Schuemann T, Mathisen J. Differential diagnosis of a sports hernia in a high-school athlete. *J Orthop Sports Phys Ther.* 2008;38:63-70.

223. Cibulka MT. The treatment of the sacroiliac joint component to low back pain: a case report. *Phys Ther.* 1992;72:917-922.

224. Cibulka MT, Delitto A. A comparison of two different methods to treat hip pain in runners. *J Orthop Sports Phys Ther.* 1993;17:172-176.

225. Hides JA, Jull GA, Richardson CA. Long-term effects of specific stabilizing exercises for first-episode low back pain. *Spine (Phila Pa 1976).* 2001;26:E243-E248.

226. Hodges PW, Richardson CA. Contraction of the abdominal muscles associated with movement of the lower limb. *Phys Ther.* 1997;77:132-142, discussion 142-144.

227. Hodges PW, Richardson CA. Delayed postural contraction of transversus abdominis in low back pain associated with movement of the lower limb. *J Spinal Disord.* 1998;11:46-56.

228. Sahrmann SA. *Diagnosis and Treatment of Movement Impairment Syndromes.* St. Louis: Mosby; 2002.

229. Watkins RG. Spinal exercise program. In: Watkins RG, ed. *The Spine in Sports.* St. Louis: Mosby; 1996:283-301.

230. Preskitt JT. Sports hernia: the experience of Baylor University Medical Center at Dallas. *Proc (Bayl Univ Med Cent).* 2011;24:89-91.

231. Kumar A, Doran J, Batt ME, et al. Results of inguinal canal repair in athletes with sports hernia. *J R Coll Surg Edinb.* 2002;47:561-565.

6

Hip Osteoarthrosis

MOREY J. KOLBER

CHAPTER OUTLINE

Evidence suggests that hip pain may affect up to 15% of the population at any given time, with trends suggesting a higher prevalence among women, sedentary cohorts, and older populations.[1-3] The underlying cause of musculoskeletal hip pain is multifactorial, ranging from pediatric soft tissue injuries to degenerative sequelae. Of the various diagnoses implicated in the etiology of hip pain, degenerative joint disease has had the greatest economic consequence and is one of the highest contributors to the global disability burden.[4] Clinical recognition and management of degenerative hip disorders require an understanding of risk factors, pathophysiology, differential diagnosis, and intervention options. Accordingly, this chapter presents an overview of epidemiologic risk factors and pathophysiology, as well as the evidence underpinning clinical and imaging-based diagnosis. Both conservative and surgical intervention strategies are discussed within the context of evidence-based practice.

Background

Osteoarthrosis

Osteoarthritis, properly referred to as osteoarthrosis (OA), is the most common type of joint disease worldwide.[5] More than 27 million persons in the United States alone are affected by this condition,[6,7] with speculation that the true prevalence is often underreported. OA represents a heterogeneous cluster of signs and symptoms consisting of histopathologic and radiologic findings that coincide with functional impairments and disability. The condition may be viewed as a degenerative disorder stemming from compromise or biomechanical breakdown of articular cartilage and subchondral bone, with evidence that inflammation, previous trauma, cytokine imbalance, and abnormal biomechanics may serve causative roles.[8-11] Synovial weight-bearing joints are primarily affected with OA; however, other joints such as the carpometacarpal joint of the thumb and acromioclavicular joint of the shoulder are not uncommonly involved among certain subgroups.

The condition of OA has historically been classified into primary and secondary variants,[12-14] although the division is somewhat nebulous. Primary OA is an imprecise type linked to age and an idiopathic (e.g., unknown) etiology. Secondary OA has been characterized as occurring from specific predisposing factors such as prior surgical intervention, trauma, and abnormal biomechanical loading patterns. For example, degenerative changes in a joint that occurs in a younger patient following trauma or as a result of dysplasia would be classified as secondary OA.

Hip Osteoarthrosis

Degenerative OA of the hip joint, also known as coxarthrosis, is one of the more common causes of hip pain among older patients. The International Classification of Diseases ninth revision (ICD-9) diagnosis codes for hip OA include the following: 715.15, osteoarthrosis localized primary; 715.25, osteoarthrosis localized secondary; 715.35, osteoarthrosis localized not specified whether primary or secondary; and 715.95, osteoarthrosis not specified whether generalized or localized. Given the outdated terminology and limited information that can be obtained from ICD-9 codes, the switch to the ICD-10 (tenth revision) system allows for more integration with modern technology. Sample ICD-10 codes for hip OA are noted in Table 6-1.[12]

Pathophysiology

The femoroacetabular joint, hereafter referred to as the hip, is a synovial ball-and-socket joint consisting of articular cartilage, subchondral bone, synovium, and a joint capsule (see Chapter 1 for a detailed review of hip cartilage anatomy). In short, the joint surface comprises articular cartilage, which is an avascular structure composed primarily of chondrocytes surrounded by a matrix that includes proteoglycans, glycos-

TABLE 6-1	International Classification of Diseases Tenth Revision—Codes for Hip Osteoarthrosis (Coxarthrosis)	
Code	**Diagnosis**
M16.1	Primary coxarthrosis, unilateral
M16.0	Primary coxarthrosis, bilateral
M16.2	Coxarthrosis resulting from dysplasia, bilateral
M16.3	Dysplastic coxarthrosis, unilateral
M16.4	Posttraumatic coxarthrosis, bilateral
M16.5	Posttraumatic coxarthrosis, unilateral
M16.7	Secondary coxarthrosis, not otherwise specified

Copyright © World Health Organization.

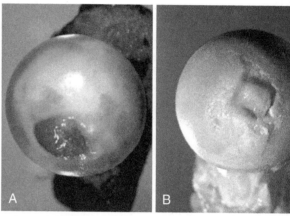

• **Figure 6-1 A,** Healthy femoral head articular cartilage. **B,** Femoral head with degenerative articular cartilage. (From Vardaxis N. *A Textbook of Pathology.* 2nd ed. Melbourne, Australia: Mosby Australia; 2010.)

aminoglycans, and collagen.[15] The articular cartilage protects the underlying subchondral bone by redistributing load and reducing friction at the joint. Healthy articular cartilage (Fig. 6-1, *A*) is sustained under conditions whereby a balance exists between synthesis and degradation. Synovial fluid, which is composed in part of hyaluronate, supplies nutrients to the joint and provides the viscosity needed to absorb loads and reduce friction. See Chapter 1 for a discussion of cartilage zones, matrix, and architecture.

On a pathologic basis, hip OA primarily affects the articular cartilage, subchondral bone, synovial fluid, and joint capsule.[8,9,13,16] Figure 6-2 illustrates the expected changes in cartilage morphology associated with OA and the corresponding histologic grade as established by the Osteoarthritis Research Society International. Independent of the associated inflammation and underlying cause, the condition is essentially the result of a complex series of events.

The earliest change seen in OA is glycosaminoglycan depletion, which leads to a more permeable and hypertrophic matrix.[15] In these early stages, swelling of the cartilage

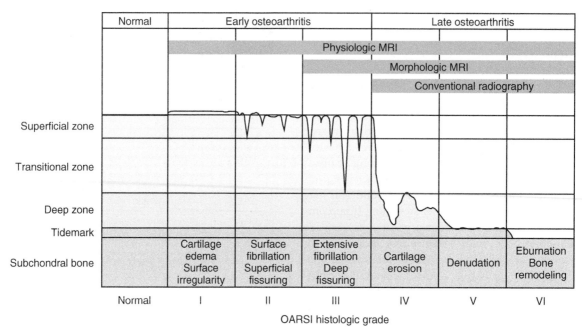

Normal	Early osteoarthritis		Late osteoarthritis		
		Physiologic MRI			
			Morphologic MRI		
			Conventional radiography		

Superficial zone

Transitional zone

Deep zone

Tidemark

Subchondral bone

	Cartilage edema Surface irregularity	Surface fibrillation Superficial fissuring	Extensive fibrillation Deep fissuring	Cartilage erosion	Denudation	Eburnation Bone remodeling
Normal	I	II	III	IV	V	VI

OARSI histologic grade

• **Figure 6-2** Diagram illustrating changes in cartilage morphology that occurs with progression of osteo-arthritis. The Osteoarthritis Research Society International (OARSI) grades are presented. *MRI,* Magnetic resonance imaging. (From Palmer AJ, Brown CP, McNally EG, et al. Non-invasive imaging of cartilage in early osteoarthritis. *Bone Joint J.* 2013;95-B:738-746.)

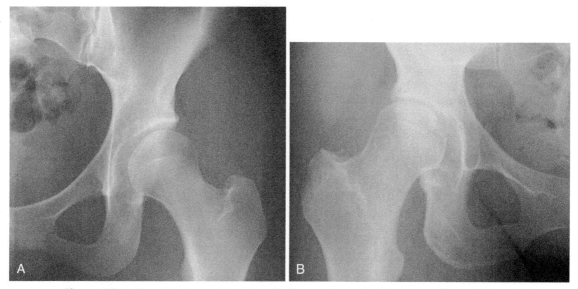

• **Figure 6-3 A,** Normal anteroposterior view. **B,** Decreased superior joint space. (From Clohisy JC, Carlisle JC, Beaulé PE, et al. A systematic approach to the plain radiographic evaluation of the young adult hip. *J Bone Joint Surg Am.* 2008;90[suppl 4]:47-66.)

occurs, usually a result of increased (albeit aberrant) proteo-glycan synthesis (e.g., increased water content), which may be an initial effort by chondrocytes to repair damaged artic-ular cartilage. This stage is often characterized by hypertro-phic repair of the articular cartilage. Although repair is hypertrophic, ensuing changes lead to reduced compressive stiffness and permeability changes.[17] At this stage, changes are radiographically elusive.[15] As the condition progresses, which may take years and may go unnoticed from a symptom perspective, the level of proteoglycans synthesized sharply declines, and the cartilage further loses elasticity.

Although collagen content is still maintained in early stages, organization is haphazard and leads to decreased elasticity and strength.[17] Further, owing to decreased strength and elasticity, the cartilage develops microscopic clefts (fissures) compromising the articular structure's integrity and ability to absorb loads. Over time, a progressive loss of cartilage, referred to as chondropenia, occurs. It is at this stage that changes may be identified on radiographs. Chondropenia results in decreased joint space, often at areas of high load such as the superior joint space (Fig. 6-3). The changes (decreased joint space at areas of high load) seen with OA

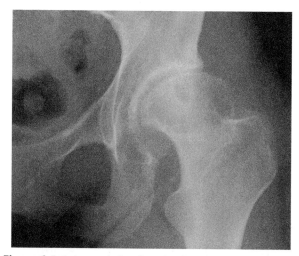

• **Figure 6-4** Anteroposterior view showing severe joint space narrowing, loss of sphericity of femoral head, and cysts in the femoral head and acetabulum. (From Clohisy JC, Carlisle JC, Beaulé PE, et al. A systematic approach to the plain radiographic evaluation of the young adult hip. *J Bone Joint Surg Am.* 2008;90[suppl 4]:47-66.)

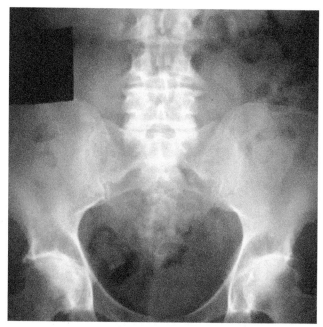

• **Figure 6-5** Bilateral anteroposterior view showing hip osteoarthrosis with the presence of osteophytosis and sclerosis at the weight-bearing regions. (From Swain J, Bush KW. *Diagnostic Imaging for Physical Therapists.* Philadelphia: Saunders; 2009.)

contrast with those of systemic inflammatory arthritides such as rheumatoid arthritis (RA) in which uniform joint space compromise is often seen. Erosion in the joint from a loss of cartilage and joint space occurs until subchondral bone is exposed and irregular (see Fig. 6-1, *B*). During this phase, denudation has occurred. The erosion leads to increased biomechanical stress to the subchondral bone, which responds with a process known as eburnation.[15] Eburnation is a condition whereby exposed subchondral bone undergoes a sclerosing process and hardens, resembling an ivory-like appearance on radiographs. The traumatized subchondral bone often experiences synovial intrusion and undergoes cystic degeneration as well. Subchondral cysts may have a diameter up to 2 cm, although frequently less, and they may be seen at the acetabulum and femoral head (Fig. 6-4). Further, at areas of high stress along the articular margin, vascularization of the subchondral marrow, osseous metaplasia of connective tissue, and ossifying cartilage lead to the outgrowth of irregular new bone in a process referred to as osteophytosis (Fig. 6-5). Fragmentation of these osteophytes may occur, resulting in the presence of loose bodies. Moreover, as degeneration progresses the femoral head may lose normal sphericity (e.g., shape). At some point during the degenerative sequelae, the pathologic changes may lead to pain and adaptive shortening of the soft tissue structures surrounding the joint. Shortening of soft tissues such as the capsule, ligaments, and musculature invariably produces impairments that perpetuate the joint's loss of function and play a vital role in the morbidity associated with hip OA.[12,18,19]

Pain experienced from OA is multifactorial and is presumed to arise from a combination of mechanisms.[8] In particular, vascular congestion of the subchondral bone leads to increased intraosseous pressure and degenerative-type changes in the synovium, which may activate the synovial nociceptors. Additionally, osteophytosis may cause pain from the associated periosteal elevation. Moreover, joint effusion from edema may stretch an already shortened capsule and be a nociceptive source. Similar to other conditions, pain from OA may be chemically induced from injury to neighboring tissue (e.g., bursa or ligament) or coexisting problems such as muscle spasm, central sensitization, and psychological factors. From an impairment perspective, ensuing joint contractures lead to pain, decreased mobility, and stiffness of the joint. Collectively, the aforementioned degenerative changes and associated impairments serve a primary role in the disability burden associated with hip OA.

Epidemiology

Prevalence and Demographic Risk Factors

More than 27 million[6,7] persons in the United States were reported to be clinically diagnosed with OA in 2005. It has been estimated that by 2030 the prevalence is expected to exceed 67 million.[20] Internationally, OA is the most common articular disease, and as in the United States its reported prevalence is influenced by how the condition is defined, as well as by those seeking care. Prevalence studies have focused primarily on radiographic disease as inclusion criteria because it is easier to define than clinical presentation. On the basis of radiologic findings alone, 80% to 90% of persons older than 65 years of age have OA.[20-22] The prevalence and incidence of OA are generally higher among women than men.[23,24] The hip ranks second among large

• BOX 6-1 Hip Osteoarthrosis: Epidemiologic and Demographic Risk Factors

Approximately one in four persons is affected by symptomatic hip OA.

Hip pain reports attributable to OA rise with advancing age.

The hip joint ranks second among large joints in body affected by OA.

Combined hip and knee OA is the eleventh highest contributor to global disability.

Women are more likely than men to be affected after the fifth decade.

Lifetime hip replacement risk is 7% for men and 12% for women.

OA, Osteoarthrosis.

joints in the body affected by OA, trailing the knee, which has the highest prevalence.[4,25] Box 6-1 presents an overview of prevalence and demographic risk factors associated with hip OA.

In regard to the hip, evidence suggests that the estimated lifetime prevalence of symptomatic OA is approximately 25%; thus, one in four persons will be affected by this condition.[6] In terms of race, hip OA seems to have no consistently reported differences.[26] As stated previously, gender differences exist, with women more likely than men to develop symptomatic hip OA.[6,23] These differences are more evident after the fifth decade of life.[23] Moreover, evidence suggests that the lifetime risk of receiving a total joint replacement for hip OA is approximately 7% for men and 12% for women.[27] The economic burden of hip OA is difficult to capture because no current population-level estimates of both indirect and direct costs are available. Although reports on the total economic burden attributable to OA do not exist, reports do indicate that direct costs attributable to hospitalization for hip replacement in the United States for 2009 were approximately $13.7 billion.[28] When combined, OA of the hip and OA of the knee rank as the eleventh highest contributors to global disability and the thirty-eighth highest in disability-adjusted life-years (measure expressed as number of years lost as a result of poor health, disability, or premature death).[4]

Unlike secondary hip OA, which has recognizable risk factors, the etiology of primary (idiopathic) OA may be elusive. Risk factors, particularly those that are modifiable, are of particular interest in reducing new incidence, in steering prevention efforts, and for attenuating disease progression. With advancing age, the incidence of hip OA rises, with most obvious increases occurring at 50 years of age and leveling off or declining by 80 years of age.[23,29] Reports of pain related to hip OA also increase with age,[26] an association that may be attributable to progression of the condition, as well as ensuing impairments and functional decline. Although age is associated with OA, age alone is not a sufficiently conclusive risk factor, nor is it a modifiable risk factor. Several genes have been directly associated with OA,

thus leading to a genetic-hereditary association. Genes in bone morphogenic protein and wingless-type signaling cascades have been implicated in the etiology of OA. Moreover, genetic factors are also important in certain hereditable developmental defects and skeletal anomalies that can cause congenital joint misalignment. Trauma or surgical procedures involving the articular cartilage or supporting structures may lead to abnormal biomechanics and cytokine imbalance, which could incite or accelerate the degenerative process. Unlike direct trauma, occupational or lifestyle factors may expose the hip to degenerative changes through a microtraumatic effect.

Risk Associated With Previous Injury

Undue loading of a previously injured joint (intraarticular) may predispose the region to degeneration as excessive forces accelerate the catabolic effects of the chondrocytes and further disrupt the cartilaginous matrix. Previous injury to the hip is a clear risk factor for OA with an odds ratio of 5.0.[30,31] Essentially, patients with a previous injury to the hip are five times more likely to develop OA when compared with persons without prior injury or trauma. In many cases, a previous injury creates changes to the articular surface, as well as biomechanical impairments that lead to an abnormal loading environment.

Modifiable Risk Factors

In regard to physical activity, evidence suggests a variable association with OA. Leisure time physical activities such as walking and cycling have been associated with a lower risk of hip replacement when compared with sedentary activity levels.[32] Overall, recreational sport participation has a low risk.[30] However, high exposure to competitive or elite sporting activity before the age of 50 years has been associated with a greater risk for hip OA.[33] Unlike recreational participation, high-impact sports such as American football, track and field, and racket sports appear to increase the risk for hip OA.[33,34] The risk among athletes is more evident among those participating at an elite level, with an odds ratio of 1.6 to 2.5.[34]

Activities such as recreational running may have a protective effect in part because of an association with reduced body mass. Most investigations have not identified an increased risk of OA in runners; however, mixed evidence exists as related to running pace and mileage.[35-37] Some evidence suggests an increased risk of hip OA among runners, particularly as related to pace, mileage, or previous injury; whereas a large cohort study reported contrasting findings (e.g., running posed no risk for hip OA). In fact, one study found that those who ran at a higher energy expenditure had a decreased risk when compared with those who exercised at a metabolic equivalent (MET) of less than 1.8 hour/day. Recognizing that 1 MET is essentially the energy cost of sitting quietly, one may interpret the aforementioned MET of less than 1.8 hour/day as that of runners who were deconditioned and possessed other inherent risks. Nevertheless, in the same study, walking in lieu of running did not decrease OA risk.[37] The investigators postulated that running has a protective effect, particularly because it attenuates weight gain, which is a known risk factor for hip OA. Given the association of running with a lower body mass index (BMI), it appears that recreational participation does not increase one's risk for hip OA and may in fact reduce one's risk profile.

Occupational activity that involves heavy lifting, squatting, climbing stairs, and long-term exposure to standing have been associated with hip OA.[31,38] Heavy versus light workloads, in particular, place persons at a three times higher risk for developing hip OA.[39] Frequent or compulsory stair climbing has a reported odds ratio of 12.5.[40] Moreover, a cross-sectional survey found that persons exposed to lifting, stooping, and vibration tools have an increased risk for hip OA.[41] Evidence suggests that lifting burdens must be at least 10 kg (22 pounds), with performance for more than 10 years, to be related to hip OA.[38] It seems logical that evidence-based recommendations for exercise among healthy persons should favor recreational running over squatting or stair climbing. Moreover, while occupational hazards could be recognized, one's choice of occupation may itself be a risk factor.

Numerous studies have identified BMI and obesity as risk factors for hip OA, with odds ratios ranging from 1.6 to 15.4.[31,42] Obesity (BMI ≥30 kg/m^2) was associated with a higher prevalence of hip OA in a sample of 1157 Australians, with an adjusted odds ratio of 2.18.[42] Of those patients with hip OA in the aforementioned study, obesity was associated with higher levels of pain, increased stiffness, decreased function, and reduced quality of life. A more recent metaanalysis reported that a 5-unit increase in BMI (e.g., 32 to 37 kg/m^2) was associated with an 11% increase risk of hip OA.[43] In addition to mechanical effects, obesity may be an inflammatory risk factor for OA because of its link with increased levels of adipokines, which may promote joint inflammation. Evidence does exist to support a relationship between obesity and risk of total hip replacement. In a study of 568 women who had reported receiving a hip replacement, those with a BMI of 35 kg/m^2 or more had a relative risk of 2.6 compared with a reference population.[44] Although it is clear that an association exists, patients with OA often adopt more sedentary lifestyles than reference populations, thus subsequently leading to increases in BMI and a perpetuation of risk.

Structural Morphology

Undue loading of a developmentally dysplastic joint may predispose the region to degeneration as excessive forces accelerate the catabolic effects of the chondrocytes and further disrupt the cartilaginous matrix. Developmental disorders such as dysplasia, congenital hip dislocation, Legg-Calvé-Perthes disease, and slipped capital femoral epiphysis have been associated with OA.[45] Chapter 7 pres-

ents a detailed discussion of the aforementioned developmental disorders.

In regard to morphology, it has been suggested that femoral acetabular impingement and lower extremity length inequality may be associated with or may increase the risk of hip OA.[46] Investigators have reported that patients with lower extremity length inequality are more likely to have hip OA, although the association is weak (adjusted odds ratio of 1.20), and it is not significantly associated with radiographic progression.[47,48] With regard to the side of involvement, OA is more common when the contralateral leg is longer than when it is shorter (e.g., right hip OA would be more common when the left leg is longer).[48] When considering the relevance of limb inequality, it should be recognized that hip OA itself may cause leg-length discrepancy, and a shortened leg may simply be the result of joint space narrowing or protrusio acetabuli (e.g., medial protrusion of the femoral head into the acetabulum), as opposed to structural length change. Independent of radiographic changes, patients with lower extremity length inequality are more likely to have hip pain, aching, and stiffness than those with symmetrical lower extremity length.[49] Although the prevalence of radiographic hip OA and symptoms seems to be higher among patients with limb-length inequality, the association is weak. Moreover, having limb-length inequality is not predictive of radiographic or symptom progression.

Femoral acetabular impingement is an established risk factor for early hip OA and joint replacement.[50-55] Mechanisms for impingement of the femoral head or neck on the acetabulum include the following: the *cam variant* (nonspherical femoral head); the *pincer variant,* which is essentially acetabular overcoverage; and a *mixed cam-pincer variant.* The cam-type morphology occurs more frequently in younger patients and is thought to cause a delaminating injury to the cartilage of the acetabulum (e.g., cartilage is sheared off bone). The pincer variant lends to labral impingement, which results in labral tears, degeneration, and ossification. Evidence suggests that patients undergoing hip arthroplasty have a high incidence of radiographic abnormalities consistent with impingement; however, early surgical intervention (see the later section on surgical treatment) is associated with good outcomes.[51,53,54] Notably, in one investigation, 80% of patients who had undergone a surgical correction procedure were able to decelerate worsening of OA and did not progress to a joint replacement operation.[53] Although outcomes are generally good, they depend on the degree of degeneration in patients with concurrent hip OA-impingement.[56] Chapter 4 presents a detailed discussion of femoral acetabular impingement and labral tears.

Summary of Risk Factors

Numerous risk factors have been associated with hip OA (see Box 6-1; Table 6-2 and Box 6-2). They include, but are not limited to, age, gender, obesity, trauma, genetics, occupational hazards, infection, congenital factors, and earlier

TABLE 6-2	Risk Factors Associated With Hip Osteoarthrosis	
Modifiable Risk Factors	**Structural or Congenital Risk Factors**	
Compulsory occupational stooping and squatting	Hip dysplasia	
Frequent stair climbing or vibration tool exposure	Legg-Calvé-Perthes disease	
Long-term exposure to heavy lifting and standing	Slipped capital femoral epiphysis	
Elite-level high-impact sport participation	Chondral defects	
Obesity or high body mass index ≥30	Femoral acetabular impingement	

TABLE 6-3	Diagnostic Utility of Pain Patterns for Hip Osteoarthrosis	
Pain Location	**Sensitivity (%)**	**Specificity (%)**
Groin	84.3	70.3
Buttock	76.4	61.1
Anterior thigh	58.8	25.9
Posterior thigh	43.7	59.9
Anterior knee	68.6	48.1
Posterior knee	50.9	44.4
Anterior leg (shin)	47.0	35.2
Posterior leg (calf)	29.4	40.7

From Khan AM, McLoughlin E, Giannakas K, et al. Hip osteoarthritis: where is the pain? *Ann R Coll Surg Engl.* 2004;86:119-121.

• BOX 6-2 Recreational and Sport Participation: Risk Association for Hip Osteoarthrosis

Sports such as American football, track and field, and racket sports may increase risk.
Frequent stair climbing may increase risk.
Recreational running does not increase risk.
Walking in lieu of running does not decrease risk.
Leisure cycling or walking does not increase risk.

• BOX 6-3 Symptoms Commonly Reported by Patients With Hip Osteoarthrosis

Gradual onset
Somatic pain often present in groin, buttock, or lateral hip
Pain with squatting, prolonged standing, side sleeping, and stair climbing
Morning stiffness lasting up to 60 minutes
Audible sounds

---

surgical interventions. Early identification of modifiable risk factors may serve as the basis for preventive programs aimed at decelerating disease progression and associated symptoms. At a minimum, habitual physical conditioning,[57] efforts to prevent obesity, and modification of occupational hazards are likely to have a positive effect on the presence of pain and physical function. Although age and developmental disorders such as dysplasia are not modifiable risk factors, improving the biomechanical environment by avoidance of aberrant loading while maintaining a reasonable level of physical activity may reduce the risk of developing OA. Furthermore, given the known risk association from earlier trauma or surgical procedures, it seems reasonable for future research to direct efforts toward surgical interventions that recreate the native joint anatomy and posttraumatic rehabilitation efforts to mitigate biomechanical abnormalities.

Clinical Presentation

The diagnosis of hip OA can be made with a reasonable degree of certainty based on the physical examination alone, although radiographic findings constitute the visual reference standard. Patients with hip OA have a characteristic history (Box 6-3) and clinical examination findings that,

combined with the presence of radiographic evidence, provide a definitive diagnosis. In the absence of diagnostic imaging, evidence-based clinical guidelines exist to help steer the diagnostic process.

History and Demographics

Patients with symptomatic hip OA are typically older than 50 years of age, although age alone is not a definitive diagnostic criteria.[58] In a majority of cases, the onset is gradual, and progression is characteristically slow, with a noticeable decline in activity that coincides with advancing age. Patients with hip OA typically report ipsilateral pain in the groin (often described as a deep ache), lateral trochanteric, or buttock regions.[59-62] Although pain location may vary as a result of different stages or periarticular adaptations, groin pain in particular possesses a degree of diagnostic utility for identifying hip OA, with a sensitivity of 0.84 and specificity of 0.70.[60] Thus, one may interpret these results as indicating that only approximately 16% of patients with hip OA will not report groin pain.[60] Pain patterns arising from hip OA are somatic, and pain may be referred to the anterior thigh and knee and in some cases below the knee (Table 6-3).[59,60] Investigators have postulated that referred patterns are potentially derived from the femoral, obturator, and saphenous branch of the femoral nerve.[60,63] Although evidence exists to suggest that patients with hip OA may have pain below the knee, it would seem logical that other conditions known for having similar pain referrals (e.g., advanced lumbar degeneration or diskogenic disorders) may coexist and thus should be included in the differential diagnosis. For example, shin (anterior leg) or calf pain, when present in patients with hip pain, has a specificity of 0.35 and 0.41, respectively, for a diagnosis of hip OA.[60] Based on this information, one could surmise that in approximately 60% of cases, leg pain (e.g., shin or calf) when present, is not necessarily referred from hip OA. When a radicular pattern is present or pain is referred below the knee, concurrent lumbar disorders or alternate diagnoses should be considered (see Chapter 10 for the differential diagnosis of hip pain).

Symptom exacerbation and functional limitations with weight-bearing activities such as squatting, walking, lifting heavy objects (because of additional loading and the mechanics of lifting), and stair climbing are common. Moreover, interrupted sleep is often reported among participants with hip OA.[64] In one study, 88% of patients with hip OA reported interrupted sleep, and the primary reason for their sleep disturbance was pain.[64] Sleeping in a supine position with legs elevated may be preferred, as opposed to side lying, which may exacerbate symptoms. Audible sounds referred to as crepitus may coexist with pain. Over time, crepitus progresses to a grating sound that coincides with joint erosion and changes in synovial viscosity. Stiffness after prolonged rest and morning stiffness lasting less than an hour may be reported. In the early stages, patients often report relief with analgesics and possibly thermal modalities such as heat.

Patients may report that weather conditions such as an impending storm influence their symptoms. These claims are supported by a small body of research showing that pain increases with changes or fluctuations in barometric pressure and relative humidity.[65,66] One common theory for these claims resides in barometric pressure. Essentially, a drop in barometric pressure precedes a storm, and when barometric pressure decreases, it allows joints to swell. This physiologic change can be observed with lower extremity swelling (feet and ankles) when sitting on a long airplane flight. Although cabins are pressurized, a pressure difference from sea level remains. Most would agree that sitting for a comparable time at a desk would not produce swelling as seen on an airplane flight. Conversely, if there is an increase in barometric pressure it would reduce the potential for swelling. Another plausible mechanism for this change in pain, albeit small, resides in the potential for atmospheric pressure–induced swelling to affect hip stability inversely.[67] Although barometric pressure and relative humidity have been shown to increase pain, the scientific basis for these changes is vague, and pain increases have equated to as low as 1%, which is clinically insignificant.[66] Perhaps additional factors contribute to these symptoms, such as a propensity to adopt a sedentary activity level during inclement weather.

Physical Examination

The physical examination often identifies gait abnormalities, a loss of hip mobility, and characteristic weakness. Gait abnormalities often result from the combined influence of pain, loss of mobility, and weakness. These impairments often manifest in a shortened stance and stride phase, decreased velocity, and reduced hip excursion, among other deviations.[68,69] Furthermore, because evidence suggests that patients with lower limb OA are at a higher risk for falls, an assessment of fall risk may be indicated.[70]

Mobility and Muscle Performance

Investigators have proposed that patients with hip OA would have a characteristic loss of mobility, with internal rotation (IR) range of motion being most limited, followed by flexion, and then abduction, referred to as a capsular pattern. Studies investigating capsular patterns of the hip have emerged to support that IR is most limited and painful; however, these studies failed to support a proportional loss of mobility that would define patients with OA.[71-74] Research does implicate a global loss of mobility among patients with radiographically confirmed hip OA, with the severity of degeneration dictating the number of restricted movement planes, as well as the degree of movement loss.[74] The specificity of a hip IR mobility loss among patients with moderate to severe OA ranges from 0.42 to 0.54, with sensitivity ranging from 0.86 to 1.0.[75] Moreover, one study compared passive range of motion among patients with hip OA with a matched asymptomatic cohort.[19] The study reported significantly less mobility in the OA group, with mean group differences of 16 degrees for IR, 18 degrees for flexion, 10 degrees for extension, and 21 degrees for external rotation.[19]

Hip OA is often associated with changes in muscle performance, size, and composition. Although variability exists among research reports, it is clear that a significant proportion of patients with hip OA will develop selective atrophy of type II muscle fibers and weakness of the hip flexors, abductors, external rotators, and adductors.[76,77] Furthermore, evidence suggests that patients with hip OA may have atrophy and weakness of the knee extensors (quadriceps), knee flexors, hip flexors, hip extensors, hip adductors, and hip abductors when compared with healthy adults without OA.[76,78,79] Although hip range of motion and muscle performance measurements are standard orthopedic assessment tools, it should be recognized that the reproducibility of these assessments may have shortcomings because weighted Kappa values (degree of interrater agreement) range from 0.52 to 0.65 (0 is chance and 1 is perfect agreement) between orthopedic and chiropractic physicians, respectively.[80] Intraclass correlation coefficient (ICC) values of 0.54 to 0.88 have been reported for physical therapists and suggest moderate to good reproducibility.[73] Efforts to standardize procedures are recommended, given the range of findings among various clinical professions and the potential for disagreement. Moreover, decreased mobility and motor weakness may be the results of activity decline or discomfort and not solely direct reflections of degenerative changes.

Functional Assessment

Functional activity assessment is an instrumental component of the hip examination. The Osteoarthritis Research Society International recommends, based on multiple-attribute consensus and global activity themes, the timed up-and-go, 30-second chair stand, 4×10 m fast-paced walk, and the 6-minute walk tests as independent measures of function to be assessed when evaluating a patient with hip OA.[81] The timed up-and-go test is common to clinical practice, requires minimal space and time, and assesses multiple activities including walking, turning, and sit-to-stand transitions, whereas the 6-minute walk test may have feasibility issues given the time allotment. Evidence suggests that patients with hip OA have a 34% slower time on the timed up-and-go test and walk 28% less distance on the 6-minute walk test when compared with healthy persons without hip OA.[76] Additional outcome instruments are available to assess multiple dimensions of pain, function, and disability among patients with hip OA. Instruments such as the Western Ontario and McMaster Universities Osteoarthritis Index (WOMAC), the Lower Extremity Functional Scale (LEFS), and the Harris Hip Score (HHS) have been validated among patients with hip OA and offer insight into patients' perceived functional limitations, as well as other attributes. The WOMAC is a self-administered 24-item index that can be used for hip or knee OA and measures 3 dimensions that include pain, stiffness, and disability. The WOMAC is available in more than 100 language forms and has been found to possess good test-retest reliability, with ICC values ranging between 0.77 and 0.94 for patients with hip OA.[82,83] The LEFS is a 20-item regional instrument that measures perceived function in the lower extremity and has been reported to have an ICC of 0.92 among community-dwelling patients with hip OA.[83] The HHS was developed primarily for the postoperative population; thus, it is often used following operations such as hip arthroplasty. The HHS has a self-administered portion, as well as sections on range of motion and the presence of structural abnormalities such as leg-length discrepancy and fixed positional deformities. The administrative burden of the HHS is greater than that of the WOMAC and LEFS; however, the HHS has the benefit of assessing clinician-measured impairments such as range of motion and positional faults.

Special Tests

Individualized clinical tests have been described to assist with the differential diagnosis of hip pain; however, a paucity of evidence exists to support the disease-specific validity of these tests for OA (see Chapter 2 for a detailed summary of examination tests). The flexion abduction external rotation (FABER) and scour tests are two of the more commonly used tests for identifying intraarticular disorders.[73,84] They may therefore be useful as adjuncts to

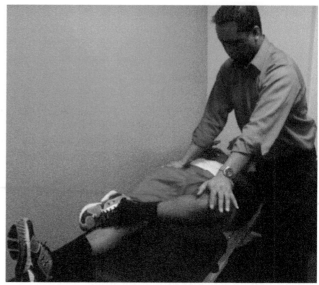

• **Figure 6-6** Flexion Abduction External Rotation (FABER)–Patrick Test. The clinician places affected hip in the abducted externally rotated position in that the lateral ankle rests on the anterior leg of the unaffected side. Once in position the examiner passively lowers the knee toward the floor. A positive response would be concordant pain or reduced mobility compared with either the unaffected side or an angle less than 60 degrees from a vertical axis.

the clinical examination when OA is suspected. The FABER test, also known as the Patrick test, involves placing the lateral malleolus of the affected lower extremity on the knee or leg of the opposite extremity while the examiner passively lowers the knee to the floor (Fig. 6-6). This test among a small cohort of patients with hip OA had a sensitivity of 0.57 and specificity of 0.71 when compared with radiographic findings.[73] The authors of the aforementioned study defined a positive test result as pain reproduction and a measureable mobility impairment based on an angle of less than 60 degrees from a vertical axis.

The scour test generally involves placing the affected hip into approximately 90 degrees of flexion, adduction, and IR (toward the opposite shoulder) with an axial load applied, followed by abduction and external rotation while slightly increasing flexion and maintaining an axial load (Fig. 6-7). Some variations of the test exist; however, the general principle is to load the hip joint while moving it in a manner that resembles a circular arc of motion. Pain in the lateral hip or groin constitutes a positive test result. The presence of crepitus or grating may also be noted and offers insight into the degenerative nature of hip OA. The sensitivity and specificity of this test have been reported at 0.62 and 0.75, respectively, when compared with radiographic findings.[73]

Diagnostic Imaging

The diagnosis of hip OA is typically based on both the physical examination and the radiographic presentation. Radiographs are the most economical imaging test available in regard to time and cost when compared with other

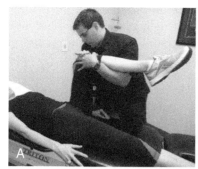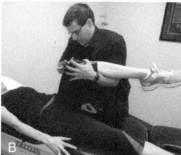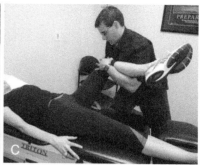

• **Figure 6-7** Scour Test. **A,** Start position requires flexion of hip to 90 degrees while applying an axial load. **B,** Add adduction and internal rotation (toward the opposite shoulder) while maintaining axial load. **C,** Move the hip in a circular arc from internal rotation and adduction to abduction and external rotation while maintaining an axial load. Pain in the lateral hip or groin constitutes a positive test result.

imaging modalities, and they serve as a first-order study. Standard radiographic views include an anteroposterior (AP) view (see Figs. 6-3 to 6-5) and a lateral view, referred to as a frog view, which closely resembles the FABER test position, as well as various specialty views (see Appendix C for radiographic views and interpretation). The radiographic findings in most cases are visible on the areas of the hip prone to load and are sensitive to moderate to advanced arthritic changes. Although multiple views may be used to improve identification and monitor structural changes, a standard AP radiograph offers considerable diagnostic utility.[29,58,85] Some practitioners prefer a weight-bearing view to accentuate joint space narrowing, but a consensus has determined that the value of a weight-bearing view lies in monitoring disease progression in patients with established OA,[29] thus it is not a strict requirement for diagnosis. It is not uncommon for radiographic findings to be bilateral in primary OA, whereas unilateral findings may be confined to individual hips with previous trauma or dysplasia. Radiographic findings suggestive of OA include joint space narrowing and sclerosis, osteophytosis, cyst formation, abnormal bone contour, and protrusio acetabuli (see Figs. 6-3 to 6-5).[58,85] Evidence suggests that joint space narrowing alone is a sufficient predictor of hip OA.[86]

The Croft grading scale is commonly used to identify minimum joint space on a weight-bearing AP view,[86] with measurements obtained from the closest point of the femoral head to the acetabular ridge. The normal superior joint space, supine or standing, is generally greater than 2.5 mm,[86,87] which is considered a grade 0 according to the Croft criteria, and a change of 0.5 mm or more represents a pathologically relevant reduction in joint space. In cases of severe OA (Croft grade 2), the joint space is decreased to a width of 1.5 mm or less.[86]

The Kellgren-Lawrence grading scale is a commonly accepted and reliable radiographic criteria for classifying degenerative changes associated with hip OA (Table 6-4), and its reliability and predictive validity exceed that of measuring minimal joint space width alone.[85,86] The scale consists of five grades and evaluates the presence of joint space narrowing, sclerosis, cysts, osteophytosis, and femoral head

TABLE 6-4	Kellgren-Lawrence Grading Scale for Hip Osteoarthrosis
Grade	**Radiographic Identifiers**
0 (None)	Normal: no evidence of joint space narrowing, osteophytes or sclerosis
1 (Doubtful)	Subtle narrowing of medial joint space and possible osteophytes around femoral head
2 (Minimal)	Definite narrowing of joint space with osteophytes and slight sclerosis
3 (Moderate)	Marked narrowing of joint space, slight osteophytes, sclerosis, cyst formation, and deformity of femoral head and acetabulum
4 (Severe)	Gross loss of joint space with sclerosis and cysts, marked deformity of femoral head and acetabulum, large osteophytes

From Kellgren J, Lawrence J. Radiological assessment of osteoarthrosis. *Ann Rheum Dis.* 1957;16:494-502.

contour (sphericity) (Fig. 6-8). Kellgren-Lawrence grades of 2 or greater are more accurately predictive of a future joint replacement than are other radiographic classification systems or individual criteria for hip OA.[87]

In cases of early hip OA, structural changes are often radiographically elusive, and more advanced imaging techniques may be indicated should the symptoms warrant. Figure 6-2 presents an overview of imaging modalities used for the detection of OA at various stages of degeneration. Magnetic resonance imaging (MRI) is the preferred modality for diagnosing avascular necrosis, osteomyelitis, neoplasm, and radiographically occult fractures. In regard to hip OA, MRI can detect similar findings identified on radiographs and can also depict soft tissue changes and provide a more definitive visualization of the articular cartilage (especially in the sagittal plane) and periarticular soft tissue.[88] Moreover, radiographs have a relatively low sensitivity (0.44) for identifying the presence of subchondral

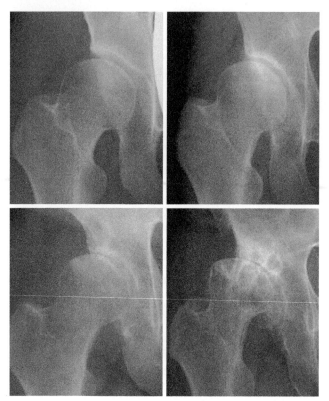

• **Figure 6-8** Kellgren-Lawrence Grading Criteria for Hip Osteoarthrosis (OA) With Grades 1 to 4 Illustrated. Grade 0 to 1, none or doubtful signs of OA *(top left);* grade 2, mild OA with mild joint space narrowing and sclerosis *(top right);* grade 3, marked narrowing of joint space and sclerosis *(bottom left);* and grade 4, gross loss of joint space with sclerosis and cysts, marked deformity of femoral head (loss of sphericity) and acetabulum, and osteophytosis *(bottom right).* (From Fugii M, Nakashima Y, Noguchi Y, et al. Effect of intra-articular lesions on the outcome of periacetabular osteotomy in patients with symptomatic hip dysplasia. *J Bone Joint Surg Br.* 2011;93:1449-1456.)

cysts when compared with MRI.[89] If OA is to be detected at its early stage to allow preemptive interventions, then MRI would seem to be the modality of choice. From a clinical perspective, advanced imaging such as MRI is not a required element for diagnosing hip OA and is often reserved for differential diagnosis and for the identification of disorders amenable to surgical repair.

Computed tomography and diagnostic ultrasound have limited roles outside of what is visualized on radiographs and MRI. Ultrasound does not have an established role in the diagnosis of hip OA, although it may be used to monitor changes in articular cartilage. Additionally, ultrasound may offer a role in guided hip injections and aspiration. Scintigraphy (bone scan) is used to identify increased localization of an injected radionucleotide to areas of subchondral remodeling and synovitis.[29] Scintigraphy may help differentiate OA from bone metastasis, systemic conditions, and osteomyelitis; however, it does not have a routine role in identifying hip OA. Arthrocentesis, the aspiration of joint fluid from the hip, is reserved for differential diagnosis and may help distinguish OA from other causes of joint pain.

Anesthetic hip injection may be used as a diagnostic tool based on the premise that pain relief following injection suggests an intraarticular disorder. In regard to the diagnostic utility of anesthetic hip injections, a metaanalysis evaluated the results of numerous case series designs and reported a sensitivity and specificity of 0.97 and 0.91, respectively.[90] Despite apparent face validity and diagnostic accuracy of case series designs, high-quality studies to support the validity of anesthetic hip injections for identifying hip OA are lacking.[90]

Differential Diagnosis

The etiology of hip pain is multifactorial, and diagnosis largely depends on collaborative information from the history, physical examination, and diagnostic imaging, as well as patients' demographics and risk factors. Numerous conditions of the hip, including inflammatory arthritides, metabolic disease, neoplasm, and osteonecrosis, as well as the neighboring spine and sacroiliac joint, may be implicated in the etiology of hip pain (see Chapter 10 for an overview of the differential diagnosis of hip pain). Clinicians should consider conditions other than hip OA when the history, physical examination, and imaging findings are not consistent with current diagnostic criteria for OA. Furthermore, when patients are recalcitrant to interventions deemed efficacious for hip OA and have limited imaging findings, an alternate diagnosis should be considered. Advanced imaging, arthrocentesis (e.g., joint aspiration), and laboratory testing serve as useful adjuncts to the examination and may provide critical information for the differential diagnosis. Inflammatory arthritides, metabolic conditions, intraarticular disorders (e.g., femoral acetabular impingement), and metastatic cancer may be responsible for hip pain and masquerade as OA in the presence of degenerative findings. When considering the differential diagnosis, clinicians should be aware of specific features that distinguish these conditions from OA.

RA is characterized by prolonged morning stiffness often lasting longer than 1 hour, unlike OA, in which the duration of morning stiffness is typically shorter. Additionally, OA of the hip is characterized by osteophytosis, in contrast to RA, which is characterized by bone erosion and the absence of osteophytosis. An additional characteristic of RA is the presence of multiple joint involvement and systemic manifestations of the disease. The metacarpophalangeal (MCP) joints of the hand as well as the wrists are often symmetrically involved in RA. This involvement contrasts with OA, which may have a unilateral presentation and rarely involves the wrist and MCP joints. Although no clear laboratory values are specifically associated with hip OA, RA is characterized by increased erythrocyte sedimentation rate (ESR), C-reactive protein (CRP), and the cyclic citrullinated peptide (CCP) antibody test, along with a positive serum rheumatoid factor. Spondyloarthropathies, characterized by their predilection for the spine, may affect the peripheral joints and be a source of hip pain. Historical variables such as interrupted sleep and reduced symptoms with activity, as well as age demographics (younger age), distinguish spondyloarthropathies from OA. Additionally, laboratory tests such as elevated ESR and CRP may be present along with a positive human leukocyte antigen B27 (HLA-B27), all of which would most likely be unremarkable in the diagnosis of OA. Metabolic conditions such as gout or pseudogout may be responsible for hip pain and would be characterized by periodic episodes of acute pain, as well as elevated uric acid levels. Additionally, radiographic imaging of gout may show a radiopaque appearance of tophi at the joint.

Metastatic or primary cancer (e.g., chondrosarcoma) of the hip may be responsible for a patient's complains of hip or pelvic pain. Factors to consider include a previous history of cancer at a region known for metastatic dissemination to bone (e.g., prostate), as well as nocturnal pain unrelieved by positioning. Neoplasms typically present as radiographic lytic or blastic changes; aggressive lesions are characterized by irregular borders and often remain on one side of the joint, unlike OA, which crosses joint spaces.

Osteonecrosis, also known as avascular necrosis, is characterized by hip pain and in the early stages may not be evident on standard radiographs. Moreover, osteonecrosis may coexist with hip OA. Early changes consistent with femoral avascular necrosis would be present on advanced imaging such as MRI, whereas latter stages are radiographically evident in regard to altered morphology of the femoral head. A history of corticosteroid use may be present; however, this is a weak diagnostic variable independent of other findings. A previous fracture of the femoral neck may be viewed as a risk factor for avascular necrosis, which often prompts the use of joint replacement in lieu of surgical hardware fixation.

Diagnosis

A structural diagnosis of hip OA is often based on imaging findings, with radiographs as the reference standard.[29,86,88] Although radiographs provide a structural dimension of the pathologic features, abnormal findings are often present among asymptomatic persons. Moreover, early-stage OA may be radiographically elusive in symptomatic patients, thus lending importance to the physical examination. Advanced imaging modalities may be used as adjuncts to diagnosis but typically are reserved for patients with suspected surgical disease or those requiring differential diagnosis.[88] Specific laboratory values offer utility for differential diagnosis only because no specific markers have been commonly associated with OA from a universally accepted perspective. A definitive diagnosis of hip OA is inclusive of both history and physical examination as well as imaging findings, with laboratory results used as adjuncts to the differential diagnosis where applicable.

The American College of Rheumatology (ACR) identified criteria, based on testing clusters, that may be used for classifying patients with hip pain into a diagnosis of OA.[58] Specifically, criteria from the history, physical examination, laboratory results, and radiographic findings were used to develop testing clusters that may aid clinical decision making. According to the ACR criteria (Fig. 6-9), patients with hip pain would be classified as having OA if they met

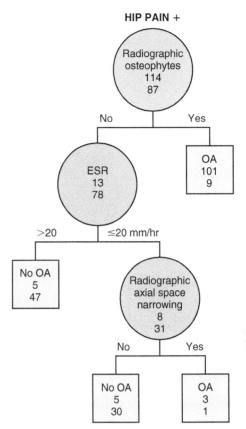

• **Figure 6-9** American College of Rheumatology Criteria Using Combined Clinical and Radiographic Criteria. Numbers within *circles* and *boxes* indicate patients in the study with osteoarthrosis (OA) versus those from the control group *(bottom numbers)*. *ESR,* Erythrocyte sedimentation rate. (From Altman R, Alarcón G, Appelrouth D, et al. The American College of Rheumatology criteria for the classification and reporting of osteoarthritis of the hip. *Arthritis Rheum.* 1991;34: 505-514.)

two of three criteria: ESR of less than 20 mm/hour, radiographic evidence of osteophytes at the femur or acetabulum, or decreased joint space. The diagnostic validity of this criterion was found to be high, with specificity of 0.91 and sensitivity of 0.89. Thus, it is reasonable to assert that the aforementioned criteria would underestimate or fail to conclude a diagnosis of hip OA in approximately 11% of patients who in fact have hip OA. Moreover, the criteria would classify 9% of patients as having hip OA who in fact have an alternate condition. A potential limitation of this testing cluster for some health care professionals may lie in the clinical utility of a classification system that depends on imaging or laboratory values.

Clinical criteria, based solely on testing clusters from the physical examination and history, have been reported as a means of accurately identifying patients with symptomatic hip OA as well.[58,73] One proposed criterion from the ACR includes hip pain with hip IR range of motion less than 15 degrees and hip flexion of 115 degrees or less. An additional testing cluster proposed by the ACR for patients with hip pain includes IR measuring 15 degrees or more that produces pain during testing, morning stiffness for 60 minutes

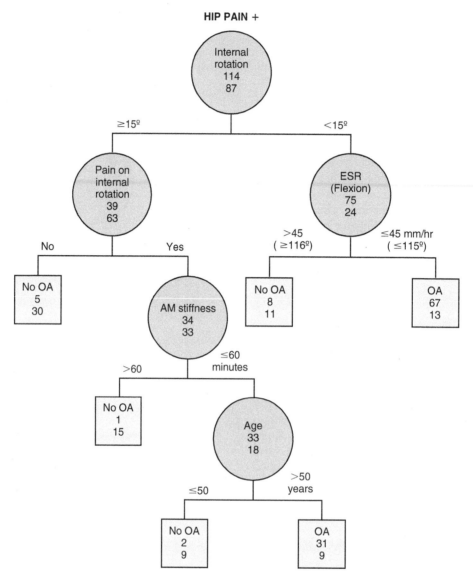

HIP PAIN +

• **Figure 6-10** American College of Rheumatology Clinical Criteria for Hip Osteoarthrosis (OA). Beginning with hip pain and knowledge of hip internal rotation, the classification tree illustrates relevant testing clusters with numbers in *circles* and *boxes* representing patients with OA and controls without hip OA *(lower numbers)*. If erythrocyte sedimentation rate (ESR) is not available, flexion mobility of 115 degrees or less may be substituted. (From Altman R, Alarcón G, Appelrouth D, et al. The American College of Rheumatology criteria for the classification and reporting of osteoarthritis of the hip. *Arthritis Rheum.* 1991;34:505-514.)

or less, and age older than 50 years. The aforementioned two clinical clusters (combined in Fig. 6-10), when compared with radiographic findings, have a reported sensitivity and specificity of 0.86 and 0.75, respectively. Thus, one could expect a 14% false-negative rate and a 25% false-positive rate. One could surmise that someone meeting more than one criterion or testing cluster is more likely to have an accurate classification of hip OA, although this assertion would need to be evaluated because overfitting may increase false-positive findings.

In addition to the ACR criteria, a clinical prediction rule was derived based on data from 72 participants, of whom 21 had hip OA with a Kellgren-Lawrence grade of 2 or higher based on radiographs.[73] This particular testing cluster identified 5 possible clinical predictors of hip OA: (1) pain

aggravated with squatting, (2) lateral or anterior hip pain with scour test, (3) active hip flexion causing lateral pain, (4) pain with active hip extension, and (5) passive hip IR range of motion up to 25 degrees (Box 6-4). A positive likelihood ratio of 5.2 was reported for patients meeting 3 of the 5 criteria. Table 6-5 provides additional diagnostic criteria interpretation based on a varying number of fulfilled predictors. This rule requires validation and impact analysis to be further accepted for clinical practice.

Prognosis

The prognosis for patients with hip OA depends on numerous variables. In a majority of cases, OA of the hip advances slowly, with joint replacement a viable end point for many

TABLE 6-5 Diagnostic Utility of the Hip Osteoarthrosis Clinical Prediction Rule Based on Number of Predictors

Present	Positive Likelihood Ratio	Negative Likelihood Ratio	Sensitivity	Specificity
5/5	7.3	0.87	0.14	0.98
4/5	24.3	0.53	0.48	0.98
3/5	5.2	0.33	0.71	0.86
2/5	2.1	0.31	0.81	0.61
1/5	1.2	0.27	0.95	0.18

• BOX 6-4 **Hip Osteoarthrosis: Clinical Prediction Rule**

Self-reported pain with squat
Lateral hip pain with active hip flexion
Scour test with adduction causing lateral hip or groin pain
Pain with active hip extension
Passive hip internal rotation ≤25 degrees

patients. Evidence suggests that age, female gender, a baseline minimum joint space of up to 2.5 mm, and a Kellgren-Lawrence scale grade of 2 or more are the strongest variables predictive of disease progression.[91,92] Furthermore, a Kellgren-Lawrence grade of 2 or more has been reported to be the strongest radiographic predictor of a future joint replacement.[87] A body of evidence, albeit small, supports the contention that exercise therapy and education may postpone the need for hip replacement.[93,94] Currently, no evidence-based interventions exist that have the ability to reverse the disease process. Rather, interventions are directed at symptom relief and surgical interventions to enable function. Patients who have undergone joint replacement interventions generally have a good prognosis. However, joint replacements performed among younger cohorts will have to be revised as time passes, depending on the patient's activity level.

Nonsurgical Interventions

Numerous consensus-based guidelines exist for the management of hip OA, with the commonality of improving outcomes and using the most efficacious evidence. Patients presenting with a clinical diagnosis of hip OA are often treated with a combination of pharmacologic and nonpharmacologic therapies, and joint replacement is reserved for those who are recalcitrant to conservative measures.

Nonsurgical management of hip OA often requires a multimodal approach, with a significant indication that the promotion of physical activity is generally efficacious, provided it is commensurate with the patient's ability to perform such activities.[95] The ACR published recommendations for pharmacologic and nonpharmacologic therapies

for patients with symptomatic hip OA who do not have comorbidities including cardiovascular, renal, or gastrointestinal problems (Table 6-6).[95] Although most of the ACR guidelines are consistent with the available consensus of evidence, individual clinical trials may offer more detailed information in regard to clinical applications.

Pharmacologic Treatment

Most authoritative guidelines recommend pharmacologic management with acetaminophen (paracetamol) as the first-line therapy, followed by nonsteroidal antiinflammatory drugs (NSAIDs) and intraarticular corticosteroid injections based on consideration of comorbidities. Acetaminophen is a pharmacologic treatment option for symptoms related to OA, particularly for those patients with a known intolerance to NSAIDs. Evidence suggests that acetaminophen is inferior to NSAIDs and superior to a placebo for improving hip pain related to OA.[96] Both NSAIDs and intraarticular corticosteroid injections have shown efficacy for the management of hip OA, particularly when they are used for flare-ups.[97] The Chronic Osteoarthritis Management Initiative of the U.S. Bone and Joint Initiative evaluated organizational recommendations and guidelines and subsequently recommended acetaminophen as the first-line pharmacologic therapy, with topical agents and oral NSAIDs as second-line agents.[98] Although NSAIDs are superior to acetaminophen for hip OA, the risk of serious events such as gastrointestinal bleeding should be considered, and the appropriate gastroprotective strategies should be employed.[99]

Intraarticular corticosteroid injections have been recommended as an intervention for hip OA.[58,98] Evidence suggests that corticosteroid injections may provide relief of hip pain lasting up to 3 months among patients with OA.[100,101] Furthermore, it appears that intraarticular corticosteroids have a comparable effect to that of viscosupplementation, and they offer a significant benefit for reducing pain during walking.[101]

Diacerein has been proposed for use as a slow-acting, symptom-modifying or disease-modifying drug for OA. The strength of evidence for the use of diacerein is low to moderate, as noted in a review published in 2014. According to the evidence, symptomatic benefits of pain reduction are minimal; however, a benefit in terms of slowing the

TABLE 6-6	American College of Rheumatology 2012 Guidelines for the Management of Hip Osteoarthritis	
Guideline	**Pharmacologic**	**Nonpharmacologic**
Strongly recommend	Opioid analgesics for patients who have been recalcitrant to other therapies and are either not a candidate or unwilling to undergo joint replacement	Cardiovascular, aquatic, and/or resistance land-based exercise Weight loss for persons overweight (includes education)
Conditionally recommend	Acetaminophen Oral NSAIDS Tramadol Intraarticular corticosteroid injection	Self-management programs Walking aids as needed Psychosocial interventions Manual therapy with exercise supervised by a physical therapist Instruction in use of thermal agents
No recommendation	Topical NSAIDs Intraarticular hyaluronate injections Duloxetine or opioid analgesics	Balance exercises Manual therapy interventions alone Tai chi
Recommend against	Chondroitin sulfate Glucosamine	*

From Hochberg MC, Altman RD, April KT, et al. American College of Rheumatology 2012 recommendations for the use of nonpharmacologic and pharmacologic therapies in osteoarthritis of the hand, hip, and knee. *Arthritis Care Res.* 2012;64:465-474.
NSAID, nonsteroidal antiinflammatory drug.
*The American College of Rheumatology did not "recommend against" any specific nonpharmacologic intervention.

progression of femoral acetabular space narrowing was identified when compared with a placebo.[102] Diarrhea is a more commonly reported side effect of this medication.

Viscosupplementation is an intraarticular injection of hyaluronic acid or its derivatives into an osteoarthritic joint. The therapeutic goal of viscosupplementation is to restore the viscoelasticity of synovial fluid and the natural protective functions of hyaluronic acid in the joint.[103,104] Recommendations for the use of intraarticular viscosupplementation are controversial as a result of insufficient or weak evidence.[98,101,103] Although few placebo-controlled trials exist and the evidence is variable, a benefit of viscosupplementation for the management of hip OA has been identified in regard to pain, disability, and a reduction in NSAID consumption.[104-106] However, a factor limiting the practicality of viscosupplementation for hip OA resides in reimbursement because it is approved by the U.S. Food and Drug Administration (FDA) only for the knee as of 2014.

Glucosamine and chondroitin are used by patients independently or in combination as an over-the-counter supplement based on the premise that these supplements can attenuate or modify cartilage loss in affected joints. Because of their safety profile and potential for increasing proteoglycan synthesis in articular cartilage, glucosamine and chondroitin have gained substantial popularity. To date, research trials have shown mixed results, and the ACR recommends against their use for hip OA.[95,98,107,108] Results from metaanalyses have noted some degree of efficacy; however, these analyses cite potential quality issues of existing research.[108,109] When used independent of chondroitin, glucosamine preparations do not offer a statistically significant benefit when compared with placebo for improving function, reducing

pain, decreasing medication use, and preserving joint space in patients with hip OA.[110,111] Furthermore, evidence suggests that the progression of hip OA is not affected by glucosamine use. Chondroitin sulfate, when used independently of glucosamine, was found to have little to no benefit for hip OA in a more recent metaanalysis.[109] Despite a paucity of evidence, glucosamine and chondroitin supplementation remains popular because of its widespread availability and safety profile.

In summary, health care providers routinely recommend pharmacologic agents as part of a multimodal approach for managing hip OA. Although nearly all clinical guidelines recommend pharmacologic interventions, their effect size is often small to medium at best, and in many cases the toxicity profile is poor compared with nonpharmacologic options. The choice of pharmacologic agent should be based on efficacy as well as safety profile. Acetaminophen (Tylenol) is recommended as a first-line agent; however, its efficacy is inferior to that of NSAIDs and corticosteroid injections. When the patient's medical history does not prohibit use, NSAIDs are a recommended second-line therapy, with corticosteroid injections reserved for flare-ups. Because the evidence for glucosamine and chondroitin is poor, their use is not recommended. Viscosupplementation appears to have a benefit; however, it is not yet approved for use in patients with hip OA.

Nonpharmacologic Interventions

Nonpharmacologic management of hip OA is multimodal and may include patient education and self-management, exercise interventions and manual therapy, weight loss

• BOX 6-5 **Recommendations for the Nonpharmacologic Management of Hip Osteoarthrosis***

Education: Limit compulsory squatting, prolonged standing, climbing, and heavy lifting.
Education: Avoid side sleeping, wear shoes with shock absorption, and avoid sitting with legs crossed.
Weight management advice and referral are provided as necessary.
Encourage low-impact aerobic activity with advancement and modification based on symptoms.
Skilled rehabilitation is indicated to address global impairments of muscle performance and mobility.
Skilled manual therapy services are indicated, to include stretching, joint distraction, and mobilization.
Balance training and ambulatory devices are provided as needed.

*Patient programs should be tailored to the individual patient and developed under the purview of the medical team.

measures, use of assistive devices regenerative medicine, and, finally, surgical interventions.[98] Box 6-5 presents general recommendations for the nonpharmacologic management of hip OA based on the available evidence.

Education and Lifestyle Modifications

A consensus of evidence-based guidelines recommends self-management programs and education as vital adjuncts to the care of patients with hip OA. Self-management measures include, but are not limited to, education on joint protection, activity modification, weight management, activities to influence self-care, and psychosocial interventions. Patient education and self-management programs have been found to decrease pain, increase function, and reduce the routine use of medications.[112-116] Moreover, evidence has found that patient education may provide greater perceived pain relief than medications for certain patients with hip OA.[116] Recommendations may include education on maintaining appropriate seat height and firmness to provide greater ease of movement during sit-to-stand transitions and advice to avoid crossing legs when sitting.[117] The use of pillows to increase seat height for transfers or as a means of limiting adduction when placed between the legs for side sleeping should be recommended.[117]

For standing, patients with hip OA should be educated on unweighting techniques for the affected side, as well as the use of appropriate footwear. Footwear recommendations often include soft soles to absorb impact, with heel pads as necessary to correct asymmetries in leg length. Heel lifts for patients with leg-length inequality may be used to achieve pelvic obliquity, although these devices have not been shown to decelerate radiographic progression of OA.[118] In the aforementioned study, pain relief was achieved with the use of a heel lift; however, a sample size of 27 is inadequate to draw a conclusive impression.[118] High heels or

prolonged standing should be avoided. Avoidance of prolonged or repetitive squatting and kneeling would seem reasonable, given its association with hip OA, as well as the biomechanical consequences of aberrant loading. Additionally, advice on weight management and referral to the appropriate dietary professional may be indicated.

Ambulation Devices

Assistive devices such as walkers, canes, and crutches may be used in patients with hip OA to reduce pain with weight bearing and to improve functional independence.[12] A cane should be used on the contralateral side as a means of reducing abductor demand and acetabular pressure on the involved side.[119,120] Assistive devices should otherwise be prescribed based on a thorough assessment of the patient's gait pattern, pain levels, and fall risk.

Manual Therapy

The use of manual therapy has been found effective, and it is recommended for short-term pain relief and to improve hip mobility and function,[12] particularly in patients with mild hip OA. Specific manual therapy interventions such as stretching to increase muscle flexibility, traction or distraction of the hip joint, and various joint mobilizations have been found to be effective for pain relief, function, perceived improvement, and range of motion.[121,122] Although evidence suggests that manual therapy offers improved patient satisfaction when compared with exercise, manual therapy interventions appear to have no additional long-term benefit when they are added to exercise interventions or are used as independent interventions. Essentially, manual therapy interventions appear to offer a short-term benefit when part of a comprehensive intervention plan.

Therapeutic Exercise

Therapeutic exercise generally includes low-impact aerobic activity, range of motion, and muscle performance activities. Most programs are multimodal and include frequent low-impact activities such as swimming, walking, or cycling, as well as progressive strengthening and range-of-motion activities, with the shared goals of improving function and decreasing pain. Although balance exercises may not be given high priority, according to the 2012 ACR recommendations, their utility should not be overlooked as a supervised intervention in patients with balance impairments.

Therapeutic exercises should generally be prescribed based on the patient's tolerance. They often commence in a non–weight-bearing or what is referred to as open kinetic chain position and then progress the degree of functional loading or weight bearing as tolerated. Muscle performance exercises should focus on the gluteal muscles, hip flexors, and quadriceps because they are most often affected in hip OA. Flexibility activities should focus on global range of motion, with specific efforts to stretch the iliopsoas, psoas, rectus femoris, adductors, and abductors. Most evidence suggests that programs should be continued well beyond the formal episode of care because patients may lose gains over time.

Land- and water-based activities are reportedly efficacious for patients with hip OA and are recommended as part of a comprehensive treatment plan.[98] The use of aquatic therapy appears to have a short-term benefit among patients with hip OA for reducing pain, improving mobility, and improving physical function and strength, as well as quality of life. The decision to incorporate aquatic therapy into the program should be based on the individual patient's presentation and on factors such as access to a temperature-controlled pool and adherence. Land-based therapies would appear to have greater functional specificity. However, aquatic therapy is a viable alternative to land-based exercises for those patients with an intolerance to weight-bearing activities.

When prescribing therapeutic exercise plans, consideration should be given to low-impact aerobic activity, as well as exercises designed to improve range of motion, flexibility, gait, and muscle performance.[12,95,98] Guidelines for exercise dosage exist, and most clinicians would agree that an efficacious routine should be inclusive of overload as well as a reasonable frequency. Of particular importance for any intervention plan is the need to address a patient's individual impairments and functional limitations (e.g., specificity of training).

Physical and Thermal Modalities

Thermal modalities such as heat may be of benefit to patients with hip OA.[95] However, therapeutic ultrasound is not recommended.[98] The 2011 Dutch Physiotherapy Guidelines[123] on hip and knee OA state that, based on limited evidence, the provision of massage, ultrasound, electrotherapy, electromagnetic field, and low-level laser therapy cannot be recommended. In the aforementioned guidelines, transcutaneous electrical stimulation and heat therapy were neither recommended nor discouraged.

Regenerative Medicine

Regenerative medicine is an emerging technology that serves to bridge the gap between conservative and surgical interventions for a wide range of musculoskeletal disorders. Various regenerative therapies alone and in combination are used in clinical practice including, but not limited to, adipose-derived or bone marrow stem cell therapies, platelet-rich plasma, and cytokines or anticytokines such as interleukin-1 antagonists and transforming growth factor. Collectively, these regenerative therapies have been postulated to have the benefit of activating growth factors that signal repair, thereby modulating the inflammatory process and supporting a vast array of events that foster healing and regeneration. Reports suggest that autologous platelet-rich plasma has the ability to attract stem cells and stimulate the release of numerous cytokines and growth factors that stimulate healing for a wide range of disorders.[124]

Stem cell therapies derived from bone marrow and adipose cells are thought to have antiinflammatory and protective effects on chondrocytes and lend to repair of damaged or degenerative tissues. Stem cell therapy is often combined with platelet-rich plasma because the latter attracts stem cells and provides much needed vascular support. Cytokine therapy serves the role of balancing the good and bad cytokines through stimulating angiogenesis, mitigating the inflammatory process at the cellular level, and supporting collagen synthesis and repair. For patients with OA, the premise for these therapies would seem to be based on restoring the histologic and biomechanical characteristic of articular cartilage. Thus, altering the course or perhaps reversing the degenerative cascade would seem to be the long-term objective, although the juried evidence of this is limited for hip OA.

Although limited research exists to evaluate the effect of these therapies for hip OA among human subjects, a body of evidence supports the use of platelet-rich plasma injections. Reports from a noncontrolled prospective study found that platelet-rich plasma therapy lends to a statistically significant short-term and long-term improvement in mean pain scores and function among patients with degenerative OA of the hip.[125,126] Unfortunately, a paucity of evidence exists to support the premise that regenerative therapies will reverse the degenerative cascade, despite what seems to be compelling physiologic justification.

Summary of Nonpharmacologic Interventions

In summary, most hip OA intervention trials have investigated drug therapies and surgical procedures.[127] To this detriment, a paucity of evidence exists to support many nonpharmacologic interventions. In light of this disparity, clinicians and researchers alike should be cognizant of the difference between an absence of high-quality evidence and evidence of ineffectiveness or harm. Most consensus-based guidelines for treating hip OA share a common perspective focusing on nonpharmacologic interventions that promote patient-driven interventions, as opposed to passive or palliative therapies delivered by health care professionals.[112,117] A compelling body of evidence and authoritative guidelines support self-management programs and education as a vital adjunct to the care of patients with hip OA. Moreover, activity that is physically tolerable and that seeks to mitigate impairments and promote functional independence serves a vital role for improving quality of life and delaying more aggressive interventions such as arthroplasty. Assistive devices and balance training should be considered based on the inclination of health care providers who have an understanding of a patient's physical status and safety, rather than external sources of data-driven evidence. Viscosupplementation appears to offer a benefit in regard to pain and function, although its use may be limited by reimbursement guidelines. When compared with viscosupplementation, the benefits of platelet-rich plasma on pain and function are comparable, although cost may present a deterrent to use. Future research on regenerative therapies may offer promise as a nonsurgical alternative. However, comparative research trials are needed to determine whether indeed these therapies are superior to other nonsurgical interventions and can deliver the vast array of postulated regenerative benefits in patients with hip OA.

Surgical Interventions

Overview

Considerable evidence exists to support the efficacy of nonsurgical interventions for improving quality of life in patients with OA, although a role in reversing or attenuating the degenerative cascade has not been established. Nonsurgical interventions are widely accepted as a means of mitigating pain and improving function; however, the long-term prognosis on disease progression is largely influenced by the amount of cartilage damage that has occurred before treatment.[128] For many patients, depending on the degree of degeneration and associated risk factors, surgical interventions present a viable end point. Referral for a surgical consultation is considered for patients who experience a significant decline in quality of life and are recalcitrant to nonsurgical interventions. Evidence suggests that early surgical management, before significant functional loss and disability have developed, is associated with better postoperative outcomes than delayed intervention.[129,130] Despite advances in surgical techniques and a greater understanding of research, considerable debate remains about the optimal surgical management of hip OA. The type of surgical procedure is often dictated by the stage of degeneration and intrinsic vulnerabilities such as age, activity level, and the presence of femoral acetabular impingement and instability. Surgical options for hip OA generally include joint replacement, as well as joint-preserving procedures designed to ameliorate etiologic risk factors such as instability and impingement.

Joint-Preserving Surgery

Joint-preserving surgical techniques are performed in an effort to prevent or decelerate the degenerative sequelae in patients with early OA, as well as in patients with established risk factors such as femoral acetabular impingement or dysplasia.[53,55,128,131] Essentially, the intentions of joint-preserving surgery are to optimize the mechanical environment of the hip and reduce aberrant loading. Surgical options generally include reorientation osteotomy for hip dysplasia, microfracture for smaller articular cartilage defects, and chondroplasty or resection for impingement.[128] Advances in surgical technology have enabled minimally invasive procedures such as arthroscopy to serve a key role in joint preservation; however, traditional open exposure with dislocation may be indicated in many cases. The prognostic efficacy of joint preservation ultimately depends on the stage of OA, because these procedures are generally not recommended for patients with advanced degenerative changes.[25] From an outcome perspective, corrective surgical

procedures for femoral acetabular impingement have been shown to decelerate OA and the progression to joint replacement surgery.[53,56]

Joint Replacement Surgery

Joint replacement (arthroplasty) is a viable surgical option for patients with advanced hip OA.[132] According to the American Academy of Orthopaedic Surgeons, approximately 230,000 joint replacement procedures of the hip, hereafter referred to as hip arthroplasty, were performed in the United States in 2008.[133,134] Because of efficacious outcomes and increased survivorship of modern prosthetic implants, a projected increase to 572,000 procedures by 2030 has been reported.[135]

Numerous types of procedures have been described in the literature, and each approach shares common goals of replacing the native joint with a prosthetic implant and restoring quality of life.[132] Surgical techniques (conventional versus minimally invasive) and implant design are determined based on the patient's demographics (age, activity level, and longevity), as well as the surgeon's preference and training.[132] Evidence pertaining to risk factors for failure and postoperative outcomes for a particular approach are often matched to patient-related characteristics as part of the decision-making process. Current arthroplasty procedures vary by choice of implant design (type of prosthesis), bearing surface, fixation method (cemented or noncemented), and surgical approach. Although postoperative outcomes and expectations are closely aligned with implant design and bearing surface, postoperative care is influenced to a greater degree by method of fixation and surgical approach.

Types of Hip Replacement Implant Design

If arthroplasty is the chosen surgical procedure, implant design options generally include traditional joint replacement (hemiarthroplasty or conventional total hip replacement) or resurfacing arthroplasty. In a conventional total hip replacement (Fig. 6-11), both the acetabulum and the femoral head are replaced by fixed prosthetic components made of metal, polyethylene, or ceramic. The acetabulum is prepared by reaming the cavity until it resembles the shape of the prosthetic component. The femoral head and neck are resected, and the stem with attached femoral head is implanted. The femoral head articulates directly with the prosthetic acetabular component and selected bearing surface, which may be metal or a polyethylene insert.

In a hemiarthroplasty procedure (Fig. 6-12), the native acetabulum is spared, and only the femoral head and neck are replaced by the prosthetic components. Indications for hemiarthroplasty include femoral head and neck fractures with an acetabulum that is free of disease. This procedure may be performed using either a unipolar or a bipolar prosthesis. The unipolar prosthesis has a monoblock design, whereas the femoral head is fixed to the stem and articulates directly with the native acetabulum. Unipolar prostheses are

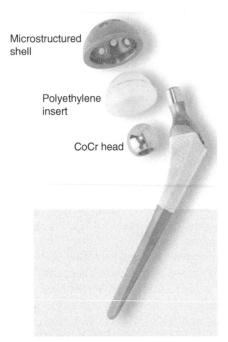

Microstructured shell

Polyethylene insert

CoCr head

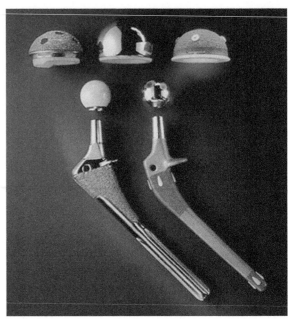

• **Figure 6-11** Conventional Total Hip Replacement Implant Components. Metal femoral stem and ball shown with a polyethylene on metal acetabular component. (From Capello WN, D'Antonio JA, Feinberg JR, Manley MT: Alternative bearing surfaces: alumina ceramic bearings for total hip arthroplasty. In Pellegrini VD, editor: *Instructional Course Lectures 54*. Rosemont, IL: American Academy of Orthopaedic Surgeons; 2005, pp 171-176.)

• **Figure 6-12** Conventional and Bipolar Hemiarthroplasty Implant Components. Metal femoral stems are shown with a ceramic ball femoral head *(left)* and a metal ball femoral head *(right)*. Note the porous acetabular cup *(left)* with a polyethylene insert, the bipolar femoral head *(center)* that articulates directly with the native acetabulum, and the cemented acetabular cup *(right)* with a polyethylene insert. (Courtesy Zimmer, Inc., Warsaw, Ind.)

rarely used because of concern over premature wear and stress to the native acetabulum. In lieu of a unipolar hemiarthroplasty, many surgeons use a bipolar prosthesis (Fig. 6-13, *right*). A bipolar hemiarthroplasty uses a polyethylene-lined metal cup that articulates externally with the native acetabulum and internally with a small femoral head (ball) fixed to the femoral stem (see Fig. 6-12, *center*). The advantage of a bipolar prosthesis over a unipolar design resides in the two articulation points, which are thought to decrease stress and wear on the native acetabulum.

Although relatively less common and often reserved for revisions, tripolar arthroplasty prosthetics exist and are composed of either a bipolar hemiarthroplasty placed inside a constrained acetabular shell or a traditional joint replacement with a dual mobility (articulation) acetabular cup (Fig. 6-14).[136] Dual mobility acetabular cups have gained attention, since their FDA approval in the United States in 2009, as a viable option for treating postoperative instability in both primary and revision surgical procedures. The dual mobility acetabular design is thought to offer superior mobility in a stable environment and reduce wear through its dual articulation design.[137] Biomechanically, this implant design allows the typical metal-on-polyethylene bearing surface movement; however, if the femoral neck and liner come in contact (impingement), a second articulation is recruited between the polyethylene liner and the acetabular shell.[137]

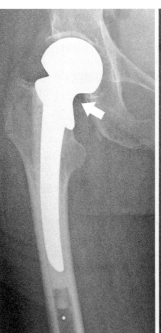
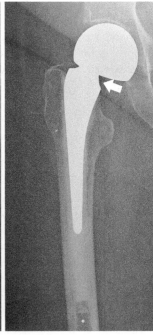

• **Figure 6-13** Anteroposterior radiographs illustrating a unipolar *(right)* and bipolar *(left)* hemiarthroplasty. Both radiographs show a cemented femoral stem. With the bipolar design, the femoral stem and ball are located within and articulate directly with the cup; therefore, they may be visualized in an eccentric position when compared with a unipolar design *(arrows)*. (From Pluot E, Davis ET, Revell M, et al. Hip arthroplasty. Part 1. Prosthesis terminology and classification. *Clin Radiol.* 2009;64:967-971.)

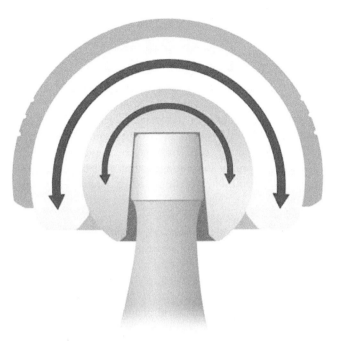

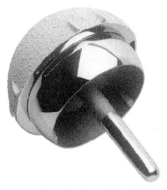

• **Figure 6-15** Resurfacing Metal-on-Metal Implant Components. (Courtesy Corin Group PLC, Cirencester, United Kingdom.)

• **Figure 6-14** A dual-mobility prosthesis, illustrated here, permits a greater range of motion prior to impingement. This tripolar design consists of two distinct articulations. One articulation is traditional and occurs between the femoral head and acetabular liner, whereas the second articulation occurs between the liner and the shell. The second articulation is recruited if the femoral neck contacts the liner. (From a presentation by Wetzel R, Puri L, Stulberg SD. *Modular Dual Mobility Acetabular Components: An Important Extension of a Proven Approach to Hip Instability.* Joint Reconstruction and Implant Service, Northwestern University Medical School, Chicago, Illinois.)

Resurfacing arthroplasty is used as an alternative to traditional joint replacement in an effort to preserve bone stock. This procedure involves replacing the articular surface of the femoral head with a metal cap that articulates with a metal acetabular component, as illustrated in Figure 6-15. The femoral head has a short stem that typically passes down into the femoral neck, unlike in traditional joint replacement, in which the stem passes into the femoral shaft. Resurfacing arthroplasty offers the advantages of bone preservation, improved mobility, and greater activity levels when compared with traditional joint replacement. Improved mobility is appreciated as a result of the metal-on-metal design that provides the opportunity for a larger femoral head. Following resurfacing arthroplasty, outcomes such as running, sports, and manual labor significantly exceed those of traditional joint replacement.[138] Despite superior activity-related outcomes, registry data have shown an increased revision rate related to implant failure when compared with traditional joint replacement.[25,139,140]

Bearing Surfaces

The articulation surface of prosthetic implants, referred to hereafter as bearing surfaces, are generally made of metal, polyethylene, or ceramic. Bearing surfaces of the acetabulum generally consist of ultrahigh-molecular-weight or highly cross-linked polyethylene, metal, or ceramic materials. Femoral heads are generally made of metals such as cobalt-chromium, molybdenum, and titanium alloys, and in fewer instances ceramic, depending on the acetabular component.[141] The type of bearing surface seems to be a key consideration for the longevity of hip implants, as well as the pursuit of an active lifestyle.[142] The most common type of bearing surface used in a total hip replacement consists of a metal-backed acetabular shell with a highly cross-linked polyethylene liner that articulates with a metal femoral head (see Fig. 6-11).[142-144] These surfaces are a good choice for the majority of patients and have a 98% survival rate at 10 years.[142] Bipolar hemiarthroplasty bearing surfaces consist of a metal ball that articulates with a polyethylene-lined femoral cup (see Fig. 6-12, *center*). The use of a polyethylene bearing surface provides a reliable, albeit susceptible, wear surface.[145] Metal-on-metal wear surfaces (see Fig. 6-15; Fig. 6-16) were developed to improve the survivorship of hip implants by decreasing the abrasive wear and particle formation seen with conventional polyethylene components. Metal-on-metal bearing surfaces are attractive in that they allow for a larger femoral head and thus may offer improved mobility and reduced dislocation propensity.[146] Current resurfacing arthroplasty implant designs incorporate metal-on-metal bearing surfaces as a means of improving mobility to allow greater activity levels among recipients. Despite benefits of metal bearing surfaces, a disadvantage when compared with ceramic or polyethylene bearing surfaces is the rate of revision.[147] Moreover, the use of metal bearing surfaces has fallen out of favor because of concerns over the systemic presence of metal ions, adverse tissue reactions, and osteolysis.[142,146,148] Ceramic bearing surfaces may be used because they have superior wear properties when compared with metal and polyethylene and metal on metal; however, audible squeaking and fracture (of ceramic component) may render their use unpopular.[142,144,149]

As expected, all implant designs and bearing surfaces have advantages and disadvantages. Therefore, an individualized selection process that balances risk against functional demands would seem to offer the best individualized outcome. Research regarding the optimal type of prosthetic design and bearing surfaces is constantly changing because of new-generation implants and changing indications. For

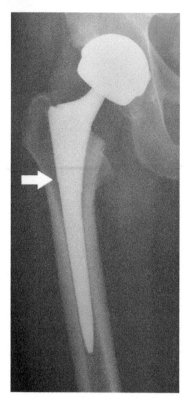

• **Figure 6-16** Anteroposterior radiograph illustrating a traditional total hip replacement with a metal-on-metal bearing surface. Note the uncemented femoral stem *(arrow)* and a relatively large metal-on-metal articulation. (From Pluot E, Davis ET, Revell M, et al. Hip arthroplasty. Part 1. Prosthesis terminology and classification. *Clin Radiol.* 2009; 64:967-971.)

the surgeon, a careful understanding of the individual patient's activity demands and comorbidities may assist in the selection process, whereas the patient should find comfort in selecting the surgeon, as opposed to muddling through outcome studies. Independent of prosthetic type and bearing surface, postoperative care largely influences outcomes following joint replacement. Moreover, the type of implant fixation and the surgical approach often dictate postoperative care.

Implant Fixation and Approach

From a procedural perspective, factors such as method of implant fixation (cemented vs. noncemented) and anatomic approach (location and level of invasiveness) have relevance in the early stages of postoperative care,[132] and to some degree they may influence long-term outcomes and revision rates. Cementless fixation is achieved by press-fitting a slightly oversized prosthetic component into a prepared cavity or surface (see Fig. 6-16).[141] When cementless fixation techniques are used, a prosthetic component is selected that allows ingrowth of bone onto a porous coated or textured surface. In some cases screw fixation is used with a press-fit acetabular component. The cemented fixation method involves a pressurized injection of cement into the space between the implant and bone (see Fig. 6-13). The cement, made of polymethylmethacrylate and other

materials, acts more like grout than glue and achieves early fixation. Hip replacements that use a cemented femoral implant paired with a noncemented acetabular component are referred to as hybrids. In particular, patients who have cemented implant fixation of the prosthesis are generally allowed to bear weight as tolerated immediately, whereas it is common for surgeons to restrict weight bearing for a period of up to 6 weeks in patients who have a noncemented implant.[150] An advantage to having noncemented fixation is thought to be longevity of the procedure, hence it is more commonly encountered in a relatively younger population.[150-152] Moreover, the choice of fixation method seems to have geographic patterns of use.

The postsurgical intervention, residual impairments, risk for revision, and precautions often depend on the type of approach (e.g., anatomic location to access the joint). Specifically, whether the procedure was performed from an "anterior," "anterolateral," "lateral," "transtrochanteric," or "posterior-posterolateral" surgical approach must be considered.[132] Generally speaking, approaches are often labeled by their proximity to the gluteus medius muscle, and each approach has advantages and disadvantages in regard to soft tissue trauma and postoperative sequelae. Although many of the approaches have evolved over time to be less invasive, newer minimally invasive procedures exist (e.g., mini-posterior), with the purported benefits of smaller incisions (typically <10 cm) and reduced soft tissue dissection. Furthermore, numerous surgical idiosyncrasies exist to the traditional and minimally invasive approaches in regard to soft tissue dissection and repair, thus reinforcing the need to view each postoperative patient as unique.

Posterior-Posterolateral Approach

Although various surgical procedures have been practiced since 2000 and regional variations exist, the posterior-posterolateral, hereafter referred to as posterolateral, approach is the most common. It is preferred by many surgeons because of its excellent joint exposure during the procedure.[153,154] Although the posterolateral approach is most common, minimally invasive techniques such as the mini-posterior and minimally invasive anterior approach are gaining popularity.[155-158] Irrespective of the chosen approach, all have similar goals of restoring joint function; however, the considerable procedural differences have direct relevance in terms of immediate postoperative and long-term precautions,[132] which should be considered.

The conventional posterolateral approach is performed through an incision that may extend up to 20 cm[159] in the posterior and lateral region of the hip (Fig. 6-17). Posterior approaches with smaller incisions (e.g., mini-posterior 5 to 6 cm) and less soft tissue dissection have been described in the literature.[160] However, a more recent metaanalysis concluded that the minimally invasive posterior approach was not superior to the traditional approach in regard to postoperative hip function and recovery.[161] The conventional procedure has been associated with positive outcomes in function and pain, but a high rate of postoperative

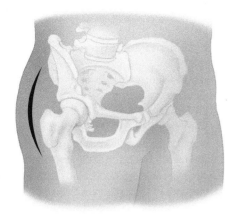

• **Figure 6-17** Standard Posterolateral Approach Incision. (Redrawn from Biomet, Inc., Warsaw, Ind.)

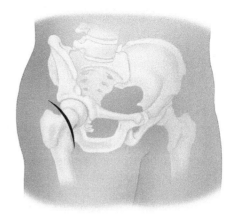

• **Figure 6-18** Direct Anterior Approach Incision. (Redrawn from Biomet, Inc., Warsaw, Ind.)

dislocation has been documented when compared with other techniques such as the minimally invasive anterior approach.[154,155,162-164] Although variations on the posterolateral approach exist, it is common practice for the surgeon to split or partially release the gluteal maximus and release the short hip external rotators (piriformis, superior and inferior gemelli, quadratus femoris, and obturator internus), as well as the hip capsule,[153,154,163] to gain access to the joint.

The posterior mini-approach is less invasive in that the piriformis is preserved intact and the gluteus maximus is split.[160] Once the joint is exposed, the hip is then dislocated by simultaneously placing the leg in flexion, IR, and adduction.[153] Once dislocated, the joint is prepared, and the prosthetic implants are inserted. The decision to use a cemented versus noncemented implant depends on the patient's needs and the surgeon's preference. Noncemented implants are generally reserved for the younger, more active patient,[150,151] because the procedure omits the risk of component loosening and premature revision surgery. Following implant insertion, the soft tissue is repaired, with a complete repair offering greater levels of stability.[153,154,163] As expected, the soft tissue requires time to heal and may render the hip unstable until it is adequately healed with sufficient strength and power.[153,163,165]

Although postoperative restrictions may vary, a period of limited hip adduction, IR, and flexion greater than 90 degrees is universally implemented to allow the repaired soft tissue to heal and mitigate dislocation risk. Furthermore, a short period of protection is indicated for the repaired musculature as well. Generally speaking, protection of repaired musculature for any approach typically involves the avoidance of dynamic resistance (to the repaired musculature) for up to 6 weeks. Functional use and submaximal isometrics of the repaired soft tissue are generally not discouraged.

Direct Anterior Approach

The minimally invasive direct anterior approach is generally performed through a small anterior incision (<10 cm) between the tensor fasciae latae and sartorius muscles (Fig. 6-18).[158,166] This procedure and the operating tables designed

to facilitate the surgical procedure are rather new compared with the posterolateral, lateral, and anterolateral approaches, and this approach is reported to be less invasive but more technically demanding on the surgeon.[167] An advantage of this technique lies in the surgical procedure because the hip muscles are not disrupted (cut or released) during the operation.[155,158,167] As a result, the hip is purported to have a reduced incidence of instability and weakness when compared with more invasive procedures such as the posterolateral approach. Surgical variations exist, and some surgeons may prefer a more invasive anterior approach that includes dissection of contractile tissue.[157] Surgical variations of this technique may shift the incision location to avoid meralgia paresthetica (injury to the lateral femoral cutaneous nerve). The decision to repair the anterior capsule is based on the surgeon's preference and has postoperative activity implications for end-range or combined extension and external rotation.

Anterolateral Approach

The anterolateral approach provides adequate exposure to the hip joint through the intermuscular plane between the tensor fasciae latae and the gluteus medius.[157] Mini-incision and conventional approaches exist for this procedure. The minimally invasive approach generally involves an 8- to 10-cm incision with little to no detachment of the gluteus medius or minimus or tensor fasciae latae musculature, whereas the traditional procedure requires an incision of 16 to 18 cm and lends to varying degrees of gluteus medius and minimus detachment.[157,168,169] Variations among surgical techniques exist for both the traditional and minimally invasive procedures. Abduction weakness is a recognizable impairment seen postoperatively with the traditional approach, although evidence suggests comparable clinical and functional benefits at a 4-year prospective follow-up when comparing the procedures.[169] Dislocation risk is relatively low compared with posterior approaches; however, some surgeons may prefer patients to limit end-range or combined hip extension with external rotation or supine bridging activities for the first 6 weeks to allow inert tissue healing. Additionally, the repaired fibers of the gluteus medius may require a short period of protection to enable healing.

Lateral and Transtrochanteric Approaches

The lateral approach is generally performed in patients at risk of postoperative dislocation (e.g., comorbidities or hyperlaxity) because this operation has a reduced risk of dislocation when compared with other approaches.[170,171] Moreover, this approach has been purported to offer an optimal environment for orientation of implants and for creating a stable hip because it allows preservation of posterior soft tissue structures.[170-172] This approach generally consists of a direct lateral incision, with splitting or partial detachment of the hip abductors (gluteus medius and minimus) to gain access to the joint.[157,170,173] Generally, the hip abductors are partially released from the greater trochanter by either a release of the functional tendon or in some cases an osteotomy.[173] The degree of soft tissue detachment varies, and to this extent repair must be protected in the postoperative phase, based on the surgeon's recommendation. An inherent disadvantage of this approach resides in the necessity of detaching the hip abductors to gain entry to the joint. Additionally, damage to the superior gluteal nerve may be a complication. From a functional expectation, short-term hip abductor weakness and a postoperative limp may be present. The benefit of this approach, however, lies in a significant reduction in the incidence of postoperative dislocation.[171] Although surgical circumstances often dictate specific postoperative management, a short period of protected hip abduction may be implemented to protect the repaired musculature. Weight bearing is often progressed as tolerated, and hip dislocation precautions are not typically necessary. When the abductors are lifted using an osteotomy, it would not be unreasonable to have a period of weight-bearing restrictions to allow bone union based on a timeline determined by the surgeon.

The transtrochanteric approach is often limited to complex and revision cases. This approach, through a trochanteric osteotomy, provides good visualization of the anterior and posterior hip, as well as the complete acetabulum.[157,174] Enhanced exposure of the hip is often necessary for complicated cases (e.g., ankylosis, protrusio acetabuli, or dysplasia) or revision procedures to facilitate removal of fixed femoral components.[157] The procedure involves an incision centered on the trochanter, generally in line with fibers of gluteus maximus. The gluteus maximus is split, and once the joint is exposed, an osteotomy of the greater trochanter is performed. The hip abductors and external rotators (excluding quadratus femoris) remain attached to the trochanteric fragment.[174] The trochanter is later reattached using wires. The advantages of this approach include a low dislocation rate (1.27%) and preservation of the abductor and external rotator muscles.[171,174] Weight-bearing and active hip abduction are often delayed for a minimum of 6 weeks to protect the surgical repair and allow bone union.[157,174] Movement precautions are generally not necessary, given the relatively low rate of dislocation and preservation of the external rotators.[174]

Preoperative Physical Therapy

The initiation of physical therapy as a preoperative intervention is often based on expectations of improved postoperative outcomes and a shorter length of stay. Many institutions consider preoperative physical therapy an integral component of a comprehensive care pathway model for patients undergoing joint replacement. The definition of what constitutes preoperative care may vary because one may assume that most patients scheduled for surgery have been recalcitrant to conservative measures, which often include some type of formal rehabilitation. Nevertheless, preoperative rehabilitation interventions (i.e., those performed within approximately 2 months of surgical admission) often include patient education about expectations, discussion of walking aids, precautions, postoperative care and recovery planning, and formal exercises to mitigate impairments. Although many facilities and surgeons have their own model of patient management, evidence does suggest that a few visits of preoperative physical therapy are associated with a significant reduction in postacute care services such as home health care, inpatient rehabilitation, and skilled nursing facility care.[175] Interestingly, evidence for reduced cost was found after adjusting for comorbidities, demographics, and procedural variables. Moreover, the results pertaining to reduced postacute use are not dose dependent; thus, a cost shift to preoperative care is not anticipated.[175] Other studies have suggested a reduced length of stay attributed to preoperative care.[176] Furthermore, evidence indicates that preoperative physical therapy may improve function even in patients with the most complicated cases.[177] The clinical interest in improving function and impairments resides in the association between preoperative variables (e.g., function and strength) and postoperative outcomes.[178-180]

Future studies are needed to determine whether a broadly recognized benefit indeed exists, such that one could state with certainty that withholding preoperative interventions is deleterious to the outcome following hip arthroplasty. Irrespective of the available levels of evidence, preoperative care appears innocuous in regard to side effects, and preliminary evidence does appear to exist on cost, length of stay, and physical function. The decision to incorporate preoperative physical therapy interventions should be individualized based on an individual patient's needs. More compelling evidence is needed to make a global recommendation about the benefit in regard to postoperative quality of life and impairments.[181,182]

Postoperative Interventions: Joint Replacement

Initial Postoperative Period

Irrespective of approach, postoperative rehabilitation is generally initiated in the first 24 hours after the procedure.[150,183] During the first day, patients generally exercise the involved lower extremity, including the ankle, knee, and hip, while ensuring that all postsurgical precautions are followed and any untoward physiologic responses are appropriately

TABLE 6-7	General Postoperative Precautions Following Hip Replacement*	
Restriction	**Consideration**
Limited weight bearing	Trochanteric osteotomy Uncemented fixation
Hip flexion >90 degrees, adduction past midline, and internal rotation	Posterolateral approach Mini-posterior approach
End-range or combined hip extension and external rotation	Direct anterior approach Anterolateral approach
Active hip abduction	Trochanteric osteotomy
Dynamic resistance training to repaired musculature	All approaches

*Specific precautions: Timelines should be based on the surgeon's preference, procedural idiosyncrasies, and risk factors.

managed.[132] Table 6-7 presents an overview of postoperative precautions.

Most patients receive anticoagulant medications as a means of ameliorating venous stasis, coagulopathy, and endothelial injury, all of which may promote deep vein thrombosis and potentially pulmonary embolism.[184] Although the optimal duration that a patient will be taking anticoagulant medications may vary, evidence suggests that extended out-of-hospital prophylaxis may continue for up to 1 month and potentially longer as a means of preventing complications.[185] Although anticoagulation therapy has known benefits for reducing complications, the health care provider must recognize the potential risks of bleeding, infection, and thrombocytopenia.[185,186] Exercise interventions and ambulation (with weight-bearing status often determined based on method of fixation) are encouraged to decrease the likelihood of deep vein thrombosis (blood clot) and other perils associated with postoperative immobility (pulmonary embolism, pneumonia, lasting effects of general anesthesia).[132] Evidence suggests that patients who receive multiple intervention sessions per day are more likely to achieve earlier functional outcomes.[187] Although twice-daily interventions improve functional outcomes, they do not translate into a shorter length of stay.[187] The inpatient (acute care) rehabilitation generally continues daily until the patient is medically stable and able to be discharged to a lower level of medical care,[132] before ultimately being discharged home.

In the United States, length of stay varies, with reports of 2 to 5 days on average following primary hip arthroplasty.[188-190] Factors influencing length of stay include age, body mass, blood management, preoperative physical function, timing of postoperative physical therapy, and surgical approach.[183,188,191-193] Evidence suggests that initiating early physical therapy, preferably on the day of the surgical procedure or within 24 hours, leads to a decreased length of stay.[183,194,195] From a physical functioning perspective, patients who had difficulty managing stairs and who required a walking device preoperatively are more likely to have a longer length of stay.[193] Moreover, preliminary evidence suggests that preoperative physical therapy may reduce length of stay.[176] However, further investigations are needed to determine a definitive benefit. Finally, a trend does exist for earlier discharge among those patients who had an anterior approach when compared with the posterolateral or mini-posterior approach.[188,196]

Residual Impairments

Postoperative outcomes have generally focused on the posterolateral and anterior approaches; therefore, much of the discussion regarding outcomes and evidence is limited to these methods. From an impairment perspective, a body of evidence suggests that clients who have had the anterior approach will progress to higher functional levels early in their rehabilitation; however, by the time of discharge from formal care, differences in function are minimal.[167,197] At the time of discharge and extending well into the next few years or longer, patients who have undergone any hip arthroplasty procedure typically have impairments; however, the degree of impairments is multifactorial and includes the premorbid status of the patient, comorbidities, and type of procedure, because more invasive procedures are associated with greater muscle morbidity.[198-202] In regard to function, evidence suggests that patients demonstrate limitations in their ability to climb stairs and present with decreased walking velocity, as well as reduced step length, for up to 2 years following the surgical procedure.[203,204] By 1 year postoperatively, only 32% of persons will use an assistive device for ambulation, and by the fifth postoperative year this use further declines to 13%.[201] Although the aforementioned evidence points to deficits persisting up to 2 years, it should be recognized that this is the terminal point of the investigations and that these deficits may persist well beyond 2 years.

From an impairment perspective, a loss of hip extension and external rotation range of motion was reported in several investigations.[197,203,205,206] These limitations may affect normal walking mechanics, as well as the ability to perform functional activities such as placing a foot on the opposite knee for donning and doffing shoes and socks or performing foot hygiene activities. A loss of flexion range of motion has not been identified as a common postsurgical impairment, and any activity exceeding 90 degrees of flexion should be avoided in most cases among those patients who have had a posterolateral approach. Muscle morbidity is most often reported as a persistent problem following hip replacement, with more invasive procedures potentially leading to greater damage.[198] One investigation using MRI, identified muscle morbidity (atrophy or decreased radiologic density) of the iliopsoas, gluteus maximus, and hip adductor and abductor groups for up to 2 years following a posterolateral approach.[199] Moreover, reports of reduced power and strength of the hip flexors, abductors, adductors, and external rotator musculature have been reported well beyond discharge from rehabilitation.[197,200,206,207] Finally, decreased postural stability of the operative leg,[208] and compromised cardiovascular fitness[209] have also been reported as persistent impairments following hip replacement. Although many studies have investigated deficits up to 2 years, evidence indicates that deficits in activities such as walking may continue to persist beyond this timeframe.[201] Moreover, evidence indicates that a time-dependent gradual decline in function begins, on average, approximately 5 years postoperatively,[201] thus substantiating the need for continued and progressive exercise-based interventions. Box 6-6 lists more common impairments that persist beyond formal care among patients who have had hip replacement procedures.

Postoperative Precautions

Health care providers and patients should remain cognizant of the proclivity for dislocation, as well as the need to restrict activities that may influence premature wear of the prosthetic components or impediment of bone union (in cases of osteotomy). Irrespective of procedure, most patients are subject to certain precautions, with the approach often dictating the nature of restrictions (see Table 6-6). Dislocation is a common complication of hip replacement and occurs in up to 11% of patients following a primary or revision procedure with a predilection toward posterolateral approaches.[171,210,211] A cumulative report of 14 studies found an average dislocation incidence of 2% following a primary posterolateral approach when the soft tissue was adequately repaired versus 4% with minimal repair.[171] Essentially, the risk of dislocation is up to six times more likely following a posterolateral approach than after an anterior, direct lateral, and transtrochanteric approach.[163,171,212] This difference in risk of dislocation is likely the result of the more invasive nature of the posterolateral approach because soft tissue (muscle and capsule) is dissected to gain entry into the joint. Approximately 50% of all dislocations occur during the first 3 months postoperatively,[210,213] and they are thought to be caused by instability ensuing from weakness of the repaired soft tissue as well as noncompliance with postoperative activity precautions.

Generally speaking, postoperative activity restrictions are physiologically derived from an understanding of the surgical approach and are generally consistent among surgeons, with only the duration of these restrictions having variability.[132] Specifically, the hip is dislocated during the operation (posterolateral approach) by combined flexion, IR, and

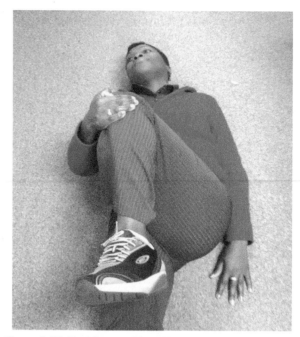

• **Figure 6-19** Combined position of flexion past 90 degrees with hip adduction and internal rotation.

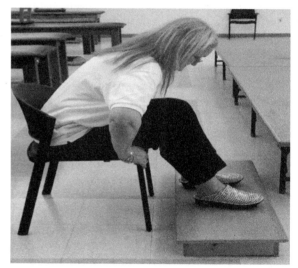

• **Figure 6-20** Functional Position of Risk for Dislocation. Note: The hip is flexed beyond 90 degrees.

adduction (Fig. 6-19); thus, performance of these motions (combined or individually) postoperatively may place a patient at risk for dislocation.[150,214,215] Moreover, activities such as flexing the hip past 90 degrees (Fig. 6-20), such as when assuming the position similar to sitting in a low chair, bending forward while seated, or squatting, are purported causes of hip dislocation following a posterolateral approach.[163,215] It would seem reasonable that the soft tissue has healed and one's risk profile for dislocation is reduced by the twelfth postoperative week. Outside of activity restrictions, evidence indicates that an increased body mass index, alcoholism, a previous dislocation, and undergoing a hip replacement for repair of a fracture are additional dislocation risk factors.[163,202,212]

Although most dislocations occur during the first 3 months, evidence suggests that dislocations may occur well beyond 5 years following the surgical procedure.[216] In light of the aforementioned evidence, it is recommended that patients be instructed to avoid individual combined motions of hip flexion greater than 90 degrees, adduction, and IR following posterolateral approach for a period of at least 12 weeks or longer, based on the surgeon's preference.[132] Moreover, patients should be instructed to avoid any activities such as squatting and kneeling that place their hip in a position of greater than 90 degrees of flexion for a similar duration. Evidence suggests that those patients who possess greater amounts of flexion, adduction, and IR mobility are more likely to experience a dislocation,[217] a finding that further substantiates recommendations to avoid efforts to increase these motions for a reasonable time following a posterolateral approach.

Unlike with the posterolateral approach, evidence suggests a substantially decreased risk of dislocation following both the minimally invasive direct anterior and the anterolateral approach. In fact, evidence suggests that postoperative mobility restrictions are generally unnecessary following a direct anterior approach.[164,218] Specifically, investigations have reported no change in the dislocation risk when precautions were not implemented following an anterior approach.[164,218] Mobility restrictions following a direct anterior approach depend on surgical factors. Surgeons who make an effort to repair the anterior capsule may have a preference for limiting extremes of hip extension and external rotation during the early postoperative phase of healing.

Generally, component failure and wear occur in a linear pattern with time since the operation, with up to 10% of patients having loosening by year 10 and increasing 17% by year 14.[201] It is accepted that wear is a function of loading; thus, the number of cycles (repetitions, also known as level of activity) and the magnitude of loading (body mass) influence the amount of wear.[219] Postoperatively, health care professionals must recognize the balance between activity needed for cardiovascular health and general fitness levels and the amount of activity that may lead to premature wear or failure of the prosthesis.[219] Many surgeons advise their patients to avoid high-level activity following hip arthroplasty to prevent premature wear and loosening of the prosthetic implants[201] because an association between activity levels and component failure has been substantiated.[201] A consensus of what constitutes "high activity" has been established among representative members of the Hip Society. Although the details of recommended activities are discussed in the exercise programming section of this chapter, activities such as jogging, rock climbing, high-impact aerobics, football, and racquetball are best avoided.[201]

Muscle Performance Exercise

Postoperative impairments such as decreased range of motion, pain, and strength have been implicated as risk factors that may prevent patients from achieving optimal outcomes.[220] Individualized exercise programs have been found to be effective in addressing both early-stage and late-phase impairments and physical function following the surgical procedure.[221] Convincing evidence indicates that both aerobic-based and resistance-based training promote favorable adaptations in this population.[221] Supporting evidence of benefits of flexibility exercise following a joint replacement procedure is currently lacking; however, a theoretical basis does exist for its inclusion in a targeted fitness routine.[132]

Resistance training that targets the lower extremity musculature is critical to restoring normal physical function postoperatively.[221] It is beneficial to initiate a progressive resistance training program as expeditiously as possible after the procedure, because investigators have suggested that muscle strength declines as much as 4% per day during the first week of immobilization.[222] In one study,[223] 24 early-stage (1 week after the surgical direct lateral approach) subjects were randomized into either a low-resistance therapy group or a group that supplemented conventional therapy with heavy resistance training. The experimental group performed 4 sets of 5 repetitions of both the angled leg press and hip abduction with resistance bands. Training was carried out at approximately 85% of 1 repetition maximum, with loads progressively increased to accommodate ongoing increases in strength. At the conclusion of this study, subjects who supplemented therapy with resistance training showed significantly greater lower body strength and rate of force development compared with those who received therapy alone. Moreover, work efficiency was significantly greater in the strength-trained group versus controls at a 6- and 12-month follow-up (by 29% and 30%, respectively).[224] No adverse effects were associated with heavy resistance training despite patients being progressed in the program before soft tissue healing. These findings are consistent with other research,[225] which reported that early-stage progressive resistance exercise increased maximal lower body strength, muscle mass, and muscle function to a greater extent than did standard rehabilitation in older subjects, as well as markedly reducing their length of hospital stay. Resistance exercise is equally important and effective for enhancing functional abilities in later-stage recovery after hip arthroplasty. Additionally, evidence suggests that a 3-month progressive resistance training program significantly increased strength, functional motor performance, and balance while reducing behavioral and emotional problems related to falls when compared with a control group following hip arthroplasty.[226]

In the early phases of rehabilitation, resistance exercises should be restricted to no more than 90 degrees of hip flexion, to help ensure that stresses do not exceed the capacity of the joint, which could potentially result in a hip dislocation.[223] Caution should be exercised when performing any lunges and squats or activities that promote concurrent hip IR or adduction past the midline of the body in patients with traditional dislocation precautions.

It also is beneficial to include abduction and external rotator exercises as part of a resistance training program. The hip abductors are essential for normal gait and prevention of falls,[223] and exercise that directly targets these muscles can help to restore normal physical function among patients following the surgical procedure. Strengthening of the external rotators is important for hip stability, as well as performance. Evidence suggests that these muscles may be impaired following posterior or posterolateral approaches as a result of surgical dissection despite successful repair. Although investigators have reported that high-intensity strength training is a viable strategy in early-stage recovery,[223] it may be too strenuous for some patients. Moreover, some clients may still be taking anticoagulant medications, which may increase their risk of bleeding in response to more strenuous exercise.[184,185] From a risk perspective, early stages of strengthening should focus on submaximal isometrics and, when tolerated, based on pain and function, advanced in a gradual manner. A more conservative approach following the submaximal isometric phase would start out at 50% of the 1 repetition maximum and then gradually increasing intensity to 80% after 6 to 8 weeks, which has been reported safe and effective in patients who have had a hip arthroplasty.[225]

Cardiorespiratory Exercise

Many patients who undergo joint replacement operation have experienced physical disability and reduced activity levels for years that have caused aerobic deconditioning.[227] Direct cardiorespiratory exercise therefore can be beneficial in helping these patients regain aerobic capacity and endurance and in improving quality of life. Studies directly evaluating exercise-related cardiovascular changes following hip arthroplasty are limited. In one investigation, significant functional improvements were reported from treadmill training (as a supplement to physical therapy) with partial body weight support for subjects in the early-phase of recovery after hip arthroplasty.[228] Subjects were evaluated by the HHS questionnaire, an assessment instrument consisting of weighted scores for pain, limping, the use of aids for mobility, maximum walking distance, competence in daily activities, and hip range of motion. After 10 days, the HHS score in patients receiving physical therapy in addition to partial body weight-supported treadmill training was more than 13 points higher (a positive finding) compared with controls receiving physical therapy alone. Further, clinically relevant improvements persisted at 3- and 12-month follow-up. Moreover, evidence suggests that pulmonary embolism is one of the more common causes of mortality following joint replacement surgery.[186] This finding emphasizes the need to reserve vigorous aerobic training judiciously only for those patients who are medically cleared for such activity. In one study, researchers demonstrated significant improvements in maximum oxygen consumption following a 6-week arm ergometry interval training compared with a nontraining control group that received traditional daily rehabilitation.[229] In addition, trained subjects covered significantly greater distances in the timed 6-minute-walk test versus controls (405 m vs. 259 m, respectively). One-year follow-up showed that the training group maintained this advantage, as well as displaying significantly lower scores on the WOMAC (indicative of a better outcome).[230]

Flexibility Exercise

Restoring functional range of motion may be a goal if mobility impairments persist following hip arthroplasty. Evidence suggests that hip extension and external rotation mobility deficits may persist postoperatively.[198,205,206] Moreover, contracture of the iliopsoas, rectus femoris, adductors, and tensor fasciae latae has been identified among patients reporting hip pain at the 2-month period following hip arthroplasty.[231] In the aforementioned descriptive study,[231] the investigators reported successfully managing 92% of these patients with a flexibility program that consisted of manual stretching during clinic visits two to five times a week and a home exercise program. A nonrandomized study of older adults after hip replacement reported no improvements in hip range of motion following a nonsupervised, at-home flexibility and strengthening protocol.[232] Given the home-based nature of this study, it could be postulated that the null results likely reflected suboptimal exercise performance or poor compliance with the routine.

The paucity of studies examining flexibility exercise following hip replacement makes it difficult to provide evidence-based recommendations. Performing slow, static stretching exercise for the hip joint to improve impaired motions to enhance functional movement would seem to have little downside.[233] As a general precaution, patients who have had a posterolateral approach arthroplasty should avoid stretches that involve combined flexion, adduction, and IR (see Fig. 6-19) because these exercises may predispose the joint to dislocation and potentially stress healing tissue if performed prematurely. Additionally, patients who have had a direct anterior or anterolateral approach may be advised to limit painful or combined hip extension and external rotation to provide adequate time for anterior soft tissue healing. As stated previously, some surgeons posit that precautions are not indicated following the direct anterior procedure. Finally, hip adduction past midline, as typically required to stretch the tensor fasciae latae, should be avoided in the early phases of healing following posterolateral, anterolateral, direct lateral, and transtrochanteric approaches, to allow adequate time for soft tissue healing.

Return to Recreational Sports, Exercise, and Work

Increased postoperative activity levels following hip replacement operations undoubtedly contribute to improved strength, power, endurance, and cardiovascular fitness.[132] Although these health benefits are well known, high-level activity participation is not without risk because prosthetic wear and component loosening are directly related to activity. Although numerous factors may contribute to failure, loosening and wear of the prosthetic components are undoubtedly related to loading magnitude and frequency.[219]

Health care professionals involved in the prescription of exercise must recognize the balance between the level of activity needed for the pursuit of fitness and the amount that may predispose a patient to prosthetic failure as a result of premature wear.[219] Although evidence-based guidelines for return to sports and higher-level activities are few, a consensus of experts in a 2007 survey of the Hip Society and the American Association of Hip and Knee Surgeons recommended a return to athletic activity 3 to 6 months postoperatively.[234] Specific guidelines from the aforementioned consensus report suggest that more than 90% of those surveyed agree that, with experience, golf, swimming, doubles tennis, hiking, road cycling, dancing, bowling, and low-impact aerobics, as well as training with treadmill, weight-machines, elliptical machine, and stationary bicycle, are acceptable activities.[165,219] Activities such as jogging, martial arts, singles tennis, contact sports, moderate- to high-impact aerobics, snowboarding, racquetball or squash, baseball, and softball were not recommended by more than 50% of those surgeons surveyed.[165,219] Despite consensus-based guidelines, it is advised that the individual patient consult with his or her team of health care providers before resuming higher level sport or exercise.

Similar to these issues of activity is that of return to work. According to a review by Kuijer and colleagues,[235] a patient's ability to return to work postoperatively reduces economic burden and improves the patient's economic situation. Tanavalee and associates[236] found that a two-incision approach (small anterior and posterior) versus a mini-posterior approach allowed for earlier return to work. Any surgical approach with postoperative restrictions is likely to lead to delayed return to work, with greater restrictions leading to a longer period out of work.[132] Moreover, discharge guidelines for early discharge had no effect, positive or negative, on return to work. On a positive note, an additional consideration of work status is that those patients with physical work were found to have lower incidence of revision related to prosthesis loosening.[237]

Postoperative Prognosis

Although no single factor determines prognosis, patients who are of advanced age, obese, and female generally have a lower functional status following hip replacement and are more likely to be discharged to a rehabilitation facility as opposed to directly home.[238] Obesity and depression are associated with higher pain levels at 2 and 5 years postoperatively. Age and gender are not associated with higher postoperative pain levels. Female gender, obesity, and depression are associated with increased use of medication for pain.[239] From a predictive perspective, preoperative function is the strongest predictive factor of postoperative function.[132,202] The literature appears to support preoperative mobility and strengthening as interventions that may lead to earlier gains in function.[180,213,220,227,240] Preoperative patient education, in person or by telephone, may lead to a shorter length of stay, reduced cost, and decreased anxiety postoperatively.[175,176,190] The use of regional anesthesia,[241,242] clinical pathways,[243-246] and smoking cessation[247] can lead to

---

> **BOX 6-7** **Risk Factors for Dislocation and Revision After Hip Arthroplasty Surgery**
>
> Use of smaller femoral heads (22 mm versus 28 mm)
> Minimally invasive or posterolateral approach when compared with alternate approaches
> Preoperative diagnosis of femoral neck fracture
> Osteonecrosis of femoral head
> Male gender

fewer incidences of complications. Many patients undergoing hip arthroplasty are of working age and are able to return to work by 3 to 7 weeks and can gradually return to athletic activity after approximately 3 to 6 months, as long as all postoperative guidelines are followed.[165,219,234,235,236]

Despite a seamless postoperative course for most patients, complications exist, and some patients require extensive rehabilitation to restore normal physical function postoperatively.[132] Strength and mobility impairments may persist well beyond discharge from formal medical care, and over-zealous activity may lead to premature revision. A conservative approach is best, with a gradual progression of program variables implemented over time based on the individual patient's response to training.[132]

Survivorship of modern prosthetic implants is generally good; an analysis of 438,733 hips indicated a 15-year survival rate of 84% to 88% when diagnosis, age, and gender were adjusted for analysis.[248] Despite generally favorable outcomes, unplanned readmission and revision surgical procedures are unfortunate necessities resulting from complications. Box 6-7 presents a summary of factors associated with revision arthroplasty for dislocation.[212] Generally speaking, aseptic loosening (19.7%), instability or dislocation (22.5%), and infection (14.8%) are the most common indications for revision.[248,249] The effect of surgical approach on dislocation risk was evaluated with pooled data indicating a 1.27% and 0.55% dislocation risk for the transtrochanteric and direct lateral approaches, respectively.[171] When compared with lateral and direct anterior approaches, minimally invasive techniques and posterolateral approaches are associated with a higher risk of revision resulting from dislocation.[171,212] In regard to bearing surfaces, metal on metal has a higher revision rate than metal on polyethylene and ceramic components.[142] Fixation method outcomes are not clear in regard to survivorship of cementless versus cemented implants.[152,248,250,251] There does seem to be clear evidence that the use of larger femoral heads is associated with a decreased risk of dislocation when compared with smaller femoral heads.[212]

In summary, joint replacement is a common surgical procedure, and its incidence is likely to increase over the coming years, with advances in prosthetic design that meet the demands of the younger, more active patient.[132] Irrespective of technique and implant selection, joint replacement has been reported as efficacious in some manner for improving the recipient's quality of life.[134,213] Outcome studies generally report patient satisfaction and reduced pain, with 90% of patients satisfied with their improvements at 15 years following the operation.[201,252,253] Because

of good outcomes and consistency of implant performance, most surgeons allow patients to return to previously performed low- to moderate-impact activities in 3 to 6 months.[201,219] Future studies are needed to determine the most efficacious postoperative management strategies.

Summary

Hip OA affects a significant proportion of the population and creates a considerable economic burden. The etiology of this disorder is multifactorial, with a consensus of evidence recognizing the role of hip dysplasia, obesity, occupational hazards, and previous trauma. The diagnosis is based on both clinical and imaging criteria, with defined testing clusters providing greater certainty. Evidence-based intervention strategies are multimodal and include both pharmacologic and nonpharmacologic treatments (Fig. 6-21). Goals for conservative care range from preventive efforts in persons at increased risk, deceleration of the degenerative cascade, and improvements in quality of life. Although research has advanced our knowledge and understanding of OA, no current nonsurgical interventions have been found efficacious for reversing the degenerative sequelae. Disease-modifying agents and regenerative medicine show future promise; however, a paucity of evidence is a barrier to widespread use. Consequently, the disease often progresses to destruction of the joint and reduced quality of life, thereby affording a critical role to surgical interventions. Joint replacement remains the mainstay of surgical interventions and is a viable option for those patients with advanced degeneration. Joint replacement outcomes are generally good irrespective of implant design and approach. Postoperative evidence supports activity-based interventions because impairments are common and at times persistent. Although variability exists in postoperative care, consistent precautions exist to ensure a good prognosis. Future research on specific exercise-based interventions, as well as manual therapies and physical agents, will be warranted if functional outcomes are to coincide with advances in surgical technology.

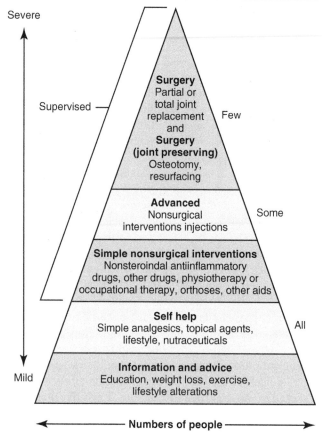

• **Figure 6-21** General Management Strategies for Hip Osteoarthrosis. (From Dieppe PA, Lohmander LS. Pathogenesis and management of pain in osteoarthritis. *Lancet.* 2005;365:965-973.)

Case Studies

Case Studies 6-1 and 6-2 illustrate two approaches to patients with hip pain and OA.

CASE STUDY 6-1

Status After Hip Arthroplasty

A 56-year-old male patient presents with a 2-year history of right hip pain. His onset of pain was gradual and progressively worsened over the past year, with progressive difficulty functioning in his occupation as a warehouse clerk. He recently moved into a two-story house and was unable to ascend stairs without considerable pain. He was recalcitrant

to nonsurgical interventions including lifestyle modifications, physical therapy, and corticosteroid injections. He underwent a posterolateral approach total hip replacement approximately 1 week ago. Based on his surgeon's recommendation, he had a cemented metal-on-polyethylene implant. His preoperative radiographs indicated that he had Kellgren-Lawrence grade

CASE STUDY 6-1

Status After Hip Arthroplasty—cont'd

3 osteoarthrosis and a superior joint space of 1 mm. His discharge body mass index (BMI) from the hospital was 35 kg/m² (obese). The patient has been discharged home from the hospital with an exercise program (ankle pumping, walking, heel slides, and general isometric squeezing of quadriceps and gluteals) and a reacher with instructions to avoid bending forward. This patient lives with spouse in a two-story home and has access to a swimming pool. At the present time he is able to ambulate without assistance and has pain that he describes as intermittent and manageable without medications. His medical history reveals hypertension and hypercholesterolemia. His surgical history is inclusive of hip arthroscopy 15 years ago for a labral tear. His present goals are to return to his previous occupation as a warehouse clerk and to resume recreational activities such as golf and racquetball. He is scheduled to follow up with his surgeon in 1 week.

Case Disposition

The patient presented with risk factors for hip osteoarthrosis that included an elevated BMI, an earlier hip operation (trauma), and occupational hazards. Surgical treatment was indicated based on the stage of osteoarthrosis determined by radiographs and progressing hip symptoms recalcitrant to conservative interventions. Moreover, the patient was experiencing an inability to function at his job and difficulty with functional activities at home. The type of hip replacement he received remains the gold standard because of its consistent performance. Given his desired activity level, current physical status, and the need to be cognizant of postoperative complications, it will be necessary that his surgeon provide some key recommendations at the follow-up visit.

At the follow-up visit, radiographs will be obtained and the incision inspected to ensure that there are no postoperative complications. Because of the procedural approach, precautions of avoiding hip flexion greater than 90 degrees, crossing legs, and internally rotating the hip are still required. At this stage, a raised toilet seat and reacher are still

necessary to avoid hip flexion beyond 90 degrees. Discontinuation of precautions would be based on the surgeon's preference and the method of closure. Although most dislocations occur in the first 3 months and soft tissue is of sufficient strength to stress at 6 weeks, many surgeons continue with precautions for a longer time period. From an evidence-based perspective, it seems that a 12-week period is a reasonable time to respect precautions, particularly when adequate surgical closure was performed, and the patient has no additional risk factors for dislocation. Referral for physical therapy is indicated to help the patient safely improve his independence with activities of daily living and return to his occupational duties. Rehabilitation measures should focus on progressive pain-free muscle performance activities that focus on hip and lower extremity musculature. Progressive strengthening is indicated given the associated muscle morbidity following hip replacement; however, exercises should be pain free, and overzealous resistance toward hip extension and external rotation should be avoided until soft tissue healing occurs. Range-of-motion exercises should be functional and focused on improving hip extension, abduction, and external rotation. Engaging in cardiorespiratory training would be beneficial, provided activities are low impact. From a functional perspective, activities that promote independent stair climbing are warranted, provided the patient is supervised in the early stages. Once the wound heals, water-based therapy may be a useful adjunct to land-based activities. From a lifestyle and occupational perspective, the patient should be counseled to address BMI because it is a factor affecting complications and outcome.

A detailed discussion of job requirements should enable safe return to work with modifications at an appropriate time. Long-term considerations should be made in regard to compulsory job requirements if heavy lifting and squatting are required. Most surgeons would agree that a return to golf is reasonable at 3 to 6 months; however, the patient must be educated to avoid higher-impact activities such as racquetball.

CASE STUDY 6-2

A 1-Year History of Hip Pain

A 66-year-old woman presents with a 1-year history of right lateral hip and groin pain. She reports hip stiffness in the morning lasting 20 to 30 minutes for the past few years; however, she had not experienced groin pain until 1 year ago. She acknowledges that pain has been minimal until 2 weeks ago, when symptoms were exacerbated while performing exercises at a local fitness facility. Specifically, she reports performing unaccustomed exercises such as squatting and stair climbing. She reports a history of sacroiliac joint pain on the right side that was successfully treated with manual therapy; however, similar treatments were not effective for her current pain. Physical examination reveals groin pain with hip internal rotation and lateral hip pain with flexion. Mobility limitations of internal rotation at 20 degrees compared with 35 degrees on the left side, and flexion is measured at

110 degrees on the right side compared with 120 degrees on the left. Strength is symmetrical, and she has no gait abnormalities outside of a shortened stance phase at the right lower extremity. A demonstration of squat performance reveals pain and an inability to maintain hip abduction on the right side. The patient declines radiographs and blood draw at this time.

Case Disposition

This patient presents with symptoms and signs of hip osteoarthrosis. Her age (>50 years) and gender increase her risk profile for osteoarthrosis. Her history reveals a gradual onset of symptoms, pain with squatting, and morning stiffness, which are all associated with osteoarthrosis. Her physical examination, albeit limited, provides evidence of

Continued

limited and painful hip internal rotation and flexion, both of which are associated with hip osteoarthrosis. Performance of the scour test may have aided in the diagnosis; however, the patient meets the American College of Rheumatology clinical criteria for hip osteoarthrosis that includes hip pain with age older than 50 years, morning stiffness lasting less than 60 minutes, and painful hip internal rotation. Given the diagnostic utility of this criterion, once could expect a false-positive diagnosis in 25% of cases. In the absence of radiographic findings, the clinical diagnosis may be further supported with the clinical prediction rule because the patient meets three of five criteria. Meeting three of five criteria has a positive likelihood ratio of 5.2 and is associated with a 14% false-positive classification. The gradual history helps support the diagnosis, and it seems apparent that

squatting and stair climbing exercises were responsible for her symptom exacerbation. Interventions at this stage would focus on first-line pharmacologic agents such as acetaminophen, lifestyle modifications such as sleeping and footwear changes as needed, fitness modifications to avoid exacerbation, formal rehabilitation to address impairments, and instruction in use of thermal agents such as heat. If symptoms are recalcitrant to conservative efforts, second-line oral pharmacologic agents such as NSAIDs or a corticosteroid injection may be of benefit. Alternately, viscosupplementation may be beneficial. Given a paucity of evidence for deceleration or regression of the disease process, regenerative medicine and complementary interventions such as oral glucosamine and chondroitin should not be advised with definitive confidence.

References

1. Christmas C, Crespo CJ, Franckowiak SC, et al. How common is hip pain among older adults? Results from the third national health and nutrition examination survey. *J Fam Pract.* 2002;51: 345-348.

2. Dawson J, Linsell L, Zondervan K, et al. Epidemiology of hip and knee pain and its impact on overall health status in older adults. *Rheumatology (Oxford).* 2004;43:497-504.

3. Thiem U, Lamsfuss R, Gunther S, et al. Prevalence of self-reported pain, joint complaints and knee or hip complaints in adults aged ≥ 40 years: a cross-sectional survey in Herne, Germany. *PLoS ONE.* 2013;8:e60753.

4. Cross M, Smith E, Hoy D, et al. The global burden of hip and knee osteoarthritis: estimates from the global burden of disease 2010 study. *Ann Rheum Dis.* 2014;73:1470-1476.

5. Neogi T. The epidemiology and impact of pain in osteoarthritis. *Osteoarthritis Cartilage.* 2013;21:1145-1153.

6. Murphy LB, Helmick CG, Schwartz TA, et al. One in four people may develop symptomatic hip osteoarthritis in his or her lifetime. *Osteoarthritis Cartilage.* 2010;18:1372-1379.

7. Lawrence R. Estimates of the prevalence of arthritis and other rheumatic conditions in the United States. Part II. *Arthritis Rheum.* 2008;58:26-35.

8. Hunter D, Guermazi A, Roemer F, et al. Structural correlates of pain in joints with osteoarthritis. *Osteoarthritis Cartilage.* 2013;21:1170-1178.

9. Mandelbaum B, Waddell D. Etiology and pathology of osteoarthritis. *Orthopedics.* 2005;28:S207-S214.

10. Abramson S, Attur M. Developments in the scientific understanding of osteoarthritis. *Arthritis Res Ther.* 2009;11:227.

11. Krasnokutsky S, Attur M, Palmer G, et al. Current concepts in the pathogenesis of osteoarthritis. *Osteoarthritis Cartilage.* 2008;16(suppl 3):S1-S3.

12. Cibulka MT, White DW, Woehrle J, et al. Hip pain and mobility deficits—hip osteoarthritis: clinical practice guidelines linked to the international classification of functioning, disability, and health from the orthopaedic section of the American Physical Therapy Association. *J Orthop Sports Phys Ther.* 2009; 39:A1-A25.

13. Lane NE. Clinical practice: osteoarthritis of the hip. *N Engl J Med.* 2007;357:1413-1421.

14. Hoaglund F, Steinbach L. Primary osteoarthritis of the hip: etiology and epidemiology. *J Am Acad Orthop Surg.* 2001;9: 320-327.

15. Palmer AJ, Brown CP, McNally EG, et al. Non-invasive imaging of cartilage in early osteoarthritis. *Bone Joint J.* 2013;95-b: 738-746.

16. Martel-Pelletier J. Pathophysiology of osteoarthritis. *Osteoarthritis Cartilage.* 2004;12:S31-S33.

17. Pearle AD, Warren RF, Rodeo SA. Basic science of articular cartilage and osteoarthritis. *Clin Sports Med.* 2005;24:1-12.

18. Palazzo C, Ravaud JF, Papelard A, et al. The burden of musculoskeletal conditions. *PLoS ONE.* 2014;9:e90633.

19. Rydevik K, Fernandes L, Nordsletten L, Risberg MA. Functioning and disability in patients with hip osteoarthritis with mild to moderate pain. *J Orthop Sports Phys Ther.* 2010;40: 616-624.

20. Hootman J, Helmick C. Projections of US prevalence of arthritis and associated activity limitations. *Arthritis Rheum.* 2006; 54:226-229.

21. Pereira D, Peleteiro B, Araújo J, et al. The effect of osteoarthritis definition on prevalence and incidence estimates: a systematic review. *Osteoarthritis Cartilage.* 2011;19:1270-1285.

22. Roberts J, Burch T. Osteoarthritis prevalence in adults by age, sex, race, and geographic area. *Vital Health Stat.* 1966;11: 1-27.

23. Oliveria SA, Felson DT, Reed JI, et al. Incidence of symptomatic hand, hip, and knee osteoarthritis among patients in a health maintenance organization. *Arthritis Rheum.* 1995;38: 1134-1141.

24. Srikanth VK, Fryer JL, Zhai G, et al. A meta-analysis of sex differences prevalence, incidence and severity of osteoarthritis. *Osteoarthritis Cartilage.* 2005;13:769-781.

25. Gandhi R, Perruccio AV, Mahomed NN. Surgical management of hip osteoarthritis. *CMAJ.* 2014;186:347-355.

26. Jordan J, Linder G, Renner J, Fryer J. The impact of arthritis in rural populations. *Arthritis Care Res.* 1995;8:242-250.

27. Culliford DJ, Maskell J, Kiran A, et al. The lifetime risk of total hip and knee arthroplasty: results from the UK General

Practice Research Database. *Osteoarthritis Cartilage*. 2012;20: 519-524.

28. Agency for Healthcare Research and Quality. *HCUPnet: national and regional estimates on hospital use for all patients from the HCUP nationwide inpatient sample (NIS). National statistics—principal procedure only. ICD-9-CM 81.54 and 81.51.* Available at <http://www.hcup-us.ahrq.gov/nisoverview.jsp>; 2011 Accessed 22.9.15.

29. Altman RD, Bloch DA, Dougados M, et al. Measurement of structural progression in osteoarthritis of the hip: the Barcelona consensus group. *Osteoarthritis Cartilage*. 2004;12:515-524.

30. Cooper C, Inskip H, Croft P, et al. Individual risk factors for hip osteoarthritis: obesity, hip injury, and physical activity. *Am J Epidemiol*. 1998;147:516-522.

31. Richmond SA, Fukuchi RK, Ezzat A, et al. Are joint injury, sport activity, physical activity, obesity, or occupational activities predictors for osteoarthritis? A systematic review. *J Orthop Sports Phys Ther*. 2013;43:515-B19.

32. Ageberg E, Engstrom G, Gerhardsson de Verdier M, et al. Effect of leisure time physical activity on severe knee or hip osteoarthritis leading to total joint replacement: a population-based prospective cohort study. *BMC Musculoskelet Disord*. 2012;13:73.

33. Vingård E, Alfredsson L, Goldie I, Hogstedt C. Sports and osteoarthrosis of the hip: an epidemiologic study. *Am J Sports Med*. 1993;21:195-200.

34. Spector TD, Harris PA, Hart DJ, et al. Risk of osteoarthritis associated with long-term weight-bearing sports: a radiologic survey of the hips and knees in female ex-athletes and population controls. *Arthritis Rheum*. 1996;39:988-995.

35. Marti B, Knobloch M, Tschopp A, et al. Is excessive running predictive of degenerative hip disease? Controlled study of former elite athletes. *BMJ*. 1989;299:91-93.

36. Walther M, Kirschner S. Is running associated with premature degenerative arthritis of the hip? A systematic review. *Z Orthop Ihre Grenzgeb*. 2004;142:213-220 [in German].

37. Williams PT. Effects of running and walking on osteoarthritis and hip replacement risk. *Med Sci Sports Exerc*. 2013;45: 1292-1297.

38. Jensen LK. Hip osteoarthritis: Influence of work with heavy lifting, climbing stairs or ladders, or combining kneeling/ squatting with heavy lifting. *Occup Environ Med*. 2008;65: 6-19.

39. Lievense A, Bierma-Zeinstra S, Verhagen A, et al. Influence of work on the development of osteoarthritis of the hip: a systematic review. *J Rheumatol*. 2001;28:2520-2528.

40. Lau E, Cooper C, Lam D, et al. Factors associated with osteoarthritis of the hip and knee in Hong Kong Chinese: obesity, joint injury, and occupational activities. *Am J Epidemiol*. 2000; 152:855-862.

41. Heliövaara M, Mäkelä M, Impivaara O, et al. Association of overweight, trauma and workload with coxarthrosis: a health survey of 7,217 persons. *Acta Orthop Scand*. 1993;64:513-518.

42. Ackerman IN, Osborne RH. Obesity and increased burden of hip and knee joint disease in Australia: results from a national survey. *BMC Musculoskelet Disord*. 2012;13:254.

43. Jiang L, Rong J, Wang Y, et al. The relationship between body mass index and hip osteoarthritis: a systematic review and meta-analysis. *Joint Bone Spine*. 2011;78:150-155.

44. Karlson EW, Mandl LA, Aweh GN, et al. Total hip replacement due to osteoarthritis: the importance of age, obesity, and other modifiable risk factors. *Am J Med*. 2003;114:93-98.

45. Jacobsen S, Rømer L, Søballe K. Degeneration in dysplastic hips: a computer tomography study. *Skeletal Radiol*. 2005;34: 778-784.

46. Gofton JP, Trueman GE. Studies in osteoarthritis of the hip. II. Osteoarthritis of the hip and leg-length disparity. *Can Med Assoc J*. 1971;104:791-799.

47. Golightly YM, Allen KD, Helmick CG, et al. Hazard of incident and progressive knee and hip radiographic osteoarthritis and chronic joint symptoms in individuals with and without limb length inequality. *J Rheumatol*. 2010;37:2133-2140.

48. Golightly YM, Allen KD, Renner JB, et al. Relationship of limb length inequality with radiographic knee and hip osteoarthritis. *Osteoarthritis Cartilage*. 2007;15:824-829.

49. Golightly YM, Allen KD, Helmick CG, et al. Symptoms of the knee and hip in individuals with and without limb length inequality. *Osteoarthritis Cartilage*. 2009;17:596-600.

50. Beck M, Kalhor M, Leunig M, Ganz R. Hip morphology influences the pattern of damage to the acetabular cartilage: femoroacetabular impingement as a cause of early osteoarthritis of the hip. *J Bone Joint Surg Br*. 2005;87:1012-1018.

51. Lafrance R, Williams R, Madsen W, et al. The prevalence of radiographic criteria of femoral acetabular impingement in patients undergoing hip arthroplasty surgery. *Geriatr Orthop Surg Rehabil*. 2014;5:21-26.

52. Leunig M, Beck M, Dora C, Ganz R. Femoroacetabular impingement: trigger for the development of coxarthrosis. *Orthopade*. 2006;35:77-84 [in German].

53. Steppacher SD, Anwander H, Zurmuhle CA, et al. Eighty percent of patients with surgical hip dislocation for femoroacetabular impingement have a good clinical result without osteoarthritis progression at 10 years. *Clin Orthop Relat Res*. 2015; 473:1274-1283.

54. Lung R, O'Brien J, Grebenyuk J, et al. The prevalence of radiographic femoroacetabular impingement in younger individuals undergoing total hip replacement for osteoarthritis. *Clin Rheumatol*. 2012;31:1239-1242.

55. Sankar WN, Nevitt M, Parvizi J, et al. Femoroacetabular impingement: defining the condition and its role in the pathophysiology of osteoarthritis. *J Am Acad Orthop Surg*. 2013; 21(suppl 1):S7-S15.

56. Philippon MJ, Schroder E, Souza BG, Briggs KK. Hip arthroscopy for femoroacetabular impingement in patients aged 50 years or older. *Arthroscopy*. 2012;28:59-65.

57. Juhakoski R, Malmivaara A, Lakka TA, et al. Determinants of pain and functioning in hip osteoarthritis: a two-year prospective study. *Clin Rehabil*. 2013;27:281-287.

58. Altman R, Alarcon G, Appelrouth D, et al. The American College of Rheumatology criteria for the classification and reporting of osteoarthritis of the hip. *Arthritis Rheum*. 1991; 34:505-514.

59. Hsieh PH, Chang Y, Chen DW, et al. Pain distribution and response to total hip arthroplasty: a prospective observational study in 113 patients with end-stage hip disease. *J Orthop Sci*. 2012;17:213-218.

60. Khan AM, McLoughlin E, Giannakas K, et al. Hip osteoarthritis: where is the pain? *Ann R Coll Surg Engl*. 2004;86:119-121.

61. Khan NQ, Woolson ST. Referral patterns of hip pain in patients undergoing total hip replacement. *Orthopedics*. 1998;21: 123-126.

62. Nakamura J, Oinuma K, Ohtori S, et al. Distribution of hip pain in osteoarthritis patients secondary to developmental dysplasia of the hip. *Mod Rheumatol*. 2013;23:119-124.

63. Deshmukh AJ, Thakur RR, Goyal A, et al. Accuracy of diagnostic injection in differentiating source of atypical hip pain. *J Arthroplasty.* 2010;25:129-133.

64. Fielden JM, Gander PH, Horne JG, et al. An assessment of sleep disturbance in patients before and after total hip arthroplasty. *J Arthroplasty.* 2003;18:371-376.

65. Brennan SA, Harney T, Queally JM, et al. Influence of weather variables on pain severity in end-stage osteoarthritis. *Int Orthop.* 2012;36:643-646.

66. Dorleijn DM, Luijsterburg PA, Burdorf A, et al. Associations between weather conditions and clinical symptoms in patients with hip osteoarthritis: a 2-year cohort study. *Pain.* 2014;155:808-813.

67. Wingstrand H, Wingstrand A, Krantz P. Intracapsular and atmospheric pressure in the dynamics and stability of the hip: a biomechanical study. *Acta Orthop Scand.* 1990;61:231-235.

68. Constantinou M, Barrett R, Brown M, Mills P. Spatial-temporal gait characteristics in individuals with hip osteoarthritis: a systematic literature review and meta-analysis. *J Orthop Sports Phys Ther.* 2014;44:291-B297.

69. Eitzen I, Fernandes L, Nordsletten L, Risberg MA. Sagittal plane gait characteristics in hip osteoarthritis patients with mild to moderate symptoms compared to healthy controls: a cross-sectional study. *BMC Musculoskelet Disord.* 2012;13:258.

70. Dore AL, Golightly YM, Mercer VS, et al. Lower limb osteoarthritis and the risk of falls in a community-based longitudinal study of adults with and without osteoarthritis. *Arthritis Care Res (Hoboken).* 2015;67:633-639.

71. Bijl D, Dekker J, van Baar M, et al. Validity of Cyriax's concept capsular pattern for the diagnosis of osteoarthritis of hip and/or knee. *Scand J Rheumatol.* 1998;27:347-351.

72. Klässbo M, Harms-Ringdahl K, Larsson G. Examination of passive ROM and capsular patterns in the hip. *Physiother Res Int.* 2003;8:1-12.

73. Sutlive TG, Lopez HP, Schnitker DE, et al. Development of a clinical prediction rule for diagnosing hip osteoarthritis in individuals with unilateral hip pain. *J Orthop Sports Phys Ther.* 2008;38:542-550.

74. Birrell F, Croft P, Cooper C, et al. Predicting radiographic hip osteoarthritis from range of movement. *Rheumatology (Oxford).* 2001;40:506-512.

75. Chong T, Don D, Kao M, et al. The value of physical examination in the diagnosis of hip osteoarthritis. *J Back Musculoskelet Rehabil.* 2013;26:397-400.

76. Judd DL, Thomas AC, Dayton MR, Stevens-Lapsley JE. Strength and functional deficits in individuals with hip osteoarthritis compared to healthy, older adults. *Disabil Rehabil.* 2014;36:307-312.

77. Sirca A, Susec-Michieli M. Selective type II fibre muscular atrophy in patients with osteoarthritis of the hip. *J Neurol Sci.* 1980;44:149-159.

78. Arokoski MH, Arokoski JP, Haara M, et al. Hip muscle strength and muscle cross sectional area in men with and without hip osteoarthritis. *J Rheumatol.* 2002;29:2185-2195.

79. Rasch A, Bystrom AH, Dalen N, Berg HE. Reduced muscle radiological density, cross-sectional area, and strength of major hip and knee muscles in 22 patients with hip osteoarthritis. *Acta Orthop.* 2007;78:505-510.

80. Poulsen E, Christensen HW, Penny JO, et al. Reproducibility of range of motion and muscle strength measurements in patients with hip osteoarthritis: an inter-rater study. *BMC Musculoskelet Disord.* 2012;13:242.

81. Dobson F, Hinman RS, Roos EM, et al. OARSI recommended performance-based tests to assess physical function in people diagnosed with hip or knee osteoarthritis. *Osteoarthritis Cartilage.* 2013;21:1042-1052.

82. Basaran S, Guzel R, Seydaoglu G, Guler-Uysal F. Validity, reliability, and comparison of the WOMAC osteoarthritis index and Lequesne algofunctional index in Turkish patients with hip or knee osteoarthritis. *Clin Rheumatol.* 2010;29:749-756.

83. Pua YH, Cowan SM, Wrigley TV, Bennell KL. The lower extremity functional scale could be an alternative to the Western Ontario and McMaster Universities osteoarthritis index physical function scale. *J Clin Epidemiol.* 2009;62:1103-1111.

84. Maslowski E, Sullivan W, Forster Harwood J, et al. The diagnostic validity of hip provocation maneuvers to detect intra-articular hip pathology. *PM R.* 2010;2:174-181.

85. Kellgren J, Lawrence J. Radiological assessment of osteoarthrosis. *Ann Rheum Dis.* 1957;16:494-502.

86. Reijman M, Hazes J, Koes B, et al. Validity, reliability, and applicability of seven definitions of hip osteoarthritis used in epidemiological studies: a systematic appraisal. *Ann Rheum Dis.* 2004;63:226-232.

87. Reijman M, Hazes JM, Pols HA, et al. Validity and reliability of three definitions of hip osteoarthritis: cross sectional and longitudinal approach. *Ann Rheum Dis.* 2004;63:1427-1433.

88. Loeuille D. When should MRI for knee or hip osteoarthritis be performed? *Rev Prat.* 2012;62:625-629.

89. Xu L, Hayashi D, Guermazi A, et al. The diagnostic performance of radiography for detection of osteoarthritis-associated features compared with MRI in hip joints with chronic pain. *Skeletal Radiol.* 2013;42:1421-1428.

90. Dorleijn DM, Luijsterburg PA, Bierma-Zeinstra SM, Bos PK. Is anesthetic hip joint injection useful in diagnosing hip osteoarthritis? A meta-analysis of case series. *J Arthroplasty.* 2014;29:1236-1242.

91. Lievense AM, Bierma-Zeinstra SM, Verhagen AP, et al. Prognostic factors of progress of hip osteoarthritis: a systematic review. *Arthritis Rheum.* 2002;47:556-562.

92. Reijman M, Hazes JM, Pols HA, et al. Role of radiography in predicting progression of osteoarthritis of the hip: prospective cohort study. *BMJ.* 2005;330:1183.

93. Svege I, Nordsletten L, Fernandes L, Risberg MA. Exercise therapy may postpone total hip replacement surgery in patients with hip osteoarthritis: a long-term follow-up of a randomised trial. *Ann Rheum Dis.* 2015;74:164-169.

94. Pisters MF, Veenhof C, Schellevis FG, et al. Long-term effectiveness of exercise therapy in patients with osteoarthritis of the hip or knee: a randomized controlled trial comparing two different physical therapy interventions. *Osteoarthritis Cartilage.* 2010;18:1019-1026.

95. Hochberg MC, Altman RD, April KT, et al. American College of Rheumatology 2012 recommendations for the use of non-pharmacologic and pharmacologic therapies in osteoarthritis of the hand, hip, and knee. *Arthritis Care Res.* 2012;64:465-474.

96. Towheed TE, Maxwell L, Judd MG, et al. Acetaminophen for osteoarthritis. *Cochrane Database Syst Rev.* 2006;(1):CD004257.

97. Trijau S, Avouac J, Escalas C, et al. Influence of flare design on symptomatic efficacy of non-steroidal anti-inflammatory drugs in osteoarthritis: a meta-analysis of randomized placebo-controlled trials. *Osteoarthritis Cartilage.* 2010;18:1012-1018.

98. Nelson AE, Allen KD, Golightly YM, et al. A systematic review of recommendations and guidelines for the management of osteoarthritis: the chronic osteoarthritis management initiative

of the U.S. Bone and Joint Initiative. *Semin Arthritis Rheum.* 2014;43:701-712.

99. Peura D, Goldkind L. Balancing the gastrointestinal benefits and risks of nonselective NSAIDs. *Arthritis Res Ther.* 2005; 7:S7-S13.

100. Lambert R, Hutchings E, Grace M, et al. Steroid injection for osteoarthritis of the hip: a randomized, double-blind, placebo-controlled trial. *Arthritis Rheum.* 2007;56:2278-2287.

101. Qvistgaard E, Christensen R, Torp-Pedersen S, Bliddal H. Intra-articular treatment of hip osteoarthritis: a randomized trial of hyaluronic acid, corticosteroid, and isotonic saline. *Osteoarthritis Cartilage.* 2006;14:163-170.

102. Fidelix TS, Macedo CR, Maxwell LJ, Fernandes Moca Trevisani V. Diacerein for osteoarthritis. *Cochrane Database Syst Rev.* 2014;(2):CD005117.

103. Richette P, Ravaud P, Conrozier T, et al. Effect of hyaluronic acid in symptomatic hip osteoarthritis: a multicenter, randomized, placebo-controlled trial. *Arthritis Rheum.* 2009;60: 824-830.

104. Migliore A, Tormenta S, Massafra U, et al. Intra-articular administration of Hylan G-F 20 in patients with symptomatic hip osteoarthritis: tolerability and effectiveness in a large cohort study in clinical practice. *Curr Med Res Opin.* 2008;24: 1309-1316.

105. Conrozier T, Vignon E. Is there evidence to support the inclusion of viscosupplementation in the treatment paradigm for patients with hip osteoarthritis? *Clin Exp Rheumatol.* 2005; 23:711-716.

106. Migliore A, Granata M, Tormenta S, et al. Hip viscosupplementation under ultrasound guidance reduces NSAID consumption in symptomatic hip osteoarthritis patients in a long follow-up: data from Italian registry. *Eur Rev Med Pharmacol Sci.* 2011;15:25-34.

107. McAlindon TE, LaValley MP, Felson DT. Efficacy of glucosamine and chondroitin for treatment of osteoarthritis. *JAMA.* 2000;284:1241.

108. Wandel S, Juni P, Tendal B, et al. Effects of glucosamine, chondroitin, or placebo in patients with osteoarthritis of hip or knee: network meta-analysis. *BMJ.* 2010;341:c4675.

109. Reichenbach S, Sterchi R, Scherer M, et al. Meta-analysis: chondroitin for osteoarthritis of the knee or hip. *Ann Intern Med.* 2007;146:580-590.

110. Rozendaal R, Koes B, van Osch G, et al. Effect of glucosamine sulfate on hip osteoarthritis: a randomized trial. *Ann Intern Med.* 2008;148:268-277.

111. Rozendaal R, Uitterlinden E, van Osch G, et al. Effect of glucosamine sulphate on joint space narrowing, pain and function in patients with hip osteoarthritis: subgroup analyses of a randomized controlled trial. *Osteoarthritis Cartilage.* 2009;17: 427-432.

112. Zhang W, Moskowitz R, Nuki G, et al. OARSI recommendations for the management of hip and knee osteoarthritis. Part II. OARSI evidence-based, expert consensus guidelines. *Osteoarthritis Cartilage.* 2008;16:137-162.

113. Callahan L, Mielenz T, Freburger J, et al. A randomized controlled trial of the people with arthritis can exercise program: symptoms, function, physical activity, and psychosocial outcomes. *Arthritis Rheum.* 2008;59:92-101.

114. Fries J, Carey C, McShane D. Patient education in arthritis: randomized controlled trial of a mail-delivered program. *J Rheumatol.* 1997;24:1378-1383.

115. Hughes S, Seymour R, Campbell R, et al. Impact of the fit and strong intervention on older adults with osteoarthritis. *Gerontologist.* 2004;44:217-228.

116. Superio-Cabuslay E, Ward M, Lorig K. Patient education interventions in osteoarthritis and rheumatoid arthritis: a meta-analytic comparison with nonsteroidal antiinflammatory drug treatment. *Arthritis Care Res.* 1996;9:292-301.

117. Bennell K. Physiotherapy management of hip osteoarthritis. *J Physiother.* 2013;59:145-157.

118. Ohsawa S, Ueno R. Heel lifting as a conservative therapy for osteoarthritis of the hip: based on the rationale of Pauwels' intertrochanteric osteotomy. *Prosthet Orthot Int.* 1997;21: 153-158.

119. Neumann D. An electromyographic study of the hip abductor muscles as subjects with a hip prosthesis walked with different methods of using a cane and carrying a load. *Phys Ther.* 1999;79:1163-1173.

120. Neumann D. Biomechanical analysis of selected principles of hip joint protection. *Arthritis Care Res.* 1989;2:146-155.

121. French HP, Cusack T, Brennan A, et al. Exercise and manual physiotherapy arthritis research trial (EMPART) for osteoarthritis of the hip: a multicenter randomized controlled trial. *Arch Phys Med Rehabil.* 2013;94:302-314.

122. Hoeksma H, Dekker J, Ronday H, et al. Comparison of manual therapy and exercise therapy in osteoarthritis of the hip: a randomized clinical trial. *Arthritis Rheum.* 2004;51:722-729.

123. Peter WF, Jansen MJ, Hurkmans EJ, et al. Physiotherapy in hip and knee osteoarthritis: development of a practice guideline concerning initial assessment, treatment and evaluation. *Acta Reumatol Port.* 2011;36:268-281.

124. Dold AP, Zywiel MG, Taylor DW, et al. Platelet-rich plasma in the management of articular cartilage pathology: a systematic review. *Clin J Sport Med.* 2014;24:31-43.

125. Sánchez M, Guadilla J, Fiz N, Andia I. Ultrasound-guided platelet-rich plasma injections for the treatment of osteoarthritis of the hip. *Rheumatology (Oxford).* 2012;51:144-150.

126. Battaglia M, Guaraldi F, Vannini F, et al. Efficacy of ultrasound-guided intra-articular injections of platelet-rich plasma versus hyaluronic acid for hip osteoarthritis. *Orthopedics.* 2013;36: e1501-e1508.

127. Zhang W, Doherty M, Arden N, et al. EULAR evidence based recommendations for the management of hip osteoarthritis: report of a task force of the EULAR Standing Committee for International Clinical Studies Including Therapeutics (ESCISIT). *Ann Rheum Dis.* 2005;64:669-681.

128. Pun SY, O'Donnell JM, Kim YJ. Nonarthroplasty hip surgery for early osteoarthritis. *Rheum Dis Clin North Am.* 2013;39: 189-202.

129. Hajat S, Fitzpatrick R, Morris R, et al. Does waiting for total hip replacement matter? Prospective cohort study. *J Health Serv Res Policy.* 2002;7:19-25.

130. Vergara I, Bilbao A, Gonzalez N, et al. Factors and consequences of waiting times for total hip arthroplasty. *Clin Orthop Relat Res.* 2011;469:1413-1420.

131. Leunig M, Ganz R. The evolution and concepts of joint-preserving surgery of the hip. *Bone Joint J.* 2014;96-B:5-18.

132. Brueilly KE, Schoenfeld BJ, Darbouze MR, Kolber MJ. Postrehabilitation exercise considerations following hip arthroplasty. *Strength Cond J.* 2013;35:19-30.

133. American Academy of Orthopaedic Surgeons. *The Burden of Musculoskeletal Diseases in the United States.* Rosemont, Ill: American Academy of Orthopaedic Surgeons; 2008.

134. Lesch D, Yerasimides J, Brosky J Jr. Rehabilitation following anterior approach total hip arthroplasty in a 49-year-old female: a case report. *Physiother Theory Pract.* 2010;26: 334-341.

135. Kurtz S, Ong K, Lau E, et al. Projections of primary and revision hip and knee arthroplasty in the united states from 2005 to 2030. *J Bone Joint Surg Am.* 2007;89:780-785.

136. Mulcahy H, Chew FS. Current concepts of hip arthroplasty for radiologists. Part 2. Revisions and complications. *AJR Am J Roentgenol.* 2012;199:570-580.

137. De Martino I, Triantafyllopoulos GK, Sculco PK, Sculco TP. Dual mobility cups in total hip arthroplasty. *World J Orthop.* 2014;5:180-187.

138. Pollard TC, Baker RP, Eastaugh-Waring SJ, Bannister GC. Treatment of the young active patient with osteoarthritis of the hip: a five- to seven-year comparison of hybrid total hip arthroplasty and metal-on-metal resurfacing. *J Bone Joint Surg Br.* 2006;88:592-600.

139. Corten K, MacDonald SJ. Hip resurfacing data from national joint registries: what do they tell us? What do they not tell us? *Clin Orthop Relat Res.* 2010;468:351-357.

140. Johanson PE, Fenstad AM, Furnes O, et al. Inferior outcome after hip resurfacing arthroplasty than after conventional arthroplasty: evidence from the Nordic Arthroplasty Register Association (NARA) database, 1995 to 2007. *Acta Orthop.* 2010;81:535-541.

141. Mulcahy H, Chew FS. Current concepts of hip arthroplasty for radiologists. Part 1. Features and radiographic assessment. *AJR Am J Roentgenol.* 2012;199:559-569.

142. Topolovec M, Milosev I. A comparative study of four bearing couples of the same acetabular and femoral component: a mean follow-up of 11.5 years. *J Arthroplasty.* 2014;29:176-180.

143. Bozic KJ, Kurtz S, Lau E, et al. The epidemiology of bearing surface usage in total hip arthroplasty in the United States. *J Bone Joint Surg Am.* 2009;91:1614-1620.

144. Huo MH, Dumont GD, Knight JR, Mont MA. What's new in total hip arthroplasty. *J Bone Joint Surg Am.* 2011;93: 1944-1950.

145. Rajpura A, Kendoff D, Board TN. The current state of bearing surfaces in total hip replacement. *Bone Joint J.* 2014;96-B: 147-156.

146. Russell RD, Estrera KA, Pivec R, et al. What's new in total hip arthroplasty. *J Bone Joint Surg Am.* 2013;95:1719-1725.

147. Smith AJ, Dieppe P, Vernon K, et al. Failure rates of stemmed metal-on-metal hip replacements: analysis of data from the national joint registry of England and Wales. *Lancet.* 2012; 379:1199-1204.

148. Amstutz HC, Le Duff MJ, Campbell PA, et al. Complications after metal-on-metal hip resurfacing arthroplasty. *Orthop Clin North Am.* 2011;42:207-230, viii.

149. Jarrett CA, Ranawat AS, Bruzzone M, et al. The squeaking hip: a phenomenon of ceramic-on-ceramic total hip arthroplasty. *J Bone Joint Surg Am.* 2009;91:1344-1349.

150. Pratt E, Gray PA. Total hip arthroplasty. In: Maxey L, Magnusson J, eds. *Rehabilitation for the Postsurgical Orthopedic Patient.* 2nd ed. St. Louis: Mosby; 2007:293-306.

151. von Schulze PC, Pellengahr C, Fottner A, et al. Uncemented arthroplasty of the hip. *Orthopade.* 2009;38:461-470 [in German].

152. Wyatt M, Hooper G, Frampton C, Rothwell A. Survival outcomes of cemented compared to uncemented stems in primary total hip replacement. *World J Orthop.* 2014;5:591-596.

153. Gilbert NF, Huo MH. Posterior surgical approach for total hip arthroplasty. *Semin Arthroplasty.* 2004;15:72-75.

154. Weeden SH, Paprosky WG, Bowling JW. The early dislocation rate in primary total hip arthroplasty following the posterior approach with posterior soft tissue repair. *J Arthroplasty.* 2003; 18:709-713.

155. Hallert O, Li Y, Brismar H, Lindgren U. Direct anterior approach: initial experience of a minimally invasive technique for total hip arthroplasty. *J Orthop Surg Res.* 2012;7:1-6.

156. Lovell TP. Single-incision direct anterior approach for total hip arthroplasty using a standard operating table. *J Arthroplasty.* 2008;23:64-68.

157. Kelmanovich D, Parks ML, Sinha R, Macaulay W. Surgical approaches to total hip arthroplasty. *J South Orthop Assoc.* 2003;12:90-94.

158. Yerasimides JG, Matta JM. Primary total hip arthroplasty with a minimally invasive anterior approach. *Semin Arthroplasty.* 2005;16:186-190.

159. Chung WK, Liu D, Foo LSS. Mini-incision total hip replacement-surgical technique and early results. *J Orthop Surg (Hong Kong).* 2004;12:19-24.

160. Procyk S. Initial results with a mini-posterior approach for total hip arthroplasty. *Int Orthop.* 2007;31(suppl 1):S17-S20.

161. Li N, Deng Y, Chen L. Comparison of complications in a single-incision minimally invasive THA and conventional THA. *Orthopedics.* 2012;35:e1152-e1158.

162. DeWal H, Maurer SL, Tsai P, et al. Efficacy of abduction bracing in the management of total hip arthroplasty dislocation. *J Arthroplasty.* 2004;19:733-738.

163. Dudda M, Gueleryuez A, Gautier E, et al. Risk factors for early dislocation after total hip arthroplasty: a case matched case-control design. *J Orthop Surg.* 2010;18:179-183.

164. Restrepo C, Mortazavi SM, Brothers J, et al. Hip dislocation: are hip precautions necessary in anterior approaches? *Clin Orthop Relat Res.* 2011;469:417-422.

165. Healy WL, Lorio R, Lemos MJ. Athletic activity after joint replacement. *Am J Sports Med.* 2001;29:377-388.

166. Oinuma K, Eingartner C, Saito Y, Shiratsuchi H. Total hip arthroplasty by a minimally invasive direct anterior approach. *Oper Orthop Traumatol.* 2007;19:310-326.

167. Moskal JT. Anterior approach in THA improves outcomes: affirms. *Orthopedics.* 2011;34:e456-e458.

168. Higuchi F, Gotoh M, Yamaguchi N, et al. Minimally invasive uncemented total hip arthroplasty through an anterolateral approach with a shorter skin incision. *J Orthop Sci.* 2003;8: 812-817.

169. Repantis T, Bouras T, Korovessis P. Comparison of minimally invasive approach versus conventional anterolateral approach for total hip arthroplasty: a randomized controlled trial. *Eur J Surg Traumatol.* 2014;24:1439-1445.

170. Pai VS. A modified direct lateral approach in total hip arthroplasty. *J Orthop Surg (Hong Kong).* 2002;10:35-39.

171. Masonis JL, Bourne RB. Surgical approach, abductor function, and total hip arthroplasty dislocation. *Clin Orthop Relat Res.* 2002;405:46-53.

172. Harding P, Holland AE, Delany C, Hinman RS. Do activity levels increase after total hip and knee arthroplasty? *Clin Orthop Relat Res.* 2014;472:1502-1511.

173. Hardinge K. The direct lateral approach to the hip. *J Bone Joint Surg Br.* 1982;64:17-19.

174. Kerboull L, Hamadouche M, Kerboull M. Transtrochanteric approach to the hip. *Interact Surg.* 2007;2:149-154.

175. Snow R, Granata J, Ruhil AV, et al. Associations between preoperative physical therapy and post-acute care utilization patterns and cost in total joint replacement. *J Bone Joint Surg Am.* 2014;96:e165.

176. Crowe J, Henderson J. Pre-arthroplasty rehabilitation is effective in reducing hospital stay. *Can J Occup Ther.* 2003;70:88-96.

177. Desmeules F, Hall J, Woodhouse LJ. Prehabilitation improves physical function of individuals with severe disability from hip or knee osteoarthritis. *Physiother Can.* 2013;65:116-124.

178. Kamimura A, Sakakima H. Preoperative predictors of ambulation ability at different time points after total hip arthroplasty in patients with osteoarthritis. *Rehabil Res Pract.* 2014;2014:861268.

179. Nankaku M, Tsuboyama T, Akiyama H, et al. Preoperative prediction of ambulatory status at 6 months after total hip arthroplasty. *Phys Ther.* 2013;93:88-93.

180. Röder C, Staub LP, Eggli S, et al. Influence of preoperative functional status on outcome after total hip arthroplasty. *J Bone Joint Surg Am.* 2007;89:11-17.

181. Ferrara PE, Rabini A, Maggi L, et al. Effect of pre-operative physiotherapy in patients with end-stage osteoarthritis undergoing hip arthroplasty. *Clin Rehabil.* 2008;22:977-986.

182. McDonald S, Page MJ, Beringer K, et al. Preoperative education for hip or knee replacement. *Cochrane Database Syst Rev.* 2014;(5):CD003526.

183. Juliano K, Edwards D, Spinello D, et al. Initiating physical therapy on the day of surgery decreases length of stay without compromising functional outcomes following total hip arthroplasty. *HSS J.* 2011;7:16-20.

184. Jameson SS, Charman SC, Gregg PJ, van der Muelen JH. The effect of aspirin and low-molecular-weight heparin on venous thromboembolism after hip replacement. *J Bone Joint Surg Br.* 2011;93:1465-1470.

185. Hull RD, Pineo GF, Stein PD, et al. Extended out-of-hospital low-molecular-weight heparin prophylaxis against deep venous thrombosis in patients after elective hip arthroplasty: a systematic review. *Ann Intern Med.* 2001;135:858-869.

186. Poultsides LA, Gonzalez Della Valle A, Memtsoudis SG, et al. Meta-analysis of cause of death following total joint replacement using different thromboprophylaxis regimens. *J Bone Joint Surg Br.* 2012;94:113-121.

187. Stockton KA, Mengersen KA. Effect of multiple physiotherapy sessions on functional outcomes in the initial postoperative period after primary total hip replacement: a randomized controlled trial. *Arch Phys Med Rehabil.* 2009;90:1652-1657.

188. Martin CT, Pugely AJ, Gao Y, Clark CR. A comparison of hospital length of stay and short-term morbidity between the anterior and the posterior approaches to total hip arthroplasty. *J Arthroplasty.* 2013;28:849-854.

189. Peterson MG, Cioppa-Mosca J, Finerty E, et al. Effectiveness of best practice implementation in reducing hip arthroplasty length of stay. *J Arthroplasty.* 2008;23:69-73.

190. Yoon R, Nellans K, Geller J, et al. Patient education before hip or knee arthroplasty lowers length of stay. *J Arthroplasty.* 2010;25:547-551.

191. Bou Monsef J, Boettner F. Blood management may have an impact on length of stay after total hip arthroplasty. *HSS J.* 2014;10:124-130.

192. Maradit Kremers H, Visscher SL, Kremers WK, et al. Obesity increases length of stay and direct medical costs in total hip arthroplasty. *Clin Orthop Relat Res.* 2014;472:1232-1239.

193. van Aalst MJ, Oosterhof J, Nijhuis-van der Sanden MW, Schreurs BW. Can the length of hospital stay after total hip arthroplasty be predicted by preoperative physical function characteristics? *Am J Phys Med Rehabil.* 2014;93:486-492.

194. Raphael M, Jaeger M. van Vlymen J. Easily adoptable total joint arthroplasty program allows discharge home in two days. *Can J Anaesth.* 2011;58:902-910.

195. Guerra ML, Singh PJ, Taylor NF. Early mobilization of patients who have had a hip or knee joint replacement reduces length of stay in hospital: a systematic review. *Clin Rehabil.* 2014;[Epub ahead of print].

196. Nakata K, Nishikawa M, Yamamoto K, et al. A clinical comparative study of the direct anterior with mini-posterior approach: two consecutive series. *J Arthroplasty.* 2009;24:698-704.

197. Pospischill M, Kranzl A, Attwenger B, Knahr K. Minimally invasive compared with traditional transgluteal approach for total hip arthroplasty. *J Bone Joint Surg Am.* 2010;92:328-337.

198. Müller M, Tohtz S, Springer I, et al. Randomized controlled trial of abductor muscle damage in relation to the surgical approach for primary total hip replacement: minimally invasive anterolateral versus modified direct lateral approach. *Arch Orthop Trauma Surg.* 2011;131:179-189.

199. Rasch A, Bystrom AH, Dalen N, et al. Persisting muscle atrophy two years after replacement of the hip. *J Bone Joint Surg Br.* 2009;91:583-588.

200. Rasch A, Dalen N, Berg HE. Muscle strength, gait, and balance in 20 patients with hip osteoarthritis followed for 2 years after THA. *Acta Orthop.* 2010;81:183-188.

201. Röder C, Parvizi J, Eggli S, et al. Demographic factors affecting long-term outcome of total hip arthroplasty. *Clin Orthop Relat Res.* 2003;417:62-73.

202. Brueilly KE, Pabian PS, Straut LC, et al. Factors contributing to rehabilitation outcomes following hip arthroplasty. *Phys Ther Rev.* 2012;17:301-310.

203. Lamontagne M, Varin D, Beaulé PE. Does the anterior approach for total hip arthroplasty better restore stair climbing gait mechanics? *J Orthop Res.* 2011;29:1412-1417.

204. Maffiuletti NA, Impellizzeri FM, Widler K, et al. Spatiotemporal parameters of gait after total hip replacement: anterior versus posterior approach. *Orthop Clin North Am.* 2009;40:407-415.

205. Perron M, Malouin F, Moffet H, McFadyen BJ. Three-dimensional gait analysis in women with a total hip arthroplasty. *Clin Biomech (Bristol, Avon).* 2000;15:504-515.

206. Häkkinen A, Borg H, Kautiainen H, et al. Muscle strength and range of movement deficits 1 year after hip resurfacing surgery using posterior approach. *Disabil Rehabil.* 2010;32:483-491.

207. Sicard-Rosenbaum L, Light KE, Behrman AL. Gait, lower extremity strength, and self-assessed mobility after hip arthroplasty. *J Gerontol A Biol Sci Med Sci.* 2002;57:47-51.

208. Trudelle-Jackson E, Emerson R, Smith S. Outcomes of total hip arthroplasty: a study of patients one year postsurgery. *J Orthop Sports Phys Ther.* 2002;32:260-267.

209. Horstmann T, Vornholt-Koch S, Brauner T, Grau S. Mündermann A. Impact of total hip arthroplasty on pain, walking ability, and cardiovascular fitness. *J Orthop Res.* 2012;30:2025-2030.

210. Meek RM, Allan DB, McPhillips G, et al. Late dislocation after total hip arthroplasty. *Clin Med Res.* 2008;6:17-23.

211. Wetters NG, Murray TG, Moric M, et al. Risk factors for dislocation after revision total hip arthroplasty. *Clin Orthop Relat Res.* 2013;471:410-416.

212. Hailer NP, Weiss RJ, Stark A, Karrholm J. The risk of revision due to dislocation after total hip arthroplasty depends on surgical approach, femoral head size, sex, and primary diagnosis: an analysis of 78,098 operations in the Swedish hip arthroplasty register. *Acta Orthop.* 2012;83:442-448.

213. Brander V, Stulberg S. Rehabilitation after hip- and knee-joint replacement: an experience- and evidence-based approach to care. *Am J Phys Med Rehabil.* 2006;85:S98-S118.

214. Nadzadi ME, Pederson DR, Yack JH, et al. Kinematics, kinetics, and finite element analysis of commonplace maneuvers at risk for total hip dislocation. *J Biomech.* 2003;36:577-591.

215. Tanino H, Ito H, Harman MK, et al. An in vivo model for intraoperative assessment of impingement and dislocation in total hip arthroplasty. *J Arthroplasty.* 2008;23:714-720.

216. von Knoch M, Berry DJ, Harmsen WS, Morrey BF. Late dislocation after total hip arthroplasty. *J Bone Joint Surg Am.* 2002;84:1949-1953.

217. Krenzel BA, Berend ME, Malinzak RA, et al. High preoperative range of motion is a significant risk factor for dislocation in primary total hip arthroplasty. *J Arthroplasty.* 2010;25:31-35.

218. Peak EL, Parvizi J, Ciminiello M, et al. The role of patient restrictions in reducing the prevalence of early dislocation following total hip arthroplasty; a randomized prospective study. *J Bone Joint Surg Am.* 2005;87:247-253.

219. Jacobs CA, Christensen CP, Berend ME. Sport activity after total hip arthroplasty: changes in surgical technique, implant design, and rehabilitation. *J Sport Rehabil.* 2009;18:47-59.

220. Sharma V, Morgan P, Cheng E. Factors influencing early rehabilitation after THA: a systematic review. *Clin Orthop Relat Res.* 2009;467:1400-1411.

221. Di Monaco M, Vallero F, Tappero R, Cavanna A. Rehabilitation after total hip arthroplasty: a systematic review of controlled trials on physical exercise programs. *Eur J Phys Rehabil Med.* 2009;45:303-317.

222. Appell HJ. Muscular atrophy following immobilization: a review. *Sports Med.* 1990;10:42-58.

223. Husby VS, Helgerud J, Bjorgen S, et al. Early maximal strength training is an efficient treatment for patients operated with total hip arthroplasty. *Arch Phys Med Rehabil.* 2009;90:1658-1667.

224. Husby VS, Helgerud J, Bjorgen S, et al. Early postoperative maximal strength training improves work efficiency 6-12 months after osteoarthritis-induced total hip arthroplasty in patients younger than 60 years. *Am J Phys Med Rehabil.* 2010; 89:304-314.

225. Suetta C, Magnusson SP, Rosted A, et al. Resistance training in the early postoperative phase reduces hospitalization and leads to muscle hypertrophy in elderly hip surgery patients: a controlled, randomized study. *J Am Geriatr Soc.* 2004;52: 2016-2022.

226. Hauer K, Specht N, Schuler M, et al. Intensive physical training in geriatric patients after severe falls and hip surgery. *Age Ageing.* 2002;31:49-57.

227. Wang AW, Gilbey HJ, Ackland TR. Perioperative exercise programs improve early return of ambulatory function after total hip arthroplasty: a randomized, controlled trial. *Am J Phys Med Rehabil.* 2002;81:801-806.

228. Hesse S, Werner C, Seibel H, et al. Treadmill training with partial body-weight support after total hip arthroplasty: a randomized controlled trial. *Arch Phys Med Rehabil.* 2003;84: 1767-1773.

229. Maire J, Dugue B, Faillenet-Maire AF, et al. Recovery after total hip joint arthroplasty in elderly patients with osteoarthritis:

positive effect of upper limb interval-training. *J Rehabil Med.* 2003;35:174-179.

230. Maire J, Dugue B, Faillenet-Maire AF, et al. Influence of a 6-week arm exercise program on walking ability and health status after hip arthroplasty: a 1-year follow-up pilot study. *J Rehabil Res Dev.* 2006;43:445-450.

231. Bhave A, Mont M, Tennis S, et al. Functional problems and treatment solutions after total hip and knee joint arthroplasty. *J Bone Joint Surg Am.* 2005;87(suppl 2):9-21.

232. Sashika H, Matsuba Y, Watanabe Y. Home program of physical therapy: effect on disabilities of patients with total hip arthroplasty. *Arch Phys Med Rehabil.* 1996;77:273-277.

233. Harvey L, Herbert R, Crosbie J. Does stretching induce lasting increases in joint ROM? A systematic review. *Physiother Res Int.* 2002;7:1-13.

234. Klein GR, Levine BR, Hozack WJ, et al. Return to athletic activity after total hip arthroplasty: consensus guidelines based on a survey of the Hip Society and American Association of Hip and Knee Surgeons. *J Arthroplasty.* 2007;22:171-175.

235. Kuijer P, de Beer M, Houdijk J, Frings-Dresen M. Beneficial and limiting factors affecting return to work after total knee and hip arthroplasty: a systematic review. *J Occup Rehabil.* 2009;19:375-381.

236. Tanavalee A, Jaruwannapong S, Yuktanandana P, Itiravivong P. Early outcomes following minimally invasive total hip arthroplasty using a two-incision approach versus a mini posterior approach. *Hip Int.* 2006;16(suppl 4):17-22.

237. Dubs L, Gschwend N, Munzinger U. Sport after total hip arthroplasty. *Arch Orthop Trauma Surg.* 1983;101:161-169.

238. dePablo P, Losina E, Phillips CB, et al. Determinants of discharge destination following elective total hip replacement. *Arthritis Rheum.* 2004;51:1009-1017.

239. Singh JA, Lewallen D. Predictors of pain and use of pain medications following primary total hip arthroplasty (THA): 5,707 THAs at 2-years and 3,289 THAs at 5-years. *BMC Musculoskelet Disord.* 2010;11:90.

240. Gilbey H, Ackland T, Wang A, et al. Exercise improves early functional recovery after total hip arthroplasty. *Clin Orthop Relat Res.* 2003;408:193-200.

241. Hu S, Zhang Z-Y, Hua Y-Q, et al. A comparison of regional and general anaesthesia for total replacement of the hip or knee. *J Bone Joint Surg Br.* 2009;91:935-942.

242. Macfarlane AJ, Prasad GA, Chan VWS, Brull R. Does regional anaesthesia improve outcome after total hip arthroplasty? A systematic review. *Br J Anaesth.* 2009;103:335-345.

243. Kim S, Losina E, Solomon D, et al. Effectiveness of clinical pathways for total knee and total hip arthroplasty: literature review. *J Arthroplasty.* 2003;18:69-74.

244. Dowsey M, Kilgour M, Santamaria N, Choong P. Clinical pathways in hip and knee arthroplasty: a prospective randomised controlled study. *Med J Aust.* 1999;170:59-62.

245. Van Herck P, Vanhaecht K, Deneckere S, et al. Key interventions and outcomes in joint arthroplasty clinical pathways: a systematic review. *J Eval Clin Pract.* 2010;16:39-49.

246. Hypnar L, Anderson L. Attaining superior outcomes with joint replacement patients. *J Nurs Adm.* 2001;31:544-549.

247. Moller AM, Villebro N, Pedersen T, Tonnesen H. Effect of preoperative smoking intervention on postoperative complication: a randomised clinical trial. *Lancet.* 2002;359:114-117.

248. Makela KT, Matilainen M, Pulkkinen P, et al. Countrywise results of total hip replacement: an analysis of 438,733 hips

based on the Nordic Arthroplasty Register Association database. *Acta Orthop.* 2014;85:107-116.

249. Bozic KJ, Kurtz SM, Lau E, et al. The epidemiology of revision total hip arthroplasty in the United States. *J Bone Joint Surg Am.* 2009;91:128-133.

250. McMinn DJ, Snell KI, Daniel J, et al. Mortality and implant revision rates of hip arthroplasty in patients with osteoarthritis: registry based cohort study. *BMJ.* 2012;344:e3319.

251. Mohaddes M, Garellick G, Karrholm J. Method of fixation does not influence the overall risk of rerevision in first-time cup revisions. *Clin Orthop Relat Res.* 2013;471:3922-3931.

252. Santaguida PL, Hawker GA, Hudak PL, et al. Patient characteristics affecting the prognosis of total hip and knee joint arthroplasty: a systematic review. *Can J Surg.* 2008;51:428-436.

253. Montin L, Leino-Kilpi H, Suominen T, Lepisto J. A systematic review of empirical studies between 1966 and 2005 of patient outcomes of total hip arthroplasty and related factors. *J Clin Nurs.* 2008;17:40-45.

7

The Pediatric and Adolescent Hip

MELISSA MORAN TOVIN, ALICIA FERNANDEZ-FERNANDEZ, AND FRAN GUARDO

CHAPTER OUTLINE

Four commonly seen childhood diseases of the hip include developmental dysplasia of the hip (DDH), congenital femoral deficiency (CFD), slipped capital femoral epiphysis (SCFE), and Legg-Calvé-Perthes disease (LCPD). Additionally, the pediatric and adolescent hip is a common site of overuse conditions, particularly in the young athlete. Left untreated, these conditions can have lasting and debilitating effects into adolescence and adulthood.[1-5] This chapter focuses on these common disorders of the hip and explores epidemiology, client profile, assessment, common mechanisms, postsurgical considerations, and rehabilitation considerations. Many of the conditions presented in this chapter have clinical presentations that are similar to each other, as well as to other conditions of the hip not addressed here. Differential diagnosis is essential and can be accomplished through up-to-date evidence-based assessments, radiographs, and other tests.

Typical Developmental Dysplasia of the Hip

DDH represents a spectrum of hip disorders ranging from a mildly dysplastic but stable hip to a severely dysplastic and frankly dislocated hip.[6] In DDH, prenatal or postnatal atypical development of the hip causes an abnormal relationship between the femoral head and acetabulum, and it can result in both subluxation and dislocation of the joint (Fig. 7-1). In a subluxated hip, the femoral head is displaced from its normal position but maintains contact with the acetabulum; in a dislocated hip, no articulation exists between the femoral head and the acetabulum.[7] An unstable hip is one that is reduced in the acetabulum but can be provoked to subluxate or dislocate.[8] Teratologic and neuromuscular types of hip dysplasia are related to the presence of other conditions such as Down syndrome, arthrogryposis, and cerebral palsy, but typical DDH generally occurs in otherwise healthy infants, children, and adolescents.[9] Typical DDH can be diagnosed in infancy, childhood, or adolescence. The clinical features and treatment approaches depend on the age of the child and severity of the abnormality. Clinical presentation can range from instability to dislocation in infancy, to asymmetry and gait deviations in childhood, to pain and early-onset osteoarthritis in adolescents and young adults.

Infancy

DDH is the most common abnormality in the neonate, with an estimated incidence ranging from 1% to 3% with

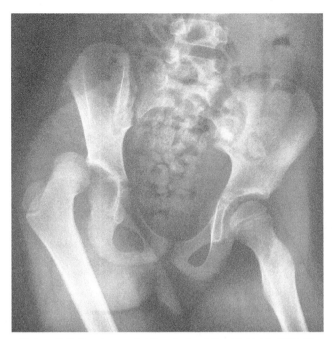

• **Figure 7-1** Developmental Dysplasia of the Right Hip With Dislocation. (From Bontrager KL, Lampignanno J. *Radiographic Positioning and Related Anatomy.* 7th ed. St. Louis: Mosby; 2010.)

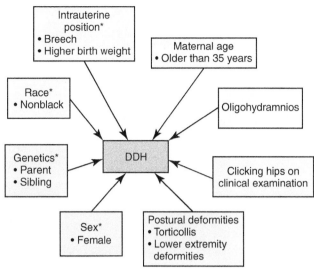

• **Figure 7-2** Risk Factors Contributing to Developmental Dysplasia of the Hip (DDH). The *asterisks* indicate critical risk factors.

clinical examination and from 4% to 5% with ultrasonic examination.[10-12] Approximately 1 of 20 full-term babies are born with some hip instability, and 2 to 3 of 1000 infants require treatment.[13] Risk factors associated with DDH in otherwise healthy infants include breech presentation, higher birth weight, older maternal age, race, female sex, family history, oligohydramnios (low amniotic fluid), and clicking hips during examination.[2,8,14] Postural deformities, such as torticollis and lower extremity deformities, are also associated with DDH.[7] Additionally, improper swaddling with the hips and knees in extension and limited abduction, as practiced in some cultures (e.g., Japanese, Native American, Turkish, and Australian cultures), has been implicated in an increased incidence of DDH (Fig. 7-2).[2,7]

Female sex, positive family history, race, and intrauterine position are the most critical risk factors.[8] Higher rates of DDH occur in female patients because they are especially susceptible to the maternal hormones relaxin and estrogen, which may contribute to ligamentous hyperlaxity resulting in instability of the hip in the neonate.[2,15] If a parent has a history of DDH, the infant is 12 times more likely to develop DDH, and the risk increases to 36% if a parent and sibling have DDH.[16] The incidence of DDH is decreased among black or African American individuals in comparison with all other races.[8] Limited movement related to intrauterine position and breech position at birth are strongly associated with DDH.[8]

Early diagnosis and treatment of DDH through hip abduction positioning devices can improve long-term outcomes (see Figs. 7-17 to 7-21).[2] Screening for DDH begins immediately following birth with identification of risk factors and physical examination of the newborn. Physical

examination includes clinical provocative tests, described in detail later in this section. Screening may also include static and dynamic ultrasound examination to detect skeletal abnormalities and instability of the hip joint. Diagnostic ultrasonography is often used to confirm the presence of DDH (Fig. 7-3). It can distinguish cartilaginous components of the acetabulum and the femoral head from other soft tissue structures, it permits multiplanar examinations to determine the position of the femoral head with respect to the acetabulum, it does not require sedation or ionizing, and it is less expensive than computed tomography (CT) or magnetic resonance imaging (MRI).[7]

The evidence to date, however, does not indicate with certainty that screening for DDH is effective.[17] Universal ultrasonic screening, in particular, is highly debated among experts. Ultrasonic examination has been implemented universally for all infants, or selectively for those infants who present with risk factors, but little evidence supports ultrasonic examination as being more efficacious than clinical examination alone. Skeptics argue that a higher potential exists for overtreatment of hips that will resolve untreated, or treatment of otherwise normal hips as a result of false-positive findings,[2,7] and that abduction treatment can potentially cause avascular necrosis of the femoral head. "The role of ultrasonography is controversial, but it generally is used to confirm diagnosis and assess hip development once treatment is initiated."[8]

A randomized controlled trial (RCT) by Laborie and associates[18] compared selective ultrasound screening, universal ultrasound screening, and clinical screening alone for DDH. This study was a maturity review of an initial RCT. The initial RCT included 11,925 infants born within a 2½-year span between 1988 and 1990. In the initial trial, the infants were randomly assigned to 3 groups: universal ultrasound screening, selective ultrasound screening, or clinical screening alone. The maturity review was conducted

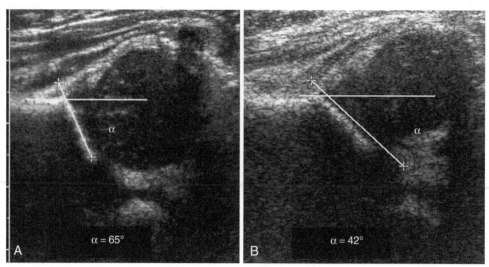

• **Figure 7-3** Normal ultrasonogram of an infant **(A)** and comparison with a case of developmental dysplasia of the hip **(B).** (From Kliegman RM, Stanton BMD, St. Geme J. *Nelson Textbook of Pediatrics.* 19th ed. Philadelphia: Saunders; 2011.)

between 2007 and 2009, and 2038 infants from the original RCT, born in 1989, were ultimately included in the review. Although more infants were identified and treated in the universal ultrasound screening group, and the least number of infants was identified and treated in the clinical examination only group, findings indicated no significant difference between groups for rates of hip reduction in radiographs at skeletal maturity, concluding that universal ultrasound screening and subsequent treatment had no significant impact on radiographic signs of dysplasia or early degenerative changes at skeletal maturity. Additionally, findings indicated a nonsignificant difference in the rate of late-presenting cases; thus ultrasonic examination did not appear to "catch" cases potentially missed during screening through clinical examination alone.[18] Nevertheless, some health systems have implemented universal ultrasound screening in an effort to reduce the rate of late diagnosis.[17] Of note is the finding that increased treatment rates in the universal ultrasound screening group were not associated with a higher incidence of avascular necrosis of the femoral head, thereby indicating no adverse effects to abduction treatment in the study subjects.[18]

Evidence supports routine clinical examination by a clinician trained and skilled in performing tests to detect hip instability in all infants.[2] Despite limited research to support the value of ultrasonic examination, some experts advocate its use through risk stratification to inform selective use for female infants born in breech position.[17] Neonatal screening using a combination of clinical examination and selected ultrasonic examination is recommended by the American Academy of Pediatrics (AAP).[15] Refer to Table 7-1 for a summary of recommendations outlined in the AAP clinical practice guidelines for early detection of DDH.

As stated previously, physical examination should take place immediately after birth, and it should begin with a general examination to detect conditions associated with DDH such as torticollis or other postural deformities.[7]

TABLE 7-1	American Academy of Pediatrics Guidelines for Early Detection of Developmental Dysplasia of the Hip in Newborns
Risk Factor Stratification	**Recommendation**
All infants	Physical examination by a properly trained health care provider (e.g., physician, pediatric nurse practitioner, physician assistant, or physical therapist)
Positive Ortolani or Barlow sign	Referral to orthopedist
Female and breech delivery	Hip imaging: ultrasound at 6 wk of age OR radiographs at 4 mo of age
Male infants born in the breech position	Hip imaging optional
Female infants with a positive family history of DDH	Hip imaging optional

From American Academy of Pediatrics Subcommittee on Developmental Dysplasia of the Hip. Clinical practice guideline: early detection of developmental dysplasia of the hip. *Pediatrics.* 2000;105(4):896-905. *DDH,* Developmental dysplasia of the hip.

Both lower extremities should be observed in the supine position, without a diaper, for the presence of femoral shortening (referred to as the Galeazzi sign), and for skinfold asymmetry (Figs. 7-4 and 7-5). Although asymmetric skinfolds are not specific to DDH, they are a common finding in unilateral hip dislocation, as is leg length discrepancy (LLD).[8] The Galeazzi sign, unequal height of the knees, is elicited by placing the child supine with both hips and knees flexed, and it is typically caused by hip dislocation or

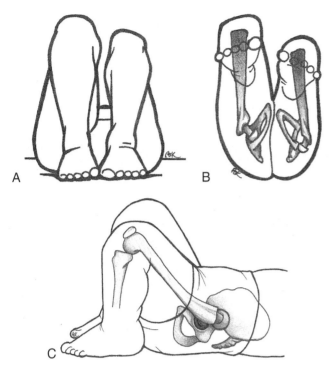

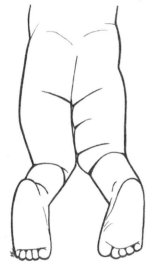

• **Figure 7-4 A** to **C,** The Galeazzi sign indicates femoral shortening, possibly from developmental dysplasia of the hip.

• **Figure 7-5** Skinfold asymmetry is common in unilateral hip dislocation.

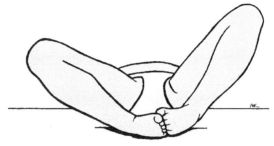

• **Figure 7-6** Limited hip abduction of less than 60 degrees may indicate hip dislocation on affected side and may be helpful in identifying patients with bilateral developmental dysplasia of the hip.

congenital femoral shortening. A higher incidence of DDH of the left hip (60%) than the right hip (20%), or of both hips (20%), is reported.[8]

Hip abduction should also be evaluated because limited hip abduction develops by 3 months of age on the affected side in infants with hip dislocation.[8] Hip abduction of less than 60 degrees on the affected hip may indicate hip dislocation. If DDH is bilateral, the infant will present with limited abduction in both hips. Limited abduction is particularly important in identifying bilateral hip dislocations because the leg lengths may appear equal, with a negative Galeazzi sign, and no apparent asymmetries[8,9] (Fig. 7-6).

Next, the Ortolani and Barlow tests should be performed on each hip separately to evaluate hip stability, by using the following steps:[15,19]

• Loosen or fully remove the diaper.
• With the newborn supine, grasp the pubic symphysis and sacrum firmly with one hand to stabilize the pelvis.
• Place the index and middle fingers along the newborn's greater trochanter with the thumb placed along the inner thigh, and the first web space anterior to the knee.
• Flex the hip to 90 degrees with the leg held in neutral rotation.
• Gently abduct the hip while lifting the leg anteriorly. With this maneuver, a "clunk" is felt as the dislocated femoral head reduces into the acetabulum. *This is a positive Ortolani sign.*
• Proceed to the Barlow test as follows:
    • Position the newborn supine and the hips flexed to 90 degrees and the same hand placement used in the Ortolani test.
    • Gently adduct while posteriorly directed pressure is placed on the knee.
    • A palpable clunk or sensation of movement is felt as the femoral head exits the acetabulum posteriorly. *This is a positive Barlow sign.*
• Each test is performed one hip at a time, with gentle force (Fig. 7-7)

High-pitched clicks are commonly elicited with flexion and extension and are inconsequential. A dislocatable hip has a rather distinctive clunk, whereas a subluxable hip is characterized by a feeling of looseness, a sliding movement, but without the true Ortolani and Barlow clunks. Separating true dislocations (clunks) from a feeling of instability and from benign adventitial sounds (clicks) takes practice and expertise.[15]

In many cases, physical and sonographic screenings result in false-positive findings, and signs of instability disappear within a few weeks. For this reason, unless examination reveals actual dislocation, the infant can be observed for 3 to 6 weeks before treatment is initiated.[7] If evidence of DDH is noted through physical and ultrasonic evaluation following the 3- to 6-week observation period, treatment is indicated.[7]

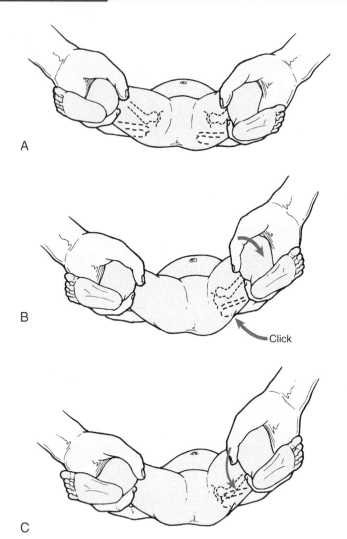

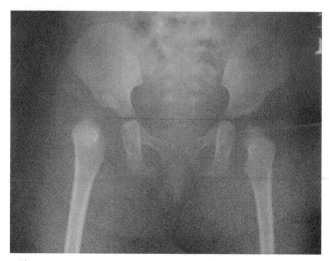

• **Figure 7-8** Developmental hip dysplasia (patient's right hip). This child, in whom the condition was detected at 2.5 years of age, was walking with a noticeable limp and had a "short" right leg appearance. (From Evans AM. *Pocket podiatry: paediatrics.* Edinburgh: Churchill Livingstone; 2010.)

• **Figure 7-7** The Ortolani Sign and the Barlow Test. **A,** In the newborn, the two hips can be equally flexed, abducted, and laterally rotated without producing a "click." **B,** The Ortolani sign or first part of the Barlow test. **C,** Second part of the Barlow test. (From Magee D. *Orthopedic Physical Assessment.* 6th ed. St. Louis: Saunders; 2013.)

Despite neonatal screening protocols and diagnostic imaging, DDH may go undiagnosed until the child is 18 months of age or older.[15] In children who are older than 3 months of age, the Ortolani and Barlow tests become difficult to perform because of soft tissue contracture. At this time, physical assessment focuses on secondary signs of hip dislocation: restricted abduction, LLD, and, once the child is walking, a Trendelenburg limp.[8] These signs may not appear until the child is older than 9 months of age, and limping in response to a weak gluteus medius muscle may be the first sign of a dislocated hip[8] (Fig. 7-8).

Prevention

The period between birth and the first few weeks of life may be the best time for prevention of DDH.[2] Parent education on proper swaddling and improper use of carrying or positioning devices may be beneficial in preventing DDH. Some swaddling practices and devices may position the infant in restricted hip abduction, with the hips and knees in extension. Proper swaddling, positioning, and carrying with the hips in abduction, with the hips and knees in flexion, may lessen the risk of DDH. Refer to Figure 7-9 for examples of improper and proper swaddling, carrying, and positioning. The triple-diaper technique, which increases abduction position of the hip in newborns, has also been used to prevent DDH, with little evidence of its success.[20]

Treatment

The goal in the management of DDH is to achieve a stable, concentric reduction of the hip to ensure that any dysplasia is adequately corrected and to avoid the complications of treatment, the most significant of which is avascular necrosis (AVN) of the femoral head.[6]

Early treatment during infancy typically consists of an abduction positioning device, the most common of which is the Pavlik harness (Fig. 7-10), introduced by Arnold Pavlik in 1946. Other abduction treatments include the von Rosen splint, the Craig splint, the Ilfeld splint, hip spica casts, and the Frejka abduction pillow, although the Pavlik harness is the most commonly used and recommended device[7,21] (Figs. 7-11 to 7-15).

The Pavlik harness is a dynamic positioning device to allow free movement within limitations imposed by lower extremity straps that restrict extension and adduction of the hips. The harness is used full time until evidence of reduction is shown using ultrasonography or other imaging. Successful reduction, or maintenance of a reduced but dysplastic hip, has been reported at rates of 80.2% to 100% using the Pavlik harness, with higher success rates if treatment is initiated when the child is younger than 7 weeks of age.[6,19] Little consensus exists regarding timing of Pavlik harness use, with concerns of overtreatment if it is initiated too early (before

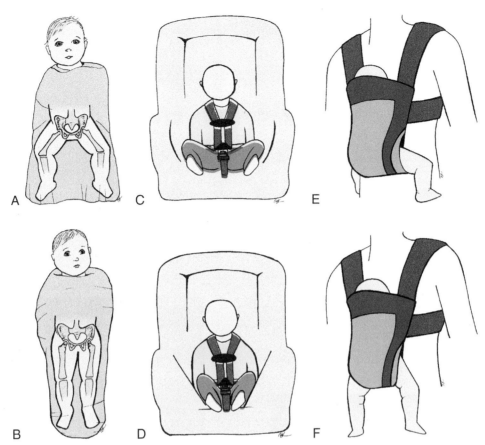

• **Figure 7-9** Proper swaddling, positioning, and carrying may be beneficial in preventing developmental dysplasia of the hip. **A,** Proper swaddling allows active hip flexion and abduction and knee flexion. **B,** Improper swaddling restricts hip active range of motion. **C,** A well-fitting car seat allows hips to abduct and externally rotate. **D,** A car seat that is too narrow or too small restricts hip abduction and external rotation. **E,** Proper positioning in a baby carrier allows for hip and knee flexion and hip abduction. **F,** Positioning in a baby carrier with the hips and knee extended should be avoided.

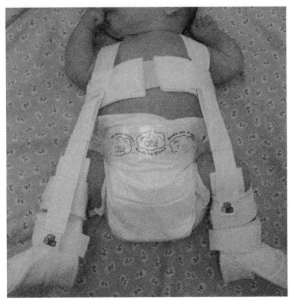

• **Figure 7-10** Pavlik Harness. (From Kliegman RM, Stanton BMD, St. Geme J. *Nelson Textbook of Pediatrics.* 19th ed. Philadelphia: Saunders; 2011.)

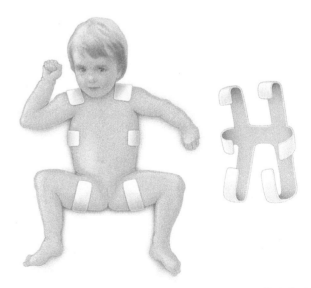

• **Figure 7-11** von Rosen Splint. (From Herring JA, ed. *Tachdjian's Pediatric Orthopaedics: From the Texas Scottish Rite Hospital for Children.* 5th ed. Philadelphia: Saunders; 2014.)

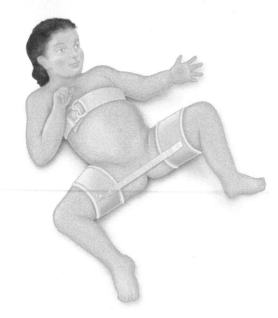

• **Figure 7-12** Craig Splint. (From Herring JA, ed. *Tachdjian's Pediatric Orthopaedics: From the Texas Scottish Rite Hospital for Children.* 5th ed. Philadelphia: Saunders; 2014.)

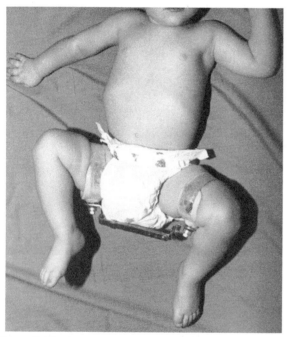

• **Figure 7-13** Ilfeld Splint. (From Hsu JD, Michael J, Fisk J. *AAOS Atlas of Orthoses and Assistive Devices.* 4th ed. St. Louis: Saunders; 2008.)

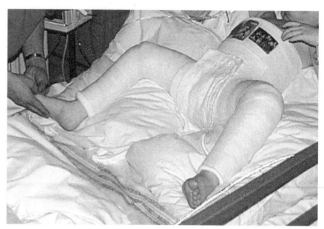

• **Figure 7-14** Hip Spica Cast. (From Price DL, Gwin JF. *Pediatric Nursing: An Introductory Text.* 11th ed. St. Louis: Saunders; 2012.)

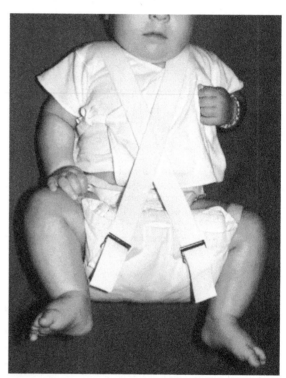

• **Figure 7-15** Frejka Abduction Pillow. (From Hsu JD, Michael J, Fisk J. *AAOS Atlas of Orthoses and Assistive Devices.* 4th ed. St. Louis: Saunders; 2008.)

6 weeks) and an increased risk of failure if it is initiated when the child is older than 4 months of age.[6] The Pavlik harness, however, is the international gold standard for children younger than 6 months of age.[19] Evidence regarding duration of harness treatment is also limited, varying from 11 to 28 weeks.[6] Nevertheless, most experts recommend surveillance during treatment with ultrasonography to determine duration based on success of treatment.[6-8]

If a dislocated hip is not reduced with harness treatment within 3 weeks, the harness should be discontinued, and an alternative treatment should be considered. In these cases, alternative treatment generally consists of closed reduction, with the patient under anesthesia, with spica casting (see Fig. 7-14); this is also the treatment of choice for children who are older than 6 months of age.[8]

Adverse effects of the Pavlik harness are uncommon and have been attributed to compliance issues from parental misunderstanding or physician misuse or issues related to the severity of the DDH.[7,22] Adverse effects include transient femoral neuropathy caused by persistent hyperflexion of the hips and avascular necrosis caused by excessive abduction; avascular necrosis is rare, with a reported incidence of less than 1%.[7,8] Another problem related to misuse of the harness occurs when a hip is not adequately reduced and rests on the posterior lip of the acetabulum for a prolonged period, thus causing blunting of the acetabulum and a form of dysplasia (termed Pavlik harness disease).[7] Close follow-up, early recognition and management of adverse effects, and parental involvement and education can minimize complications and improve success of treatment (Fig. 7-16).

In the event that closed reduction treatment is not successful, open reduction should be considered. Open reduction of the hip in a child with DDH involves lengthening tendons, removing obstacles to reduction, and tightening the hip capsule once reduction is obtained.[8] Complications include femoral head necrosis and repeat dislocation. In older children, open reduction becomes more complex, and by 18 months of age, femoral osteotomies with or without pelvic osteotomies may be necessary.[8]

Childhood and Adolescence

Patients diagnosed with DDH are routinely monitored for residual dysplasia into adolescence. In some cases, children who are treated in infancy for DDH may present with dysplasia after skeletal maturity, and others may not show signs and symptoms of DDH until adolescence.[12,23] Evidence indicates that adolescent DDH and infantile DDH are two distinct conditions with different etiologic factors: in a study of 541 patients with acetabular dysplasia, demographic differences were found between patients with infantile DDH and adolescent-onset of DDH.[23] The infancy-diagnosed group had higher rates of environmental factors associated with dysplasia (i.e., left-side hip involvement, breech presentation, and first-born birth). The adolescent-diagnosed and adult-diagnosed group (9 to 51 years old) had a higher male incidence, increased bilateral hip involvement, and a first-order family history of total hip arthroplasty before age 65 years, thus indicating a separate disease process. According to the findings, adolescent-diagnosed dysplasia is not detected until symptoms develop; this feature suggests the need for screening younger family members of patients with osteoarthritis to identify those at risk.[23]

The most common symptom of DDH in adolescents is an insidious onset of hip pain. Thorough review of the child's medical and family history can identify factors associated with DDH and can rule out other causes of hip instability.[9] Differential diagnosis can be accomplished through provocative tests including the impingement test for acetabular lesions, the apprehension test for instability, and the bicycle test for abductor insufficiency.[1,15] Positive test findings indicate the need for confirmation through imaging.

MRI is preferable to radiographs or CT in children and adolescents to evaluate acetabular morphologic features before closure of the triradiate cartilage, which occurs at 12

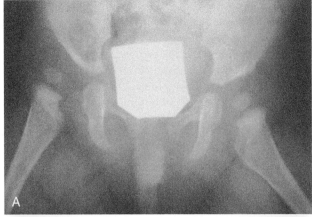

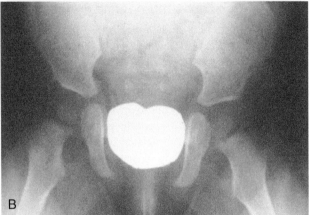

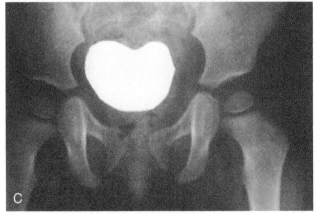

• **Figure 7-16 A,** At 4 months of age: right hip dislocated, severe acetabular dysplasia. **B,** At 7 months of age: treated full time with a Pavlik harness for 3 months. The right hip is reduced, and acetabular dysplasia remains present. The patient continued Pavlik harness treatment for 3 more months, part time (night and naps only). **C,** At 15 months of age: both hips centered in the acetabula with good acetabular development bilaterally. (From Campbell SK, Palisano RJ, Orlin MN, eds. *Physical Therapy for Children.* 4th ed. St. Louis: Saunders; 2011.)

years in girls and at 14 years in boys. The posterior wall of the acetabulum develops late in a predictable fashion. If the posterior wall is not fully developed, a higher rate of false-positive results may result from the radiographic appearance of acetabular retroversion and a hypoplastic posterior wall.[24]

Untreated hip dysplasia may cause early degenerative hip arthritis. Intervention for moderate or severe hip dysplasia in adolescents or young adults is generally surgical, to restore joint stability and mechanics and delay the onset of osteoarthritis.[1] Several surgical approaches to adolescent typical developmental dysplasia are used, including acetabular osteotomy,[25] Ganz osteotomy,[26] and Bernese periacetabular osteotomy.[3] Symptomatic patients with closed triradiate cartilage and no or minimal arthritis benefit from periacetabular osteotomy. Bernese periacetabular osteotomy is recommended and has good results in these patients.[3] For patients who already have severe arthritis and cartilage damage, more conservative treatment including nonsteroidal antiinflammatory medication and physical therapy is recommended until total hip replacement is necessary.[1]

Rehabilitation Considerations and Programming

Rehabilitation after surgical intervention depends on the procedure performed. Immediately following Bernese periacetabular osteotomy, the patient is typically on bed rest, with the knee and hip flexed, and can begin touch-down weight-bearing with crutches by day 2.[3] Patients usually increase weight bearing at approximately 6 to 8 weeks and are off crutches after 3 or 4 months postoperatively.[3,26]

In cases of total hip arthroplasty, home physical therapy is effective in improving hip muscle strength and function when the therapy is practiced at least three times per week, although compliance with the exercises may be an issue for the adolescent patient that can delay return of preoperative strength.[26] Immediate postoperative full weight bearing and intense physical therapy appear to reduce the time to return to preoperative strength.[26] Some evidence indicates that the addition of hippotherapy to a traditional physical therapy program may improve motor functioning in a child with DDH.[27]

Teratogenic and Neuromuscular Hip Dysplasia

Teratologic hip dysplasia refers to the more severe, fixed dislocation that occurs prenatally, usually in children with genetic or neuromuscular disorders.[8,15] Diagnosis and management of teratologic and neuromuscular hip dysplasia differ from those of typical DDH.

Children with neuromuscular disorders may develop dysplasia because of muscular imbalances and abnormal muscle tone that cause the joint to become unstable. Children with spasticity often have movement patterns of adduction and internal rotation, and they present with lower extremity scissoring and internal rotation during functional positions, mobility, and, in those who are ambulatory, walking. These persistent posturing and movement patterns may cause the femoral head to translate over the posterior edge of the acetabulum. This posterolateral, and even global, acetabular deficiency seen in neuromuscular or teratologic DDH is in contrast to the anterosuperior acetabular deficiency seen in typical DDH.[28] Pelvic osteotomies that address the acetabular deficiency and optimize coverage of the femoral head may become necessary to improve hip stability in these patients. Conservative

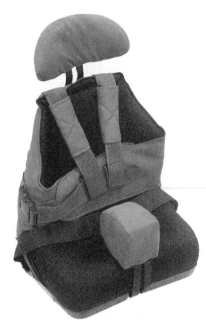

• **Figure 7-17** Positioning Seat. (Courtesy Drive Medical, Port Washington, NY.)

management, including physical therapy, may delay or prevent the need for surgical treatment in patients with teratologic and neuromuscular dysplasia.

Physical therapy assessment and treatments to address and maintain proper hip position can prevent the development of hip dysplasia and can manage existing dysplasia in children with teratologic and neuromuscular conditions. The identification of flexibility and strength imbalances is important to allow the child to obtain and maintain neutral positions of the hip and lumbopelvis. Adequate hip range of motion (ROM) must be achieved through a stretching program, and it should be supported through use of positioning and orthotic devices and an appropriate seating support system that encourages a neutral hip position (Figs. 7-17 to 7-21). Additionally, the therapist should address postural control and balance responses to maintain alignment during functional movements. For ambulatory children, alignment during weight bearing and gait is particularly important. In fact, walking has been shown to be beneficial in hip development in children with cerebral palsy.[29] These strategies can keep an unstable hip from becoming fully dislocated, or they can prevent secondary hip problems from developing in children with abnormal muscle tone and can improve the quality of life for children and their families.[30,31]

Congenital Femoral Deficiency

CFD is a rare birth defect that was formerly known as proximal femoral focal deficiency (PFFD), and it encompasses a spectrum of severity of femoral deficiency, deformity, and discrepancy. Patients with CFD have a degree of lack of integrity and stability of the hip and knee (deficiency), malorientation and malrotation of the femur with

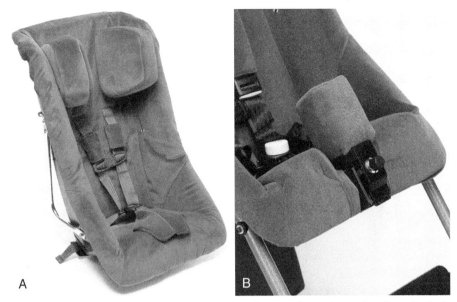

• **Figure 7-18 A,** Car seat. **B,** Swing Away abductor. (Courtesy Columbia Medical, Santa Fe Springs, Calif.)

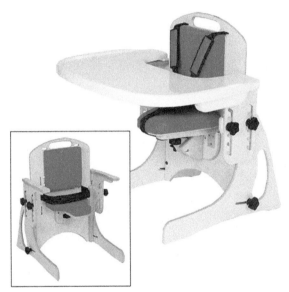

• **Figure 7-19** Hip Spica Chair. (Courtesy Smirthwaite USA, LLC, New York, NY.)

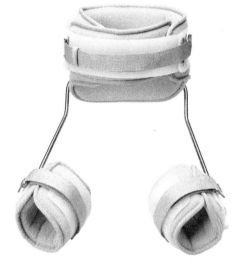

• **Figure 7-20** The Sitting Walking and Standing Hip Orthosis (SWASH) prevents hip adduction in sitting, standing, and walking. (Courtesy Allard USA, Inc., Rockaway, NJ.)

soft tissue contractures (deformity), and femoral shortening (discrepancy). The incidence ranges from 1 in 40,000 live births to 1 in 100,000 live births for those cases associated with fibular hemimelia,[32] and it can manifest unilaterally or in both femora.

Etiology and Classification

The etiology of CFD is not entirely known, but it does not seem to be associated with hereditary factors. Some toxins such as thalidomide exposure in early pregnancy are known to cause the disorder.[33] Other theories that have been proposed include sclerotome subtraction postulating an injury to the neural crest, and more recently it has been hypothesized that a defect in the maturation of chondrocytes at the growth plate may be responsible for the development of CFD.

Two major classifications of CFD are used. The Paley classification addresses radiologic and soft tissue presentations of the condition and is based on factors that will influence reconstruction and limb lengthening (Fig. 7-22).[32] The Aiken classification is descriptive, based solely on radiologic factors,[34] and it is primarily focused on factors associated with amputation or prosthetic reconstruction of the limb.[32] The treatment discussed in this chapter uses the Paley classification system and its recommendations.

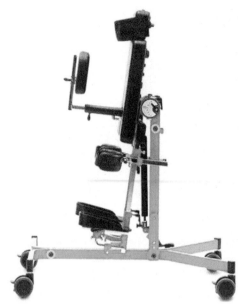

• **Figure 7-21** Snug Seat Gazelle PS Stander. (Courtesy R82, Inc. [formerly Snug Seat, Inc.], Matthews, NC.)

Surgical Considerations

Patients with most forms of CFD do very well with reconstruction and limb lengthening. A surgical reconstruction life plan is important for planning and should be given by the surgeon at the first visit. In very severe forms, Paley type 3, pelvic support osteotomy and foot amputation may be recommended when the family finds a rotationplasty to be an unacceptable option or when the foot is severely dysplastic.[35] Otherwise, with Paley type 3 CFD, in which the foot and ankle are stable, a rotationplasty is recommended to use the strength of the gastrocnemius muscles to extend the prosthetic limb forward (Fig. 7-23). LLD can be predicted,[36] using the Paley growth application software for smartphones.

If reconstruction and lengthening are recommended, an initial preparatory surgical procedure will be performed to stabilize the hip and the knee. To lengthen any segment safely, the proximal and distal joints must be stable.[37] The stabilization operations vary with the Paley classification type, and full explanation is beyond the scope of this

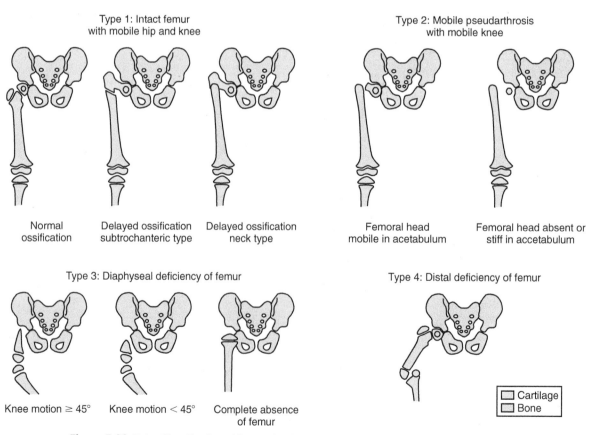

Type 1: Intact femur with mobile hip and knee

Normal ossification   Delayed ossification subtrochanteric type   Delayed ossification neck type

Type 2: Mobile pseudarthrosis with mobile knee

Femoral head mobile in acetabulum   Femoral head absent or stiff in accetabulum

Type 3: Diaphyseal deficiency of femur

Knee motion ≥ 45°   Knee motion < 45°   Complete absence of femur

Type 4: Distal deficiency of femur

☐ Cartilage
☐ Bone

• **Figure 7-22** Paley Classification of Congenital Femoral Deficiency. (Redrawn from Paley D, Guardo F. Lengthening reconstruction surgery for congenital femoral deficiency. In: Kocaoglu M, Tsuchiya H, Eralp L, eds. *Advanced Techniques in Limb Reconstruction Surgery.* Berlin: Springer; 2015:247.)

chapter, but the surgical procedure can take place as early as 18 to 24 months of age. The surgical procedure to stabilize the hip is referred to as a systematic utilitarian procedure for extremity reconstruction (SUPER) hip one or SUPER hip two; similarly, the knee stabilization operation is referred to as a SUPER knee. Both can be accomplished at the same time, although not all children will need both.[38] Lengthening of the femur can begin as early as 3 years of age, once the child has fully recovered from the stabilization procedure (Fig. 7-24).

The initial lengthening requires an external fixator that will span at least the length of the femur and cross the knee to the tibia to prevent posterior subluxation of the tibia during the lengthening process (see Case Study 7-2, at the end of the chapter). Multiple pins are inserted into the femur through the skin above and below the site of the osteotomy to stabilize and distract the bone. This works as an external scaffolding and allows for weight bearing as tolerated in patients with normal sensation. A hinge at the knee allows for ROM and stretches to be performed. Some patients with a hip joint that requires further stabilization during lengthening have external fixation that extends to the pelvis, and they may or may not have a hinge to allow hip motion. Botulinum toxin is often injected into the quadriceps muscle to minimize spasms and facilitate knee ROM throughout the lengthening process.

The lengthening process has three phases: (1) latency, (2) distraction, and (3) consolidation. Latency phase is the time

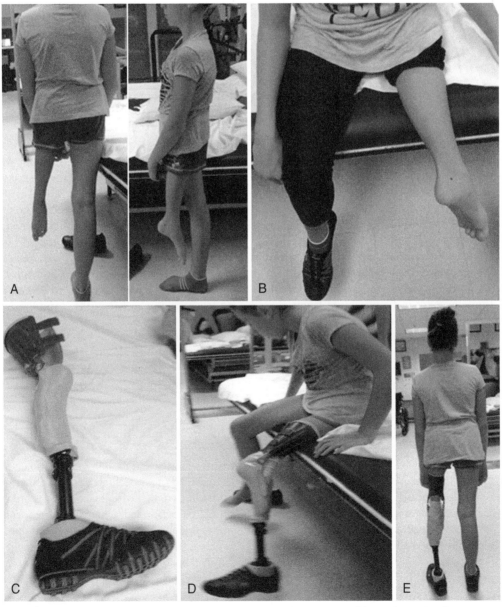

• **Figure 7-23** **A** and **B,** An 11-year-old patient with congenital femoral deficiency, 3 months after rotationplasty. **C** to **E,** Prosthesis worn following rotationplasty.

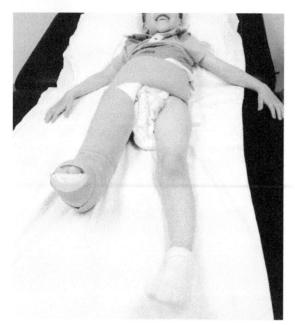

• **Figure 7-24** Four-Year-Old Child, 2 Weeks Following SUPER Hip and Knee Operation. He is in a removable spica cast to allow for gentle range-of-motion exercises and stretches.

between the osteotomy procedure and the beginning of the distraction, and it results in the initial callus formation of the bone. The latency period lasts 1 to 7 days. Distraction is the phase where the bone is slowly pulled apart (0.25 mm, four times per day, for a total rate of 1 mm per day), thereby stretching the bone callus that will form the bone regenerate. The distraction phase continues until the goal is met or the lengthening is stopped because of complications. The rate of distraction can be slowed to address decreasing passive ROM. Typically, 8 cm is the maximum length that can be achieved safely with each femoral lengthening. Consolidation is the phase when the distraction stops and the regenerate fills in, thus allowing the bone to heal and strengthen to support the full weight of the body.[37] This phase is typically as long as the distraction phase in children, and it is 1.5 times the distraction phase in adults.

For subsequent lengthening procedures, the child may be a candidate for an internal device if the length and shape of the femur are adequate for insertion of the telescoping rod (see Case Study 7-2, for PRECICE [Ellipse Technologies, Inc., Aliso Viejo, Calif.] lengthening nail images). Lengthening procedures are recommended at 4- to 6-year intervals, depending on the total length that the child requires if external fixation is used. When using implantable devices for lengthening, shorter lengthening procedures at more frequent intervals are recommended.[35] Another option is epiphysiodesis to the unaffected side, strategically planned to stop growth to allow the CFD side to catch up and decrease the number of lengthening procedures needed.

Rehabilitation Considerations and Programming

Physical therapy is a key part of the limb reconstruction process.[33] The rate of distraction, or bone growth during lengthening, is much faster than physiologic growth and results in muscle spasm when the muscles reach the end of their extensibility. Uncontrolled spasms can lead to further muscle shortening, joint contracture, nerve compression, and joint subluxation if aggressive stretches and skilled physical therapy are not performed. The philosophy of therapy during lengthening is very different from that of most orthopedic procedures. Typically, after an orthopedic operation, the patient is at his or her worst immediately following the surgical procedure and gradually improves over time. During lengthening, however, the patient is at his or her best ROM 1 to 2 weeks after the surgical procedure, and as the distraction of the bone progresses, the muscles and soft tissue become tighter, and the ROM decreases. Once the distraction ends, during the consolidation phase, the muscles begin to soften with continued stretches, and the typical pattern of recovery is seen.

In the Paley Advanced Limb Lengthening Institute (West Palm Beach, Fla.)[37] treatment protocols for patients in the distraction phase, physical therapy sessions begin with active warm-up, which is accompanied, or followed by, moist heat application to the thigh. Warm-up activities include closed-chain activities to encourage weight acceptance and hip and knee ROM. These activities are followed by open-chain activities using active, active-assisted, and passive ROM. Some of the specific exercises performed include active and passive hip flexion and extension, hip abduction and adduction (not to exceed neutral adduction to minimize risk of subluxation), knee flexion and extension with the hip flexed and extended, and ankle ROM. Electrical stimulation is used as needed to address pain or increase muscle recruitment. Kinesio (Kinesio Precut, Albuquerque, NM) tape can be used as needed to decrease knee pain and facilitate knee motion.

The therapist also performs soft tissue mobilization and progressive stretches. One-joint muscles should be stretched before performing the more aggressive two-joint muscle stretches (e.g., seated knee flexion stretch performed before prone knee flexion stretch). Important muscles that should be stretched three times per day include hip adductors, hamstrings, quadriceps to include rectus femoris, and gastrocnemius. Patellar mobilization is also helpful, because the patella tends to ride high as the rectus femoris becomes increasingly tighter with increased bone growth. All stretches should be performed using short lever arms to reduce the risk of fracture. An important consideration postoperatively is that if the child has had the SUPER hip procedure, the iliotibial band has been removed, and the tensor fasciae latae has been sutured to the greater trochanter to serve as a stronger abductor. If the patient has had a SUPER knee, the iliotibial band has been used to construct extraarticular anterior and posterior cruciate ligaments.

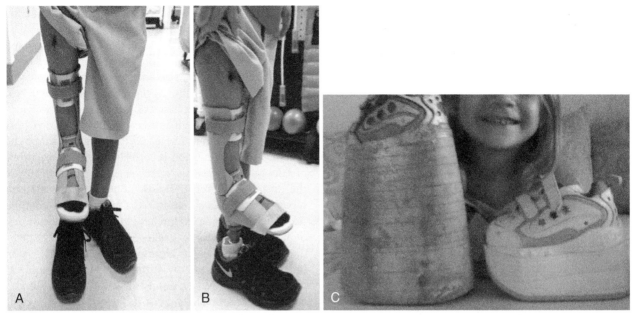

• **Figure 7-25 A** and **B,** Example of a "prosthosis" worn with large leg length discrepancy. **C,** Difference in shoe height following SUPER hip and knee operation and one femoral lengthening.

It is important to monitor shoe lift height during therapy and adjust it accordingly during the lengthening, to encourage knee extension with gait and standing. A shoe lift is typically recommended for LLD of less than 10 cm, whereas a pylon and false foot combination is more appropriate for greater discrepancies (Fig. 7-25). However, these parameters have not been addressed in the literature, are more anecdotal, and are based on many years of work with this specialized population.[32] The "prosthosis," which consists of a laminated ankle-foot orthosis (AFO) with a pylon and a prosthetic foot, is sometimes referred to in practice as a cross between a prosthesis and an orthosis. The prosthosis allows for more of a dynamic response during ambulation and is better tolerated by active patients. Use of an AFO may be needed with larger lifts, particularly if the patient also has fibular hemimelia and an unstable ankle. To allow for foot clearance, the lift should be at least 1 cm less than the LLD. The lift should be constructed with a rocker sole to assist forward progression, and a flare at the base allows for greater stability. Multiple tunnels can be drilled into the lift to minimize the weight of a large shoe lift.

Frequency of formal physical therapy during the distraction phase of lengthening is a minimum of five times per week, with each session lasting approximately 1 hour, based on Paley Advanced Limb Lengthening Institute protocols. During femoral lengthening for CFD, the muscles most at risk to limit hip and knee ROM are the two-joint muscles. The passive ROM of the hip should ideally be 0 to 90 degrees of extension to flexion and abduction of 0 to 30 degrees, and the knee measured in prone should demonstrate full knee extension and as close to 90 degrees of flexion as possible. If knee passive ROM drops to less than 45 degrees of flexion, or if knee extension to 0 degrees is lost, the lengthening will be slowed or halted because joint function should

never be sacrificed for length. If the rate of distraction is slowed by a loss of passive ROM, as previously mentioned, the frequency or duration of physical therapy may also be increased to facilitate lengthening of the soft tissues and allow for continued distraction of the bone. The majority of the time during physical therapy is spent on obtaining knee flexion and maintaining knee extension. Although both active and passive ROM is performed throughout, passive ROM is more important than active ROM during the distraction phase. During the consolidation phase, active ROM and strengthening must be progressed. The weakest muscles during lengthening are the antigravity muscles (quadriceps, gluteus maximus and medius, and plantarflexors), and gait deviations will result if they are not strengthened. The strengthening program should include progressive open-chain exercises against gravity and closed-chain activities within the patient's weight-bearing restrictions.

Once bone consolidation has reached an acceptable level to support body weight, if the patient has undergone leg lengthening with an external fixation device, it will be removed, and a rod may be inserted in the femur to prevent fracture. The patient will have limited weight bearing and no passive ROM or stretches for 4 weeks following removal because the pin sites are inherently weak, and stress can result in fracture. If an internal device was used for the lengthening, the weight-bearing status will be progressed to weight bearing as tolerated. This can be determined only by radiographic review by the orthopedic physician. After 1 year, the internal device is removed.

Slipped Capital Femoral Epiphysis

SCFE is a separation or slippage of the femoral head from the femoral neck resulting from a loss of integrity at the growth plate (Fig. 7-26). The overall incidence in the United States is 10.8 cases per 100,000,[39] making it the most common hip disorder in adolescents.[40] It typically occurs during growth spurts between 10 and 15 years of age, with an average age of presentation of 12.0 years for boys and 11.2 years for girls.[41] Boys have approximately double the cases as girls, and a higher incidence is reported in Asians or Pacific Islanders and in blacks or African Americans.[41]

Common Mechanisms

The displacement of the femoral head at the growth plate seems to be related to localized weakness or excessive stress on the area that eventually results in instability of the plate and subsequent slippage. The incidence of bilateral cases varies widely, but it could be as high as 50% to 60%.[41,42] In unilateral cases, the left hip is involved more often than the right hip. Contributing factors to the occurrence of SCFE may include obesity, hormonal factors, the presence of torsional or alignment issues at the hip, or a history of trauma.[40,41] More rarely, SCFE can occur after radiation therapy and chemotherapy.[43]

Client Profile and Diagnosis

A typical client profile for SCFE would be an obese adolescent boy who presents with the following signs and symptoms: intermittent hip or knee pain, limping or avoidance of weight bearing, external rotation of the hip, and decreased internal rotation ROM. A classic sign is obligatory external rotation during hip flexion (Drehmann sign).[40] Recognizing this cluster of signs as indicators of a potential SCFE case is extremely important because it will expedite the diagnostic process and proper management of a displaced epiphysis, thus reducing the risk for complications. Differential diagnosis may include ruling out femoral fractures, avascular necrosis of the femoral head in older adolescents, LCPD in

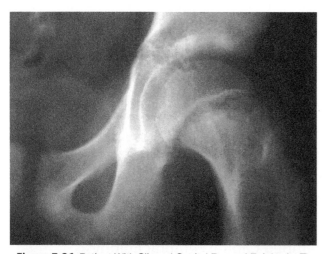

• **Figure 7-26** Patient With Slipped Capital Femoral Epiphysis. The radiograph clearly shows an increase in width of the growth plate, as well as inferior displacement of the femoral head at the medial aspect of the growth plate. (From Swain J, Bush KW. *Diagnostic Imaging for Physical Therapists.* St. Louis: Saunders; 2009.)

younger children, osteomyelitis, septic arthritis, ischial bursitis, and muscle strain, among other disorders.

Diagnosis of SCFE is made by clinical and radiographic examination, and classification is based on several factors: ability to bear weight, duration of symptoms, and radiographic assessment. A clinical classification into stable versus unstable considers the patient's ability to bear weight; in stable SCFE, the patient can bear weight with or without crutches; whereas in unstable SCFE, the patient cannot bear weight. This classification is correlated with the occurrence of femoral osteonecrosis, which is approximately 50% for the unstable hip versus almost nonexistent for the stable hip.[42] Because this classification is prognostic of complications, it has become the preferred clinical classification for SCFE. A second way to classify SCFE clinically is based on duration of clinical symptoms: acute (<3 weeks), chronic (>3 weeks), and acute on chronic (chronic with exacerbation). This classification seems to be falling into disuse in current clinical practice, given its lack of predictive ability for complications and its lack of correlation with overall prognosis.

Radiographic assessment provides a qualitative and quantitative manner to diagnose and classify SCFE, with several complementary measurements that can inform diagnosis and prognosis. Measurements of the amount of displacement of the proximal femoral epiphysis can be classified as grade I or mild (<33% displacement of the epiphysis with respect to neck width), grade II or moderate (33% to 50%), and grade III or severe (>50%). Another useful measurement is the Southwick angle (Fig. 7-27), which is the angle between the epiphysis and the shaft in a frog-leg lateral radiograph, and it can be classified as mild (<30 degrees), moderate (30 to 50 degrees), and severe (>50 degrees).[40] Grade I displacements (<33%) and mild angles (<30 degrees) are associated with improved prognosis and fewer complications such as avascular necrosis, acetabular impingement, or adult hip osteoarthrosis.[40] Another useful diagnostic tool in radiographic assessment is the Klein line (Fig. 7-28): a line drawn along the superior aspect of the neck of the femur should cross the femoral head.[44] If the femoral head is flush with or does not touch the line, this is indicative of SCFE. The terminology "positive Trethowan sign" is used when the Klein line is above the femoral head. Classification schemes for SCFE, along with their prognostic value, are summarized in Table 7-2.

Long-term sequelae of SCFE can cause serious compromise to the hip joint and can alter its stability and function because the damage to chondral tissue following deformity is cumulative and irreversible.[4] As a result, early detection and treatment are crucial to minimize later complications caused by sustained joint deformity and abnormal mechanical patterns, such as femoroacetabular impingement and hip osteoarthrosis.[4,45]

Postinjury and Surgical Considerations

Possible approaches to the management of SCFE include conservative and surgical methods. Although some reports have noted the use of casting in addressing SCFE,[46] little evidence exists on the effectiveness of conservative interventions in SCFE, including traction, rest, or orthotic management. Conservative treatment is also deterred by the problem that the risk of further slipping continues for as long as the growth plate is open. Therefore, the main focus of SCFE treatment is surgical, often as soon as possible after diagnosis. The goals of surgical intervention are to stabilize the epiphysis, prevent further slippage, and avoid complications such as avascular necrosis and chondrolysis.[42]

The simplest surgical approach is stabilization by screw fixation or pinning, followed by a period of immobilization and activity reduction.[47] Care must be taken during the fixation procedure to ensure that the screw tip does not penetrate the joint space, because this would increase the risk of chondrolysis. To ensure proper placement, fixation operations may be performed with concurrent imaging, such as fluoroscopy. Revision surgical procedures may be needed after periods of significant growth to ensure that the joint continues to be stable, so patients are followed up radiologically on a periodic basis until growth is completed. In some cases, fixation of the asymptomatic contralateral femur is performed prophylactically as a result of the high incidence of bilateral presentation, although the practice remains controversial because of the risk of iatrogenic damage.[42,48] Alshryda and colleagues[49] described some of the factors that should be considered in making the decision to pin the uninvolved side prophylactically. These include the age of the child and the etiology of the slip (children who are younger than 10 years of age and patients with SCFE with an endocrine or renal origin have a higher risk of

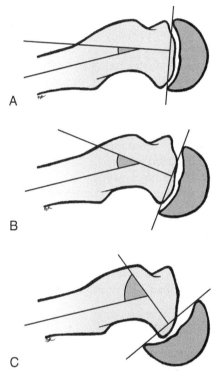

• **Figure 7-27** In slipped capital femoral epiphysis, the angle between the epiphysis and the shaft can be classified as mild (**A,** <30 degrees), moderate (**B,** 30 to 50 degrees), or severe (**C,** >50 degrees).

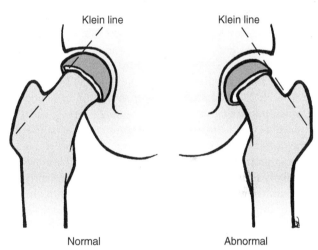

• **Figure 7-28** The line of Klein *(dashed)* is used to detect slipped capital femoral epiphysis (SCFE). In a normal hip *(left),* the line that follows the superior edge of the neck of the femur intersects a portion of the epiphysis in the anteroposterior view. In SCFE *(right),* the line passes above the epiphysis (Trethowan sign).

TABLE 7-2	Clinical and Radiologic Classification Schemes for Slipped Capital Femoral Epiphysis		
Classification Scheme	**Source**	**Level**	**Prognostic Value**
Stability	Clinical	Stable (can bear weight), unstable	Yes; unstable classification associated with osteonecrosis
Timeline	Clinical	Acute (<3 wk), chronic, acute on chronic	No association with prognostic factors
Amount of epiphyseal displacement	Radiologic	Grade I (mild, <1/3), grade II (moderate), or grade III (severe, >1/2)	Yes; grade I displacements associated with improved prognosis and fewer complications
Angle between epiphysis and shaft (Southwick angle)	Radiologic	Mild (<30 degrees), moderate, or severe (>50 degrees)	Yes; mild displacements associated with improved prognosis and fewer complications

bilateral involvement), the compliance of the child and family, and the nature of the current slip (a severe and rapidly progressing case may justify prophylactic contralateral pinning). Severe cases may not be amenable to pinning or screw fixation because of deformity, and they may require advanced surgical procedures such as osteotomies with or without surgical dislocations to restore normal alignment, or even hip arthroplasty.[40]

Emerging techniques in the surgical management of SCFE include computer-assisted fixation and arthroscopic-assisted osteoplasty.[42] Whereas traditional open surgical approaches are associated with significant morbidity and have long recovery times, arthroscopic surgical procedures provide a less invasive treatment method with shorter recovery periods, and more recent reports show promising outcomes for arthroscopic surgery in the management of childhood hip disorders including SCFE.[50]

Rehabilitation Considerations

Physical therapy in the postsurgical period is focused on progressive gait training, pain reduction, weight-bearing activities, core and lower extremity strengthening, ROM, proprioception, endurance training, and return to functional activities. The plan of care must be progressed cautiously to allow for healing after the surgical procedure; aggressive ROM and strengthening should be avoided in the initial postoperative period, depending on the patient's tolerance as well as the surgeon's recommendations, based on the severity of the injury and the surgical procedure used. The appropriate level of activity in the postoperative period, particularly related to weight bearing, is somewhat controversial and may depend on the severity of the slip. In a survey of European orthopedic surgeons, Sonnega and associates[47] found that 17% of respondents did not place restrictions on weight bearing after surgical treatment of mild stable SCFE. However, in most cases, a more cautious approach is preferred. Patients typically remain toe-touch weight bearing with crutches for 6 to 8 weeks, and they may return to full weight bearing once evidence shows healing during radiographic assessment, usually approximately 8 to 10 weeks postoperatively.[51]

During the postsurgical period, activity is increased gradually, along with progressive ROM and strengthening exercises and amplified weight-bearing demands. Progressive and balanced strengthening of hip muscles is important for subsequent stabilization of the joint and full recovery of functional abilities. ROM exercises of the hip should emphasize hip flexion, internal rotation, and abduction; and full knee and ankle ROM should be maintained or regained. Strengthening of the lower extremities within weight-bearing restrictions and trunk and abdominal strengthening are important precursors to progressively demanding functional training. Care must be placed during gait training to ensure that the patient is able to safely negotiate different surfaces as needed for ambulation and participation in the community, while following

appropriate precautions and avoiding deviations or improper alignment habits that could have a long-term impact on the patient's gait. In the final period before return to full activity, including return to sports if applicable, the patient will benefit from advanced coordination, balance, and agility training. As a general consideration, and given that obesity has been identified as one of the precipitating factors of SCFE (more than half the patients with SCFE exceed the 95th percentile weight for age),[41] it is important to address overall conditioning in the late postoperative period for any patient who is obese, regardless of his or her earlier level of involvement in sports.

Legg-Calvé-Perthes Disease

LCPD is an idiopathic form of osteonecrosis of the capital femoral epiphysis that can lead to femoral head abnormalities and permanent deformity. It is named after three doctors who first identified the disease independently in the early twentieth century. The overall incidence of LCPD in the United States is between 4 and 15.6 per 100,000 children.[52] Bilateral presentation occurs in approximately 10% to 20% of cases.[52] LCPD is more frequent in white male patients (5 males:1 female),[53] and it typically manifests between the ages of 2 and 14 years, with an average age of diagnosis of 5 to 7 years.[52,53] Younger patients tend to have a better prognosis and fewer long-term complications, and clinical studies demonstrate better outcomes in children younger than 6 years of age compared with older children.[54] In patients older than 15 years of age, the disease is typically considered an adolescent form of avascular necrosis of the femoral head, which has a worse prognosis than LCPD but a better prognosis than adult avascular necrosis.

Common Mechanisms

The main mechanism for LCPD is an interruption of flow to the femoral head epiphysis through the superior and inferior retinacular arteries (see Chapter 1). The exact cause of this interruption is not always known, although LCPD has been associated with several factors including repetitive mechanical trauma, a history of synovitis that increases intracapsular pressure, coagulopathies, congenital vascular deformities, marked growth spurts during which bone growth may outpace vascular growth, disorders that increase blood viscosity (e.g., sickle cell disease), a history of low birth weight, steroid use, leukemia, graft-versus-host disease, Stickler syndrome, DDH, and SCFE, among others.[52,53,55] The apparent association between LCPD and abnormal growth patterns, both in utero and during childhood, has led some investigators to discuss the importance of environmental factors that could affect normal growth and development. Examples of factors currently under investigation include manganese deficiency and exposure to second-hand smoke, although no strong associations have been found so far between these factors and LCPD.[53]

Client Profile and Diagnosis

Diagnosis of LCPD is based on clinical presentation and medical tests including radiography or other forms of imaging, ultrasound to rule out synovitis, and blood tests to rule out infection.[55]

A typical client profile for LCPD is a child of elementary school age who presents with hip, groin, thigh, or knee pain along with an antalgic gait, a positive Trendelenburg sign, muscle spasms in the iliopsoas and hip adductors with hip contracture in flexion and adduction, and decreased ROM in hip extension, abduction, and internal rotation.[55] A Drehmann sign (obligatory external rotation during hip flexion) may also be present. A child with this constellation of signs and symptoms should be referred to a pediatric orthopedic specialist for further evaluation. Differential diagnosis includes femoral fractures, SCFE, septic arthritis, osteomyelitis, ischial bursitis, and muscle strain, among others.

The first symptoms of LCPD may not develop until several months after the initial interruption of flow to the femoral head that triggers the osteonecrotic episode. Osteonecrosis reduces the ability of the femoral head to sustain loads, and it causes accumulation of microscopic damage in bone areas that are poorly equipped to repair this insult, with deformation of the femoral head secondary to subchondral fractures.[54] Subsequent revascularization and reabsorption of the necrotic bone are biologically intended as a repair mechanism and make the disease self-limiting, which is a positive development in the natural history of LCPD. However, this repair process actually has the undesirable side effect of contributing to further deformity (Fig. 7-29), because of the imbalance between bone resorption and

formation.[56] As a result, the natural healing mechanisms that are activated in response to the original loss of vascularization essentially perpetuate some of the mechanical dysfunction caused by the disease.

Prognostic Factors

The natural history of LCPD is self-limited and includes four stages of progression based on radiologic findings (known as Waldenström's classification).[56] The stages are as follows:

1. The initial stage or condensation stage, in which the femoral head becomes necrotic after loss of vascularization, with mild flattening and increased radiodensity of the ossific nucleus, and widening of the medial joint space
2. The fragmentation stage or resorptive state, with increased flattening and fragmented appearance of the ossific nucleus in response to increased osteoclastic activity
3. The reossification stage or healing stage, with appearance of new bone deposited by osteoblasts and disappearance of radiodense fragments
4. The residual stage, with normal radiodensity of the femoral head and remodeling of the head and the acetabulum. In this stage, the shape of the femoral head may still change throughout the process of skeletal maturation.

Long-term outcomes are determined by remodeling of the femoral head and the acetabulum and by the combined biomechanics of the end products of this remodeling. The remodeling process may not be finalized until up to 5 years after the initial episode, and skeletal maturation also has an influence on the ultimate outcome.[54] Based on the need to guide intervention in the earlier stages to prevent severe deformity, other investigators have created prognostic classification systems that can be applied at the fragmentation stage to predict possible outcomes and guide management. Examples include the Salter-Thompson classification, the Catterall classification, and the lateral pillar classification, among others. The Salter-Thompson classification is guided by the observation of a crescent sign indicating a subchondral fracture, and it classifies femoral head involvement in the fracture as group A (<50% involvement) or group B (>50% involvement), with group A best suited for noninvasive treatment.[54] In the Catterall classification (Fig. 7-30), the extent of femoral head involvement is labeled by groups I through IV, which signify up to 25%, 50%, 75%, and complete femoral head involvement, respectively. Groups III and IV are associated with poor outcomes.[54] In the lateral pillar classification (Fig. 7-31), the lateral pillar is defined as the lateral 15% to 30% of the epiphysis. Then, the height of the lateral pillar is used to label imaging observations into group A (no loss of height), B (< 50% height loss), or C (>50% height loss), with an optional B/C group border that labels 50% height loss. Groups B and C have worse outcomes than group A. Some studies report that the lateral pillar and Salter-Thompson classification methods are better predictors of outcomes at

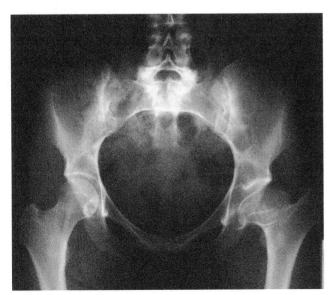

• **Figure 7-29** Patient With Legg-Calvé-Perthes Disease. Compare the healthy right femoral head (*left side* of the image) with the affected left femoral head (*right side* of the image). (From Swain J, Bush KW. *Diagnostic Imaging for Physical Therapists*. St. Louis: Saunders; 2009.)

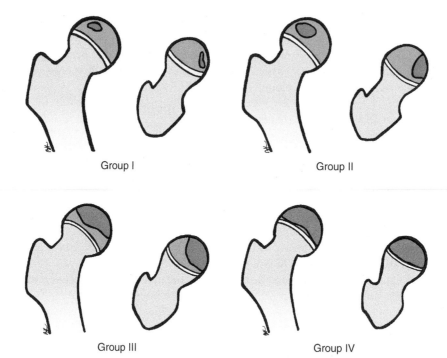

• **Figure 7-30** Catterall Classification of Legg-Calvé-Perthes Disease. Involvement of the femoral head is progressively classified into groups I through IV (<25%, <50%, <75%, complete involvement).

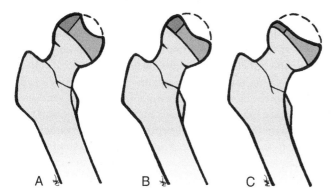

• **Figure 7-31** Lateral Pillar Classification of Legg-Calvé-Perthes Disease, Based on the Height of the Lateral 15% to 30% of the Epiphysis. The *dashed line* represents the complete shape of a healthy capital femoral epiphysis for comparison. **A,** Group A has no loss of height. **B,** Group B has less than 50% height loss. **C,** Group C has more than 50% height loss.

skeletal maturity than the Catterall method.[54,57] However, controversy remains regarding which classification system can best guide management.[58]

An important conundrum of these prognostic classification systems is that although they can guide treatment, one must be able to observe damage to make an appropriate classification based on the radiograph. In the case of the Salter-Thompson classification, the crescent sign can already be observed at the initial fragmentation stage, but it may be transient and easy to miss.[54] Use of the Catterall and lateral pillar classifications is possible only later in the disease, because significant fragmentation must have

occurred to classify patients properly into their corresponding groups. As a result, in waiting to make a classification, the window of opportunity for early treatment may be missed. Current efforts in classification are geared toward using other forms of imaging that may provide earlier clues to guide treatment choices.

Several studies have looked at other prognostic factors that can help indicate whether to choose watchful waiting or direct intervention. In general, age seems to be a strong predictor of outcomes, with children younger than 6 years of age having better outcomes and children older than 10 years of age having poorer outcomes. In a 5-year study done in Norway,[59] risk factors for poor outcome included age of 6 years or older at diagnosis, degree of femoral head necrosis, height of the lateral pillar of the epiphysis less than 50% of normal height, and femoral head coverage less than 80%. The investigators concluded that most children younger than 6 years of age do not need special treatment, and surgical containment in older children is indicated only when an additional two or more of the foregoing risk factors are present. Although prognosis is better in younger patients, poor outcomes can be observed even in patients younger than 6 years of age who have large necrotic areas. In another study, Nakamura and associates[60] followed 100 patients from younger than 6 years of age (mean age, 4.5 years) to skeletal maturity. The patients had been diagnosed with unilateral or bilateral LCPD and subsequently underwent repair of the epiphysis. The investigators determined that lateral pillar classification (odds ratio, 3.6) and hip abduction range (odds ratio, 4.0) were strong prognostic factors in patients' outcomes.

Surgical and Rehabilitation Considerations

The natural course of the disease is self-limiting, and eventual revascularization and remodeling occur. Therefore, treatment is needed only in those children who are likely to experience femoral deformity during the revascularization process, which occurs over several years.[61] As previously mentioned, the remodeling process itself is intimately related to the development and perpetuation of deformity. Treatment is aimed at helping minimize damage to the joint during the recovery process, reducing pain, and decreasing the likelihood of long-term complications such as severe deformity and osteoarthritis. Treatment approaches may include ROM, limiting weight bearing, containment, and distraction. ROM interventions and reductions in weight bearing have limited benefits when applied in isolation. However, evidence indicates that these approaches are beneficial when they are applied in combination with containment and that appropriate ROM, obtained by physical therapy, short-term traction, or casting, is a prerequisite for successful containment.[61,62]

Containment is indicated in children older than 8 years of age or in a child of any age who shows signs of femoral head extrusion; this treatment should be provided in the early stages of fragmentation.[62] Containment has the goal of maintaining appropriate contact and proper load distribution between the capital femoral epiphysis and the acetabulum, to reduce stresses on the epiphysis.[62] This involves placing the femur in abduction and internal rotation, or abduction and flexion, and it can be accomplished with orthotics (e.g., Petrie casts or A-frame orthoses) or surgically. In general, the trend has been toward a reduction in orthotic management based on lack of evidence of effectiveness, although this is controversial.[63-65] In younger children (up to 8 years old), orthotic and surgical outcomes seem to be more comparable, whereas for older children, surgical outcomes are clearly superior.[61] Surgical approaches may include varus osteotomies of the femoral head, pelvic osteotomies to modify the orientation of the acetabulum, or creation of a bony shelf over the epiphysis.[62] In patients with severe cases in which the femoral head is significantly deformed, extensive reconstructive surgery may be necessary to restore the shape of the femoral head and ensure congruency with the acetabulum,[66] and soft tissue release may be necessary to optimize outcomes. Physical therapy is an important adjuvant to both orthotic and surgical approaches to containment. In the preintervention period, it is paramount to obtain adequate ROM and to reduce iliopsoas and adductor spasms and their associated contractures for the containment process to be successful. In the postcontainment period, rehabilitation programming includes progressive gait training and weight-bearing activities, pain reduction, strengthening with special emphasis on retraining gluteus medius and stabilizers of the hip, ROM of the hips in all planes, core conditioning, and training for return to functional activities.

The Cincinnati Children's Hospital Medical Center has published evidence-based guidelines for the management of children 3 to 12 years old after surgical treatment of LCPD.[67] In the initial phase of outpatient rehabilitation (0 to 2 weeks after cast removal), physical therapy services are typically provided 2 to 3 times per week, with the goals to reduce pain, maintain skin integrity, improve functional mobility, increase or maintain ROM (hip, knee, and ankle in all planes), and strengthen the hip (3/5 or greater in flexion, abduction, and extension) and the knee and ankle (3+/5 or greater). In the intermediate phase (2 to 6 weeks after cast removal), the goal is to increase the strength of the hip and knee to 60% of the healthy lower extremity, with the exception of the hip abductors, which should be strengthened to 50%. At this time, the patient can begin closed-chain exercises with little resistance (<50% body weight on affected side) as long as weight-bearing status permits. In the advanced phase (6 to 12 weeks after removal), ambulation without an assistive device is typically possible, and functional training can be progressed to more challenging activities.

Distraction is another approach that can be successfully used when surgical containment is not possible because of restrictions in ROM at the hip.[68] Hosny and associates[69] followed 29 patients (8 to 14 years old, 76% male, all with unilateral cases of LCPD) for a minimum of 2.5 years after they underwent distraction. The investigators found that 93% of patients showed ROM improvement, and 86% of patients had a significant improvement in pain. Distraction is applied with an external fixator that can be monolateral or circular and whose rotating axis is aligned with the axis of motion for hip flexion and extension.[68] Patients can start bearing partial weight 2 days after the insertion of the fixator, and distraction commences on day 3 at a rate of 1 mm per day.[68] Physical therapy during the distraction process is key to maintaining mobility and supporting tissue lengthening, and it is typically provided daily. Possible complications of the distraction process include pin infections, breakage, or subluxation.[68]

Other promising approaches to the management of LCPD include core decompression and transfemoral head–neck tunneling or transphyseal neck–head drilling. In these procedures, drilling through the femoral head and neck is performed to remove necrotic bone, relieve pain, and improve vascularization. A shelf acetabuloplasty is typically also performed to provide better coverage for the femoral head.[70]

Current research on novel strategies to treat LCPD includes a focus on pharmaceutical and biologic interventions based on available knowledge of the pathophysiology of the disease.[71] An example is the use of combinations of bone morphogenetic proteins (BMPs) and bisphosphonates, which act synergistically in repairing bone. Cheng and colleagues[72] reported that in a piglet model, simultaneous administration of BMP and bisphosphonates resulted in a significant reduction in deformity of the femoral head, reduction in number of osteoclasts, and increase in formation of trabecular bone; however, some instances of capsular heterotopic ossification occurred as a side effect. Other novel agents currently under investigation include sclerostin antibody and tumor necrosis factor-alpha.[71]

A final thought regarding management of LCPD in children is the need to consider long-term outcomes observed in adulthood. Although treatment is successful in many cases by using one or several of the approaches described earlier, and children who had LCPD are able to achieve good functional outcomes and a full recovery, the femoral head may eventually collapse or become osteoarthritic in young adults who had LCPD as children.[73] In such cases, total hip resurfacing or total hip arthroplasty may be the only treatment option available to these patients.

Overuse and Sports-Related Injuries of the Hip

Approximately 40 million boys and girls participate in organized youth sports in the United States each year.

Children and adolescents may be more prone to sports-related injury than adults because of physical and physiologic differences.[74,75] Bone growth occurs at a faster rate than muscle tendon growth, with resulting lack of flexibility and increased stress on tendons, musculotendinous junctions, and apophyses that predispose adolescents to injury during sports.[74] Open physes and growing cartilage are also susceptible to injuries, early physeal closure, and fractures.[75] This section briefly describes the overuse injuries commonly seen in the young athlete. Most of the injuries presented are discussed in great detail in other chapters within this book (i.e., Chapters 8 and 11), and thus our focus is on etiology, differential diagnosis, and special considerations specific to the pediatric and adolescent population.

It is important to differentiate between intraarticular and extraarticular hip disorders in the young athlete.[75,76] Refer to Figure 7-32 for a list of common intraarticular and extraarticular injuries to the young athlete, including causes, signs, and symptoms. Extraarticular injuries are more common in this population. Extraarticular injuries

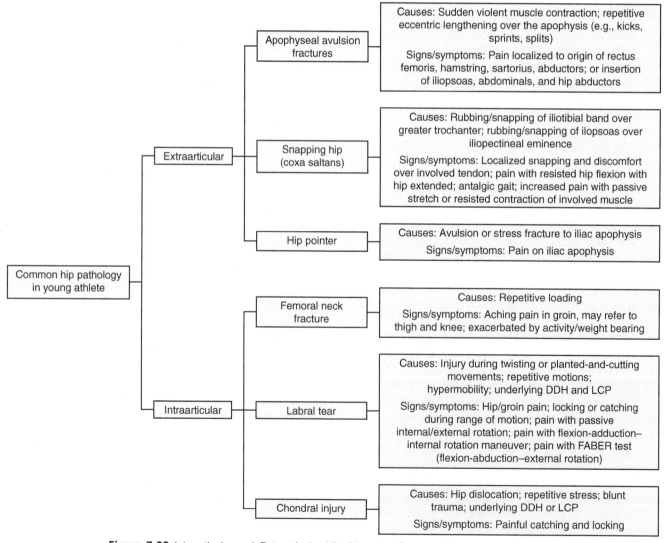

• **Figure 7-32** Intraarticular and Extraarticular Hip Disorders Common in Young Athletes. *DDH,* Developmental dysplasia of the hip; *LCP,* Legg-Calvé-Perthes disease.

commonly seen include apophyseal avulsion fracture, snapping hip (coxa sultans), and hip pointers.

The source of snapping hip pain may be the iliotibial band snapping (external) over the greater trochanter during hip movement from flexion to extension, or the iliopsoas snapping (internal) over the iliopectineal eminence (see Chapters 3 and 8 for detailed discussions on snapping hip syndrome).

"Hip pointer" is a general term for pain on the iliac apophysis caused by avulsion, stress fracture, or hematoma.[76] It is often seen in sports such as rugby, football, or other contact sports, and it is caused by a direct blow to the iliac crest that produces bruising of both bony and soft tissue. Refer to Chapter 11 for more information about diagnosis and management of hip pointers.

Intraarticular sources of hip pain commonly seen in young athletes include femoral neck stress fracture, ligamentum teres disorders, labral tears, chondral injuries (with or without loose bodies), and SCFE. SCFE is discussed in detail earlier in this chapter and thus is not addressed in this section. Intraarticular hip disorders may be difficult for the young athlete to describe, and symptoms may be vague and less localized: the patient may make a "C" shape around the hip with his or her hand when asked to identify the location of the pain.[75,76]

Labral tears in young athletes are typically caused by injury during twisting, or planting and cutting motions, or by repetitive stress, and they are commonly seen in runners and dancers.[74,76] They may also be caused by an underlying abnormal relationship between the femoral head and the acetabulum that is caused by DDH or LCPD.[76] Femoroacetabular impingement, labral tears, and chondral injury are discussed in Chapters 4 and 8. DDH and LCPD are addressed in detail earlier in this chapter.

Femoral neck fractures are caused by repetitive activity and microtrauma. Femoral neck stress fractures are most commonly seen in runners and young military recruits.[74,76] Girls and women are at greater risk, particularly those with the female athlete triad of amenorrhea, premature osteoporosis, and eating disorder.[76-80] Symptoms include groin ache-like pain, with possible referral into the thigh or knee, that is exacerbated by activity and weight bearing and relieved by rest. Physical signs include limited hip ROM and antalgic gait.[76]

Case Studies

Examples of pediatric conditions are provided in Case Studies 7-1 to 7-4.

CASE STUDY 7-1

Hip Dysplasia: Importance of Positioning and Equipment in Postural Alignment and Progressive Deformity in a Child With Dystonic Cerebral Palsy*

Thomas was a bright, articulate, 6-year-old boy with a diagnosis of dystonic cerebral palsy. He was first seen by his current physical therapist for the first time when his family had recently moved from another state. He was very proficient using his manual wheelchair, which he primarily pushed with left hand while intermittently using his right hand to guide the opposite wheel (Fig. 7-33).

The family reported that Thomas received his first wheelchair at 4 years of age. At first glance, the wheelchair had the positive features of a cute, small, lightweight frame, which was easily maneuvered by the patient. However, after looking more closely, some features were noted that may have been less than optimal and could potentially be problematic for the patient over time. The narrow seat resulted in a narrow base of support, which challenged the patient's balance in sitting. The short seat depth, with no trunk or hip guides or anterior chest support for stability, resulted in rounded thoracic spine and asymmetric alignment (Fig. 7-34).

Thomas also had increased dystonic posturing when he was self-propelling because of the effort of pushing and controlling the wheelchair. This resulted in increased trunk rotation to the left and windswept posturing to the right as he tried to stabilize his trunk and limbs to move the chair efficiently.

When Thomas was laid in the supine position, he immediately assumed a windswept posture to his right (Fig. 7-35, *A*). When asked to correct his alignment to a "straight" position, he was able to do so temporarily (Fig. 7-35, *B*). However, with activity, emotion, or discomfort, he consistently

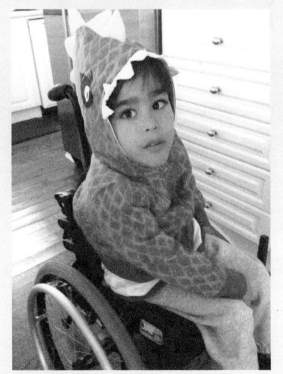

• **Figure 7-33** Thomas, a 6-Year-Old Boy With Dystonic Cerebral Palsy. (Permission for use of case photos granted by parent.)

Continued

Hip Dysplasia: Importance of Positioning and Equipment in Postural Alignment and Progressive Deformity in a Child With Dystonic Cerebral Palsy—cont'd

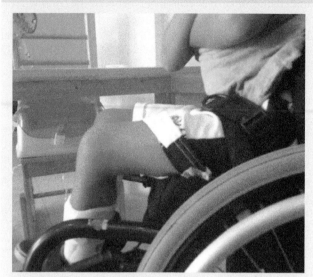

• **Figure 7-34** Close-up of the Side of Thomas' Wheelchair. This view reveals a short seat depth, lack of hip and trunk lateral supports, and a narrow base of support.

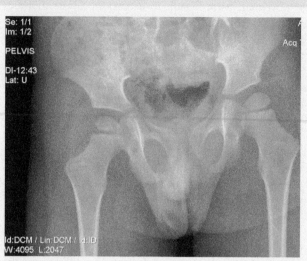

• **Figure 7-36** Radiograph of Thomas at 4 Years of Age. The radiograph shows mild left hip dysplasia with less than 25% subluxation.

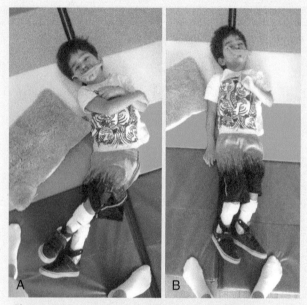

• **Figure 7-35** Typical Unsupported Postural Alignment in the Supine Position. **A,** Windswept posture to the right. **B,** Self-corrected alignment to "straight."

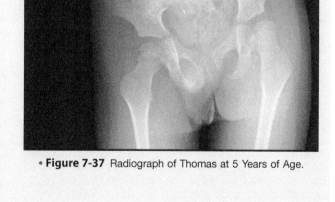

• **Figure 7-37** Radiograph of Thomas at 5 Years of Age.

returned to the typical right windswept position. Thomas' only bracing equipment consisted of his bilateral ankle-foot orthoses (AFOs).

Review of Annual Radiographs

A review of Thomas' annual radiographs, from 4 to 8 years of age, showed progressive hip dysplasia. His dysplasia had progressed from mild left hip dysplasia with less than 25% subluxation at 4 years of age to advanced dysplasia of more than 50% subluxation with acetabular deformation and flattening by 6 years of age (Figs. 7-36 to 7-39).

Interestingly, the progression of this patient's hip dysplasia coincided with the timing of his first wheelchair. The wheelchair should not be considered a causative factor in this patient's hip dysplasia because he was already predisposed to hip subluxation as a result of his asymmetry. However, it is possible that the patient's unsupported position in the wheelchair, combined with the frequency of its use, and the pattern of propulsion that the patient learned to use while trying to control his dystonia, may have all been contributing factors to the rapid progression of his hip subluxation.

CASE STUDY 7-1

Hip Dysplasia: Importance of Positioning and Equipment in Postural Alignment and Progressive Deformity in a Child With Dystonic Cerebral Palsy—cont'd

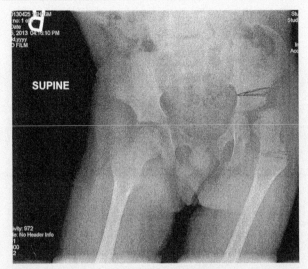

• **Figure 7-38** Preoperative Radiograph of Thomas at 6 Years of Age. The radiograph shows advanced dysplasia of more than 50% subluxation with acetabular deformation and flattening.

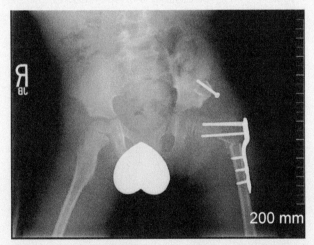

• **Figure 7-39** Postoperative Radiograph of Thomas at 7 Years of Age.

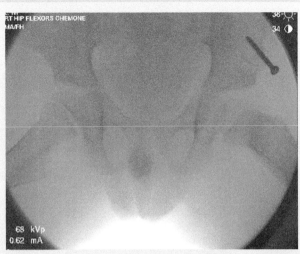

• **Figure 7-40** Postoperative Radiograph of Thomas at 8 Years of Age.

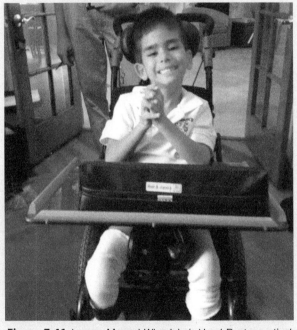

• **Figure 7-41** Loaner Manual Wheelchair Used Postoperatively. Note the wide base of support, hip and trunk lateral supports, and a tray to give upper body support.

Surgical Intervention for Left Hip Dysplasia

The patient required surgical intervention at 6½ years of age, shortly after moving from another state. A femoral varus derotation osteotomy with acetabular reconstruction was performed (see Fig. 7-39), and he was released home 1 week postoperatively, with hips braced in a Maple Leaf hip abduction brace (Becker Orthopedic, Troy, Mich.) versus a spica cast, to allow for ease of hygiene and early passive range of motion. Unfortunately, because of the dystonia, Thomas had great difficulty tolerating the brace and had high levels of pain related to the constant motion. One year later, a second, minor surgical procedure was performed to remove the femoral hardware, although the acetabular pin was left in place (Fig. 7-40). The patient felt a great deal of relief after the hardware

was removed because of the sensitivity of the hardware under his skin during positioning and rolling.

Physical Therapy and Adaptive Equipment

As soon as tolerated, the patient began using a loaner manual wheelchair with a wide base of support, hip and trunk lateral supports, and a tray to give upper body support, to achieve symmetric alignment (Fig. 7-41). After 6 months, a power

Continued

CASE STUDY 7-1

Hip Dysplasia: Importance of Positioning and Equipment in Postural Alignment and Progressive Deformity in a Child With Dystonic Cerebral Palsy—cont'd

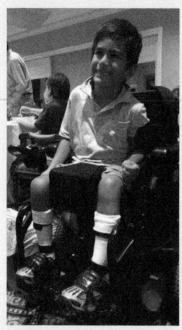

• **Figure 7-42** Power Wheelchair With Custom Seating System.

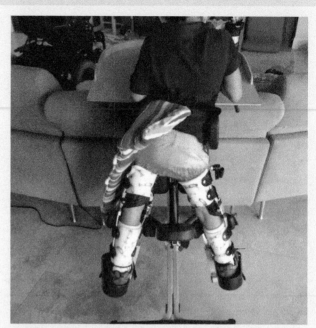

• **Figure 7-43** Thomas Standing With Hips Abducted. The Snug Seat Gazelle Stander is being used.

wheelchair with a similar custom seating system was then ordered to allow Thomas independent mobility without excessive effort, which reduced his dystonia and asymmetric posturing (Fig. 7-42).

Thomas wore the hip abduction brace full time (with the exception of bathing and passive range-of-motion activities) for 2 months postoperatively, until he was given orthopedic clearance to begin a weaning schedule and to begin weight bearing. Recommendations were made by the orthopedist to be in a stander at least 2 hours per day. The Snug Seat Gazelle Stander (Snug Seat, Inc., Matthews, NC) was selected because it is designed for standing with the hips maintained in abduction (Fig. 7-43). He also was fitted with a Rifton Pacer Gait Trainer (Rifton Equipment, Rifton, NY) and a Freedom Concepts Adaptive Tricycle (Freedom Concepts, Costa Mesa, Calif.) for home use.

Current Status

Two years postoperatively, Thomas continues with his daily standing program and wearing the hip abduction brace at night as a means of maintaining optimal alignment and preventing asymmetric posturing. He also participates in therapeutic horseback riding and aquatic therapy weekly, in addition to a 3-week summer intensive therapy program using the TheraSuit (TheraSuit, LLC, Largo, Fla.), as well as Dolphin-Assisted Therapy. He attends regular second grade, and his academic scores are above average. Adaptations at school include a standing desk and mobile prone stander to allow him to remain on peer level in the classroom, use of arm weights and a slant board for improved fine motor control using a pencil and an iPad, and an adaptive toilet that he uses at the nurse's office. His primary means of mobility is his power wheelchair (Fig. 7-44).

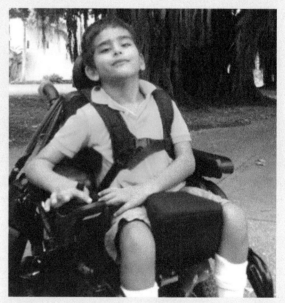

• **Figure 7-44** Thomas, at 8 Years of Age, in His Power Wheelchair.

Goals for the Future

Thomas will need to be monitored for growth, and adaptive equipment will require regular modification and adjustment to maintain optimal alignment. Otherwise, therapy and home programs will be focused on maintaining passive range of

CASE STUDY 7-1

Hip Dysplasia: Importance of Positioning and Equipment in Postural Alignment and Progressive Deformity in a Child With Dystonic Cerebral Palsy—cont'd

motion, improving strength, maintaining alignment, and providing suggestions for age-appropriate physical activity to promote overall fitness. His dystonia fluctuates daily and remains a barrier to independent standing and ambulation activities. Use of medications and botulinum toxin (Botox) has been somewhat helpful in controlling the patient's dystonia; however, he is being evaluated for deep brain stimulation at this time. Deep brain stimulation has not been well documented in children, but the family hopes it may offer relief and improved motor control.

*The authors would like to thank Mary B. Pengelley for providing pictures and information for this case.

CASE STUDY 7-2

Congenital Femoral Deficiency

Bella was diagnosed at birth with congenital femoral deficiency and mild fibular hemimelia (Fig. 7-45). Consultations with orthopedic surgeons in the patient's home state all recommended amputation of the lower leg at 1 year of age and subsequent prosthetic fitting. The family did not accept this prognosis and sought a consultation at the Paley Advanced Limb Lengthening Institute (West Palm Beach, Fla.), where they were given the option of surgical treatment to stabilize the hip and knee, followed by femoral lengthening. Bella underwent the stabilization procedure with the systematic utilitarian procedure for extremity reconstruction (SUPER) hip and SUPER knee at 2 years of age, with an excellent result (Fig. 7-46).

At 3 years of age, Bella presented for the first femoral lengthening, with an external fixator to the femur crossing the knee to the tibia and hinged at the knee (Fig. 7-47). This type of fixation protects the knee and allows for safe range of motion (ROM) to be performed. Her leg length discrepancy was 10 cm (3.9 inches) and was predicted to be 25 cm (9.8 inches). Hardware from the SUPER hip was also removed at the time of surgical treatment. An osteoplasty was performed in the femur for lengthening, botulinum toxin (Botox) was injected into the right quadriceps muscle, and an arthrogram was performed of the right knee. Bella was in the hospital for 3 days, and there she received physical therapy (PT) on postoperative day 1 to get her out of bed and encourage mobility. Bella was allowed to bear weight as tolerated, and she ambulated with a pediatric rolling walker.

The next day after discharge, Bella was seen for outpatient PT including active ROM (AROM) exercises, as well as progressive passive ROM (PROM) and stretches of the hip, knee, and ankle. Gait and functional training were also performed. Bella's family was trained over the course of therapy in home stretches to be performed three times daily. At the 4-week follow-up visit, it was discovered that Bella's femur had consolidated. A surgical procedure to reosteotomize the femur to continue lengthening was performed on an outpatient basis.

Bella attended PT five times per week for 3 months during the distraction phase. Although the hip adductors, hamstrings, and quadriceps muscles became tight as she gained 8.5 cm of new bone in the right femur, PROM at the knee was maintained at 0 to 75 degrees, and the hip remained well covered. After the distraction phase ended, Bella returned to her home state, and PT continued at five times per week, but it quickly faded as the family continued with the home program. Bella was able to walk with both feet on the ground without a shoe lift for the first time in her life.

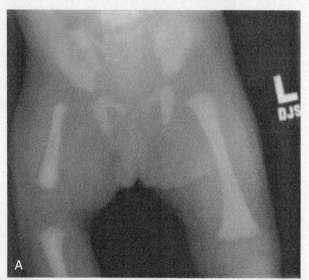

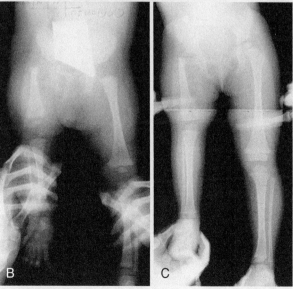

• **Figure 7-45** Bella was diagnosed with congenital femoral deficiency and mild fibular hemimelia at birth. Radiographs at birth (**A**), at 4 months (**B**), and at 17 months of age (**C**). (Courtesy Paley Advanced Limb Lengthening Institute, West Palm Beach, Fla.)

Continued

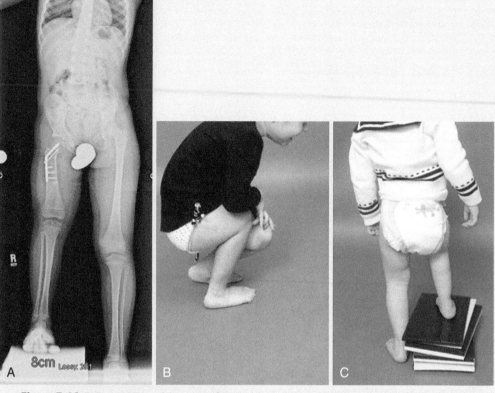

• **Figure 7-46** Bella at 3 Years of Age, After SUPER Hip and Knee Operation and Before Lengthening. (Courtesy Paley Advanced Limb Lengthening Institute, West Palm Beach, Fla.)

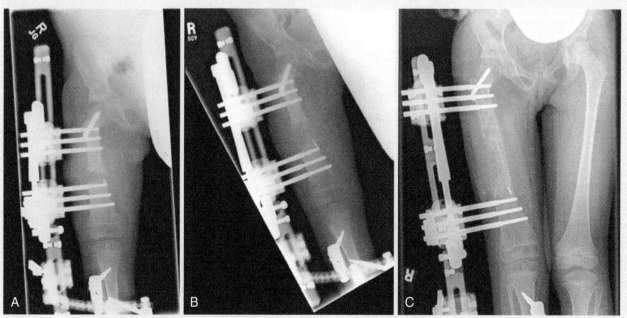

• **Figure 7-47** **A** to **C,** Bella at the distraction phase of lengthening, with the modular rail system of external fixation. (Courtesy Paley Advanced Limb Lengthening Institute, West Palm Beach, Fla.)

CASE STUDY 7-2

Congenital Femoral Deficiency—cont'd

Nine months after Bella's initial surgical procedure, the bone had fully consolidated, and the external fixator was removed. The femur was osteoporotic, and a slight lateral defect was detected, resulting in a high risk of fracture, so Bella received a prophylactic intramedullary rush rod. A 4-week rest from PT and PROM was granted to allow the pin sites to consolidate. She resumed PT three times per week, and PT faded in frequency as indicated over the next year.

At 8 years of age, Bella returned for another lengthening of the right femur, this time with the internal PRECICE rod (Ellipse Technologies, Inc., Aliso Viejo, Calif.) (Fig. 7-48). Her leg length discrepancy was 7.4 cm. She was in the hospital 3 days postoperatively, and PT was initiated there as with the first lengthening. She was fitted with a custom hip-knee-ankle-foot orthosis in 10 degrees of hip abduction with a drop-lock knee to prevent hip adduction and knee flexion contracture. She was instructed to wear the brace with the knee locked at night. Bella was allowed to bear 50 pounds of weight on her right leg and was able to walk with one crutch.

As before, outpatient PT began 1 day after discharge from the hospital. PT continued as after the first lengthening, with an emphasis on increasing tissue length of the musculature of the right hip and thigh muscles and a focus on the two-joint muscles. Although ROM continued to be well within the functional range for hip abduction, the first signs of slight hip subluxation were noted at 6 weeks of lengthening. The rate of distraction was slowed, and hip stretches were increased. Despite these efforts, the hip showed increasing signs of subluxation at the 10-week follow-up visit, and the lengthening was stopped to avoid further complications. The use of a hip brace was increased. She gained 6.2 cm of new bone. Currently, Bella is recovering nicely and has had no further progression of hip subluxation.

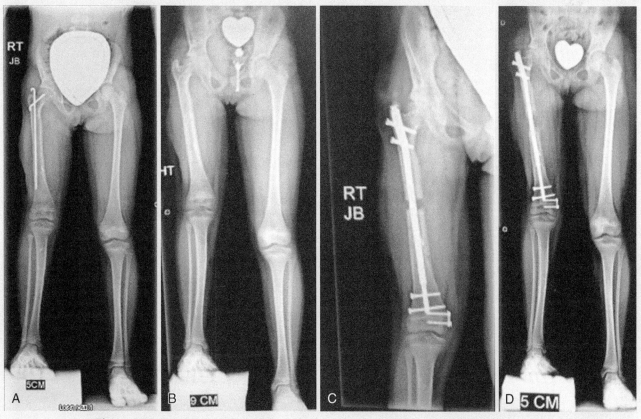

• **Figure 7-48 A,** Bella, at 3 years of age, after external fixation. **B** to **D,** Bella, at 8 years of age, before and after lengthening with the PRECICE nail. (Courtesy Paley Advanced Limb Lengthening Institute, West Palm Beach, Fla.)

A 13-Year-Old Boy With Slipped Capital Femoral Epiphysis

Luke, a 13-year-old, morbidly obese, African American boy presented to the emergency department after reporting anterior left upper thigh pain for 2 weeks without any instance of trauma noted. Luke described it as shocklike pain going down his leg, and he reported that he initially felt movement in his hip. The pain increased over time and was much worse with weight bearing. Review of radiographs revealed slipped capital femoral epiphysis (SCFE) of the left hip (Fig. 7-49). He had no history of any orthopedic injury or vitamin D deficiency. Luke's weight at the time was 116 kg (255.74 pounds).

The physician explained to the family that SCFE is a disease of increased prevalence in adolescents who have recently experienced rapid growth, is more common in overweight boys, and has a fourfold higher incidence in black or African American children.[81] Patients also have a high risk of developing SCFE on the other side. Initial treatment of bilateral percutaneous pinning of the femoral head and neck was recommended for Luke. The family was also informed of a 50% chance of requiring a more invasive surgical procedure in the future to realign the femoral head and neck. The family opted for left hip pinning only, and the surgical procedure was performed the same day (Fig. 7-50).

Five months later, it was determined that a more aggressive surgical procedure would be needed to treat the SCFE and to decrease the risk of SCFE on the right side. The family agreed, and Luke underwent left side surgical dislocation, open reduction and internal fixation of the slipped capital epiphyseal fracture, greater trochanteric advancement, and right-sided percutaneous pinning of the femoral head and neck (Fig. 7-51).

Luke remained in the hospital for 4 days, and he began physical therapy (PT) the day after the operation. He was allowed to bear weight as tolerated on the right and to touch-down bear weight on the left. A custom-molded hip-knee abduction brace was provided before Luke was allowed out of bed.

He began outpatient PT 48 hours after discharge from the hospital. PT consisted of passive range of motion of the left hip into gentle flexion and extension of 0 to 90 degrees and abduction to 30 degrees. Extremes of motion were not to be pushed at end range on the left hip. Right hip active and passive range of motion was performed with more aggressive stretches. PT was scheduled five times per week for 4 weeks, with a plan to fade in frequency as goals were met and as the family became proficient with stretches. At 6 weeks after the operation, Luke was allowed to progress to 50% weight bearing. Attendance to PT sessions was sporadic, however, and home exercises were not performed as directed. Ultimately, Luke was discharged from PT because of noncompliance.

Luke returned 15 months later for removal of the internal hardware. His weight had increased to 136.01 kg (300 pounds). He had significant loss of motion of the left hip into all planes and was stuck into external rotation. Remarkably, Luke was pain free. To assess whether a fracture or further slip had occurred, it was decided that before removal of hardware, he would undergo a manipulation under anesthesia with imaging. Luke demonstrated passive range of motion within functional limits under anesthesia, and removal of hardware was performed bilaterally without incident.

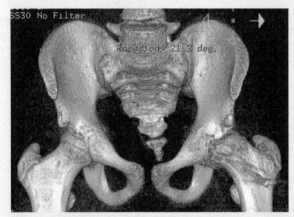

• **Figure 7-49** Pretreatment Image of Luke, a 13-Year-Old, Morbidly Obese, African American Boy Diagnosed With a Slipped Capital Femoral Epiphysis of the Left Hip. (Courtesy Paley Advanced Limb Lengthening Institute, West Palm Beach, Fla.)

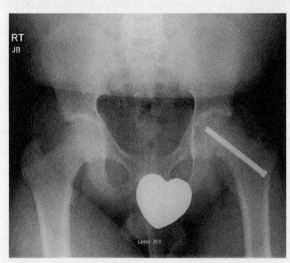

• **Figure 7-50** Luke, After Pinning of the Slipped Capital Femoral Epiphysis. (Courtesy Paley Advanced Limb Lengthening Institute, West Palm Beach, Fla.)

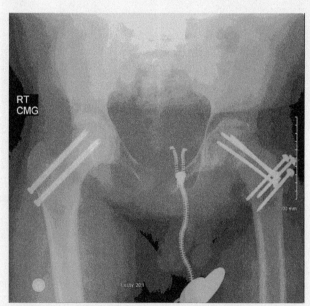

• **Figure 7-51** Luke, After Open Reduction and Internal Fixation of the Left Slipped Capital Femoral Epiphysis and Prophylactic Pinning of the Right Hip. (Courtesy Paley Advanced Limb Lengthening Institute, West Palm Beach, Fla.)

CASE STUDY 7-4

A 9-Year-Old Boy With Unilateral Legg-Calvé-Perthes Disease

Sam, a 9-year-old boy, presented to the Paley Advanced Limb Lengthening Institute (West Palm Beach, Fla.) for a second opinion 6 months after the onset of left hip pain and decreased range of motion. Radiograph revealed Legg-Calvé-Perthes disease of the left hip with subluxation and coxa magna, as well as changes in the femoral head (Fig. 7-52). Clinically, Sam was noted to have adduction and flexion contractures.

Sam underwent the following procedures: arthrogram of the left hip; application of a multiplanar external fixator to the left pelvis and femur for acute distraction of the femoral head from the acetabulum; tenotomies of the adductor longus, gracilis and psoas; and decompression of the femoral nerve. The external fixator had a hinge at the hip to allow for flexion and extension (Fig. 7-53). Sam began physical therapy (PT) in the hospital on postoperative day 1. He was discharged from the hospital 3 days after the surgical procedure and began outpatient PT 24 hours following discharge. His plan of care consisted of the following: active and passive range of motion of hip (flexion and extension), knee, and ankle; gait training (50% weight bearing); and parent and patient education for home stretches. The family was provided videos to assist with home program compliance. Sam attended PT five sessions per week for the first month, three times per week for the second month, and two times per week for the third month until fixator removal. Sam and his family continued to perform home stretches three times daily.

Sam's external fixator was removed 4 months after his initial surgical procedure. He underwent removal of the external fixator and had an arthrogram of the left hip. A unilateral hip abduction brace was ordered, weight bearing was limited to 50%, and he resumed PT to introduce active and very gentle passive range of motion exercises of the left hip in all directions except adduction. At 6 weeks, weight bearing was progressed to weight bearing as tolerated. He continued PT with fading frequency, and he was released from all treatment at 9 months with clearance to resume all activities (Fig. 7-54). Sam's mother sent a video of him scoring a goal in a soccer game the next weekend.

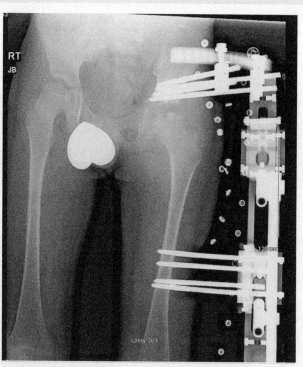

• **Figure 7-53** Postoperative View of Sam With Left Hip Distraction With External Fixation. (Courtesy Paley Advanced Limb Lengthening Institute, West Palm Beach, Fla.)

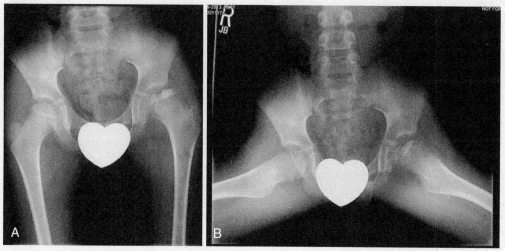

• **Figure 7-52 A** and **B,** Pretreatment views of Sam, a 9-year-old boy with left hip Legg-Calvé-Perthes disease. (Courtesy Paley Advanced Limb Lengthening Institute, West Palm Beach, Fla.)

Continued

CASE STUDY 7-4

A 9-Year-Old Boy With Unilateral Legg-Calvé-Perthes Disease—cont'd

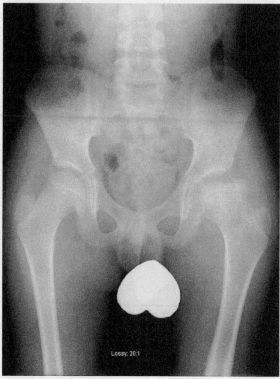

• **Figure 7-54** Sam, After Successful Treatment. (Courtesy Paley Advanced Limb Lengthening Institute, West Palm Beach, Fla.)

Acknowledgments

The authors would like to thank Elizabeth (Betsy) Kreymer, physical therapy student and graphic artist, for contributing drawings for this chapter.

References

1. Spence DD, Kelly DM, Mihalko MJ, Guyton JL. Adolescent and young adult hip dysplasia. *Curr Orthop Pract*. 2013;24(6): 567-575.
2. Price CT, Ramo BA. Prevention of hip dysplasia in children and adults. *Orthop Clin North Am*. 2012;43(3):269-279.
3. Dede O, Ward WT. Bernese periacetabular osteotomy in the surgical management of adolescent acetabular dysplasia. *Oper Tech Orthop*. 2013;23(3):127-133.
4. Millis MB, Lewis CL, Schoenecker PL, Clohisy JC. Legg-Calve-Perthes disease and slipped capital femoral epiphysis: major developmental causes of femoroacetabular impingement. *J Am Acad Orthop Surg*. 2013;21(suppl 1):S59-S63.
5. Wenger DR, Hosalkar HS. Principles of treating the sequelae of Perthes disease. *Orthop Clin North Am*. 2011;42(3):365-372.
6. Cooper AP, Doddabasappa SN, Mulpuri K. Evidence-based management of developmental dysplasia of the hip. *Orthop Clin North Am*. 2014;45(3):341-354.
7. Clarke NM, Castaneda P. Strategies to improve nonoperative childhood management. *Orthop Clin North Am*. 2012;43(3): 281-289.
8. Storer SK, Skaggs DL. Developmental dysplasia of the hip. *Am Fam Physician*. 2006;74:1310-1316.
9. Rosenfeld SB Developmental dysplasia of the hip: clinical features and diagnosis. *UpToDate* [online journal]. Feb 4, 2014. Available at: <http://www.uptodate.com/contents/developmental-dysplasia-of-the-hip-clinical-features-and-diagnosis?source>. Accessed June 29, 2014.
10. Hosalkar HS, Mubarak SJ, Sink EL, et al. *Infantile developmental hip dysplasia*. 2010. Published on the website for the International Hip Dysplasia Institute. Available at: <http://www.hipdysplasia.org/wp-content/uploads/2010/01/IHDI-Ortho-Presentation-Web.pdf>. Accessed June 29, 2014.
11. Peled E, Eidelman M, Katzman A, Bialik V. Neonatal incidence of hip dysplasia: ten years of experience. *Clin Orthop Relat Res*. 2008;466:771-775.
12. Sankar WN, Weiss J, Skaggs DL. Orthopaedic conditions in the newborn. *J Am Acad Orthop Surg*. 2009;17(2):112-122.
13. International Hip Dysplasia Institute. *What is hip dysplasia?* 2012. Available at: <http://hipdysplasia.org/>. Accessed June 23, 2015.
14. de Hundt M, Vlemmix F, Bais JM, et al. Risk factors for developmental dysplasia of the hip: a meta-analysis. *Eur J Obstet Gynecol Reprod Biol*. 2012;165(1):8-17.

15. American Academy of Pediatrics Subcommittee on Developmental Dysplasia of the Hip. Clinical practice guideline: early detection of developmental dysplasia of the hip. *Pediatrics*. 2000; 105(4):896-905.

16. International Hip Dysplasia Institute. *What causes hip dysplasia?* 2012. Available at: <http://hipdysplasia.org/developmental-dysplasia-of-the-hip/causes-of-ddh/>. Accessed June 23, 2015.

17. Shipman SA, Helfand M, Moyer VA, Yawn BP. Screening for developmental dysplasia of the hip: a systematic literature review for the US Preventive Services Task Force. *Pediatrics*. 2006;117: e557-e576.

18. Laborie LB, Engesæter IO, Lehmann TG, et al. Screening strategies for hip dysplasia: long-term outcome of a randomized controlled trial. *Pediatrics*. 2013;132:492-501.

19. Godley DR. Assessment, diagnosis, and treatment of developmental dysplasia of the hip. *JAAPA*. 2013;26(3):54-58.

20. Clarke N, Castaneda P. Strategies to improve nonoperative childhood management. *Orthop Clin North Am*. 2012;43(3): 281-289.

21. Kitoh H, Kawasumi M, Ishiguro N. Predictive factors for unsuccessful treatment of developmental dysplasia of the hip by the Pavlik harness. *J Pediatr Orthop*. 2009;29(6):552-557.

22. Murnaghan ML, Browne RH, Sucato DJ, Birch J. Femoral nerve palsy in Pavlik harness treatment for developmental dysplasia of the hip. *J Bone Joint Surg Am*. 2011;93(5):493-499.

23. Lee CB, Mata-Fink A, Millis MB, Kim YJ. Demographic differences in adolescent-diagnosed and adult-diagnosed acetabular dysplasia compared with infantile developmental dysplasia of the hip. *J Pediatr Orthop*. 2013;33(2):107-111.

24. Fabricant PD, Hirsch BP, Holmes I, et al. A radiographic study of the ossification of the posterior wall of the acetabulum: implications for the diagnosis of pediatric and adolescent hip disorders. *J Bone Joint Surg Am*. 2013;95(3):230-236.

25. Huang S, Zhao D, Yang L. New approach to the treatment of adolescent hip dysplasia. *Med Hypotheses*. 2013;81(1):122-124.

26. Sucato DJ, Tulchin K, Shrader MW, et al. Gait, hip strength and functional outcomes after a Ganz periacetabular osteotomy for adolescent hip dysplasia. *J Pediatr Orthop*. 2010;30(4): 344-350.

27. Aldridge R, Schweighart F, Easley M, Wagoner B. The effects of hippotherapy on motor performance and function in an individual with bilateral developmental dysplasia of the hip (DDH). *J Phys Ther*. 2011;2(2):54-63.

28. Rebello G, Zilkens C, Dudda M, et al. Triple pelvic osteotomy in complex hip dysplasia seen in neuromuscular and teratologic conditions. *J Pediatr Orthop*. 2009;29(6):527-534.

29. Terjesen T. Development of the hip joints in unoperated children with cerebral palsy: a radiographic study of 76 patients. *Acta Orthop*. 2006;77(1):125-131.

30. Pountney TE, Mandy A, Green E, Gard PR. Hip subluxation and dislocation in cerebral palsy: a prospective study on the effectiveness of postural management programmes. *Physiother Res Int*. 2009;14(2):116-127.

31. Arvanitis H. Pediatric hip dysplasia and positioning. *Exceptional Parent*. 2013;43(3):22-25.

32. Paley D, Standard SC. Treatment of congenital femoral deficiency. In: Flynn DM, Wiesel SW, eds. *Operative Techniques for Pediatric Orthopaedics*. Philadelphia: Lippincott Williams & Wilkins; 2011:177-198.

33. Paley D. Problems, obstacles and complications of limb lengthening by the Ilizarov technique. *Clin Orthop Relat Res*. 1990; 250:81-104.

34. Torode IP, Gillespie R. The classification and treatment of proximal femoral deficiencies. *Prosthet Orthot Int*. 1991;15(2): 117-126.

35. Dror P, Shawn CS. Lengthening reconstruction surgery for congenital femoral deficiency. In: Rozbruch SR, Ilizarov S, eds. *Limb Lengthening and Reconstruction Surgery*. New York, NY: Informa Healthcare; 2006:393-428.

36. Sabharwal S, Paley D, Bhave A, Herzenberg JE. Growth patterns after lengthening of congenitally short lower limbs in young children. *J Pediatr Orthop*. 2000;20(2):137-145.

37. Paley Advanced Limb Lengthening Institute. <http://paleyinstitute.org/>. Accessed June 23, 2015.

38. Paley D. Lengthening reconstruction surgery for congenital femoral deficiency. In: Herring J, Birch J, eds. *The Child with a Limb Deficiency*. Rosemont, Ill: American Academy of Orthopaedic Surgeons; 1998:113-132.

39. Lehmann CL, Arons RR, Loder RT, Vitale MG. The epidemiology of slipped capital femoral epiphysis: an update. *J Pediatr Orthop*. 2006;26(3):286-290.

40. Gholve PA, Cameron DB, Millis MB. Slipped capital femoral epiphysis update. *Curr Opin Pediatr*. 2009;21(1):39-45.

41. Loder RT, Skopelja EN. The epidemiology and demographics of slipped capital femoral epiphysis. *ISRN Orthop*. 2011;2011: 486512.

42. Peck K, Herrera-Soto J. Slipped capital femoral epiphysis: what's new? *Orthop Clin North Am*. 2014;45(1):77-86.

43. Liu SC, Tsai CC, Huang CH. Atypical slipped capital femoral epiphysis after radiotherapy and chemotherapy. *Clin Orthop Relat Res*. 2004;426:212-218.

44. Wu GS, Pollock AN. Slipped capital femoral epiphysis. *Pediatr Emerg Care*. 2011;27(11):1095-1096.

45. Ganz R, Leunig M, Leunig-Ganz K, Harris W. The etiology of osteoarthritis of the hip. *Clin Orthop Relat Res*. 2008;466: 264-272.

46. Pinheiro PC. Nonoperative treatment of slipped capital femoral epiphysis: a scientific study. *J Orthop Surg Res*. 2011; 6:10.

47. Sonnega RJA, van der Sluijs JA, Wainwright AM, et al. Management of slipped capital femoral epiphysis: results of a survey of the members of the European Paediatric Orthopaedic Society. *J Child Orthop*. 2011/12/01 2011;5(6):433-438.

48. Kocher MS, Bishop JA, Hresko MT, et al. Prophylactic pinning of the contralateral hip after unilateral slipped capital femoral epiphysis. *J Bone Joint Surg Am*. 2004;86(12):2658-2665.

49. Alshryda SJ, Tsang K, Al-Shryda J, et al. Interventions for treating slipped upper femoral epiphysis (SUFE). *Cochrane Database Syst Rev*. 2013;(2):CD14010397.

50. Rudd J, Suri M, Choate W, et al. Outcomes of arthroscopically treated femoroacetabular impingement in children and adolescents with slipped capital femoral epiphysis and Legg-Calve-Perthes disease. *Arthroscopy*. 2014;29(12):e209-e210.

51. Leunig M, Ganz R, Zaltz I, Tibor LM. Slipped capital femoral epiphysis and its variants. In: Haddad FS, ed. *The Young Adult Hip in Sport*. London, United Kingdom: Springer; 2014: 47-58.

52. Tran VT, Ha BY. Legg-Calve-Perthes disease. In: Daldrup-Link HE, Newman B, eds. *Pearls and Pitfalls in Pediatric Imaging: Variants and Other Difficult Diagnoses*. Cambridge, United Kingdom: Cambridge University Press; 2014.

53. Perry DC, Hall AJ. The epidemiology and etiology of Perthes disease. *Orthop Clin North Am*. 2011;42(3):279-283.

54. Kim HK, Herring JA. Pathophysiology, classifications, and natural history of Perthes disease. *Orthop Clin North Am.* 2011;42(3):285-295.

55. Dole RL, Chafetz R. *Peds Rehab Notes.* Philadelphia: FA Davis; 2010.

56. Kim HK. Legg-Calve-Perthes disease: etiology, pathogenesis, and biology. *J Pediatr Orthop.* 2011;31(2 suppl):S141-S146.

57. Kuo K, Wu K-W, Smith P, et al. Classification of Legg-Calve-Perthes disease. *J Pediatr Orthop.* 2011;31(2 suppl):S168-S173.

58. Agus H, Kalenderer O, Eryanlmaz G, Ozcalabi IT. Intraobserver and interobserver reliability of Catterall, Herring, Salter-Thompson and Stulberg classification systems in Perthes disease. *J Pediatr Orthop B.* 2004;13(3):166-169.

59. Terjesen T, Wiig O, Svenningsen S. The natural history of Perthes' disease. *Acta Orthop.* 2010;81(6):708-714.

60. Nakamura J, Kamegaya M, Saisu T, et al. Outcome of patients with Legg-Calve-Perthes onset before 6 years of age. *J Pediatr Orthop.* 2015;35(2):144-150.

61. Price CT, Thompson GH, Wenger DR. Containment methods for treatment of Legg-Calvé-Perthes disease. *Orthop Clin North Am.* 2011;42(3):329-340.

62. Joseph B, Price CT. Principles of containment treatment aimed at preventing femoral head deformation in Perthes disease. *Orthop Clin North Am.* 2011;42(3):317-327.

63. Hardesty C, Liu R, Thompson G. The role of bracing in Legg-Calve-Perthes disease. *J Pediatr Orthop.* 2011;31(2 suppl): S178-S181.

64. Rich MM, Schoenecker PL. Management of Legg-Calvé-Perthes disease using an A-frame orthosis and hip range of motion: a 25-year experience. *J Pediatr Orthop.* 2013;33(2):112-119.

65. Kamegaya M. Nonsurgical treatment of Legg-Calvé-Perthes disease. *J Pediatr Orthop.* 2011;31(2 suppl):S174-S177.

66. Paley D. The treatment of femoral head deformity and coxa magna by the Ganz femoral head reduction osteotomy. *Orthop Clin North Am.* 2011;42(3):389-399.

67. Lee J, Allen M, Hugentobler K, et al. Evidence-based care guideline for management of Legg-Calve-Perthes disease stages 1 to 4 post-surgical intervention in children aged 3 to 12 years. In: *Occupational Therapy and Physical Therapy Evidence-Based Care Guidelines, Cincinnati Children's Hospital Medical Center.* Cincinnati, Ohio: Cincinnati Children's Hospital Medical Center; 2013 guideline 41:1-18.

68. Hosny GA. Articulated distraction. *Orthop Clin North Am.* 2011;42(3):361-364.

69. Hosny G, El-Deeb K, Fadel M, Laklouk M. Arthrodiastasis of the hip. *J Pediatr Orthop.* 2011;31(2 suppl):S229-S234.

70. Herrera-Soto J, Price C. Core decompression and labral support for the treatment of juvenile osteonecrosis. *J Pediatr Orthop.* 2011;31(2 suppl):S212-S216.

71. Little DG, Kim HK. Future biologic treatments for Perthes disease. *Orthop Clin North Am.* 2011;42(3):423-427.

72. Cheng TL, Murphy CM, Cantrill LC, et al. Local delivery of recombinant human bone morphogenetic proteins and bisphosphonate via sucrose acetate isobutyrate can prevent femoral head collapse in Legg-Calve-Perthes disease: a pilot study in pigs. *Int Orthop.* 2014;38(7):1527-1533.

73. Costa CR, Johnson AJ, Naziri Q, Mont MA. Review of total hip resurfacing and total hip arthroplasty in young patients who had Legg-Calvé-Perthes disease. *Orthop Clin North Am.* 2011;42(3): 419-422.

74. Kovacevic D, Mariscalco M, Goodwin RC. Injuries about the hip in the adolescent athlete. *Sports Med Arthrosc.* 2011;19(1): 64-74.

75. Frank JS, Gambacorta PL, Eisner EA. Hip pathology in the adolescent athlete. *J Am Acad Orthop Surg.* 2013;21(11): 665-674.

76. Weiss JM, Ramachandran M. Hip and pelvis injuries in the young athlete. *Oper Tech Sports Med.* 2006;14:212-217.

77. Boles C, Ferguson C. The female athlete. *Radiol Clin North Am.* 2010;48:1249-1266.

78. Haddad FS, Bann S, Hill RA, Jones DH. Displaced stress fracture of the femoral neck in an active amenorrhoeic adolescent. *Br J Sports Med.* 1997;31(1):70-72.

79. Okamoto S, Arai Y, Hara K, et al. A displaced stress fracture of the femoral neck in an adolescent female distance runner with female athlete triad: a case report. *Sports Med Arthrosc Rehabil Ther Technol.* 2010;2:6.

80. Barrack MT, Gibbs JC, De Souza MJ, et al. Higher incidence of bone stress injuries with increasing female athlete triad-related risk factors: a prospective multisite study of exercising girls and women. *Am J Sports Med.* 2014;42(4):949-958.

81. Walter K, Young C, Lin D, et al. Slipped capital femoral epiphysis. *OrthoInfo: AAOS.* 2013. Available at: <http://orthoinfo.aaos.org/topic.cfm?topic=a00052>. Accessed November 18, 2014.

8

The Dancer's Hip

MELISSA MORAN TOVIN AND WHITNEY CHAMBERS

CHAPTER OUTLINE

Dance is an art form that has evolved considerably over the past several decades. Dance is also a sport—many styles require high levels of athleticism, skill, and highly specialized physical training. As such, dancers are at risk for sports-related injury, requiring the expertise of rehabilitation professionals with working knowledge of dance requirements and training. Dance medicine, an extension of sports medicine,[1] uses many of the same orthopedic assessment strategies and interventions, but with special consideration of the positions, movements, skills, and training regimens unique to dance.

As a foundation joint for dance movement and expression, the hip can sustain injuries that can be "exceptionally debilitating in both the long and short term,"[2] and they have resulted in loss of time from the sport for competitive dancers, as well as lost time, lost wages, and increased health-related costs for professional dancers.[3,4] Therefore, proper and early diagnosis and treatment of hip disorders are essential for this population.

The incidence of lower extremity injuries sustained by dancers falls between 60% and 88% of all dance injuries.[3-8] Although the most common sites of musculoskeletal injuries in these athletes are the foot and ankle,[3,5,9] dancers are particularly vulnerable to injuries of the hip.[2,10] Types of hip injuries typically seen in dancers are also common in other athletic populations. These include snapping hip syndrome (coxa sultans), hip tendinopathy, femoral acetabular impingement (FAI), avulsion injuries, and labral disorders.[11-17] The dancer's hip, however, is at risk for pathologic conditions caused by some factors unique to dance. Dance type and technique, training regimens, and the kinesiology of the hip joint during dance movements may result in unique mechanisms of injury and, at times, an atypical clinical presentation. This chapter focuses on the differential diagnosis, evaluation, treatment, and prevention of hip injury in dancers. Table 8-1 is a glossary of dance-related terms, many of which are used throughout this chapter.

TABLE 8-1	Glossary of Dance-Related Terms
Turnout	External rotation of the hips to place the anterior aspect of the lower extremities toward the frontal plane
First position	Standing with legs adducted, heels together, and hips externally rotated
Second position	Feet separated in a wide stance position in turnout with the feet farther apart than the hips
Third position	Adduction with the heel of one foot aligned with the midfoot of the rear foot but with no space between the legs
Fourth position	Adduction with the heel of one foot aligned with the midfoot of the rear foot but with space between the legs
Fifth position	Complete adduction with feet overlapping with heel of one leg aligned with the first metatarsal head of the other foot
Gesturing leg	Open kinetic chain motion to establish an esthetic line or prepare to accept weight
Supporting leg	Closed kinetic chain motion (weight support, jumps)
Plié	"Bending"—a squatting movement, performed in a turnout position
Grand plié	"Large bending"—deep squat in turnout
Ronde de jambe	Clockwise or counterclockwise hip circumduction with hip external rotation (turnout)
Ronde de jambe en l'aire	Ronde de jambe performed at higher levels of hip flexion with complete circumduction and pelvic motion allowed to create a circular action of the gesture leg
Grand battement	Large kicking where the gesture leg is raised in a straight position to the highest level the dancer is able to achieve, often is performed in flexion with slight abduction
Tendu battement	"Stretched beating"—keeping the toes on the ground, the working leg slides from first or fifth position to fourth or second position; both legs are kept straight
Passé	Gesture leg is flexed at the knee and hip while in the turnout position with the foot in plantarflexion to about knee height
Développé	Gesture leg is extended at the knee from a passé position maintaining turnout
Arabesque	Unilateral stance with the gesture leg extended at the hip as high as possible while keeping both hips and shoulders square
Attitude	Similar to an arabesque, but the gesture leg is flexed at the knee and can be anterior or posterior to the body

From Dunleavy K. Outcomes of hip resurfacing in a professional dancer: a case report. *Physiother Theory Pract.* 2012;28(2):142-160.

Unique Factors That Contribute to Hip Injuries in the Dancer

Emphasis on Turnout

The term turnout refers to an externally (lateral) rotated orientation of both lower extremities during dance positions and movements. Lower extremity excessive turnout, also called overturning, is emphasized in some styles of dance, including classical ballet and the many styles that build on ballet technique. Classical ballet has five basic positions, each of which requires excessive external rotation of the hip to achieve the desired turnout position (Fig. 8-1). These positions are fundamental in classical ballet training because many basic ballet movements begin and end in one of these positions.

External rotation of the leg with both feet positioned at 90 degrees laterally from parallel (i.e., both feet aligned within the frontal plane, thus creating a 180-degree angle) is considered "perfect" turnout (see Fig. 8-1, *A*). Although turnout should ideally come primarily from the hip, most of the dancer's functional turnout is accomplished by rotational components at the hip, knee, foot, and ankle joints. If hip external rotation is not sufficient, the dancer will compensate by forcing turnout by using compensatory strategies in weight bearing such as excessive pronation, foot abduction, knee flexion, external rotation torsion at the knees, and increased lumbar lordosis (Fig. 8-2). Compensated turnout is associated with nontraumatic musculoskeletal injuries in dancers, including anterior hip pain secondary to tendinopathy or FAI.[18-20]

Several factors or anatomic variations can contribute to, or limit, the amount of turnout achieved at the hip joint: angle of femoral version, orientation of the acetabulum, shape of the femoral neck, and elasticity of the iliofemoral ligament, as well as flexibility and strength balance of the

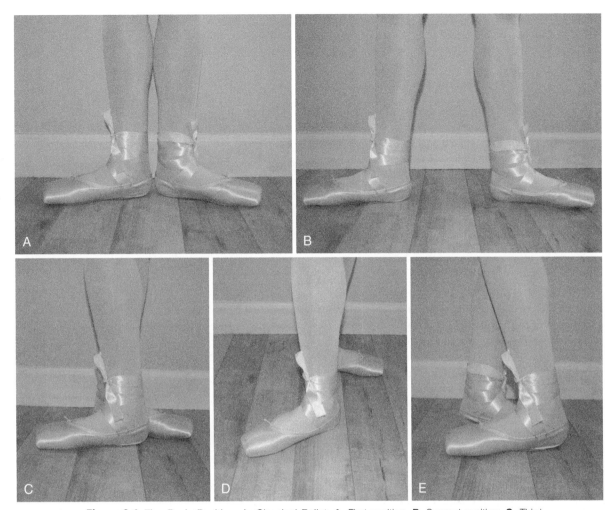

• **Figure 8-1** Five Basic Positions in Classical Ballet. **A,** First position. **B,** Second position. **C,** Third position. **D,** Fourth position. **E,** Fifth position.

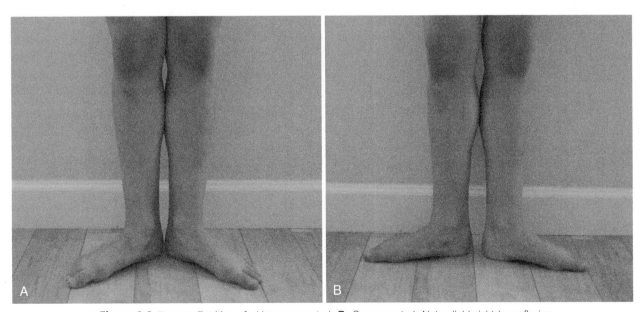

• **Figure 8-2** Turnout Position. **A,** Uncompensated. **B,** Compensated. Note slight right knee flexion, pronation (rolling in), and foot abduction to achieve greater turnout.

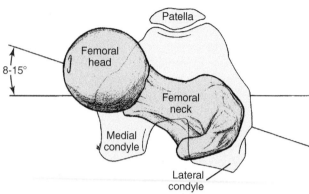

• **Figure 8-3** Femoral version refers to the angular measurement of the axis of the femoral neck in relation to the femoral condyles at the distal femur. The femoral head is normally angled anteriorly in relation to the transcondylar axis, in a position of femoral anteversion.

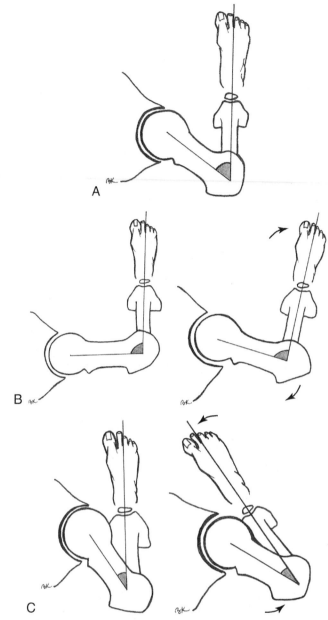

• **Figure 8-4** Femoral version can greatly influence the amount of turnout a dancer can achieve at the hip. **A,** Normal anteversion results in a neutral position of the femur, lower leg, and foot. **B,** Excessive femoral retroversion results in external rotation of the femur and can lead to "out-toeing." **C,** Excessive femoral anteversion results in internal rotation of the femur and can lead to "in-toeing."

musculature surrounding the hip joint. Individual differences in bony anatomy and structural alignment of the hip can also leave some dancers more susceptible to hip injury.

Femoral version refers to the angular measurement of the axis of the femoral neck in relation to the femoral condyles at the distal femur (Fig. 8-3). The femoral head is normally angled anteriorly in relation to the transcondylar axis, and this is referred to as femoral anteversion. At birth, femoral version measures approximately 35 to 40 degrees of anteversion, and by skeletal maturation, it measures on average between 8 and 15 degrees[21-23] of anteversion, which is considered normal range. At skeletal maturity, however, some variations in femoral version angles occur; some persons have up to 30 degrees of anteversion, whereas others have 10 to 15 degrees of femoral retroversion.[21] Femoral retroversion refers to a posterior position of the femoral head in relation to the transcondylar axis.

The amount of femoral version can greatly influence the amount of turnout a dancer can achieve at the hip (Fig. 8-4). One study found that average femoral neck anteversion in dancers (11.9 degrees) was similar to that in the average population.[23] Excessive femoral anteversion, however, results in internal rotation of the femur to position the head of the femur in the acetabulum, and it can lead to "in-toeing" (see Fig. 8-4, *C*). Increased femoral anteversion is associated with restricted hip external rotation, attributed to early contact of the neck of the femur with the lateral edge of the acetabulum.[24] Femoral anteversion affects alignment throughout the lower extremity and results in increased lumbar lordosis, an increased Q angle, patella-femoral disorders, and excessive pronation of the feet.[25] An excessively anteverted position of the femur is not desirable for the dancer because it significantly limits the dancer's ability to assume positions, maintain lower extremity and trunk alignment, and achieve the level of flexibility needed for many forms of dance. Conversely, femoral retroversion can lead to 'out-toeing,' which is desirable for the dancer (see Fig. 8-4, *B*). Retroversion is associated with increased external rotation range of motion, and it allows a dancer to

achieve greater turnout of the lower extremities with fewer compensatory strategies in the pelvis, knee, and foot.

Femoral version is typically established by 11 to 12 years of age as a result of bony maturity and cannot be influenced through training.[7] However, evidence indicates that dance training for 6 or more hours a week between the ages of 11 and 14 years can enable dancers to achieve greater turnout with fewer compensatory strategies by eliciting adaptive osseous changes and reducing femoral torsion.[26]

Anatomic deviations of the femoral neck or acetabulum may negatively influence hip joint articulation and available

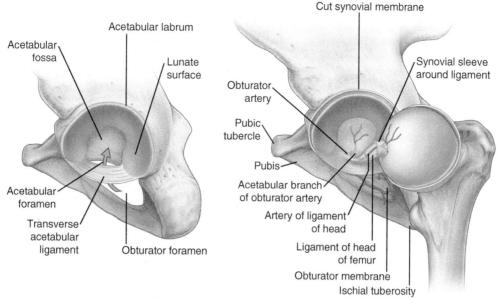

• **Figure 8-5** Acetabulum Anatomy. (From Drake R, Vogl AW. *Gray's Anatomy for Students.* 4th ed. Philadelphia: Churchill Livingstone; 2015).

range of motion, and they may predispose a dancer to injury. The acetabulum is cup shaped, providing a deep socket for the head of the femur (Fig. 8-5). Orientation, or depth and shape, of the acetabulum can affect the extent of turnout possible for a dancer. An acetabulum that is shallow (e.g., in hip dysplasia) and laterally oriented increases the external rotation range of motion available at the hip because contact between the femur and the acetabulum occur at a later point in the motion. Conversely, an acetabulum that is unusually deep and anteriorly oriented limits the amount of external rotation available as a result of earlier contact of joint surfaces (i.e., the femur contacts the edge of the acetabulum sooner during the motion).[24] Chapters 1 and 4 contain additional discussion of the anatomy and orientation of the acetabulum, the effects on lower extremity alignment and range of motion, and associated risk of injuries.

The shape and length of the femoral neck can also affect the extent of turnout achieved by a dancer. A longer femoral neck with a more concave shape allows greater amounts of abduction and external rotation at the hip, whereas a less concave and shorter femoral neck limits the end ranges of motion as a result of femoral acetabular abutment.[24] Continued and repeated abutment may lead to FAI, discussed later in this chapter, as well as in Chapter 4.

The surrounding musculature, joint capsule, and associated ligamentous structures of the hip can also greatly affect available turnout for the dancer. A detailed discussion of structure and function of ligaments of the hip is provided later in this chapter, as well as in Chapter 1. The joint capsule and, in particular, the iliofemoral ligament become taut at the end ranges of external rotation. As such, extensibility of these structures can improve a dancer's turnout. Similarly, tight musculature, particularly those with antago-

nist actions on external rotation, can also limit potential for turnout. Finally, strength of the external rotators of the hip, particularly at the end ranges, can help a dancer achieve his or her available turnout potential. Specific exercises designed to increase end-range strength and flexibility to improve turnout are presented later in this chapter.

Thorough evaluation of the dancer should include assessment of hip external rotation range of motion and limiting factors, functional turnout, and contribution of compensatory strategies to achieve turnout. Evidence supports proper and accurate assessment of turnout and compensatory factors in dancers to predict or prevent injury,[25] as well as to determine the amount of turnout available, or turnout capacity.[27] An association exists between reduced and compensated turnout and lower extremity injuries in dancers.[18,23,28] Dancers who demonstrate excessive use of compensatory strategies to compensate for insufficient hip external rotation to achieve maximal desired turnout may be at greater risk of injury.[28,29]

Assessing Turnout

Clinical assessment of turnout in dancers is an important component of evaluation and treatment of hip injury in this population. A critical review of the literature provides various methods of measuring turnout, and components of turnout, in dancers (e.g., passive versus active, weight bearing versus non–weight bearing, hip in extension versus flexion). Some of these methods are further discussed and presented in this section.

Previous studies indicated hip external rotation range-of-motion average values in dancers of 40 to 50 degrees passively[30] and at 30 to 40 degrees actively.[18,31,32] Up to 60 degrees of functional turnout (i.e., turnout during dance positions and movements) occurs exclusively through hip external rotation range of motion, with the rest contributed by the lower leg, thus achieving 69 to 87 degrees of functional turnout through compensatory strategies.[18,29,33] This potential for using compensatory strategies to forcefully achieve desired turnout may increase a dancer's susceptibility to musculoskeletal injury not only of the hip, but also of other joints of the lower extremity.[20]

Findings of a study by Negus and associates[18] underscore the importance of assessing turnout as a potential contributor to overuse injuries in ballet dancers. The study examined relationships between components of turnout and injury history in 29 ballet dancers, as well as the clinical utility of 3 turnout assessment methods (active and passive external rotation in supine and standing functional turnout). Results indicated a significant difference between static and dynamic turnout control. The researchers concluded that functional measures of turnout are more relevant to the prevalence of nontraumatic injuries, and therefore measurement of hip external rotation range of motion alone is insufficient.[18] Other studies supported clinical assessment of turnout in standing, incorporating the entire lower extremity in the turnout measurement.[27,30,34] Assessment of functional turnout, also referred to as total turnout, is useful for clinicians, as well as dance teachers, to identify potential limitations in turnout, risk for injury as a result of compensation, and turnout capacity.[24,27,31,34] Three recommended methods to assess functional (total) turnout include passive supine turnout, standing static turnout, and standing dynamic turnout.

Passive supine turnout, as described by Grossman and associates,[34] is measured with a goniometer with the dancer lying in the supine position with the knees and hips extended. The examiner passively dorsiflexes the foot while attempting to control hindfoot and forefoot alignment (to prevent pronation and foot abduction) because these factors can contribute to turnout. The dancer is cued to limit pelvic rotation by keeping the pelvis flat on the examining table and to maintain knee extension. The moving arm of the goniometer is placed along the second metatarsal, and the stationary arm is maintained in a vertical position, perpendicular to the table. The examiner passively rotates the lower extremity until motion is restricted by a capsular end feel (Fig. 8-6).

Standing static turnout is measured with the dancer standing on a whiteboard or white paper. The dancer is asked to position himself or herself actively in turnout, and the angle is measured with a goniometer directly under the foot, or by using tracings.[27,34] The stationary arm is aligned with the sagittal plane, and the moving arm is aligned with the second metatarsal (Fig. 8-7). Dancers can use friction of the floor to gain turnout in standing, and this may increase total turnout.[18]

Dynamic standing turnout is considered more functional, and therefore is more relevant than hip external rotation range of motion to prevalence of nontraumatic dance injuries.[18] This method is performed actively, and friction is eliminated by using rotational disks. The dancer

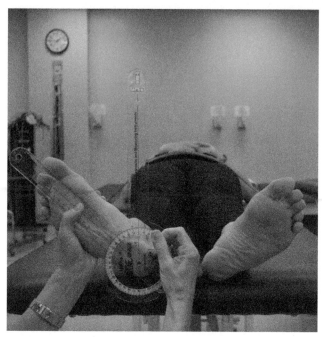

• **Figure 8-6** Passive Supine Turnout Measurement Using a Goniometer.

stands on the rotational disks with the medial and lateral malleoli placed along the central diameter of each disk. The second metatarsal is marked, and a measurement of the turnout angle is taken at the greatest range of active turnout by using markings on the surface, or a digital photograph (Fig. 8-8). Some research indicates that active turnout measurements may be significantly lower than passive total turnout measurements, and this information may be particularly important when treating a dancer for injuries most likely caused by compensatory strategies.[18,27,34]

Although functional turnout is clinically useful, it is important to address all contributing factors of turnout in the evaluation and treatment of the dancer's hip. Several components for clinical evaluation of the turnout are recommended: hip external rotation range of motion, passive functional turnout, standing static functional turnout, standing active functional turnout, and femoral anteversion.

To determine the hip's external rotation contribution to turnout, the clinician should use basic goniometric measurement techniques described in the orthopedic literature and the dance medicine literature.[35-37] Standard goniometric measurement of active and passive hip external rotation should be performed with the hip in flexion (sitting) or extension (prone). Each position provides the clinician with valuable information because turnout during dance is performed in a variety of hip positions, with both a closed chain and an open chain (see also Chapter 2 for hip external rotation range of motion assessment).

For prone goniometric measurement, position the dancer prone with both legs extended at shoulder width apart. The pelvis may be stabilized with a belt to keep the anterior-superior iliac spine on the surface of the table. Maintain the testing leg in 90 degrees of knee flexion. Passively externally

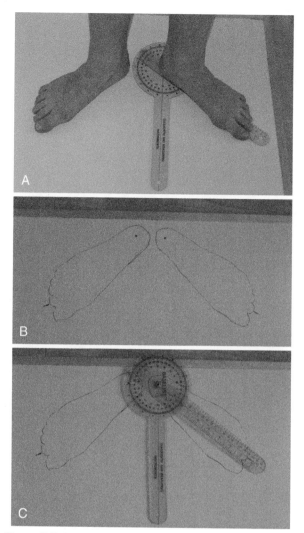

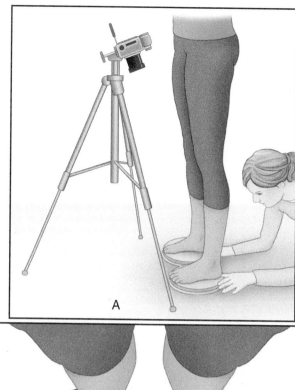

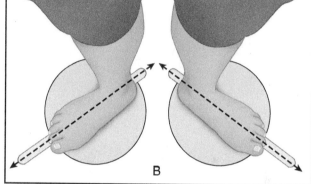

• **Figure 8-7** Standing static turnout is measured with the dancer standing in turnout, and the angle is measured with a goniometer directly under the foot **(A)** or using tracings **(B and C).**

• **Figure 8-8** Measurement of Dynamic Standing Turnout Using Rotational Disks. (Redrawn from Welsh TM, Rodriguez M, Beare LW, et al. Assessing turnout in university dancers. *J Dance Med Sci.* 2008;12(4):138.)

rotate the testing leg to the end range, with care taken to limit compensatory pelvic tilt or knee motion. Place the axis of the goniometer on the patella tendon, with the stationary arm perpendicular to the floor, and the moving arm along the tibia (Fig. 8-9, *A*).

For sitting goniometric measurement, position the dancer sitting with knees and hips flexed at 90 degrees, and allow the lower legs to hang over the edge of the table. The pelvis may be stabilized with a belt to keep weight evenly distributed on both sides. Passively externally rotate the testing leg to the end range, taking care to limit compensatory pelvic tilt or knee motion. Place the axis of the goniometer on the patella tendon, the stationary arm perpendicular to the floor, and the moving arm along the tibia (Fig. 8-9, *B*).

Clinical assessment of femoral anteversion also provides valuable information about structural limitations to turnout, as well as the potential for sustaining injury secondary to compensatory strategies to achieve greater turnout. A technique for clinical assessment, Craig test, correlates closely

(within 4 degrees) with intraoperative measurement values.[38] With the patient prone with the knee flexed at 90 degrees, the examiner palpates the greater trochanter while internally rotating the hip. At the point of maximum trochanteric prominence (i.e., when the neck of femur is parallel to the floor), the angle between the tibia midshaft and true vertical is measured with a goniometer (Fig. 8-10). This measurement represents femoral anteversion.[38] As stated earlier, normal range in the general population is 8 to 15 degrees. In the dance population, the lower the amount of femoral anteversion, the greater is the potential for achieving desirable turnout. Conversely, the greater the amount of femoral anteversion, the more limited the dancer will be in achieving desirable turnout, regardless of flexibility and strength of the hip.

Styles of Dance

In recent years, dance has become more diverse, with many different styles and contemporary interpretations of

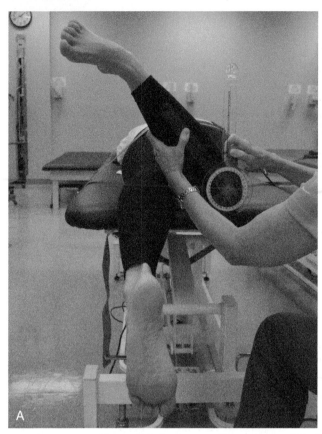
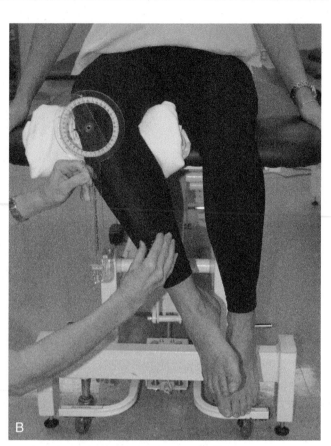

• **Figure 8-9** Goniometric Measurement of Hip External Rotation Range of Motion. **A,** In prone. **B,** In sitting.

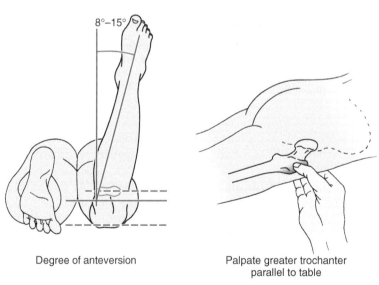

8°–15°

Degree of anteversion

Palpate greater trochanter parallel to table

• **Figure 8-10** Craig Test. (From Magee DJ: *Orthopedic Physical Assessment.* 6th ed. St. Louis: Saunders; 2014.)

traditional types of dance. Additionally, new and ethnic forms of dance have gained popularity in the mainstream dance circuit. In addition to ballet, jazz, and tap, it is not uncommon to locate community dance studios that offer classes in modern dance, Irish dance, Scottish highland dance, hip hop, capoeira, acro, salsa, flamenco, jumpstyle, belly dance, and more. Each dance genre requires specific

and stylistic movements that may increase risk for injuries to the hip.[9,39-41]

Excessive turnout is emphasized in some forms of dance, including ballet and Irish dance. In Irish dance, for example, excessive turnout and overcrossed legs are emphasized. In this form of dance, powerful jumps and stylistic maneuvers begin and end with the lower extremities externally rotated

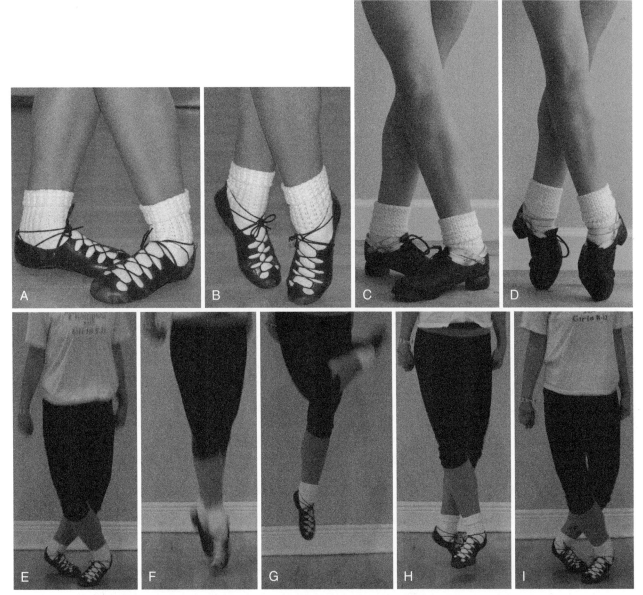

• **Figure 8-11** External rotation and overcrossing (adduction) is emphasized in Irish dance. **A** to **D,** Irish step dancers emphasize 'fifth position' with overcrossed ankles throughout most of their movements, whether dancing with soft shoes or hard shoes. **E** to **I,** In a signature ballistic movement referred to as a 'cut,' Irish dancers jump up from fifth position, further rotate one hip externally and simultaneously flex the knee to bring the foot to the opposite hip, and return to fifth position. It is important for the examiner to understand stylistic requirements of dance to identify risks and mechanisms of injury to the hip.

and adducted, which can lead to strength and flexibility imbalances that predispose the dancer to hip and other lower extremity injuries, some of which are discussed later in this chapter (Fig. 8-11).

Some forms of dance, however, do not emphasize extreme turnout, and the dancer will feel less pressure to achieve the excessive turnout position. These dance styles include jazz, modern, and tap. Evidence supports that these dancers achieve a lower mean turnout position than do ballet dancers.[42]

Early Excessive Training in Young Dancers

Not unlike in other athletic or performing arts populations, long hours of practice and the sometimes competitive or compulsive nature of the athlete may lead him or her to ignore early warning signs of injury. The dancing culture embodies this mentality, with a perception that injuries in dance are inevitable, and that dancing requires a stoic attitude toward pain, thus leading most dancers to "work through the pain."[43-45] Many dancers fear that physicians or other health providers will advise them to stop dancing,[46]

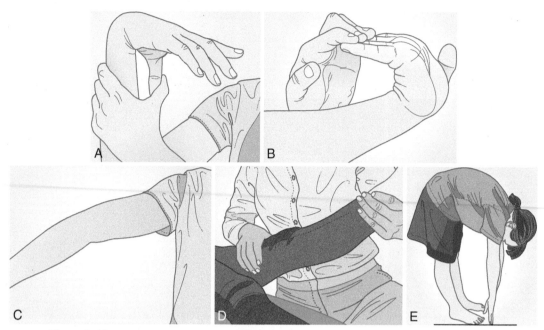

• **Figure 8-12 A** to **E,** Beighton scale movements diagram. (From Evans AM. *Pocket Podiatry: Paediatrics.* Edinburgh, United Kingdom: Churchill Livingstone; 2010:183-205.)

or they believe that health practitioners do not understand dance technique and lack training in dance injuries.[47] Evidence suggests that dancers may not comply with treatment protocols over the long term "if they perceive that such compliance would interfere with their training or performance."[48] Nonetheless, studies are encouraging, with findings indicating that physical therapists are viewed more favorably than other health providers by dancers and are seen as providing high-quality information during therapy.[48] The literature underscores the importance of being a therapist who is knowledgeable about general dance technique, specific dance style, training regimens, and dance injuries to establish an effective rapport and improved outcomes when working with this population.[50,51]

Muscle fatigue from overtraining can also lead to injury.[45] Previous studies indicated that more dance-related injuries are caused by overuse, rather than a defined traumatic injury.[3-5,9,15,16,52] Additionally, a sudden increase in training without the necessary increases in muscle strength and muscle endurance can precede the development of injuries, including stress fractures.[53] This finding underscores the need for proper training to minimize compensatory strategies, emphasis on correct technique, and education of both dancers and teachers on the importance of early identification and treatment of overuse injuries. Additional evidence suggests that periods of rest may be important in the prevention of injuries related to fatigue or overtraining. Previous research findings revealed that 90% of dancers felt tired when their injuries occurred, and 67% reported sustaining injuries toward the end of the season (performance or competition).[54] Another study found that fitness levels were lower at the end of the dancer's season, and they improved after the summer off-season.[55] This finding strengthens the

argument for periodization or rest periods for recovery. In some competitive or performance dance troops, however, no rest seasons exist, and training is year round. This is an important point of education for dancers, teachers, and directors in the prevention of dance injuries.

Joint Hypermobility and Stability

Epidemiologic studies suggest that the rate of hypermobility among dancers can be as high as 44%, particularly in students.[56] General joint hypermobility does not appear to be a factor that contributes to injury in dancers.[33,57] Rather, it is the lack of specific ranges of mobility, or core and stabilizing strength and control surrounding hypermobile joints, that may predispose dancers to injury.

Evidence indicates that joint hypermobility syndrome, a genetically inherited disorder of the connective tissue, has been correlated with increased injury in dancers.[57] The clinical presentation of this disorder consists of local or widespread musculoskeletal symptoms and joint hypermobility. Dancers with hypermobility and musculoskeletal symptoms can be screened to determine the presence of joint hypermobility syndrome or general joint hypermobility by using the Beighton scoring and Brighton criteria.[57] Although neither method was specifically designed for use in the dance population, and some criticisms of their applicability and validity in dancers and across various styles of dance have been expressed,[58] these measures are widely used clinically and in research. The Beighton scoring system of 1973,[59] a nine-point test consisting of active and passive movements, is a reliable indicator of general joint hypermobility[60] (Fig. 8-12 and Table 8-2). A score of 4 or more suggests general joint hyperlaxity

TABLE 8-2	Beighton Scoring System	
Movement		**Score**
Passive extension of the fifth finger beyond 90 degrees		1 point each side
Passive flexion of the thumb to touch the forearm		1 point each side
Hyperextension of the elbows beyond 10 degrees		1 point each side
Hyperextension of the knees beyond 10 degrees		1 point each side
Forward flexion of the trunk in standing with knees fully extended and palms of the hands flat on the floor		1 point

Data from Beighton P, Solomon L, Soskolne CL. Articular mobility in an African population. *Ann Rheum Dis.* 1973;32(5):413-418.

TABLE 8-3	Brighton Criteria	
Major Criteria		**Minor Criteria**
A Beighton score of 4 or greater Arthralgia for >3 months in 4 or more joints		A Beighton score of 1, 2, or 3 Arthralgia (>3 months' duration) in 1-3 joints or back pain (>3 months' duration) or spondylosis, spondylolysis, spondylolisthesis Dislocation or subluxation in >1 joint or in 1 joint on >1 occasion >3 soft tissue lesions (e.g., epicondylitis, bursitis) Marfanoid habitus Skin striae, hyperextensibility, thin skin, abnormal scarring Ocular signs (e.g., drooping eyelids, myopia) Varicose veins, hernia, or uterine or rectal prolapse Mitral valve prolapse

Requirements for diagnosis (presence of any 1 of the following conditions):
2 major criteria
1 major plus 2 minor criteria
4 minor criteria
2 minor criteria and unequivocally affected first-degree relative

Data from Grahame R, Bird HA, Child A. The revised (Brighton 1998) criteria for the diagnosis of benign joint hypermobility syndrome (BJHS). *J. Rheumatol.* 2000;27(7):1777-1779.

throughout the body. The Brighton criteria provide a measure of joint hypermobility syndrome based on validated criteria.[61] These criteria include the Beighton test score, symptoms, and signs of connective tissue deficiency[61] (Table 8-3).

For dancers with joint hypermobility syndrome, education and conditioning to improve neuromuscular control are crucial to preventing dance-related injury.[62,63] Hypermobility-related injury is discussed later in this chapter.

Nutrition and Female Athlete Triad

Poor nutrition and its impact on bone health in dancers have been topics of discussion and research for decades. Most forms of dance emphasize aesthetics of body movement and shape. This focus can lead to a preoccupation with body image and an increased risk for developing an eating disorder.[64] Stress fractures are associated with a more restrictive diet.[65] In a study published in 1990, Frusztajer and colleagues[65] found that dancers demonstrated energy restriction accompanied by decreased protein and fat intake, as well as deficient intake of minerals and vitamins that are crucial to optimal bone health; 70% of the dancers studied consumed less than 85% of the recommended dietary allowances for calories, and 60% presented with deficient protein intake. In 2000, Merrilees and associates[66] studied the effects of dairy food supplements on bone mineral density (BMD) in girls 15 to 18 years old. Results of this study indicated that daily supplemental calcium significantly improved BMD at the trochanter, femoral neck, and lumbar spine.

Deficiencies in nutrients, particularly bone-building nutrients such as calcium, magnesium, iron, and vitamins D, K, and C may limit new bone formation.[67] Sustained energy deficit, inadequate caloric intake relative to energy

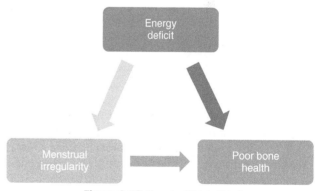

• **Figure 8-13** Female Athlete Triad.

expenditure through exercise, can disrupt hormone balance. This disruption, in turn, can lead to decreased osteoblast activity, increased bone resorption, and reduced ability to repair microdamage.[68-71] Nutritional deficits compromise bone by increasing susceptibility to fractures.[31] Lack of adequate nutrition can also affect muscular strength.[72]

The female athlete triad (FAT) is a syndrome of three interrelated disorders: energy deficits (disordered eating), menstrual irregularities, and decreased bone density (Fig. 8-13). Energy availability is the cornerstone of FAT.[11] All three disorders of FAT are associated with inadequate energy reserves.[73] Female athletes with disordered eating are more than twice as likely to have menstrual irregularities than female athletes without disordered eating.[74] Athletes with menstrual irregularity have significantly lower BMD.[75]

Female athletes, particularly those involved in a sport with an aesthetic component (e.g., dance, figure skating, gymnastics), are at greater risk for developing FAT.[11] In a study comparing elite professional female dancers and recreationally active female nondancers, the dancers experienced delayed menarche, decreased energy intake, and abnormal eating behaviors, exhibiting symptoms of the three conditions of FAT.[76] As mentioned previously, lack of nutrition from disordered eating can contribute to poor bone health and result in increased risk for stress fracture.[17] A relationship exists between components of FAT and stress fracture in dancers.[77,78] Additionally, a positive correlation is seen specifically between menstrual dysfunction and stress fractures.[79] Barrack and associates[80] studied the effect of single or combined risk factors (defined by FAT) with bone stress injuries in 259 female adolescents and young women. FAT risk factors included low body weight, low body mass index, high-volume exercise (>12 hours/week of purposeful exercise), elevated dietary restraint, pathogenic weight control behavior, participation in a leanness sport, late age of menarche, oligomenorrhea or amenorrhea, and low BMD. Findings indicate that cumulative risk for bone stress injury increases as the number of FAT-related risk factors accumulates.

The effects of nutrition, dance exposure, and pubertal delay on BMD were examined in 127 female preprofessional ballet dancers, 15 to 17 years old,[81] and the findings supported the importance of a balanced diet including calcium from dairy sources as a positive determinant for bone development. The number of years since menarche was also positively correlated with bone development.[81] In this study, the weight-bearing activity of dance appeared to protect BMD in weight-bearing bones. Similarly, in a controlled study, Friesen and colleagues[82] examined body composition, BMD, eating behaviors, and menstrual dysfunction in 31 collegiate modern dancers who were 18 to 25 years old. Compared with controls, the dancers reported a higher prevalence of disordered eating and menstrual dysfunction. Bone mass in the dancers was higher for weight-bearing bones, attributed to the weight-bearing aspects of modern dance training.[82] However, evidence indicates that although the weight-bearing aspects of dance appear to increase BMD of the lumbar spine and femoral neck, amenorrheic dancers have significantly lower BMD at the femoral neck and spine compared with their eumenorrheic counterparts.[81,83] This decreased BMD puts amenorrheic dancers at risk for fracture. Dancers have a higher incidence of bone stress injuries to the lower extremities, including the femur, acetabulum, and sacrum.[8,78,84,85]

Disordered eating, menstrual irregularities, and low BMD are important health issues for all dancers regardless of skill level.[86] Despite the evidence to support the importance of proper nutrition and energy intake for dancers, most dance programs do not initiate nutrition education with young dancers and their parents. Yet, the aesthetics and desirable thin physique of dancers is continuously reinforced in the culture of dance. Proper nutrition and eating habits should be developed alongside dance technique, particularly for young and adolescent dancers, to prevent the development of FAT and its associated risk for bone stress injuries.

Snapping Hip Syndrome (Coxa Saltans)

General Information and Common Mechanisms

Snapping hip, or coxa saltans, manifests as an audible or palpable extraarticular snapping that occurs around the hip during movement. Although often painless, it may be associated with pain or discomfort. Snapping hip occurs in approximately 10% of the general population, but it is especially prevalent in athletes, including dancers.[87] Many variables are associated with the onset of snapping hip, including muscle imbalance, muscle fatigue, muscular weakness, inadequate warmup, suboptimal training, age, and previous injury to the same muscle tissue.[33,88]

Snapping hip is particularly common in dancers, and it accounts for approximately 43.8% of hip problems in ballet dancers.[89] To diagnose and treat snapping hip properly, it is important to identify the cause. The causes of extraarticular snapping hip can be divided into two categories: external snapping hip syndrome (ESHS) and internal snapping hip syndrome (ISHS). These disorders are discussed in the context of dance-related causes and rehabilitation. For more detailed information about snapping hip syndrome, please see Chapter 3.

External Snapping Hip Syndrome

External snapping is attributed to the iliotibial band (ITB) or gluteus maximus snapping over the greater trochanter. Dancers with ESHS often describe a snapping sound from their lateral hip that occurs during movement transitions. This snap, or clunk sound, typically occurs when returning the leg from an extended, abducted, and externally rotated alignment.[90]

The onset of ESHS occurs between 14 and 16 years of age for approximately 50% of dancers, and it coincides with the age when a dancer develops the strength and flexibility to achieve and maintain their extensions at or above 90 degrees.[91] It is associated with adaptive shortening of the hip abductors and external rotators, which may result from an increase in the intensity and frequency of dance training, and it may be perpetuated by faulty dance technique as the dancer is developing new skills.[91] Factors that increase the risk of external snapping hip include a wide pelvis, prominent greater trochanter, ligamentous

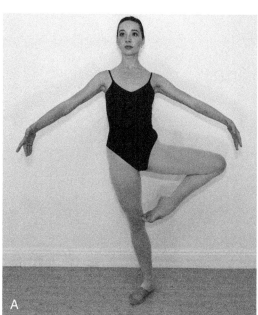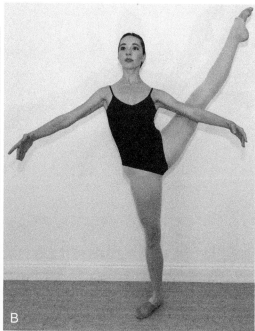

• **Figure 8-14** Ballet Positions That Flex, Abduct, and Externally Rotate the Hip. **A,** Développé to passé. **B,** Développé in second.

hyperlaxity, weakness of the hip abductors, and tightness of the ITB.[92,93]

Internal Snapping Hip Syndrome

In ISHS, the iliopsoas tendon snaps over a bony prominence, typically the iliopectineal eminence, femoral head, anterior capsule, or lesser trochanter. The tendon is susceptible to injury when the hip is flexed, abducted, and externally rotated. In dance, several positions require this motion repetitively. For example, in ballet, dancers access this motion when they move into *développé to passé* or *développé in second* positions (Fig. 8-14). These positions have been theorized to cause the psoas tendon to pull into a "U" shape as it passes below the inguinal ligament.[94]

The majority of research on snapping hip syndrome in dancers has focused specifically on ballet dancers. Currently, no studies have specifically investigated snapping hip syndrome in other types or styles of dance. This gap in research may reflect the ability to study large subject populations in ballet schools and professional ballet academies.

Assessment

The dancer's symptoms greatly assist in the diagnosis of snapping hip syndrome. In a study of ballet dancers, Winslow and Yoder found that 90% reported a history of experiencing a hip that "cracks, pops, snaps, or clicks," with 16.7% of symptoms specifically occurring at the lateral hip.[91] In the majority of cases, however, the dancers were unable to localize the source of the noise. Some degree of pain was reported with the snap at the greater trochanter by 58.4% of those dancers, and 59% could voluntarily reproduce the snap.[91]

It may be valuable to have the dancer demonstrate the motions that provoke the snapping to differentiate the source of the snapping. Provocation tests applied by the clinician to produce a palpable snap are not necessary when voluntary snapping is present. In the presence of voluntary snapping, the snapping is palpable to the clinician. The specific dance movements that commonly cause the snap involve the dancer in the *second position*, with the leg approaching or passing 90 degrees of abduction in the turned-out position (Fig. 8-15). This movement has been implicated in iliopsoas snapping.[95] Two other movements have been linked to ITB snapping: the front kick (grand battement) and a forward bend (Fig. 8-16).[95] A small number of dancers found that by snapping the hip on purpose, they could obtain pain relief.[92]

Dancers are known for their high degree of flexibility, but repetition of specific motions (e.g., to achieve desired turnout) can lead to imbalances in flexibility and compensatory soft tissue tightness. A tight tensor fasciae latae (TFL) and ITB, specifically, may contribute to snapping hip, and they should be evaluated. ITB flexibility can be assessed in the Ober position (Fig. 8-17, *A*). Psoas flexibility measured in the Thomas position (Fig. 8-17, *B*) can often reveal iliopsoas restriction, as well as compensatory tightness in the TFL. TFL tightness is indicated if the test leg remains in external rotation or abducts at the full hip extension position (Fig. 8-17, *C*). The iliopsoas is a deep structure, and isolating the tendon by manual palpation is difficult. Chapter 2 has further details on these test positions.

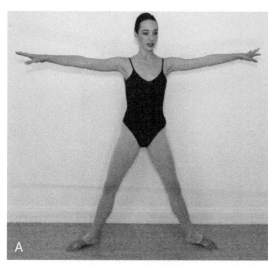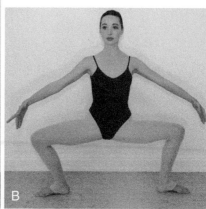

• **Figure 8-15** Dance Movements That Commonly Cause Snapping. **A**, Second position. **B,** The leg approaching or passing 90 degrees of abduction in second position.

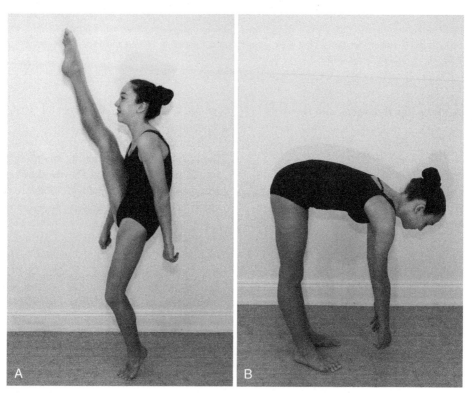

• **Figure 8-16** Movements Linked To Iliotibial Band Snapping. **A**, The front kick (grand battement). **B,** The forward bend.

Assessment of strength in the muscles surrounding the hip is also important. A study by Bennell and colleagues[31] found that dancers generally have less hip muscle strength in their flexors and abductors than do their athlete or nonathlete counterparts. Additionally, dancers in the study ranked in the lower 77th strength percentile when compared with other female athletes that included soccer players, weight lifters, and runners. This relative strength deficiency may be a contributing factor to the high incidence of snapping hip in the dance population.[31]

Rehabilitation and Treatment Considerations

Snapping hip may not be problematic for all dancers, but it may cause a varying degree of pain or discomfort at some point during their dance career. Rehabilitation of snapping hip dysfunction of either the ISHS or the ESHS must consider the following key issues:

1. Optimize technique for improved anatomical alignment and reduce compensation.
2. Identify soft tissue and myofascial restrictions that impair normal movement.

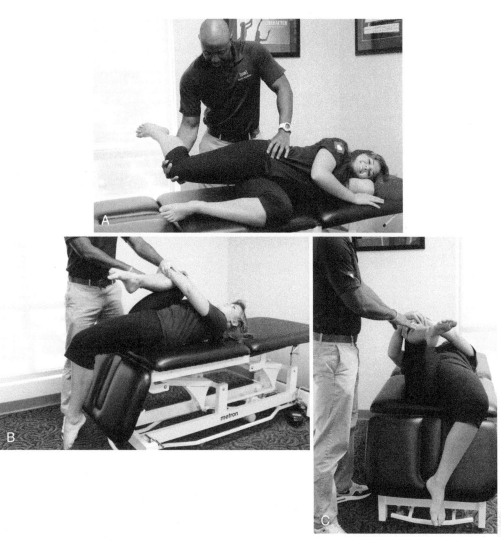

• **Figure 8-17** Assessing Flexibility. **A,** Iliotibial band flexibility should be tested in the Ober position. **B,** Psoas flexibility measured in the Thomas position **C,** The Thomas test can also reveal tensor fasciae latae tightness if the test leg remains in external rotation or abducts at the full hip extension position.

3. Improve muscle imbalances at the hip and knee.
4. Increase core and pelvic stability.

Research specific to rehabilitation of the dancer with snapping hip syndrome is lacking. Nevertheless, strength and flexibility imbalances contribute to the development of snapping hip in dance,[93] and they should be a focus of assessment and rehabilitation. Treatment should first be directed toward correcting alignment and releasing myofascial restrictions before any strengthening and neuromuscular reeducation program is undertaken. Exercises designed to restore muscle balance, increase proprioceptive control at the hip, and facilitate core stabilization can be achieved through eccentric strengthening and functional multiplanar motions that promote neutral force distribution through the lower extremity. Strengthening the deep external rotators, hip abductors, and core stabilizers to maintain full turnout with the pelvis supported over their base of support will often benefit the dancer during rehabilitation of this condition (Figs. 8-18 and 8-19).

Focal Rotatory Laxity

Common Mechanisms

Focal rotatory laxity refers to the development of localized adaptive increased laxity of the hip ligaments that is the result of repetitive rotational stresses to the hip joint. Dancers often subject their hips to the extremes of passive hip range of motion, particularly the combination of external rotation and extension. In a sample of 49 professional dancers (37 women and 12 men) who were 15 to 32 years old, Drężewska and colleagues[97] found that the range of flexion, extension, and external rotation was significantly greater in the dancers, particularly those with more than 10 years of dance experience, and that hip mobility was greater in female dancers. Findings also revealed a significantly greater range of flexion, abduction, and external rotation in dancers who had an earlier injury to their hip joints.[97] Repeated and aggressive stretching in these positions often

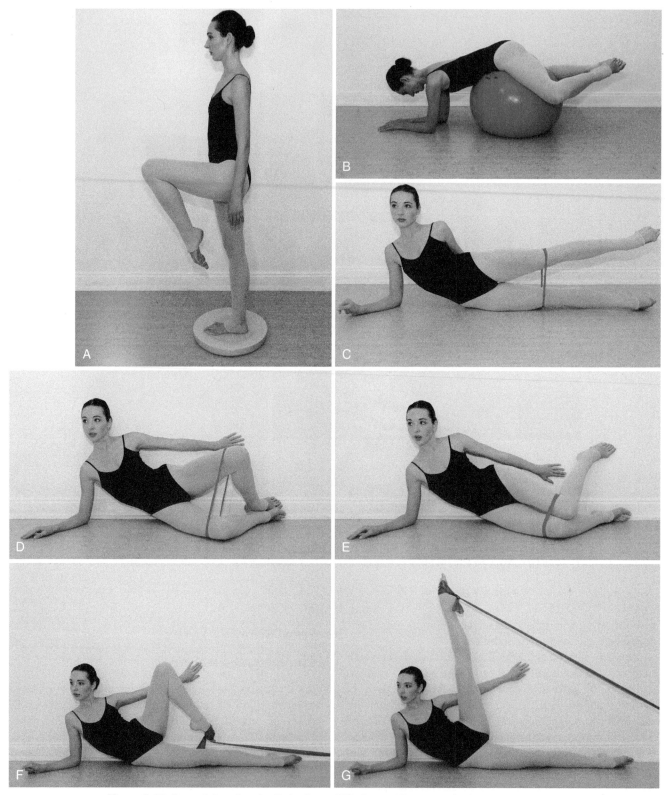

• **Figure 8-18** Strength Exercises for Abduction and Hip External Rotator Activation. **A,** Proprioceptive balance exercise. **B,** Prone over ball with hip external rotator isometric activation. **C,** Side-lying abduction. **D,** Clam shell. **E,** Clam shell with internal rotation and attempted abduction. **F,** Combination abduction and external rotation with resistance (passé). **G,** Abduction and external rotation with resistance (full développé).

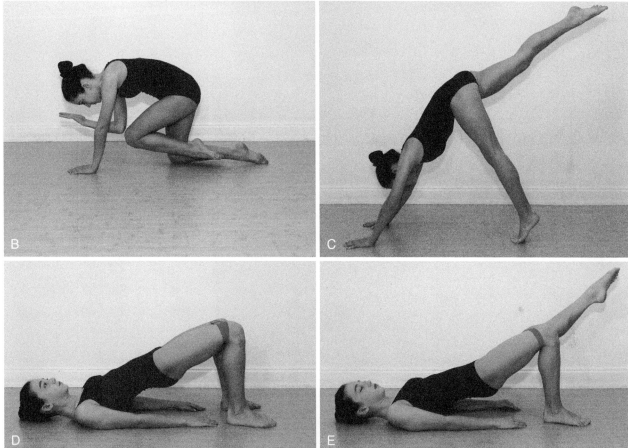

• **Figure 8-19** Core Strengthening Exercises. **A,** Quadruped opposite extremity extension. **B,** Quadruped opposite flexion. **C,** Inverted-V hip extension. **D,** Bridge with resisted band. **E,** Single leg bridge with resisted band for abduction and external rotation.

results in a significant discrepancy between a dancer's active and passive hip range of motion. The imbalance between the excessive passive motion and insufficient active strength in that same direction can contribute to joint instability and the development of focal rotatory laxity. Figure 8-20 illustrates the difference between the passive mobility and active control of the hip joint in functional dance positions.

Increased ligamentous laxity can contribute to focal rotary laxity. The hip is supported by four ligaments: the iliofemoral ligament, the ischiofemoral ligament, the pubofemoral ligament, and the ligamentum teres (Table 8-4). The combined support provided by the first three ligaments functions to limit excessive external rotation and hyperex-

tension of the hip. The iliofemoral ligament prevents excessive extension of the hip joint and also supports upright posture. The pubofemoral ligament limits excessive hip extension and also prevents excessive abduction of the hip. The pubofemoral and ischiofemoral ligaments also contribute to limit hyperabduction. The ischiofemoral ligament is the weakest of these ligaments, and it helps stabilize extension of the hip. The ligamentum teres contributes to hip stability by preventing excessive external rotation during flexion of the hip. Chapter 1 contains further discussion of the ligaments surrounding the hip joint.

Several positions, motions, and stretches common to dancers can compromise the ligamentous stability of the hip

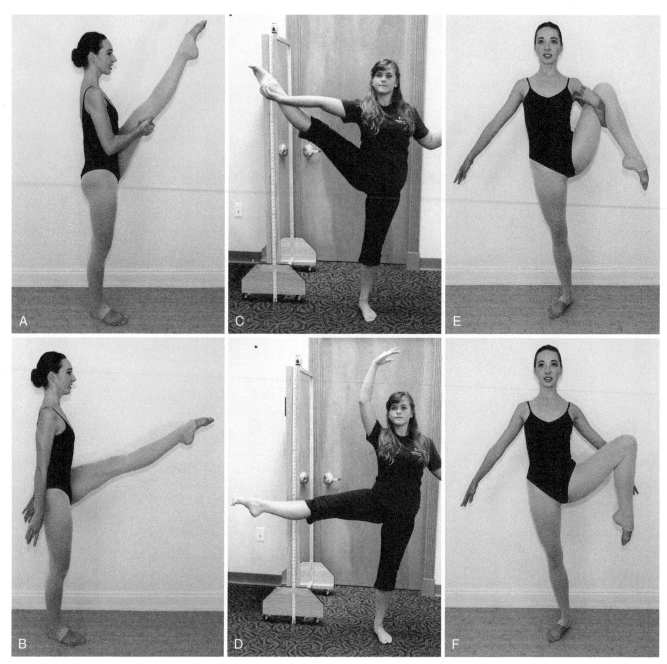

• **Figure 8-20** Functional Assessment of Dance-Specific Passive and Active Hip Mobility. **A,** Passive hip flexion with knee extension. **B,** Active hip flexion with knee extended. **C,** Passive abduction and external rotation. **D,** Active abduction and external rotation (développé). **E,** Passive abduction and external rotation with knee flexion. **F,** Active abduction and external rotation with knee flexion.

joint. The iliofemoral ligament is a strong ligament that connects the pelvis to the femur at the front of the joint (Fig. 8-21). It is considered one of the strongest ligaments in the body. It resembles a Y in shape and stabilizes the hip by limiting hyperextension. The split position in dance requires significant flexibility in the iliofemoral ligament. In the split position, the rear leg is hyperextended, placing stress on the iliofemoral ligament (Fig. 8-22). To achieve a complete split alignment, many dancers compensate by externally rotating the rear leg. The addition of external rotation in the presence of passive hyperextension places

more strain on all four hip ligaments. This type of compensation (in a split) is distinguished by the rear knee pointing out laterally (Fig. 8-23). Repetitive, passive overstretching in this end-range position can result in the development of acquired ligamentous hyperlaxity with anterior capsular distention. Associated symptoms of localized instability may include hip flexor spasms and quadratus lumborum spasms, thus giving the dancer a false illusion of hip tightness. The dancer may then attempt to stretch the musculature further, and this can cause additional capsular elongation. It is important to cue the dancer to develop the flexibility in a

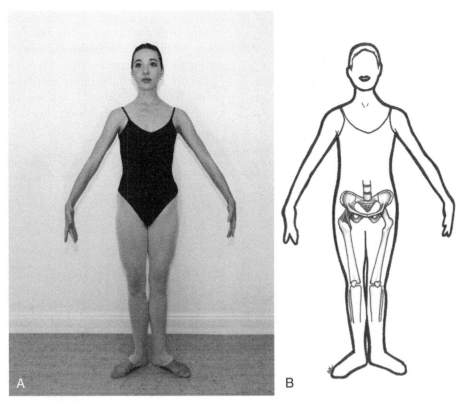

• **Figure 8-21 A** and **B,** The iliofemoral ligament connects the pelvis to the femur at the front of the joint in a Y shape and stabilizes the hip by limiting hyperextension.

TABLE 8-4	Ligaments of the Hip
Ligament	**Function**
Iliofemoral ligament	Stabilizes hip joint during extension Restricts excessive hip external rotation Restricts hip hyperextension Restricts hip hyperabduction Supports upright posture
Ischiofemoral ligament	Restricts excessive external rotation Restricts hip hyperextension Restricts hip hyperabduction
Pubofemoral ligament	Restricts excessive external rotation Restricts hip hyperextension Restricts hip hyperabduction
Ligamentum teres	Prevents excessive external rotation during hip flexion

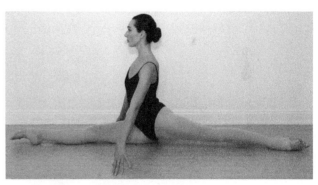

• **Figure 8-22** In the split position, the rear leg is hyperextended, placing stress on the iliofemoral ligament.

split to allow the hips to remain in a squared, or neutral, position. In this split position, referred to as a pure extension front split, the rear leg is in an extended position with the patella pointing straight down in contact with the ground. In a pure extension split, the dancer should be able to flex the rear knee and the lower leg would point straight to the ceiling (Fig. 8-24).

Additionally, the front leg of a split position places the ligamentum teres on stretch. Often, the dancer has to rotate the front leg externally to achieve the full expression of the position. The combination of repetitive stress during dynamic dance activities and a focus on passive stretching to achieve extreme ranges of flexibility can result in the development of focal rotatory laxity of the hip joint and, in extreme cases, can lead to instability of the joint.

Positions and motions in extreme ranges are often desirable aesthetically in dance. One such position is the *oversplit*. To achieve an oversplit, the dancer places the heel of the front leg on an elevated surface (see Fig. 8-23). This position requires a significant increase in the length of the ligamentum teres. Once this ligament is passively lengthened to such an extreme, it may lose its ability to provide stability during axial loading and external rotation. Injuries to the ligamentum teres have been a documented source of intractable hip pain in athletes, including ballet dancers.[98]

Other ligaments can become compromised during a split. The functions of the pubofemoral ligament are to prevent hyperextension and overabduction and to limit external rotation. The rear leg of a front split requires the pubofemoral ligament to tighten, but this action serves a less important limiting role in comparison with the ilio-femoral ligament in the hip joint. The pubofemoral ligament is considered a supporting element of the joint capsule, by reinforcing the inferior and anterior capsule. It is placed under the greatest amount of stress with a center straddle split position (Fig. 8-25). In the center straddle split position, both hips are hyperabducted and externally rotated. Repetitive overstretching in the center straddle split will affect this ligament, further contributing to focal rotatory laxity around the hip joint.

Turnout alignment that is used in dance requires a great deal of flexibility in the iliofemoral ligament (Y ligament). Many dancers are unable to attain the perfect turnout because of limitations around the hip. As described earlier in this chapter, dancers with limited hip motion may resort to compensation to achieve desired turnout. The most common compensation of the pelvis during turnout is increased anterior tilt (Fig. 8-26). By tilting the pelvis forward, the anterior ligaments become slack and allow for more hip external rotation. Some dancers compensate by moving into a posterior pelvic tilt. Posteriorly tilting the pelvis alters the femoral-acetabular dynamics, thereby adding additional stress to all hip structures. Posterior tilting essentially forces a full turnout position with increased stress on the ligaments. Although it is rare to observe a dancer who defaults to a posterior tilt, this compensation has the

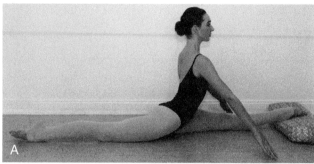
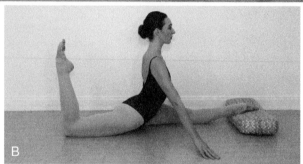

• **Figure 8-24** Pure Extension Front Split. **A,** In a pure extension front split, the rear leg is in an extended position with the patella pointing straight down in contact with the ground. **B,** In a pure extension front split, the dancer should be able to flex the rear knee and the lower leg would point straight to the ceiling.

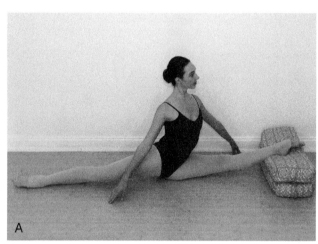
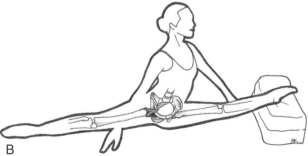

• **Figure 8-23 A,** To achieve a complete split alignment, many dancers compensate by externally rotating the rear leg. **B,** The addition of external rotation in the presence of passive hyperextension places more strain on all four hip ligaments.

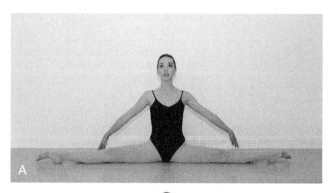
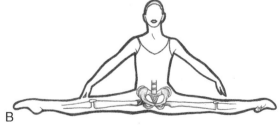

• **Figure 8-25 A** and **B,** The pubofemoral ligament is placed under the greatest amount of stress with a center straddle split position.

greatest stress on the ligaments that support hip stability in turnout. This malalignment limits the actual range of motion of the hips and activates the external rotator muscles. It also places strain on the hip flexor muscles and anterior hip labral complex. Loading a labral-deficient hip can cause significant elongation of the iliofemoral ligament.[99] These compensations put the dancer at risk of developing chronic focal rotatory instability of the hip, with increased load on the other structures of the hip joint.

Instability of the hip is often a complaint in high-level athletes participating in sports that involve the combination of repetitive hip rotation and axial loading (i.e., golf, figure skating, football, gymnastics, ballet, baseball, and martial arts).[100] Several common dance positions combine these motions: arabesque stance leg (Fig. 8-27), side tilt, and leaps. The excessive repetitive movements in these non-physiologic positions during dance can result in very high loads that strain the muscles and ligaments.[101]

Although tears of the ligamentum teres can be the result of traumatic dislocation in any sport, they more commonly have an insidious onset. During dance movements resulting in high external rotatory and axial distraction forces, the function of the ligamentum teres is thought to provide secondary stabilization of external rotation. Repetitive external rotation of the hip and axial loading may cause increased capsular laxity. Because of the subsequent instability, excess stress is placed on the ligamentum teres, and tears may occur. Ligamentum teres injuries are most commonly treated with arthroscopic débridement.[102]

Assessment

In athletes with hip instability, the most valuable information for diagnosis comes from the patient's ability to describe or demonstrate the motion that reproduces the symptoms. Patients may complain of feeling the leg "give out" during gait and sport activities.[99] In physical examination, athletes with instability often present with an audible, painful "pop" when the hip is brought from flexion to extension or with axial distraction. Most patients with capsular laxity have increased passive range of motion of the joint. This is evident when the dancer is supine with legs extended in a relaxed position; the symptomatic lower extremity may have more external rotation compared with the other side. The result of the flexion adduction internal rotation (FADIR) test may also be positive for pain from impingement because of underlying joint hypermobility (Fig. 8-28).[103]

Rehabilitation Considerations

To optimize alignment, the dancer should be cued to bring the tailbone down, thus achieving a neutral alignment of the lumbar spine, and activate the core by drawing the navel to the spine. The clinician should educate the dancer to stretch in proper alignment and to dedicate the time after practice to gain flexibility. Improving joint stability can be

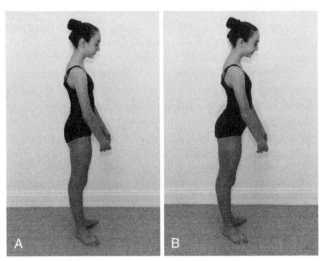

• **Figure 8-26 A,** Corrected turnout with neutral alignment. **B,** Excessive anterior pelvic tilt in turnout.

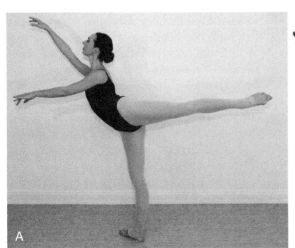
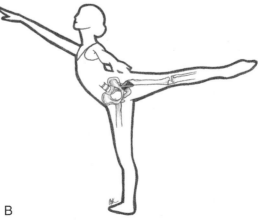

• **Figure 8-27 A** and **B,** Arabesque position places stress on the ligaments.

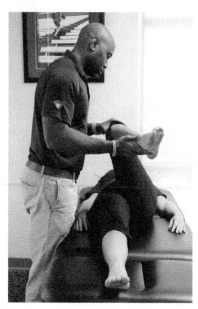

• **Figure 8-28** Results of the flexion adduction internal rotation (FADIR) test may be positive for pain from impingement resulting from underlying joint hypermobility.

achieved through weight-bearing proprioceptive exercises and exercises to increase rotational strength of the hip joint. Figure 8-29 illustrates suggested exercises to improve hip proprioception and rotational strength in dancers with focal rotary instability.

Extreme ranges of motion and repetitive forces placed through the hip are required in most forms of dance. This requirement can make rehabilitating these athletes a challenge. It is valuable to develop an understanding of dance postures and their associated biomechanical demands. This understanding can help the examiner identify the clinical origin of the dancer's injury and allow for a successful rehabilitation process.

Labral Disorders

Epidemiology

Dance often requires a combination of high volumes of training intensity and the repetition of extreme ranges of motion. With these demands, it is not surprising that many dancers complain of hip pain related to the labrum.[18] Kocher and associates[104] reported that 50% of dancers seen in their dance medicine clinic over a 3-year period came for assessment and treatment of hip pain, and 40% of those dancers were found to have a labral tear. In the general population, the prevalence of labral tears in patients presenting with hip pain has been reported to be 22% to 55%.[105]

Labral tears are associated with painful and unpredictable catching sensations in the groin, especially with internal rotation at 90 degrees of hip flexion and abduction.[104] If the labrum tears, it may act pathologically as a flap that results in intraarticular impingement limiting rotation.

Dance-Specific Biomechanics and the Kinematics of the Labrum

Specific sports, including ballet, have been linked to labral injury in previous studies.[106,107] Crawford and colleagues[108] studied the effects of labral lesions on hip kinematics at the extremes of hip joint motion. These investigators found that in the position of hip extension with abduction and external rotation, a large strain was placed on the anterior labrum at the acetabular interface where labral lesions are commonly found. This combination of movement is fundamental and is frequently accessed in all styles of dance.

FAI results from abnormal contact between the proximal femur, typically the anterosuperior femoral head neck junction, and the acetabular rim. A study by Charbonnier and associates[109] revealed that subluxation of the hip occurs frequently during extreme range of motion in dance and that all these subluxations occurred in conjunction with impingements. The study identified two specific sites of impingement; the first site was located in the superior quadrant of the acetabulum, and the second site of impingement was the posterosuperior acetabulum. These findings were confirmed on magnetic resonance imaging (MRI). Several specific dance movements appeared to produce the greatest stress on the hip. The front développé produced the highest frequency of subluxation (39%) (Fig. 8-30, *A*). The gesture leg of side développé had the highest frequency of femoroacetabular impingement (70%) (Fig. 8-30, *B*). Grand plié in second had the highest depth of penetration and the most femoroacetabular translations (Fig. 8-30, *C*).

Another study of dancers, by Safran and colleagues,[110] revealed that when the hip was externally rotated, the posterior labrum underwent significantly increased strain. Dancers have to maintain the hip in external rotation while dancing (i.e., the turnout position). This could explain why lesions were found in superior and posterosuperior positions. In an effort to preserve the hip structures, it may be beneficial to limit the number of times a dancer performs these movements during rehearsals and training to reduce repetitive stress and progressive weakening of the labrum in these areas that are prone to injury.[108]

Joint hypermobility may also be associated with FAI.[111] In a study of 55 patients 18 to 55 years old with a diagnosis of FAI, the self-reported Beighton score was feasible and reliable in determining the presence of joint hypermobility.[112] The presence of joint hypermobility in the subjects was high (i.e., 50% of the female and 24.3% of the male patients who participated in the study), a finding suggesting that joint hypermobility may be an underlying cause of FAI.[112] The dancer's desire for the aesthetics of hyperflexibility, coupled with the demands for extreme range of motion in some forms of dance, may put the dancer at risk for FAI and labral tear.

Athletic movements that require repetitive pivoting on a loaded femur are also associated with labral injury, and this is a common motion for most forms of dance. Duthon and colleagues[112a] identified labral tears with MRI in 18 of 20

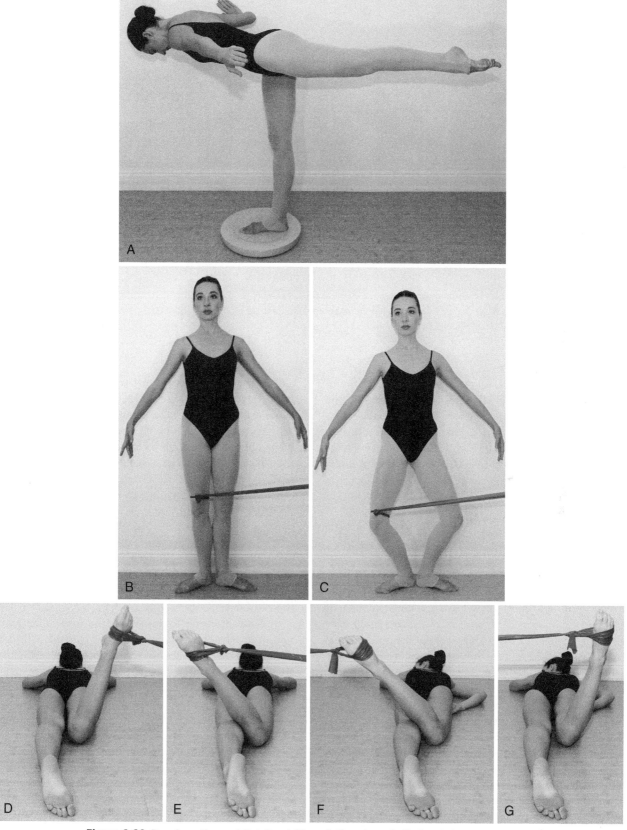

• **Figure 8-29** Proprioceptive and Rotational Strength Exercises. **A,** Airplane balance proprioceptive exercise. **B** and **C,** Plié from first position with resisted external rotation. **D** and **E,** Resisted external rotation. **F** and **G,** Resisted internal rotation.

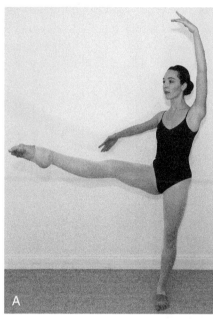
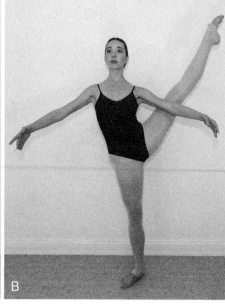
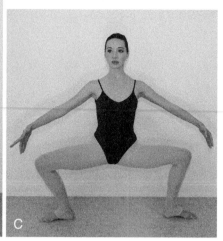

• **Figure 8-30** Dance Positions That Increase Impingement. **A,** Front développé. **B,** Side développé. **C,** Grand plié in second position.

professional ballet dancers. All the labral lesions were found in the superior aspect or posterosuperior aspect of the labrum. Previous research, conducted in the general population, overwhelmingly reported lesions in the anterior or anterosuperior labrum.[113] The high incidence of labral tears in dancers appears to reflect the extreme compression forces placed on the labrum during dance activities, which accelerate deterioration.[105]

Client Profile, Objective Findings, and Symptoms

The dancer with a labrum tear often presents with complaints of a deep, aching-type pain. Pain localized to the anterior groin has been reported in approximately 92% of patients with confirmed labral tears.[114] Patients often have a delay of 2 years or more in seeking care because dancers frequently seek medical care only after pain becomes severe enough that it interferes with participation.[104] Approximately 50% of patients with labral tears also describe mechanical symptoms such as clicking, catching, or giving way.[115] Night pain has also been identified as a frequent complaint.[116] Magnetic resonance arthrography (MRA) is particularly useful for evaluating the presence of labral disorders.[117] The Beighton score, discussed earlier, is helpful during clinical assessment by providing information about the presence of joint hypermobility.

Medical Management and Rehabilitation Considerations

The available research on the current management of labral tears has not been directly applied to a dance population,

although most of the data are relevant to providing treatment for dancers.[118] The current medical management of labral tears in dancers is based on similar recommendations for the general population. Conservative and surgical treatment options exist. One of the difficulties in determining the efficacy of treatment for labral tears is that researchers have used different measures to assess outcomes. For outcome measurement tools to be used with dancers, the extremes of range of motion used and the lengthy hours of participation required of this population must be considered.[118] The Hip Outcome Score (HOS) has the largest amount of evidence to support its use in dancers, but the Harris Hip Score is the most common outcome measure currently used by clinicians and researchers for dancers with hip disorders.[119]

If the dancer opts to pursue a conservative management option to rehabilitate a labral injury, he or she will have to modify dance activities to reduce stress on the labrum. Activity modification is a particularly important component of conservative management.[120] Avoidance of pain-provoking motions helps to reduce inflammation. In addition to activity modification, developing core strength (e.g., lower abdominal and transverse abdominal muscles) is valuable, as is improving hip joint stability by increasing synergistic recruitment of the deep hip rotators, abductors, and adductors. In a study of four patients with clinical evidence of an acetabular labrum tear, all patients responded well to a nonsurgical program that emphasized hip and lumbopelvic stabilization, correction of muscular imbalance, and sport-specific functional progression.[121] These results may suggest that patients with clinical evidence of an acetabular labral tear can show meaningful improvement with conservative intervention. Avoiding passive stretching at the end range of hip extension can possibly help to reduce strain across the anterior capsule and protect the labrum from further weakening.

Research on appropriate nonsurgical physical therapy intervention for those with suspected labral tears is limited. Further research is necessary to determine the short-term and long-term effectiveness of this approach in the management of suspected labral injuries in dancers.

Patients with confirmed labral tear and pain that persists after activity modification and a physical therapy trial may consider surgical correction. Many of these abnormalities can now also be corrected with arthroscopy. Arthroscopic surgery for labrum repair and FAI had outcomes equal to or better than those with open dislocation or mini-open methods, with a lower rate of major complications.[122]

Surgical labral repair requires lengthy rehabilitation and a period of limited weight bearing. When cam or pincer lesions are present, osteoplasty may be required to avoid recurrence. If an anatomic abnormality is found to be the cause of the labral damage, correction of this irregularity is recommended to prevent recurrence. Although few cases of cam- or pincer-type impingement or dysplasia have been noted in preprofessional or professional dancers, recreational dancers may have an incidence rate similar to that of nondancers.[118]

Return to high-level dance activity after labral surgical procedures is possible, but it can take 7 to 12 months for a dancer to return to full capacity.[105] Dancers may be hesitant to undergo these procedures because of the increased length of time for return to dance activities. Medical professionals must inform the dancer of the risk of accelerated degeneration of the joint when the labrum is débrided. In most cases, medical advice is to preserve as much of the remaining cartilage as possible to reduce risk of joint degeneration. A good understanding of the potential risks and benefits of all treatment options can assist the dancer in making an informed decision based on his or her individual circumstances.[122]

Chapter 4 has a more detailed discussion including rehabilitation considerations.

Other Musculoskeletal Injuries of the Hip Common in Dancers

Piriformis Syndrome

The piriformis muscle is responsible for external hip rotation in standing and is actively used by dancers to achieve turnout. This muscle becomes an internal rotator when the hip is flexed greater than 90 degrees. The piriformis muscle originates from the anterior surface of the sacrum, exits through the sciatic notch after bridging the anterior surface of the sacroiliac joint, and then inserts into the upper border of the greater trochanter. It is the strongest of the deep hip rotators, and because of its close proximity to neurovascular structures such as the sciatic nerve, irritation or spasms of the piriformis muscle can result in radiating pain down the posterior hip, along the sciatic nerve. Although sciatic nerve pain is more often associated with compression of lower spinal nerve roots from disk herniation or spondylolisthesis, the presence of this type of pain as a result of pure piriformis syndrome is a diagnosis of exclusion.

Epidemiology

A primary cause of piriformis syndrome is compression of the sciatic nerve attributed to spasms, shortening, irritation, or adhesions resulting from direct trauma, postsurgical injury, overuse, or prolonged sitting.[123,124] Another theory described in the literature centers on muscle imbalances in the hip. Patients with piriformis syndrome often present with hip abductor weakness.[125-128] Tonley and associates[127] posited that the piriformis muscle may either function in an elongated position or is subjected to high eccentric loads resulting from weak agonist muscles. Thus, weak gluteus maximus or medius muscles cause the hip to adduct and internally rotate excessively during weight-bearing activities and shift the eccentric load to the piriformis muscle. Repetitive eccentric overlengthening demands result in sciatic nerve compression or irritation.[127]

Muscle imbalances surrounding the hip joint, such as extensive recruitment of external rotation coupled with inadequate internal rotator strength and progressive posterolateral soft tissue tightness, may be contributing factors in piriformis syndrome in dancers. Poor technique may also result in compensatory overuse of the piriformis muscle. For example, excessive activation of the upper deep external rotator muscles (piriformis) and insufficient use of the lower deep external rotation muscles (i.e., obturator internus or externus, gemellus, and quadratus femoris) can lead to overuse.[129] Overtraining and postural fatigue can also result in compensatory patterns. As the dancer becomes fatigued, he or she may tilt the pelvis anteriorly to try to achieve greater turnout. Piriformis syndrome is also associated with sacroiliac dysfunction.[35]

Client Profile, Objective Findings, and Symptoms

Signs and symptoms of piriformis syndrome include a history of trauma to the sacroiliac and gluteal regions, point tenderness in the region of the greater sciatic foramen that may radiate down the limb and result in gait dysfunction, pain aggravated by sitting, and a positive straight leg raise test result. Gluteal atrophy may be present if the syndrome has been chronic. Physical examination tests involve lower limb manipulation to elicit buttock pain characteristic of sciatica. Passive internal rotation of the hip that reproduces buttock or sciatic pain is a positive indicator of piriformis syndrome.[121] The FADIR test is also useful because it requires the examiner to stretch the piriformis muscle by rotating the patient's hip internally while in flexion (see Fig. 8-28). In this test, the hip is placed in 90 degrees of flexion and then adduction and internal rotation. Although this test is often used to clinically diagnose FAI, piriformis pain can be reproduced in the same testing position, which can support or negate a diagnosis of piriformis syndrome.[103]

Medical Management and Rehabilitation Considerations

Initial management is often addressed with conservative therapy to reduce pain and spasm; this treatment may include nonsteroidal antiinflammatory drugs, muscle relaxants, and physical therapy.[125,126,130] Initial physical therapy may include certain modalities (e.g., hot packs, ultrasound, cold spray, soft tissue mobilization) to reduce spasm.[126,130,131] Once symptoms are reduced, physical therapy should progress to a focused rehabilitation program that balances strength and flexibility of the soft tissues surrounding the hip. Strengthening the core (Fig. 8-31, *A* and *B*) and improving muscle balance of the hip external rotators (e.g., "clamshell": see Fig. 8-18, *D* and *E*), abductors, and extensors (Fig. 8-31, *C* and *D*) should be implemented during the rehabilitation process,[127] as well as exercises to adduct and internally rotate the hip to stretch the piriformis muscle (Fig. 8-31, *E* and *F*).[131] Exercises to improve flexibility of the piriformis are also important (Fig. 8-31, *G* and *H*). For long-term treatment success and full return to dance training, it is important to identify and correct any technique errors or malalignments that contribute to piriformis tightness and overuse.[127] In cases that are not responsive to conservative management strategies, injections (i.e., corticosteroid, anesthetic, botulinum toxin [Botox]) or surgical release may be indicated.[125,126,130,132-134]

Stress Fractures

Female athletes, particularly dancers, are at increased risk for stress fractures.[135-137] Evidence indicates that engaging in high-impact sports increases stress fracture risk in preadolescent and adolescent girls.[53] Some forms of dance (e.g., Irish dance) are high impact in nature. In a study of 255 Irish dancers, 10% of reported injuries were stress injuries, and the majority of injuries affected the lower extremity and hip.[9] Stress injuries are twice as common in girls who participate in sports for 8 or more hours a week.[53] Stress fractures of the hip are easily overlooked and, if undetected, may progress to complete fractures.[138] Femoral neck stress fractures are rare, representing only approximately 5% of all stress fractures.[139] They are, however, extremely important because they are difficult to diagnose and have a high incidence of fracture nonunion, complete fracture, or avascular necrosis, which may result in an unrecoverable injury. Radiographs or bone scans are often required to identify stress fractures correctly.

Treatment for stress injury consists of rest from activity, the length of which depends on the location and severity of the injury. It is also important to identify the cause of the stress injury (e.g., overuse, malalignments, faulty technique, strength and flexibility imbalances, overtraining, suboptimal flooring) and the risk for future stress injury. Prevention strategies include screening for FAT, promoting early participation in activities that promote bone health, reducing the number of hours spent in high-impact sports, engaging in nutritional strategies to improve bone health,[140] and using a sprung floor for training.[9]

Hip Injury Prevention in Dance

Although most young women who are involved in dancing are recreational dancers of a young age (8 to 16 years old), we know very little about risk factors related to injury prevalence in this age group.[141] Current knowledge of risk factors pertains primarily to professional adult dancers and therefore may not be applicable to young recreational dancers. This limited information on major risk factors in young dancers may expose them to injury, affect their long-term physical health, and negatively affect their future careers as dancers. The high rate of injury among recreational dancers attests to the strong need for preventive action.[18]

Core strengthening for core stability and endurance is particularly recommended to manage and prevent dance-related injury.[142,143] Decreased core stability may negatively affect lower extremity joint motion and lumbar control during dance, thus resulting in an increased risk of injury.[143] Core stability and endurance can be challenging areas to develop for the dancer. Pilates is a form of exercise that focuses on developing control of the core and emphasizes proper form. It offers many exercise variations and progressions that are relevant for dancers. Pilates is often practiced by professional dancers to supplement their dance training. It can be used as a primary intervention for core stabilization or as a supplement during or after the rehabilitation process is complete. A study by Sabo[51] surveyed physical therapists who specialize in dance medicine ($n = 29$). These therapists were asked to identify specific interventions that they found to be effective when working with dancers. A total of 59 interventions were mentioned in the survey, and Pilates was the most frequently cited intervention (58.6%).[51] Understanding the potential relationship between core stability and injury risk is important to help reduce dance injury incidence and improve performance.[143] Future research should investigate specific relationships between core endurance and lower extremity dance injuries, to validate clinical efficacy and its role in injury prevention for dancers.

Overall fitness assessment can identify components of fitness that may be lacking. A balance of core stability, sensory integrity (i.e., proprioception), flexibility, power, strength, and muscular endurance not only can prevent compensations that result in injury, but also may improve dance performance.[144,145] Education regarding proper warmup, including a combination of dynamic and static stretches, is also advised to improve range of motion and prevent injury.[146] Some evidence indicates that reduced muscular power of the lower extremities is associated with severity of injuries in female contemporary dancers.[147] Training programs to improve overall fitness should include exercises that address not only strength, but also power, of the lower extremities.

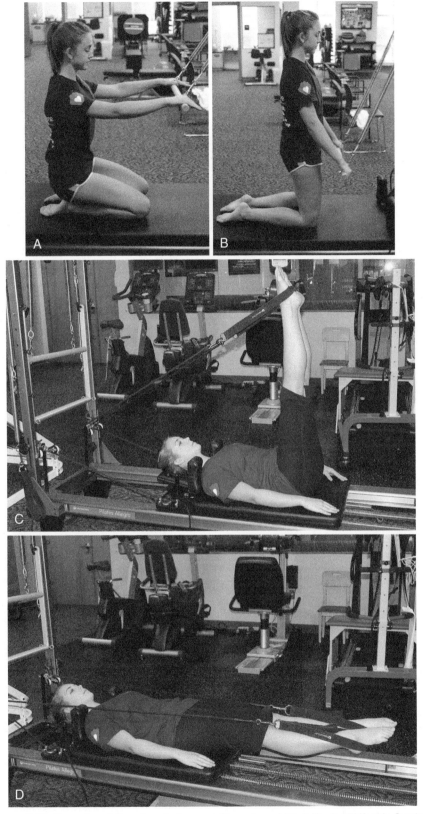

• **Figure 8-31** Examples of Exercises to Improve Strength and Flexibility for Piriformis Syndrome. **A** and **B,** Strengthening the core. **C** and **D,** Strengthening hip extensors.

Continued

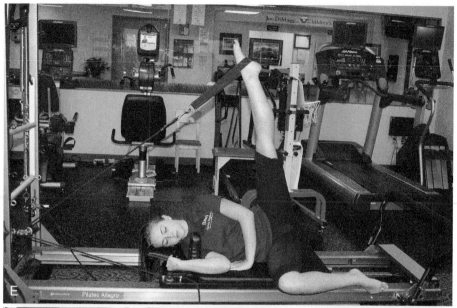

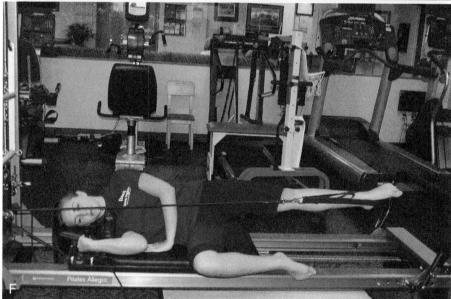

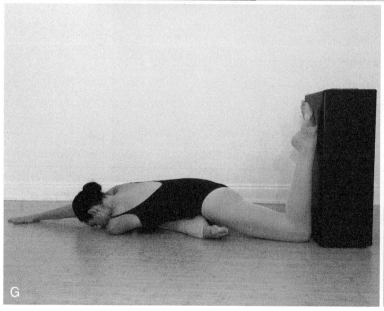

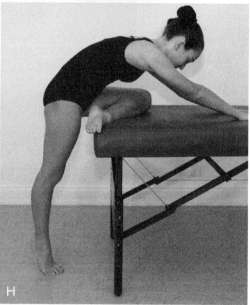

• **Figure 8-31, cont'd** **E** and **F,** Strengthening hip adductors and internal rotators to stretch the piriformis. **G,** Advanced stretch variation for tight external rotators. **H,** Modified external rotation stretch for the soft tissues.

Prevention is possible only if major risk factors are identified. Routine physical screening of young female recreational dancers should be mandatory for identifying existing injury and for decreasing the risk of future injury. This screening can serve as a means for increasing the dancers' awareness of their physical abilities and can assist in the selection of exercises that can help overcome physical limitations by addressing compensatory patterns resulting from inadequate muscle strength. Finally, physical screening may assist in correcting poor techniques, by preventing the use of compensation.[148] Screening programs have been developed in many parts of the globe, and they all share the same goals[149,150]:

- Relate the physical fitness and physical features (e.g., range of motion) of the dancer to the extreme demands of dance practice and to specific dance forms.
- Determine the correct level of practice, and suggest exercises to overcome areas of weakness.
- Identify compensations for specific positions.
- Identify risk factors for injury.
- Increase the dancers' self-awareness of their physical limitations.
- Identify any existing injuries.

Communication between therapists and dance instructors is valuable in preventing dance injury by identifying and addressing biomechanical stressors in choreography. Having an understanding of a dancer's training and skills, and paying early attention to physical complaints, can allow health professionals and teachers to identify overuse injuries before they become serious.[3,4] Communication with other individuals who can support the dancer's overall health and injury prevention is also important. These individuals include the artistic director,[50] choreographer, parents, and other health professionals with whom the dancer may interact.

Specific Considerations for Assessment of Hip Injuries in Dancers

Clinical evaluation of a dancer should begin with a thorough medical history. Additional questions, specific to dance, should be incorporated in the assessment interview. Box 8-1 provides examples of dance-specific interview questions.

Assessment and treatment of dancers, as well as preventive strategies, should focus on the strength and control of hip external rotation in functional positions, rather than on flexibility. Patterns of motor recruitment, muscle imbalances, and isometric strength at low levels of maximum voluntary contraction may be more relevant for the dancer, in terms of treatment and prevention of chronic or recurrent injury. As previously mentioned, education of dancers and teachers may also play a role in reducing the prevalence and severity of nontraumatic dance injuries. Dancers need to be encouraged to achieve turnout positions that are realistic for each individual, based on their available passive range of motion and alignment. Doing so could decrease the need

> **• BOX 8-1 Dance-Specific Questions for a Thorough History**
>
> 1. How many years have you been dancing?
> 2. In what types or styles of dance have you primarily trained?
> 3. At what age did you begin dancing?
> 4. Do you participate in any other sports or exercise classes?
> 5. How many hours of dance training do you do per week?
> 6. What does your dance training regimen involve? Do you have a warm-up or cool-down routine?
> 7. Is training all year round or seasonal? Do you have breaks in training?
> 8. Have you recently had an increase in training intensity or hours? Recent change in choreography?
> 9. Have you had any past back, hip, leg, or foot injuries?
> 10. Have you begun menstruating? At what age? Is your menstruation regular?
> 11. Are you on a restrictive diet?
> 12. Do you have any clicking or snapping in your hip? Is there pain with the snapping or clicking? Can you point to it? What provokes or relieves the symptoms?

for turnout compensation and the resultant chronic tissue overload.[18]

The need for rehabilitation specialists and therapists to perform an assessment of the entire kinetic chain is well documented and generally practiced because many musculoskeletal injuries occur higher or lower than the actual dysfunction. This is particularly important in dance, given the artistic nature and level of athleticism required for dancers to excel in their art form. Hip disorders may be attributed to improper flooring, impairments in foot biomechanics, shoe wear, strength and flexibility imbalances, and poor technique. In the case of recurring injuries, the therapist should reevaluate the entire kinetic chain, both statically and dynamically, with special attention to the dancer's biomechanics. Time observing the dancer during his or her typical dance class or practice routine is highly suggested.

Foot deformities and compensatory strategies can affect the alignment and mechanics of the hip. It is important to evaluate all dance shoes, as well as street shoes. Wearing shoes that are too small is common practice in some forms of dance, and the ramifications of this practice should be explained to the dancer, parent, and teacher. Many dance shoes do not accommodate orthotic inserts, and dancers may resist wearing these inserts. Nevertheless, encouraging dancers to wear a well-fitting sport shoe with orthotic inserts when not dancing is helpful.[7]

Finally, and as indicated earlier in this chapter, assessment of the dancer's nutritional status, menstrual irregularities, and identification of risk factors of the FAT can help the clinician determine other factors that may contribute to injury in the dancer.

As mentioned previously, psychosocial aspects of dance are also critical to understand and assess. In our experience, dancers who train at a performance or competitive level tend to be perfectionists, are accustomed to working through injuries, and are reluctant to take time off from dance training. These observations are supported by the dance literature.[45-47,151] Acknowledging the dancer's feelings and fears and encouraging modification of training when possible, rather than restricting dance activity altogether, may be key to achieving short-term and long-term adherence, as well as a trusting relationship between dancer and clinician.

Conclusion

Although injuries to the hip account for only 10% of injuries in dancers, hip injuries can be debilitating, difficult to overcome, and ultimately career ending. Dancers with hip

pain can be a challenge to treat. Many of the hip injuries discussed in this chapter are multifactorial. These injuries often include a combination of joint hypermobility, increased ligamentous laxity, muscle imbalances, and bony abnormalities, combined with improper technique, repetitive stress, and overuse. Thorough assessment, as well as understanding the mechanics of dance movement, dance-specific anatomy, and the clinical origin of their injuries, will allow for optimal treatment and long-term success.[50,152]

Case Studies

Examples of hip conditions in dancers are provided in Case Studies 8-1 and 8-2.

CASE STUDY 8-1

14-Year-Old Dancer With Snapping Hip Syndrome

History

The patient is a 14-year-old female dancer referred to rehabilitation by her orthopedic specialist with a diagnosis of right hip flexor tendinitis. She presents with complaints of snapping with pain in the front of her right hip. She started noticing the gradual onset of symptoms 3 months ago during dance class. The symptoms seem to be exacerbated when she returns her leg back to standing from a front or side leg motion or battement (kicking motion that is in >90 degrees of hip flexion). It also worsens with deep squatting motions, such as a grand plié in second position. She reports that she can reproduce the snap voluntarily and occasionally feels relief with the crack. She sometimes feels a crack in the left hip, but no pain. At times she feels that she is popping her right hip joint in and out of its socket. She is able to get through 50% of her dance practice without pain. As she progresses through her class, the pain progressively increases. She is currently dancing 2 to 3 hours/day, 6 days/week. She participates in several styles of dance (jazz, contemporary, and tap), but ballet seems to irritate the right hip the most. The onset of the symptoms coincided with an increase in the amount of her training in preparation for a holiday ballet performance in which she had the lead role. Part of the choreography included repetitive high kicking or battement (similar to the signature choreography of the Rockettes). She continued to practice despite the increasing symptoms.

She is also reporting that she was recently diagnosed with left Achilles tendinitis by a chiropractic physician. She has been receiving modality treatments (ultrasound and electrical stimulation) for her left ankle over the past 3 weeks, with minimal improvement.

Physical Therapy Examination

Earlier diagnostic imaging: Pelvic radiographs were normal.
Posture: Postural alignment was observed in her natural standing position from the anterior, posterior, and lateral

perspectives. She stands in a natural turnout alignment (lower extremities externally rotated). The lateral view revealed increased anterior pelvic tilt, increased lumbar lordosis with turnout position, pes planus bilaterally, and left calcaneal valgus.
Range of motion (ROM):

Joint Passive Range Of Motion (PROM)*	Left (degrees)	Right (degrees)
Prone hip internal rotation (IR)	50	30
Prone hip external rotation (ER)	55	60
Standing turnout	75	80
Compensated turnout	20	20
Ankle dorsiflexion (DF)	15	10
First metatarsal phalangeal (MTP) extension	80	90

*PROM: Tight right IR (30 degrees) versus left (50 degrees), tight posterior lateral hip soft tissue musculature (piriformis, hip ER), excessive passive hip ER (60 degrees) right versus left (55 degrees).

Strength:

Manual Muscle Testing (MMT)	Left	Right
Hip flexion	5/5	3/5 with 5/10 pain
Hip abduction	5/5	3/5
Gastrocnemius	5/5 with 3/10 pain at end range plantar flexion	5/5
Posterior tibialis	3/5 with 5/10 pain	5/5
Flexor hallucis longus (FHL)	3/5 with 5/10 pain	5/5

CASE STUDY 8-1

14-Year-Old Dancer With Snapping Hip Syndrome—cont'd

Functional Strength Testing	Left	Right
Single leg squat test	Normal, able to squat 65 degrees of knee flexion in neutral lower extremity alignment	Abnormal, able to squat to depth of 50 degrees of knee flexion; observed progressive dynamic valgus collapse alignment with deeper flexion
Single leg stance balance (30 seconds)	Normal	Positive Trendelenburg sign evident at 20 seconds
Core strength: forearm plank (timed)	15 seconds before a decline in form, progressive lumbar lordosis	

Weak (3/5) and painful (5/10) with resisted right hip flexion, positive Trendelenburg sign with right single leg squat for longer than 30 seconds, right hip abduction 3/5, core weakness, and inability to maintain pelvis in neutral during single leg squat on the right; the functional test revealed genu valgus dynamic collapse at 50 degrees of knee flexion, gastrocnemius strength on the left 5/5 but painful (3/10) with end-range weight-bearing plantar flexion (relevé). Weakness and pain (5/10) noted at the left posterior tibialis and FHL (3/5).

Flexibility: A positive Thomas test result was noted on the right (with abduction and external rotation [ER]), as well as a positive Ober test result on the right.

Positions of provocation: Movement of the right hip from flexion abduction/ER to extension/adduction/internal rotation (IR) elicited the painful snap. Pain increased after développé and grand plié in second position.

Hip joint accessory motion: Increased inferior and anterior glide of the right femoral head was noted. In the supine position, the tight hip/lower extremity positions were in excessive ER compared with the left lower extremity.

Special testing: The flexion-adduction-IR (FADIR) test was performed, and the right hip was positive for pain.

Physical Therapy Assessment

The patient presents with right internal snapping hip syndrome with iliopsoas tendinosis. This appears to be the result of overuse, fatigue, and development of compensatory strategies. She also has left posterior tibialis tendinosis. This has resulted from excessive weight shift through the left lower extremity to avoid pain in the right hip, exhibited through her plié and turnout positions. When she shifted her weight toward the left ankle, she would lose her intrinsic arch control and overrecruit her posterior tibialis and flexor hallucis longus.

She has poor recruitment of the right hip flexor in greater than 90 degrees of flexion. The compensation pattern that she demonstrated was to recruit her tensor fasciae latae (TFL) and rely on this muscle to raise the hip into greater ranges of flexion, thus overriding the iliopsoas. Even through the TFL is an internal rotator, she had excessive ER mobility in her hip joint, indicative of focal hyperlaxity that allowed this compensation to develop. A weak gluteus medius and ineffective core stability contributed to a lack of a stable base of support in the pelvis during single leg stance and perpetuated inefficient recruitment patterns.

Intervention

She was instructed to have a period of relative rest from hip flexion and abduction of more than 90 degrees for 2 weeks (in open and closed chain) to reduce irritation in the iliopsoas (hip flexor). She modified her dance activities to avoid the provoking positions. Modalities were used to reduce pain in her right hip flexor and left posterior tibialis.

Correction of the right hip muscle imbalance was achieved through soft tissue mobilization and foam rolling (TFL/iliotibial band [ITB]). Iliopsoas, ITB, and piriformis stretching activities were emphasized, to be done at the end of her dance practice. Education included teaching the dancer to perform stretching in the plane of the muscle, instead of the extreme range of the joint. Manual iliopsoas release was incorporated to reduce soft tissue restrictions over the anterior hip. Quadruped rocking was incorporated to facilitate posterior femoral glide and optimize centering of the femoral head in the acetabulum.

Rehabilitation exercise strategies emphasized hip and lumbopelvic stabilization and equal weight shift through her lower extremities, with core stabilization while supine seated and in functional dance-specific positions. Emphasis was placed on neutral control at the lumbar spine and neuromuscular reeducation for optimizing proper lumbopelvic dissociation movement patterns. To improve her biomechanical control further, she worked on improved pelvic stabilization control through gluteus medius strengthening, proprioception, and closed-chain stability activities. She worked on intrinsic strength for her left foot control and stretching of her first metatarsophalangeal joint to reduce strain at the medial foot. Once active hip flexion at more than 90 degrees was pain free, a home exercise program focused on gradual progression of iliopsoas strengthening exercises was implemented in dance-specific patterns. Education was critical to her recovery. She learned how to identify her specific compensation patterns, applied corrective exercises, and was able to work with the dance instructor to optimize technique.

10-Year-Old Female Dancer With Low Back Pain and Lateral Hip and Medial Patellofemoral Pain

History

The patient is a 10-year-old female dancer with low back pain and lateral hip and medial patellofemoral (PF) pain. She has been taking ballet since the age of 6 years. When she was a toddler, she walked with a toe-in gait pattern; this has improved over the past 3 years. She occasionally turns in slightly with the right foot when she walks, and according to her mother, it is noticeable only when the patient is fatigued. The pain started gradually in the past 6 months. She has grown 2 inches during that time. She trains at a ballet academy 10 hours/week and takes 2 hours of technique classes weekly.

Her pediatrician referred her to a pediatric orthopedic specialist because of suspected scoliosis. Spine radiographs were normal. The specialist did diagnose her with moderate femoral anteversion (20 to 25 degrees). The physician referred her to physical therapy out of concern for the recent onset of pain and for strategies for gaining a better natural turnout in the presence of femoral anteversion.

Discussion

Although it is possible to improve turnout in the presence of femoral anteversion, it is also the origin of her compensation during turnout that is contributing to her pain. The degree of anteversion may restrict her ability to achieve a desired turnout. During her turnout, she anteriorly tilts her pelvis, thus creating a greater degree of hip flexion, which allows the Y ligament to slacken and permits access to more rotation. This anterior tilt results in increased lumbar lordosis. Lordosis is aesthetically undesirable and potentially damaging. Her lumbar paraspinal muscles are overrecruited, and her transversus abdominal muscles are inhibited. This position places the iliopsoas muscle into a shortened position, and snapping across the iliopectineal eminence can result in inflammation and pain.

When the pelvis is in an anterior tilt, it positions the deep external rotator muscles at a disadvantage. This postural alignment makes it a challenge to access the potential strength of these muscles to aid with turnout alignment. Instead, she should stabilize her spine and pelvis in neutral and then strengthen the deep external rotator muscles to activate a more efficient turnout. Another area that is compensating is through her knee joint. Inadequate hip external rotation (ER) requires the knee joint to function beyond its role as a hinge joint; it begins to generate excessive tibial external torsion. Increased external torsion of the tibia leads to increased medial PF strain. External torsion of the tibia places the tibial tubercle in a lateral alignment and strains the medial structures of the knee joint. The anterior pelvic tilt places increased anterior weight shift and an anterior shear force over the PF joint. The final area of compensation is in her midfoot. With all the compensations occurring in the spine, hips, and knees, the midfoot responds by pronating to stabilize the position. This alignment overstretches her medial arch support and inhibits her dynamic intrinsic arch control.

Overall, she is relying more on passive compensatory acquired joint motion through her joints and has inefficient muscle recruitment patterns. She will benefit from a combination of core, deep hip ER and intrinsic foot and ankle strengthening, in addition to proper stretching techniques (adduction, psoas and hip extension, ER). This regimen will enable her to achieve their maximal turnout potential and reduce compensatory strain and pain in her back, hips, and knees.

The actual degree of external hip rotation from the joint may not improve significantly, but she can gain the ability to use what range of motion she has to her maximum capacity. She really must learn how to use the rotation from her hips correctly, and this takes time, growth, and maturity.

Acknowledgments

We would like to thank Elizabeth Kreymer, physical therapy student and graphic artist, for contributing drawings for this chapter.

References

1. Kravitz S. Dance medicine. *Clin Podiatry.* 1984;1(2):417-430.
2. Peterson JR. Hip pain in dancers: introduction. *J Dance Med Sci.* 2011;15(4):147-148.
3. Ojofeitimi S, Bronner S. Injuries in a modern dance company effect of comprehensive management on injury incidence and cost. *J Dance Med Sci.* 2011;15(3):116-122.
4. Bronner S, Ojofeitimi S, Rose D. Injuries in a modern dance company: effect of comprehensive management on injury incidence and time loss. *Am J Sports Med.* 2003;31(3):365-373.
5. Leanderson C, Leanderson J, Wykman A, et al. Musculoskeletal injuries in young ballet dancers. *Knee Surg Sports Traumatol Arthrosc.* 2011;19(9):1531-1535.
6. Baker J, Scott D, Watkins K, et al. Self-reported and reported injury patterns in contemporary dance students. *Med Probl Perform Art.* 2010;25(1):10-15.
7. Schoene LM. Biomechanical evaluation of dancers and assessment of their risk of injury. *J Am Podiatr Med Assoc.* 2007;97(1):75-80.
8. Teitz CC. Hip and knee injuries in dancers. *J Dance Med Sci.* 2000;4(1):23-29.
9. Stein CJ, Tyson KD, Johnson VM, et al. Injuries in Irish dance. *J Dance Med Sci.* 2013;17(4):159-164.
10. Chow AH, Morrison WB. Imaging of hip injuries in dancers. *J Dance Med Sci.* 2011;15(4):160-172.
11. Boles C, Ferguson C. The female athlete. *Radiol Clin North Am.* 2010;48:1249-1266.
12. Chang GH, Paz DA, Dwek JR, Chung CB. Lower extremity overuse injuries in pediatric athletes: clinical presentation, imaging findings, and treatment. *Clin Imaging.* 2013;37(5):836-846.

13. Frank JS, Gambacorta PL, Eisner EA. Hip pathology in the adolescent athlete. *J Am Acad Orthop Surg*. 2013;21(11):665-674.

14. Kovacevic D, Mariscalco M, Goodwin RC. Injuries about the hip in the adolescent athlete. *Sports Med Arthrosc*. 2011;19(1):64-74.

15. Gamboa J, Maring J, Roberts L, Fergus A. Injury patterns in elite preprofessional ballet dancers and the utility of screening programs to identify risk characteristics. *J Orthop Sports Phys Ther*. 2008;38(3):126-136.

16. Jacobs CL, Hincapié CA, Cassidy JD. Musculoskeletal injuries and pain in dancers: a systematic review update. *J Dance Med Sci*. 2012;16(2):74-84.

17. Motta-Valencia K. Dance-related injury. *Phys Med Rehabil Clin N Am*. 2006;17(3):697-723.

18. Negus V, Hopper D, Briffa N. Associations between turnout and lower extremity injuries in classical ballet dancers. *J Orthop Sports Phys Ther*. 2005;35(5):307-318.

19. Coplan JA. Ballet dancer's turnout and its relationship to self-reported injury. *J Orthop Sports Phys Ther*. 2002;32:579-584.

20. Micheli LJ, Gillespie WJ, Walaszek A. Physiologic profiles of female professional ballerinas. *Clin Sports Med*. 1984;3(1):199-209.

21. Koerner J, Patel N, Yoon R, et al. Femoral version of the general population: does "normal" vary by gender or ethnicity? *J Orthop Trauma*. 2013;27(6):308-311.

22. Toogood PA, Skalak A, Cooperman DR. Proximal femoral anatomy in the normal human population. *Clin Orthop Relat Res*. 2009;467(4):876-885.

23. Bauman P, Singson R, Hamilton W. Femoral neck anteversion in ballerinas. *Clin Orthop Relat Res*. 1994;302:57-63.

24. Clippinger K. Biomechanical considerations in turnout. In: Solomon R, Minton S, Solomon J, eds. *Preventing Dance Injuries*. 2nd ed. Champaign, Ill: Human Kinetics; 2005:135-150.

25. Cimelli S, Curran S. Influence of turnout on foot posture and its relationship to overuse musculoskeletal injury in professional contemporary dancers: a preliminary investigation. *J Am Podiatr Med Assoc*. 2012;102(1):25-33.

26. Hamilton D, Aronsen P, Løken J, et al. Dance training intensity at 11-14 years is associated with femoral torsion in classical ballet dancers. *Br J Sports Med*. 2006;40:299-303.

27. Welsh TM, Rodriguez M, Beare LW, et al. Assessing turnout in university dancers. *J Dance Med Sci*. 2008;12(4):136-141.

28. Jenkins J, Wyon M, Nevil A. Can turnout measurements be used to predict physiotherapist-reported injury rates in dancers? *Med Probl Perform Art*. 2013;28(4):230-235.

29. Khoo-Summers L, Prather H, Hunt D, Van Dillen L. Predictors of first position turnout in collegiate dancers. *Am J Phys Med Rehabil*. 2013;92(2):136-142.

30. Gilbert CB, Gross M, Klug K. Relationship between hip external rotation and turnout angle for the five classical ballet positions. *J Orthop Sports Phys Ther*. 1998;27:339-347.

31. Bennell K, Khan KM, Matthews B, et al. Hip and ankle range of motion and hip muscle strength in young female ballet dancers and controls. *Br J Sports Med*. 1999;33:340-346.

32. Khan K, Roberts P, Nattrass C, et al. Hip and ankle range of motion in elite classical ballet dancers and controls. *Clin J Sport Med*. 1997;7:174-179.

33. Hamilton WG, Hamilton LH, Marshall P, Molnar M. A profile of the musculoskeletal characteristics of elite professional ballet dancers. *Am J Sports Med*. 1992;20(3):267-273.

34. Grossman G, Waninger K, Voloshin A, et al. Reliability and validity of goniometric turnout measurements compared with MRI and retro-reflective markers. *J Dance Med Sci*. 2008;12(4):142-152.

35. Clippinger K, ed. The pelvic girdle and hip joint. In: *Dance Anatomy and Kinesiology*. Champaign, Ill: Human Kinetics; 2007.

36. Norkin CC, White DJ. *Measurement of Joint Motion: A Guide to Goniometry*. 4th ed. Philadelphia: F.A. Davis; 2009.

37. Clarkson HM. *Joint Motion and Function Assessment: A Research-Based Practice Guide*. Philadelphia: Lippincott Williams & Wilkins; 2005.

38. Ruwe PA, Gage JR, Ozonoff MB, DeLuca PA. Clinical determination of femoral anteversion: a comparison with established techniques. *J Bone Joint Surg Am*. 1992;74(6):820-830.

39. Ojofeitimi S, Bronner S, Woo H. Injury incidence in hip hop dance. *Scand J Med Sci Sports*. 2012;22(3):347-355.

40. Echegoyen S, Acuña E, Rodríguez C. Injuries in students of three different dance techniques. *Med Probl Perform Art*. 2010;25(2):72-74.

41. Mayers L, Bronner S, Agraharasamakulam S, Ojofeitimi S. Lower extremity kinetics in tap dance. *J Dance Med Sci*. 2010;14(1):3-10.

42. Trepman E, Gellman RE, Solomon R, et al. Electromyographic analysis of standing posture in demi plie in ballet and modern dancers. *Med Sci Sports Exerc*. 1994;26(6):771-782.

43. Rivaldi C, Vannacci A, Bolognesi E, et al. Gender role, eating disorder symptoms, and body image concern in ballet dancers. *J Psychosom Res*. 2006;64(4):529-535.

44. Wainwright SP, Williams C, Turner BS. Fractured identities: injury and the balletic body. *Health (London)*. 2005;9(1):49-66.

45. Murgia C. Overuse, tissue fatigue, and injuries. *J Dance Med Sci*. 2013;17(3):93-100.

46. Mainwaring LM. Psychological issues in dance medicine. Part one. *J Dance Med Sci*. 2001;5(4):104.

47. Krasnow D, Kerr G, Mainwaring L. Psychology of dealing with the injured dancer. *Med Prob Perform Art*. 1994;9(1):7-9.

48. Lai R, Krasnow D, Thomas M. Communication between medical practitioners and dancers. *J Dance Med Sci*. 2008;12(2):47-53.

49. Reference deleted in review.

50. Liederbach M. Perspectives on dance science rehabilitation understanding whole body mechanics and four key principles of motor control as a basis for healthy movement. *J Dance Med Sci*. 2010;14(3):114-124.

51. Sabo M. Physical therapy rehabilitation strategies for dancers: a qualitative study. *J Dance Med Sci*. 2013;17(1):11-17.

52. Hincapié CA, Morton EJ, Cassidy JD. Musculoskeletal injuries and pain in dancers: a systematic review. *Arch Phys Med Rehabil*. 2008;89(9):1819-1829.

53. Field A, Gordon C, Pierce L, et al. Prospective study of physical activity and risk of developing a stress fracture among preadolescent and adolescent girls. *Arch Pediatr Adolesc Med*. 2011;165:723-728.

54. Liederbach M, Compagno JM. Psychological aspects of fatigue-related injuries in dancers. *J Dance Med Sci*. 2001;5(4):116-120.

55. Koutedakis Y, Myszkewycz L, Soulas D, et al. The effects of rest and subsequent training on selected physiological parameters in professional female classical dancers. *Int J Sports Med*. 1999;20(6):379-383.

56. Day H, Koutedakis Y, Wyon MA. Hypermobility and dance: a review. *Int J Sports Med.* 2011;32(7):485-489.

57. Ruemper A, Watkins K. Correlations between general joint hypermobility and joint hypermobility syndrome and injury in contemporary dance students. *J Dance Med Sci.* 2012;16(4): 161-166.

58. Foley E, Bird HA. Hypermobility in dance: asset, not liability. *Clin Rheumatol.* 2013;32(4):455-461.

59. Beighton P, Solomon L, Soskolne CL. Articular mobility in an African population. *Ann Rheum Dis.* 1973;32(5):413-418.

60. Remvig L, Jensen DV, Ward RC. Are diagnostic criteria for general joint hypermobility and benign joint hypermobility syndrome based on reproducible and valid tests? A review of the literature. *J Rheumatol.* 2007;34(4):798-803.

61. Grahame R, Bird H, Child A. The revised Brighton 1998 criteria for the diagnosis of benign joint hypermobility syndrome. *J Rheumatol.* 2000;27(7):1777-1779.

62. Simpson MR. Benign joint hypermobility syndrome: evaluation, diagnosis, and management. *J Am Orthop Assoc.* 2006; 106(9):531-536.

63. Simmonds J, Keer R. Hypermobility and the hypermobility syndrome. *Man Ther.* 2007;12(4):298-309.

64. Abraham S. Eating and weight controlling behaviours of young ballet dancers. *Psychopathology.* 1996;29(4):218-222.

65. Frusztajer NT, Dhuper S, Warren MP, et al. Nutrition and the incidence of stress fractures in ballet dancers. *Am J Clin Nutr.* 1990;51(5):779-783.

66. Merrilees MJ, Smart EJ, Gilchrist NL, et al. Effects of dairy food supplements on bone mineral density in teenage girls. *Eur J Nutr.* 2000;39(6):256-262.

67. Weaver CM. Adolescence: the period of dramatic bone growth. *Endocrine.* 2002;17(1):43-48.

68. Hilton LK, Loucks AB. Low energy availability, not exercise stress, suppresses the diurnal rhythm of leptin in healthy young women. *Am J Physiol Endocrinol Metab.* 2000;278(1): E43-E49.

69. Ihle R, Loucks AB. Dose-response relationships between energy availability and bone turnover in young exercising women. *J Bone Miner Res.* 2004;19(8):1231-1240.

70. Lawson EA, Donoho D, Miller KK, et al. Hypercortisolemia is associated with severity of bone loss and depression in hypothalamic amenorrhea and anorexia nervosa. *J Clin Endocrinol Metab.* 2009;94(12):4710-4716.

71. Meyer F, O'Connor H, Shirreffs SM. Nutrition for the young athlete. *J Sports Sci.* 2007;25(suppl 1):S73-S82.

72. Koutedakis Y, Clarke F, Wyon M, et al. Muscular strength: applications for dancers. *Med Probl Perform Art.* 2009;24(4): 157-165.

73. Nattiv A, Loucks AB, Manore MM, et al. American College of Sports Medicine position stand: the female athlete triad. *Med Sci Sports Exerc.* 2007;39(10):1867-1882.

74. Nichols JF, Rauh MJ, Barrack MT, et al. Disordered eating and menstrual irregularity in high school athletes in lean-build and nonlean-build sports. *Int J Sport Nutr Exerc Metab.* 2007; 17(4):364-377.

75. Nichols JF, Rauh MJ, Lawson MJ, et al. Prevalence of the female athlete triad syndrome among high school athletes. *Arch Pediatr Adolesc Med.* 2006;160(2):137-142.

76. Doyle-Lucas AF, Akers JD, Davy BM. Energetic efficiency, menstrual irregularity, and bone mineral density in elite professional female ballet dancers. *J Dance Med Sci.* 2010;14(4): 146-154.

77. Barrack MT, Ackerman KE, Gibbs JC. Update on the female athlete triad. *Curr Rev Musculoskelet Med.* 2013;6(2):195-204.

78. Thomas JJ, Keel PK, Heatherton TF. Disordered eating and injuries among adolescent ballet dancers. *Eat Weight Disord.* 2011;16(3):e216-e222.

79. Barrow GW, Saha S. Menstrual irregularity and stress fractures in collegiate female distance runners. *Am J Sports Med.* 1988; 16(3):209-216.

80. Barrack MT, Gibbs JC, De Souza MJ, et al. Higher incidence of bone stress injuries with increasing female athlete triad-related risk factors: a prospective multisite study of exercising girls and women. *Am J Sports Med.* 2014;42(4):949-958.

81. Burckhardt P, Wynn E, Krieg M-A, et al. The effects of nutrition, puberty and dancing on bone density in adolescent ballet dancers. *J Dance Med Sci.* 2011;15(2):51-60.

82. Friesen KJ, Rozenek R, Clippinger K, et al. Bone mineral density and body composition of collegiate modern dancers. *J Dance Med Sci.* 2011;15(1):31-36.

83. Keay N, Fogelman I, Blake G. Bone mineral density in professional female dancers. *Br J Sports Med.* 1997;31:143-147.

84. Thienpont E, Simon J-P. Stress fracture of the acetabulum in a ballet dancer: a case report. *Acta Orthop Belg.* 2005;71(6): 740-742.

85. Noon M, Hoch AZ, McNamara L, Schimke J. Injury patterns in female Irish dancers. *PM R.* 2010;2(11):1030-1034.

86. Hincapié CA, Cassidy JD. Disordered eating, menstrual disturbances, and low bone mineral density in dancers: a systematic review. *Arch Phys Med Rehabil.* 2010;91(11):1777-1789.e1771.

87. Lee KS, Rosas HG, Phancao J-P. Snapping hip: imaging and treatment. *Semin Musculoskelet Radiol.* 2013;17(3):286-294.

88. Weber A, Bedi A, Tibor L, et al. The hyperflexible hip: managing hip pain in the dancer and gymnast. *Sports Health.* 2015;7(4):346-358.

89. Reid DC, Burnham RS, Saboe LA, Kushner SF. Lower extremity flexibility patterns in classical ballet dancers and their correlation to lateral hip and knee injuries. *Am J Sports Med.* 1987;15(4):347-352.

90. Lewis CL. Extra-articular snapping hip: a literature review. *Sports Health.* 2010;2(3):186-190.

91. Winslow J, Yoder E. Patellofemoral pain in female ballet dancers: correlation with iliotibial band tightness and tibial external rotation. *J Orthop Sports Phys Ther.* 1995;22(1): 18-21.

92. Winston P, Awan R, Cassidy JD, Bleakney RK. Clinical examination and ultrasound of self-reported snapping hip syndrome in elite ballet dancers. *Am J Sports Med.* 2007;35(1):118-126.

93. Deleget A. Overview of thigh injuries in dance. *J Dance Med Sci.* 2010;14(3):97-102.

94. Sammarco J. The dancer's hip. In: Ryan A, Stephens R, eds. *Dance Medicine: A Comprehensive Guide.* Chicago: Pluribus Press; 1987.

95. Micheli LJ, Solomon R. Treatment of recalcitrant iliopsoas tendinitis in athletes and dancers with corticosteroid injection under fluoroscopy. *J Dance Med Sci.* 1997;1:7-11.

96. Reference deleted in review.

97. Dreżewska M, Gałuszka R, Sliwiński Z. Hip joint mobility in dancers: preliminary report. *Ortop Traumatol Rehabil.* 2012; 14(5):443-452.

98. Byrd JW, Jones KS. Traumatic rupture of the ligamentum teres as a source of hip pain. *Arthroscopy.* 2004;20:385-391.

99. Tsai Y-S, McCrory JL, Sell TC, et al. Hip strength, flexibility, and standing posture in athletes with an acetabular labral tear. *J Orthop Sports Phys Ther.* 2004;34:A55-A56.

100. Philippon MJ. The role of arthroscopic thermal capsulorrhaphy in the hip. *Clin Sports Med.* 2001;20:817-829.

101. Nilsson C, Leanderson J, Wykman A, Strender LE. The injury panorama in a Swedish professional ballet company. *Knee Surg Sports Traumatol Arthrosc.* 2001;9(4):242-246.

102. Schenker ML, Martin RR, Weiland DE, et al. Current trends in hip arthroscopy: a review of injury diagnosis, techniques, and outcome scoring. *Curr Opin Orthop.* 2005;16:89-94.

103. Wang W-G, Yue D-B, Zhang N-F, et al. Clinical diagnosis and arthroscopic treatment of acetabular labral tears. *Orthop Surg.* 2011;3(1):28-34.

104. Kocher MS, Solomon R, Lee BM, et al. Arthroscopic debridement of hip labral tears in dancers. *J Dance Med Sci.* 2006;10(3–4):99-105.

105. Groh MM, Herrera J. A comprehensive review of hip labral tears. *Curr Rev Musculoskelet Med.* 2009;2(2):105-117.

106. McCarthy JC, Noble PC, Schuck MR, et al. Aufranc award: the role of labral lesions to development of early degenerative hip disease. *Clin Orthop Relat Res.* 2001;393:25-37.

107. Mason JB. Acetabular labral tears in the athlete. *Clin Sports Med.* 2001;20(4):779-790.

108. Crawford MJ, Dy CJ, Alexander JW, et al. The biomechanics of the hip labrum and the stability of the hip. *Clin Orthop Relat Res.* 2007;455:16-22.

109. Charbonnier C, Kolo FC, Duthon VB, et al. Assessment of congruence and impingement of the hip joint in professional ballet dancers: a motion capture study. *Am J Sports Med.* 2011;39(3):557-566.

110. Safran MR, Giordano G, Lindsey DP, et al. Strains across the acetabular labrum during hip motion: a cadaveric model. *Am J Sports Med.* 2011;39(suppl):92S-102S.

111. Philippon MJ, Briggs KK, Fagrelius T, Patterson D. Labral refixation: current techniques and indications. *HSS J.* 2012;8(3):240-244.

112. Naal FD, Hatzung G, Müller A, et al. Validation of a self-reported Beighton score to assess hypermobility in patients with femoroacetabular impingement. *Int Orthop.* 2014;38:2245-2250.

112a. Duthon V, Charbonnier C, Kolo F, et al. Correlation of clinical and magnetic resonance imaging findings in hips of elite female ballet dancers. *Arthroscopy.* 2013;29(9):411-419.

113. Neumann G, Mendicuti AD, Zou KH, et al. Prevalence of labral tears and cartilage loss in patients with symptoms of the hip: evaluation using MR arthrography. *Osteoarthritis Cartilage.* 2007;15:909-917.

114. Martin HD, Kelly BT, Leunig M, et al. The pattern and technique in the clinical evaluation of the adult hip: the common physical examination tests of hip specialists. *Arthroscopy.* 2010;26(2):161-172.

115. Tibor LM, Sekiya JK. Differential diagnosis of pain around the hip joint. *Arthroscopy.* 2008;24(12):1407-1421.

116. Burnett RS, Della Rocca GJ, Prather H, et al. Clinical presentation of patients with tears of the acetabular labrum. *J Bone Joint Surg Am.* 2006;88(7):1448-1457.

117. Ziegert AJ, Blankenbaker DG, De Smet AA, et al. Comparison of standard hip MR arthrographic imaging planes and sequences for detection of arthroscopically proven labral tear. *AJR Am J Roentgenol.* 2009;192:1397-1400.

118. Kern-Scott R, Peterson JR, Morgan P. Review of acetabular labral tears in dancers. *J Dance Med Sci.* 2011;15(4):149.

119. Lodhia P, Slobogean GP, Noonan VK, Gilbart MK. Patient-reported outcome instruments for femoroacetabular impingement and hip labral pathology: a systematic review of the clinimetric evidence. *Arthroscopy.* 2011;27(2):279-286.

120. Wisniewski SJ, Grogg B. Femoroacetabular impingement: an overlooked cause of hip pain. *Am J Phys Med Rehabil.* 2006;85(6):546-549.

121. Yazbek PM, Ovanessian V, Martin RL, Fukuda TY. Nonsurgical treatment of acetabular labrum tears: a case series. *J Orthop Sports Phys Ther.* 2011;41(5):346-353.

122. Matsuda DK, Carlisle JC, Arthurs SC, et al. Comparative systematic review of the open dislocation, mini-open, and arthroscopic surgeries for femoroacetabular impingement. *Arthroscopy.* 2011;27(2):252-269.

123. Magee DJ. *Orthopedic Physical Assessment.* 5th ed. St. Louis: Saunders; 2007.

124. Papadopoulos EC, Kahn SN. Piriformis syndrome and low back pain: a new classification and review of the literature. *Orthop Clin North Am.* 2004;35:65-71.

125. Byrd JW. Piriformis syndrome. *Oper Tech Sports Med.* 2005;13(1):71-79.

126. Boyajian-O'Neill LA, McClain RL, Coleman MK, Thomas PP. Diagnosis and management of piriformis syndrome: an osteopathic approach. *J Am Osteopath Assoc.* 2008;108(11):657-664.

127. Tonley JC, Yun SM, Kochevar RJ, et al. Treatment of an individual with piriformis syndrome focusing on hip muscle strengthening and movement reeducation: a case report. *J Orthop Sports Phys Ther.* 2010;40(2):103-111.

128. Durrani Z, Winnie AP. Piriformis muscle syndrome: an under-diagnosed cause of sciatica. *J Pain Symptom Manage.* 1991;6(6):374-379.

129. Martinez N, Mandel S, Peterson JR. Neurologic causes of hip pain in dancers. *J Dance Med Sci.* 2011;15(4):157-159.

130. Childers MK, Wilson DJ, Gnatz SM, et al. Botulinum toxin type A use in piriformis muscle syndrome: a pilot study. *Am J Phys Med Rehabil.* 2002;81(10):751-759.

131. Fishman LM, Dombi GW, Michaelsen C, et al. Piriformis syndrome: diagnosis, treatment, and outcome—a 10-year study. *Arch Phys Med Rehabil.* 2002;83(3):295-301.

132. Fishman LM, Konnoth C, Rozner B. Botulinum neurotoxin type B and physical therapy in the treatment of piriformis syndrome: a dose-finding study. *Am J Phys Med Rehabil.* 2004;83(1):42-50.

133. Misirlioglu TO, Akgun K, Palamar D, et al. Piriformis syndrome: comparison of the effectiveness of local anesthetic and corticosteroid injections: a double-blinded, randomized controlled study. *Pain Physician.* 2015;18(2):163-171.

134. Benzon HT, Katz JA, Benzon HA, Iqbal MS. Piriformis syndrome: anatomic considerations, a new injection technique, and a review of the literature. *Anesthesiology.* 2003;98(6):1442-1448.

135. Wentz L, Liu P, Haymes E, Ilich J. Females have a greater incidence of stress fractures than males in both military and athletic populations: a systemic review. *Mil Med.* 2011;176:420-430.

136. Feingold D, Hame S. Female athlete triad and stress fractures. *Orthop Clin North Am.* 2006;37:575-583.

137. Bennell KL, Brukner PD. Epidemiology and site specificity of stress fractures. *Clin Sports Med.* 1997;16(2):179-196.

138. Steinberg N, Siev-Ner I, Peleg S, et al. Injuries in female dancers aged 8 to 16 years. *J Athl Train*. 2013;48(1):118-123.

139. Sanderlin BW, Raspa RF. Common stress fractures. *Am Fam Physician*. 2003;68(8):1527-1532.

140. Chen Y-T, Tenforde AS, Fredericson M. Update on stress fractures in female athletes: epidemiology, treatment, and prevention. *Curr Rev Musculoskelet Med*. 2013;6(2):173-181.

141. Nunes N, Haddod J, Bartlett D, Obright KD. Musculoskeletal injuries among young recreational, female dancers before and after dancing in pointe shoes. *Pediatr Phys Ther*. 2002;14:100-106.

142. Kline JB, Krauss JR, Maher SF, Qu X. Core strength training using a combination of home exercises and a dynamic sling system for the management of low back pain in pre-professional ballet dancers: a case series. *J Dance Med Sci*. 2013;17(1):24-33.

143. Rickman AM, Ambegaonkar JP, Cortes N. Core stability: implications for dance injuries. *Med Probl Perform Art*. 2012;27(3):159-164.

144. Koutedakis Y, Metsios G, Stavropoulos-Kalinoglou A. The significance of muscular strength in dance. *J Dance Med Sci*. 2005;9(1):29.

145. Angioi M, Metsios GS, Koutedakis Y, Wyon MA. Fitness in contemporary dance: a systematic review. *Int J Sports Med*. 2009;30(7):475-484.

146. Morrin N, Redding E. Acute effects of warm-up stretch protocols on balance, vertical jump height, and range of motion in dancers. *J Dance Med Sci*. 2013;17(1):34-40.

147. Angioi M, Koutedakis Y, Metsios GS, et al. Medical problems in performing arts: physical fitness and severity of injuries in contemporary dance. *J Dance Med Sci*. 2010;14(2):74.

148. Steinberg N, Sievner I, Peleg S, et al. Extrinsic and intrinsic risk factors associated with injuries in young dancers aged 8-16 years. *J Sports Sci*. 2012;30(5):485-495.

149. Liederbach M, Spivak J, Rose D. Scoliosis in dancers: a method of assessment in quick-screen settings. *J Dance Med Sci*. 1997;1:107-112.

150. Liederbach M. Screening for functional capacity in dancers designing standardized, dance-specific injury prevention screening tools. *J Dance Med Sci*. 1997;1(3):93-106.

151. Mainwaring LM, Krasnow D, Kerr G. And the dance goes on: psychological impact of injury. *J Dance Med Sci*. 2001;5(4):105-115.

152. Moser BR. Hip pain in dancers. *Curr Sports Med Rep*. 2014;13(6):383-389.

9

The Female Hip and Pelvis

DARLA BOWEN CATHCART

CHAPTER OUTLINE

Both female and male patients can experience symptoms of pelvic myofascial dysfunction. Urinary and anal incontinence, pelvic pain, and pelvic girdle dysfunction are not gender specific. Although only women can develop gynecologic pelvic organ prolapse, men may also experience perineal descent or rectal prolapse. However, the focus of this chapter is on female pelvic structure, function, and signs and symptoms of dysfunction. As described later in the chapter, the anatomy and functional needs of the female pelvis predispose women to many of these pelvic dysfunctions. Other special considerations for development of pelvic symptoms in women relate to the hormonal, physiologic, and anatomic changes that occur with pregnancy, labor and delivery, and menopause.

International Classification of Diseases (ICD) codes related to female pelvic health are summarized in Table 9-1.[1] Ninth ICD revision (ICD-9) codes were adopted on October 1, 2008. Proposed by October 1, 2015, the U.S. Centers for Medicare & Medicaid Services require transition to the updated tenth revision ICD (ICD-10) codes. Some of the more common codes used by pelvic health therapists for billing and reimbursement related to musculoskeletal dysfunction or symptoms in the pelvic region include the following: ICD-9 724.2 Lumbago/Low back pain (ICD-10 M54.5), because many pregnant women experience low back pain, and many women with poor pelvic diaphragm muscle function also have back pain symptoms; ICD-9 719.45 Pain in joint, pelvic region, and thigh (ICD-10 M25.559 Pain in unspecified hip) may be used for patients experiencing general pelvic, hip, and thigh region pain; ICD-9 728.85 Muscle spasm (ICD-10 M62.838) and ICD-9 781.3 Lack of coordination (ICD-10 R27.9) are both often used in relation to the levator ani and surrounding trunk, hip, and thigh musculature because they contribute to pelvic pain, incontinence, and core stability problems. Other ICD codes relating to sprain of various pelvic and lumbosacral joints may be used in relation to acute pelvic girdle dysfunction and pain. Additionally, ICD-9 728.84 Diastasis of muscle (ICD-10 M62.00 Separation of muscle [nontraumatic], unspecified site) may be used to describe diastasis rectus abdominis (DRA). Although an all-inclusive list is not given here, these codes do highlight some of the coding that may be used in many pelvic health physical therapy practices.

Anatomy of the female pelvis opens this chapter, with descriptions of pelvic viscera, bony and ligamentous structures, muscles, perineum and genitalia, and nerves. A description of connections between the hip and pelvis follows this anatomy review. The International Continence Society's standardized terminology of pelvic muscle function is explained and provides the terminology used throughout the chapter. Evidence that relates pelvic diaphragm muscle and urinary dysfunction to symptoms of low back, pelvic girdle, and hip pain is summarized. The chapter then offers more in-depth details of the specific symptoms of chronic pelvic pain (CPP) and of pregnancy and postpartum-related musculoskeletal problems. At the conclusion of this chapter, collaboration with pelvic health physical therapists and other practitioners is summarized. Case studies provide pictures of pelvic symptoms in a younger woman with pregnancy-related pelvic girdle pain and in an older woman with urinary incontinence.

Anatomy of the Female Pelvis

The typical female pelvis has bony differences compared with the male pelvis, and these are discussed briefly later in

---

Male Pelvis and Male Pelvic Health

The male pelvis and male pelvic health deserve attention in their own right. Men may experience some pelvic health conditions that are similar to those that women experience and others that are unique to the male population. Although the focus of this chapter is the female pelvis, some structural makeup of the pelvis is the same (e.g., the components of the levator ani muscles), and differing structures share similarities. Specific to men is hypertrophy of the prostate that occurs with aging and related urinary symptoms, such as urinary hesitancy, frequency, or difficulty voiding. Urinary incontinence (UI) risk factors in community-dwelling men include severe physical limitations, cognitive impairments, history of stroke, urinary tract infections, prostate disease, and diabetes.[2] The prevalence of UI in men increases with age and functional dependency, and the development of UI often coincides with development of other urinary symptoms (e.g., urgency and frequency).[2] Additionally, fecal incontinence may coincide with UI.[2] Postprostatectomy UI is reported in up to 87% of men,[3] and sexual dysfunction is reported in up to 75% of men after radical prostatectomy.[4] Male-specific sexual problems may include UI during intercourse, pain with intercourse, premature ejaculation, and erectile dysfunction (ED). ED primarily affects men older than 40 years of age, with reported causes including diabetes mellitus, hypertension, obesity, lack of physical exercise, and lower urinary tract symptoms.[5] One large study reported ED is more prevalent in men with increasing age, prostatitis-like symptoms, and chronic prostatitis.[6] Men may also experience chronic pelvic pain (CPP), termed chronic prostatitis/CPP syndrome (CP/CPPS), a diagnosis of exclusion.[7] CP/CPPS is urologic or pelvic pain that may be associated with urinary symptoms and sexual dysfunction and has lasted for at least 3 of the previous 6 months.[7] A diagnosis of CP/CPPS may occur after ruling out active infections, cancer, neurologic diseases, or defined urethral diseases or dysfunctions. CP/CPPS accounts for 90% to 95% of cases of male pelvic pain.[7]

---

the chapter. The female pelvic viscera require anatomic support to have normal physiologic function (Fig. 9-1).[8] Lack of appropriate pelvic support may cause the following: pelvic organ prolapse; bladder and anal incontinence; or sexual, voiding, and defecatory dysfunction.[8] The female pelvis contains the convergence of the urologic (located most anteriorly), reproductive (located between the urologic and gastrointestinal), and gastrointestinal systems (located most posteriorly).[9]

Female Pelvic Viscera

The urologic viscera include the bladder, inferior portions of the ureters, and urethra.[9] The bladder is located anterior to the uterus, just superior and posterior to the pubic bone and symphysis. Fibrous ligaments connect the bladder anteriorly to the pubic symphysis. The urachus runs from the bladder to the umbilicus. The ureters, beginning at the renal calyxes, lie on the anterior side of the psoas muscle just lateral to the ovarian vessels and vena cava, cross the pelvic brim over the common iliac arteries, and run into the pelvis along the lateral pelvic sidewall. The ureters then enter

| | TABLE 9-1 | International Classification of Disease Codes in Pelvic Health (ICD-9 and ICD-10) |

ICD-9 Code	ICD-10 Code	Description
		Urinary Symptoms
788.31	N39.41	Urinary urgency (female or male)
625.6	N39.3	Urinary stress incontinence (female)
788.32	N39.3	Urinary stress incontinence (male)
788.33	N39.46	Mixed (stress and urge) urinary incontinence
788.63	R39.15	Urgency of urination
788.41	R35.0	Urinary frequency
788.34	N39.42	Incontinence without sensory awareness
788.35	N39.43	Postvoid dripping ("dribbling")
788.37	N39.45	Continuous leakage
788.43	R35.1	Nocturia
788.36	N39.44	Nocturnal enuresis
		Bladder Disorders
595.1	—	Chronic interstitial cystitis
N30.10	—	Chronic interstitial cystitis without hematuria
N30.11	—	Chronic interstitial cystitis with hematuria
788.20	R33.9	Urinary retention
788.64	R39.11	Urinary hesitancy
		Bowel Disorders
787.60	R15.9	Fecal incontinence
564.00	K59.00	Constipation
787.91	R19.7	Diarrhea
455.6	K64.9	Hemorrhoids
		Organ Prolapse
618.01	N81.11	Cystocele midline
618.02	N81.12	Cystocele lateral
618.04	N81.6	Rectocele
618.00	—	Prolapse of vaginal walls unspecified
N81.9	—	Female genital prolapse, unspecified
618.03	N81.0	Urethrocele
618.05	N81.81	Perineocele
618.1	—	Uterine prolapse
618.2	N81.2	Uterovaginal prolapse, incomplete
618.3	N81.3	Uterovaginal prolapse, complete
569.1	K62.3	Rectal prolapse
K62.2	—	Anal prolapse
		Pelvic Pain and Dysfunction
625.0	N94.1	Dyspareunia
625.1	N94.2	Vaginismus
625.71	N94.810	Vulvar vestibulitis

Continued

TABLE 9-1 International Classification of Disease Codes in Pelvic Health (ICD-9 and ICD-10)—cont'd

ICD-9 Code	ICD-10 Code	Description
		Urinary Symptoms
625.70	N94.819	Vulvodynia, unspecified
569.42	K62.89	Anal or rectal pain
724.79	—	Disorders of coccyx
M53.3	—	Sacrococcygeal disorders
564.6	K59.4	Anal spasm
625.3	N94.6	Dysmenorrhea
		Musculoskeletal Symptoms
724.2	M54.5	Lumbago/low back pain
719.45	—	Pain in joint, pelvic region, and thigh
M25.559	—	Pain in unspecified hip
728.85	M62.838	Muscle spasm
781.3	R27.9	Lack of coordination
846.0	—	Sprain lumbosacral joint or ligament
S33.8XXA	—	Sprain of other parts of lumbar spine and pelvis, initial encounter
846.1	—	Sprain of sacroiliac ligament
S33.6XXA	—	Sprain of sacroiliac joint, initial encounter
847.3	—	Sprain of sacrum
848.5	—	Sprain of pelvic
728.84	—	Diastasis of muscle
M62.00	—	Separation of muscle (nontraumatic), unspecified site

Copyright © World Health Organization.
ICD-9, International Classification of Diseases ninth revision; *ICD-10,* International Classification of Diseases tenth revision.
See ICD-10 Code Translator (AAPC), <https://www.aapc.com/icd-10/codes/>

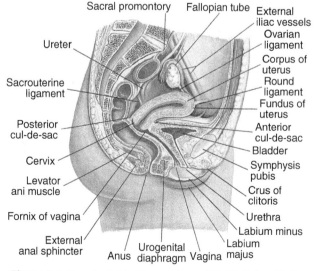

• **Figure 9-1** Female Pelvic Viscera. (From Ball JW, Dains JE, Flynn JA, et al. *Seidel's Guide to Physical Examination.* 8th ed. St. Louis: Mosby; 2015.)

the bladder's trigone region (the triangular portion of the bladder base).[9]

The gynecologic viscera include the uterus, fallopian tubes, and ovaries.[9] These organs lie centrally between the bladder and rectosigmoid colon. The three segments of the uterus are the fundus (superior portion), lower segment, and cervix. Most commonly, the uterus is anteverted (meaning the cervix angles forward) and anteflexed (the body of the uterus flexes forward) in relation to the vagina and cervix, a position that leads the uterus to rest just above the bladder. At term, a pregnant uterus increases to 20 times its usual size and weight (Fig. 9-2). After menopause, the uterus atrophies and becomes smaller than in the woman of childbearing age. The cervix is dense and fibromuscular, and it separates the uterus from and extends into the vagina.[9] The cervix and upper vagina lie suspended over the pelvic diaphragm muscles at the level of the ischial spines and fifth sacral vertebra (S5).[8] The fallopian tubes are bilateral structures, usually less than 1 cm thick, that extend 10 to 14 cm in length from the superior-lateral portion of the uterus.[9] The distal portion of the fallopian tube is the infundibulum, with finger-like projections extending freely from this end of the tube. The ovaries lie in the peritoneum in the ovarian fossa positioned closely to the iliac vessels and ureters.[9]

The uterus projects several ligamentous structures (Fig. 9-3).[9] The round ligaments are fibrous and muscular, located on the uterus just anterior to the fallopian tubes. The round ligaments extend laterally, pass the external iliac vessels, run into the internal inguinal ring, and finally extend into the labia majora.[9] The broad ligament is a folding of the peritoneum that covers the round ligaments.[8,9] The round and broad ligaments provide minimal support to the uterus.[8,9] During development of a female fetus, the round ligament guides the ovaries into their correct location. Later in life, the round ligament provides a pull of the bladder in an anterior direction above the uterus. The broad ligament, a folded sheet of peritoneum covering the uterus, uterine tubes, and ovaries, divides the pelvic cavity to create the vesicouterine fossa (anterior to the uterus) and the recto-uterine fossa (posterior to the uterus). The main support for the uterus and cervix is from the cardinal ligament, which attaches from the cervix laterally to the endopelvic fascia (which is attached to the pelvic bone).[9] The uterosacral ligaments begin at the superior-posterior portion of the cervix and pass around the rectum bilaterally to attach to the sacral vertebrae (first through fifth) to provide some support to the cervix.[9]

The portion of the gastrointestinal viscera in the pelvis is the rectum, which lies along the curvature of the sacrum posterior to the uterus. The posterior cul-de-sac between the uterus and rectum may be occupied by pathologic conditions such as endometriosis, cancer, or pelvic adhesions.[9]

Dynamic support for the all viscera housed in the pelvis occurs through muscles, ligaments, vessels, and nerves.[9] External openings of the pelvis occur through the urethra (bladder), vagina (uterus), and anus (rectum). Appropriate functioning of these systems offers bladder and bowel continence and at the same time voluntary defecation and urination. The dynamic support may undergo severe stressors, including vaginal labor and delivery[9] and chronic intraabdominal pressure (e.g., chronic constipation or long-term heavy lifting).

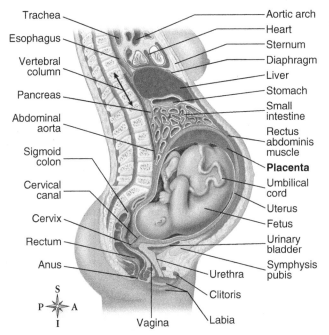

• **Figure 9-2** Pregnant Uterus. (From Patton KT. *Anatomy and Physiology*. 9th ed. St. Louis: Mosby; 2016.)

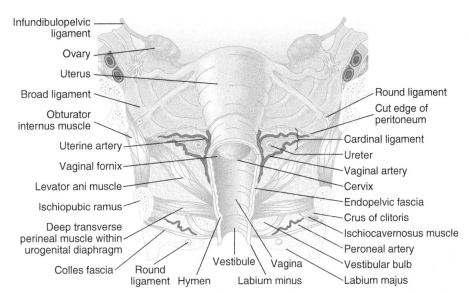

• **Figure 9-3** Coronal Section of the Pelvis Showing the Ligaments Supporting the Uterus. (From Hacker NF, Gambone JC, Hobel CJ, eds. *Hacker and Moore's Essentials of Obstetrics and Gynecology*. 5th ed. Philadelphia: Saunders; 2010.)

Bony Female Pelvis

The bony pelvis is a ring formed by the bilateral innominate bones (ilium, ischium, and pubis bones), the sacrum, and the coccyx.[8,9] The acetabulum of the innominate (hip bone) articulates with the femoral head.[8] In Chapter 1, discussion and images are provided that contrast the male and female pelvis (see Fig. 1-15 in Chapter 1). Here the focus is on the female pelvis and on describing the various pelvic shapes (Fig. 9-4). The bony pelvis may have a gynecoid, anthropoid, android, or platypelloid shape.[10] Fifty percent of women have a gynecoid pelvic shape, the classic female pelvis shape: round inlet, straight sidewalls, average prominence of ischial spines, well-rounded sacrosciatic notches, well-curved sacrum, and spacious subpubic arches (>90 degree angle). The gynecoid shape is more spacious and thus ideal for delivering babies. Thirty percent of women have an android shape, with a triangular inlet (in which arrest of descent during labor and delivery is common). The android shape is a classic male pelvis shape. Twenty percent of women have an anthropoid shape, which is oval and causes the fetal head to engage in occipitoposterior position during delivery (occipitoanterior is the desirable position). The platypelloid shape is found in approximately 3% of females, and it is a flattened gynecoid shape.[10] Because of its bony morphology, the classic male pelvis is inherently more stable than the female pelvis; the shape of the female pelvis promotes mobility for labor and delivery.

Pelvic Ligaments

The pelvic ligaments vary in composition and function from strong supporting connective tissues to smooth, muscular, fibrous, and areolar tissues with no significant supportive role[8] (see Fig. 1-17 in Chapter 1). The sacrospinous and sacrotuberous ligaments form the greater and lesser sciatic foramina,[9] which allow passage of neurovascular structures from within the pelvis to the lower extremity and genital region.[9] These two ligaments, along with the anterior longitudinal ligament of the sacrum, are dense and contribute to stability of the pelvic joints.[8] The ligaments projecting from uterine structures are discussed previously in relation to the gynecologic viscera.

Muscles of the Pelvis

The muscles of the pelvis include the "pelvic diaphragm" and the pelvic wall muscles (Fig. 9-5).[8,9]

The pelvic diaphragm muscles include the levator ani (puborectalis, pubococcygeus, and iliococcygeus) and the coccygeus.[8,9] These muscles provide the central and critical support mechanism for the pelvic viscera.[8,9] These muscles begin at the lateral pelvic wall and run downward and medially to fuse centrally and posteriorly.[9] Anteriorly, the levator hiatus is an opening within these muscles to allow the passage of the urethra, vagina, and anus.[9] The pelvic diaphragm muscles are predominantly type I (slow twitch) fibers and normally maintain constant tone to provide support for abdominopelvic contents against intraabdominal forces.[8,9] By doing so, these muscle prevent chronic strain to the pelvic ligaments and fascia.[8] Type II (fast twitch) fibers of the pelvic diaphragm muscles enable performance of quick contractions to provide support with sudden increases in abdominal pressure (e.g., when coughing, sneezing, or jumping).[8] When contracting (voluntarily or involuntarily), these muscles elevate superiorly; this action flexes the anorectal canal for fecal continence and voluntary control of the bladder. Relaxation of these muscles occurs only briefly and intermittently[8] to allow anorectal canal straightening for fecal emptying, bladder empting, and directing of the fetal head during delivery.[9] The muscles in the pelvis are hybrid (smooth and striated muscle tissue) with S2 to S4 nerve root innervation.[9] The perineal membrane and perineal body are inferior to the pelvic diaphragm muscles (more superficial) and contribute to the diaphragm of the pelvis.[8]

The pelvic wall muscles include the piriformis and obturator internus (see Fig. 9-5). These muscles are striated, and their fasciae partially cover the posterior, lateral, and inferior pelvic walls.[8] From the anterior-lateral surface of the sacrum, the piriformis muscle originates to fill part of the posterior-lateral pelvis wall. The piriformis leaves the pelvic cavity by traveling through the greater sciatic foramen and inserting onto the greater trochanter of the femur. The sidewalls of the pelvis are partly occupied by the obturator internus, which originates from the ilium, ischium, and obturator membrane inside the pelvis. The obturator internus leaves the pelvis through the lesser sciatic foramen, where it makes a turn and travels on to insert onto the

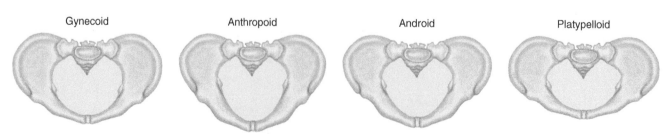

| Gynecoid | Anthropoid | Android | Platypelloid |

• **Figure 9-4** Female Bony Pelvis Shapes. (From Murray SS, McKinney ES. *Foundations of Maternal-Newborn and Women's Health Nursing.* 6th ed. St. Louis: Saunders; 2014.)

greater trochanter of the femur. On the surface of the obturator internus is a thickening of fascia, the arcus tendineus levator ani (ATLA), which provides the site of origin for portions of the levator ani muscles. Another fascial thickening, the arcus tendineus fascia pelvis (ATFP), covers the medial side of the obturator internus and levator ani muscles, runs from the inner pubic bones to the ischial spines, and provides a lateral place of attachment for the anterior vaginal wall.[8]

Female Perineum and Genitalia

The female perineum is the subcutaneous tissue that is connected superiorly (deeply) to the levator ani muscles and inferiorly (superficially) by the skin (Fig. 9-6).[9] The perineum lies centrally between the ischial spines, ischiopubic rami and pubis, and coccyx. The perineum is divided into two triangles: the urogenital triangle and the anal triangle[9]; these two triangles are separated by an imaginary line running between the two ischial tuberosities and through the perineal body (located between the distal posterior vaginal wall and the anus).[8] The perineal body serves as a fibrous attachment for the superficial perineal muscles (bulbocavernosus, superficial transverse perineal, and external anal sphincter) and the superficial portion of the levator ani that aid in genital hiatus closure.[8,9] The perineal body also provides support to the distal vagina and rectum; care in repairing the perineal body is therefore important after

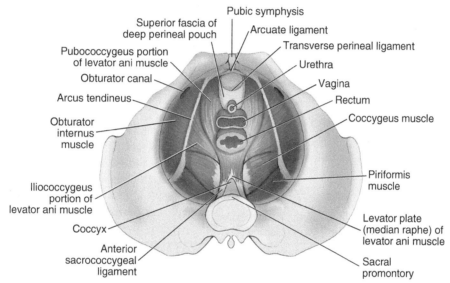

• **Figure 9-5** Female Pelvic Diaphragm. (From Falcone T, Goldberg JM. *Basic, Advanced, and Robotic Laparoscopic Surgery: Female Pelvic Surgery Video Atlas Series* (Female Pelvic Video Surgery Atlas Series). Philadelphia: Saunders; 2010.)

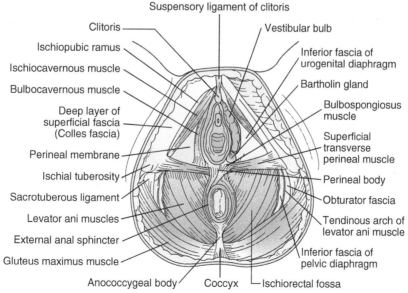

• **Figure 9-6** Female Perineum. (From Shaw RW, Luesley D. *Gynaecology.* 4th ed. Edinburgh: Churchill Livingstone; 2011.)

episiotomies and perineal lacerations and during perineal reconstructive procedures.[8]

The external female genitalia are the mons pubis, labia majora, labia minora, clitoris, and vaginal vestibule (Fig. 9-7).[9] The mons pubis is a fatty area that lies over the pubic bones and symphysis. The labia majora run longitudinally as two skin folds from the mons pubis toward the perineal body (just lateral to the labia minora). The labia minora are hairless and without fat; anteriorly, they meet to form the clitoral prepuce and frenulum. The clitoris lies within the clitoral prepuce and is homologous to the male penis. Innervation to the clitoris can be compromised with injury to the ilioinguinal nerve during lower abdominal transverse incisions. The vaginal vestibule is the area between the labia minora and holds the openings of the urethra and vagina.[9]

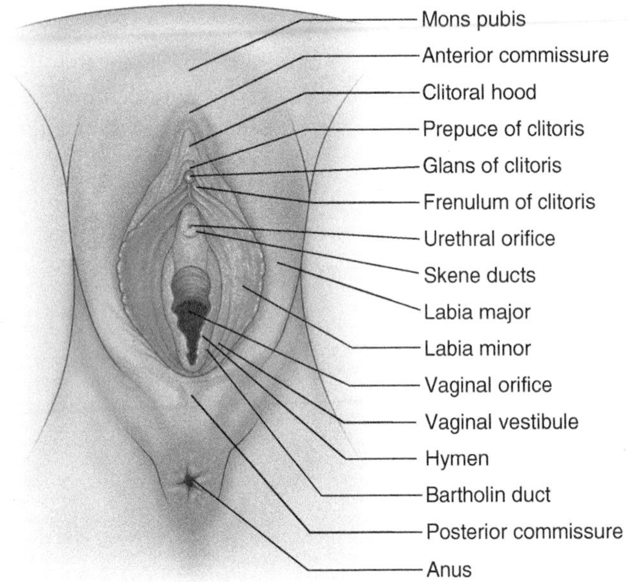
Mons pubis
Anterior commissure
Clitoral hood
Prepuce of clitoris
Glans of clitoris
Frenulum of clitoris
Urethral orifice
Skene ducts
Labia major
Labia minor
Vaginal orifice
Vaginal vestibule
Hymen
Bartholin duct
Posterior commissure
Anus

• **Figure 9-7** Female External Genitalia. (From Warren RJ, Neligan PC. *Plastic Surgery,* vol 2: *Aesthetic Surgery.* 3rd ed. London: Saunders; 2013.)

Nerves of the Pelvis

Innervation of the pelvis involves supradiaphragmatic and infradiaphragmatic portions.[9] Superior to the diaphragm (supradiaphragmatic) involves control of the bladder, uterus, and rectum (including autonomic nervous system regulation of urethral and anal sphincter tone). Sympathetic input generally allows the bladder and rectum to store urine and feces (respectively) as smooth muscle sphincters contract. Sympathetic innervation arises from hypogastric plexuses (majority) and sacral sympathetic trunk (minority). Parasympathetic input causes relaxation of the bladder outlet, urethral sphincters, and anal sphincters for release of urine and stool. Parasympathetic innervation arises from the sacral spinal nerves. The autonomic nerve structures can be damaged in labor and delivery or during surgical procedures (pelvic or spinal). The infradiaphragmatic motor innervation is almost fully somatic through the pudendal nerve and its branches. The pudendal nerve arises from S2 to S4 nerve roots (Fig. 9-8). It exits the pelvis through the greater sciatic foramen, runs posterior to the sacrospinous ligament, reenters the pelvis in the lesser sciatic foramen, and then travels through the pudendal canal (along the ischiorectal fossa)

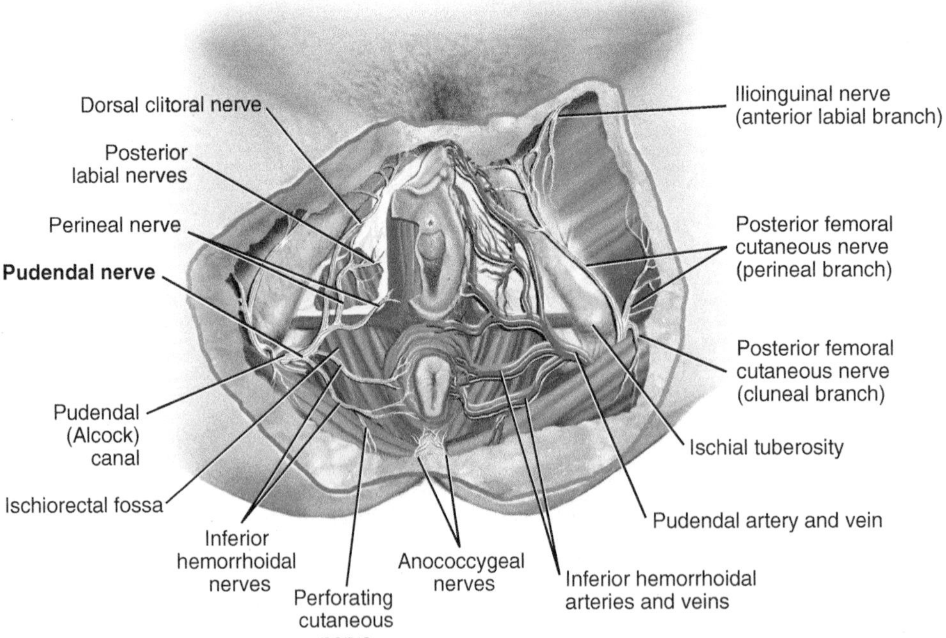
Dorsal clitoral nerve
Posterior labial nerves
Perineal nerve
Pudendal nerve
Pudendal (Alcock) canal
Ischiorectal fossa
Inferior hemorrhoidal nerves
Perforating cutaneous nerve
Anococcygeal nerves
Inferior hemorrhoidal arteries and veins
Pudendal artery and vein
Ischial tuberosity
Posterior femoral cutaneous nerve (cluneal branch)
Posterior femoral cutaneous nerve (perineal branch)
Ilioinguinal nerve (anterior labial branch)

• **Figure 9-8** Pudendal Nerve in Female. (From Baggish MS, Karram MM. *Atlas of Pelvic Anatomy and Gynecologic Surgery.* 3rd ed. St. Louis: Saunders; 2011.)

with the internal pudendal artery and vein. The space between the sacrospinous and sacrotuberous ligaments is a site of potential pudendal nerve compression. The pudendal nerve branches to provide cutaneous innervation of the external genitalia, motor innervation of the urogenital diaphragm, and innervation of the striated muscles of the urethra and anus.[9] These three pudendal nerve branches include the inferior rectal branch, the perineal branch, and the anterior (clitoral) branch. The nerve to the pelvic diaphragm muscles, or levator ani nerve, travels on the superior surface of the coccygeus muscle just medial to the ischial spine.[8]

Anatomic Connections Between the Pelvis and Hip

The bony pelvis provides the major mechanism for transferring weight and forces of the trunk and upper limbs to the lower limbs.[8] Additionally, it provides sites of attachment for the muscles of the lower extremities and trunk that may contribute to pain and dysfunction of the hip and pelvis.[8] Understanding of the muscles that attach into the pelvis and hip joint and lower extremity is helpful in clinical management and appropriate referral of patients with pelvic and hip pain or other dysfunction[8,11] (Table 9-2).

The anterior fascial compartment of the thigh holds the sartorius, iliopsoas, pectineus, and quadriceps femoris muscles (refer to Fig. 1-27).[8] The anterior superior iliac spine (ASIS) serves as the origin for the sartorius as it crosses the hip and runs distally to attach to the medial tibial surface. The anterior inferior iliac spine (AIIS) and the ilium just superior to the acetabulum are the sites of origin for the rectus femoris, which then inserts onto the patella and converges with other quadriceps tendons to insert on the tibial tuberosity. The iliac fossa provides the origin of the iliacus, which unites with the psoas to form the iliopsoas, which passes under the inguinal ligament and attaches to the lesser trochanter of the femur. The pectin pubis is the origin site for the pectineus, which also inserts on the lesser trochanter of the femur.[8]

The medial compartment of the thigh contains the gracilis, obturator internus, and adductor longus, brevis, and adductor portion of the adductor magnus (pubofemoral portion) muscles.[8] From the inferior pubic ramus and ramus of the ischium, the gracilis arises and inserts into the medial tibia. The obturator membrane and pubic and ischial rami serve as origin sites for the obturator internus, which then inserts into the greater trochanter of the femur. The pubic ramus and ischial tuberosity are the origin sites for the adductors.[8]

The posterior compartment of the thigh is occupied by the biceps femoris, semitendinosus, semimembranosus, and hamstring portion of the adductor magnus (ischiocondylar portion) muscles[8] (see Fig. 1-28). The ischial tuberosity provides the origin of all these muscles. The biceps femoris inserts into the head of the fibula, the semitendinosus onto the medial tibia, the semimembranosus onto the medial

tibial condyle, and the hamstring portion of the adductor magnus onto the adductor tubercle of the femur.[8] Additionally, the gluteus medius and minimus, piriformis, gemellus superior and inferior, obturator internus, and quadratus femoris travel from the pelvis to attach into the superior femur and trochanter.

In considering the muscular connections between the hip and pelvis, physiologic differences between female and male muscular systems are worth noting (Table 9-3). Adolescence brings hormonal changes that cause an increase in lean muscle mass for boys, but an increase in fat deposits for girls, without an increase in muscle mass.[12] This fat deposition leads to female breast development and widening of the hips during puberty. By the mid-teen years, girls have approximately 75% of the strength that boys have.[12] Additionally, women have a higher proportion of type I fibers (slow twitch) compared with men.[13] Muscle performance differences have been noted that may contribute to a higher risk of certain injuries in girls and women. Female athletes demonstrate contraction of quadriceps with anterior tibial perturbation, as opposed to boys and men, who contract the hamstrings.[14] Girls and women also have less ability to contract muscles around the knee when loaded internal rotation is occurring,[15] and women are less able to stabilize the knee in an anterior-posterior plane.[16,17] Higher rates of anterior cruciate ligament injuries are associated with a variety of factors, including poor hip-knee control with landing from a jump.[12] Patellofemoral pain may be associated in differences in quadriceps activity (timing, intensity, torque production).[12]

A final consideration in the connection between the hip and pelvis is related to neural connections. Several nerves travel from the lower trunk and pelvis to the hip, thigh, and perineal structures (refer to Fig. 1-6). The ilioinguinal, iliohypogastric, lateral femoral cutaneous, and femoral nerves exit laterally from the psoas muscle. The genitofemoral nerve travels through the belly of the psoas. The obturator nerve exits medially from the psoas muscle to travel through the obturator foramen. Each of these nerves can become compressed and irritated with iliopsoas tightness or involvement,[11] or with anatomical changes during pregnancy.[18] Additionally, the sciatic nerve passes superiorly, through, or inferiorly to the piriformis muscle; piriformis spasm or strain may result in sciatic nerve irritation.[11] Compression of the lateral femoral cutaneous nerve can occur with compression between the inguinal ligament and abdomen or tight clothing, with resulting paresthesia of the lateral thigh.[11] Neural connections between the hip and pelvis are discussed further in this chapter in relation to specific conditions.

Standardized Terminology of Pelvic Muscle Function

The International Continence Society formed the Pelvic Floor Clinical Assessment Group, which published

TABLE 9-2	Muscles With Attachment in the Pelvis and in Lower Extremity

Muscle	Pelvis Attachment*†	Lower Extremity Attachment*†	Action†
		Anterior Fascial Compartment of Thigh	
Sartorius	ASIS	Medial tibial surface	Flexes, abducts, and externally rotates hip Flexes and internally rotates knee
Rectus femoris	AIIS and ilium	Patella	Flexes hip Extends knee
Iliacus	Iliac fossa	Lesser trochanter of femur	Flexes and externally rotates hip
Psoas	T12-L4 vertebral bodies/disks; L1-L5 costal processes		
Pectineus	Pectin pubis		Adducts, externally rotates, and slightly flexes hip Stabilizes pelvis in coronal and sagittal planes
		Medial Compartment of the Thigh	
Gracilis	Inferior pubic ramus, ramus of ischium	Medial tibia	Adducts and flexes hip Flexes and internally rotates knee
Obturator internus	Intrapelvic surfaces of obturator membrane, pubic and ischial rami	Greater trochanter of femur	Externally rotates, adducts, and extends hip Stabilizes hip joint
Adductors	Pubic ramus, ischial tuberosity		Adducts hip Flexes hip (up to 70 degrees of flexion) Extends hip (past 80 degrees of flexion) Stabilizes pelvis in coronal and sagittal planes
		Posterior Compartment of the Thigh	
Gluteus maximus	Sacrum, ilium, thoracolumbar fascia, sacrotuberous ligament	Iliotibial tract and gluteal tuberosity	Extends and externally rotates hip Upper fibers abduct hip Lower fibers adduct hip
Gluteus medius Gluteus minimus	Ilium	Greater trochanter	Abducts hip Stabilizes pelvis in coronal plane Anterior portion flexes and internally rotates hip Posterior portion extends and externally rotates hip
Piriformis	Anterior surface of sacrum	Greater trochanter (apex)	Externally rotates, abducts, and extends hip Stabilizes hip joint
Tensor fasciae latae	Anterior superior iliac spine	Iliotibial tract	Tenses fascia latae Abducts, flexes, and internally rotates hip
Biceps femoris, long head	Ischial tuberosity	Head of fibula	Extends hip Stabilizes pelvis in sagittal plane Flexes and externally rotates knee
Semitendinosus Semimembranosus		Medial tibia Medial tibial condyle	Extends hip Stabilizes pelvis in sagittal plane Flexes and internally rotates knee
Ischiocondylar portion of adductor magnus		Adductor tubercle of the femur	Adducts, extends, and slightly flexes hip Stabilizes pelvis in coronal and sagittal planes

AIIS, Anterior inferior iliac spine; *ASIS*, anterior superior iliac spine.
*Data from Corton MM. Anatomy of the pelvis: how the pelvis is built for support. *Clin Obstet Gynecol.* 2005;48:611-626.
†Data from Gilroy AM. *Anatomy: An Essential Textbook.* Thieme: New York; 2013:107, 319, 324-326.

TABLE 9-3	Physiologic Differences Between Male and Female Muscle Systems	
Feature	Male	Female
Adolescent hormonal changes	Increase in lean muscle mass	Increase in fat deposits: breast development, widening of hips No increase in muscle mass
Strength	Greater strength development	75% of the strength that males have
Muscle type	Higher proportion of type II fibers (fast twitch)	Higher proportion of type I fibers (slow twitch)
Stabilization	Contract hamstrings with anterior tibial perturbation More ability to contract surrounding knee muscles with loaded internal rotation More ability to stabilize the knee in anterior-posterior plane	Contract quadriceps with anterior tibial perturbation Less ability to contract muscles around the knee with loaded internal rotation Less ability to stabilize knee in anterior-posterior plane
Pain and injury		Higher rates of patellofemoral pain Higher rates of anterior cruciate ligament injuries

Data from references 12 to 17.

standardized terminology related to pelvic diaphragm muscles in 2005.[19] The intent was to develop terms related to pelvic muscle function that could be used across health care providers and facilitate clear communication among these different groups of practitioners. A multidisciplinary group was involved in establishing this terminology.

The term *pelvic floor muscles* describes the muscular layer of the pelvic outlet, extending from the peritoneum of pelvic viscera (most cranial) to the skin of the vulva, scrotum, and perineum (most caudal). However, in this chapter, this muscular layer is referred to as the "pelvic muscle diaphragm," as described previously.[8,9] The term *diaphragm* versus *floor* is chosen here because floor likely creates an image of a static and flat structure, whereas diaphragm contributes to the image of a bowl or funnel-shaped structure that has dynamic features. Healthy pelvic diaphragm muscles are in fact not flat, but have sturdy thick layers of bowl or funnel shapes that, when functioning properly, are very dynamic in their ability to elevate and support the contents of the trunk and pelvis while also providing continence and stabilizing the pelvic girdle joints and lower

spine. This funnel of muscle normally lies horizontally, to give "floor" support when the pelvis and spine are in a neutral position (with normal lordosis).

Terminology was also established to describe pelvic diaphragm muscle function (Table 9-4). Normal pelvic diaphragm muscle function occurs when these muscles are able to contract and relax on command.[19] Additionally, the muscles respond appropriately to an increase in intraabdominal pressure. For instance, if a patient coughs, sneezes, or exerts force with the trunk and upper body (as when lifting a heavy item), then the pelvic diaphragm muscles will contract to provide closure of pelvic outlets (urethra and anus, to maintain continence) and provide support to the trunk and pelvis as a deep core stabilizing muscle. With normal function, a strong and normal voluntary contraction is observed with internal pelvic muscle examination. A normal involuntary contraction is also observable and palpable as appropriate, such as with instruction to cough during examination. The ability to relax the muscle completely on command is also noted.[19] With normal function of the pelvic diaphragm muscles, a person will report normal bladder, bowel, and sexual function.

Underactive pelvic diaphragm muscle function causes the muscles to be unable to contract adequately or at all on command or as needed for function.[19] Thus, the muscles do not provide adequate closure to pelvic outlets, potentially resulting in urethral leakage of urine or anal leakage of feces, liquid, mucus, or gas. Additionally, the muscle may not provide adequate support to the pelvic organs, and this situation may result in pelvic organ prolapse (descent of a pelvic organ below its normal location).[19] Various types of pelvic organ prolapse can occur and may involve the bladder, urethra, rectum, lower intestine, cervix, uterus, or perineum (Table 9-5). This lack of muscular support may also contribute to low back pain, pelvic girdle pain, and inadequate core muscle control for a variety of functions.[20] Finally, lack of adequate pelvic muscle contraction may contribute to a decrease in sexual function because contraction of the pelvic diaphragm muscles contributes to sexual sensation and orgasm.[21,22] However, sexual function is multifactorial, and other factors may result in or contribute to a lack of desired sexual function.

Overactive pelvic diaphragm muscle function causes the muscles to be unable to relax adequately or at all for necessary functions that require a "release" of the muscles and an opening of the pelvic outlets.[19] This lack of relaxation may cause the urethra to have an inadequate opening to release urine, possibly resulting in hesitancy of the start of the urinary stream, "staccato" urination in which the stream stops and starts, a weak or "spraying" urinary stream, urinary urgency, or incomplete emptying of the bladder. In extreme cases, overactive muscles can cause complete obstruction of urination, although this is most likely to result after trauma to the pelvic muscles and urethral structures. Anal and bowel function can also be affected because the overactive muscles obstruct the lower rectum and anal region, thus possibly resulting in difficulty

TABLE 9-4 **Pelvic Diaphragm Muscle Function: Standardized Terminology From the International Continence Society**

Pelvic Muscle Term	Description of Muscle Function	Signs and Symptoms
Normal muscle function	Able to contract on command Able to relax on command Able to contact and relax in response to changes in intraabdominal pressure as appropriate	Normal or strong voluntary and involuntary contraction Complete relaxation on command Normal bladder, bowel, and sexual functioning
Underactive muscle function	Unable to contract adequately (or at all) on command or when required for function	Absent or weak voluntary and involuntary contraction Urinary or anal incontinence Pelvic organ prolapse Loss of sexual function or sensation Pelvic girdle or low back pain[20]
Overactive muscle function	Unable to relax fully or adequately as needed	Partial or absent voluntary muscle relaxation Obstructed urination or defecation Dyspareunia or vaginismus Pelvic pain
Nonfunctioning muscle	No muscle contraction palpable with internal vaginal or rectal examination	No signs of muscle contraction or relaxation Any dysfunctional symptom may be present

Data from Messelink B, Benson T, Berghmans B, et al. Standardization of terminology of pelvic floor muscle function and dysfunction: report from the pelvic floor clinical assessment group of the International Continence Society. *Neurourol Urodyn.* 2005;24:374-380.

TABLE 9-5 **Types of Pelvic Organ Prolapse in Female Patients**

Prolapse Type	Description
Apical prolapse	Descent of cervix and uterus inferiorly into vaginal canal (causing vaginal canal to invert on itself); in extreme cases, cervix and uterus may protrude externally through vaginal opening
Cystocele	Descent of bladder into anterior vaginal wall
Urethrocele	Descent of urethra into anterior vaginal wall; typically occurs with cystocele
Rectocele	Descent of rectum into posterior vaginal wall
Enterocele	Descent of lower intestine into vaginal wall (variable locations)
Anal prolapse	Descent of anal tissues externally through anus
Rectal prolapse	Descent of rectal tissues externally through anus (causing inversion of rectum on itself)
Perineal descent	Bulging of perineal tissues inferiorly away from pelvis and trunk

releasing gas or feces, chronic constipation, or incomplete evacuation of feces. Finally, overactivity can cause muscle tension, myofascial pain and trigger points leading to pelvic pain symptoms, and obstruction of the vaginal opening (introitus) leading to vaginismus. Vaginismus, as described later, is a condition in which entry into the vaginal opening and canal is painful, and in some cases impossible, such as for insertion of a tampon or of a penis for sexual activity. Similar to vaginismus is dyspareunia, which is pain with sexual activity. Dyspareunia is often associated with pain during intercourse, but it can also occur with arousal or orgasm without sexual penetration. This pain with sexual activity may also occur in areas away from the vagina and pelvis, such as the lower abdomen, low back, buttocks, hips, and thighs.

The Connection: Pelvic Diaphragm Muscles and Low Back, Pelvic Girdle, and Hip Pain and Conditions

This section of the chapter begins to examine the various patient populations in which the female pelvis is a factor in lumbopelvic-hip complex dysfunction and symptom development. The different patient classifications that are described through the remainder of the chapter are summarized in Table 9-6.

As described previously, many structural and nervous connections exist between the hip joint and pelvis region, with additional connections from these two areas to the lower trunk (lumbar spine and lower abdomen) and the thigh and lower leg. Thus, the potential for impairments in one region may reasonably contribute to those in an adjacent region. Trigger point referral patterns have also been described in which intrapelvic muscles may refer pain outside the pelvis and vice versa.[23] The coccygeus muscle can refer pain not just to the coccyx, but also to the gluteus maximus region; additionally, trigger points in this muscle can create sensations of bowel fullness and discomfort (even when the bowel is empty). The piriformis muscle, which originates within the bony pelvis and travels laterally to the greater trochanter, may cause pain in the sacroiliac joint, the hip joint region, and the hamstrings. Trigger points in the obturator internus muscle, which also originates within the pelvis then exits to attach into the greater trochanter, may create a sensation of rectal fullness and cause pain in the coccyx, hamstrings, posterior thigh, urethra (including sensation of bladder urgency), vagina, and vulva. The adductor magnus can refer pain to the perineum and bladder and may also create a sensation of fullness in the rectum.[23]

Urinary Incontinence Connection With Low Back Pain and Other Trunk Impairments

Evidence suggests that patients with urinary incontinence may experience lack of proper function in lumbopelvic and levator ani muscles,[24-27] breathing difficulties,[27,28] (tendency toward use of secondary breathing muscles, shallow breathing, breath-holding, and incoordination between breathing diaphragm and deep core muscles), and low back pain.[25,26,28,29] Impaired balance has also been demonstrated in a small study comparing ground reaction force plate measurements in women with stress urinary incontinence (having a greater center of pressure

TABLE 9-6 **Summary of Chapter Key Findings in Female Patients With Lumbopelvic-Hip Complex Dysfunctions***

Patient Classification	Patient Profile	Common Mechanisms	Interventions, Rehabilitation, and Programming
Connection: pelvic diaphragm muscles and low back, pelvic girdle, and hip pain	Lack of research to identify common demographics May or may not have bladder, bowel, or sexual symptoms Symptoms also may occur in pelvis or refer to distal structures	Aging sacroiliac joint referral Obturator internus muscle contribution to anterior groin or posterolateral hip pain and to bladder urgency or frequency Pelvic diaphragm muscle involvement in pelvic girdle symptoms Poor pelvic diaphragm muscle recruitment or substituting Valsalva for muscle contraction	Addressing deep stabilizing core muscles with nonspecific low back pain (transversus abdominis, multifidus, pelvic diaphragm muscles, breathing diaphragm): focus on slow, controlled contraction with body awareness Avoiding cues for "bracing" or "drawing in" toward umbilicus (inhibits deep core muscles) Progressing muscle training to functional movement and positions Addressing posture and positions: optimal neutral or "tall" postures promote core muscle function
Chronic pelvic pain	4%-20% of women Ages 15-50 yr Up to 60% have not received a specific diagnosis Up to 20% have not had diagnostic testing Risk factors: psychosocial issues, miscarriage, long menstrual cycles, pelvic inflammatory disease, abuse history (sexual, psychological, physical) Altered postural habits	33%-35% of diagnostic laparoscopies reveal no pathologic features Pain may arise from musculoskeletal, gynecologic, urologic, gastrointestinal, or neurologic systems Increased sensitization in the nervous system Musculoskeletal and neural focus: intrapelvic compression or injury of nerves Pelvic diaphragm muscle underactivity causing decreased support of joints and structures Pelvic diaphragm muscle overactivity causing trigger points, decreased introital size Sacrococcygeal joint injury or strain Surgical trauma	Reduction of stressors to involved neural structures (postures, positions, use of cushions) Education in chronic pain development and pain science Encouraging multidisciplinary team approach to address physical and psychological factors Encouraging holistic approach (e.g., including stress management, sleep hygiene, relaxation techniques, diet) Muscle training and reeducation to address motor control problems: core muscle focus with normalized breathing patterns Progression of muscle training to dynamic movement and functional movements Physical agents and manual therapy used as needed, with care for patient to not become "dependent" on passive treatments Neural mobilization techniques and reduction of stress to neural tissues with positioning education

Continued

TABLE 9-6 Summary of Chapter Key Findings in Female Patients With Lumbopelvic-Hip Complex Dysfunctions—cont'd

Patient Classification	Patient Profile	Common Mechanisms	Interventions, Rehabilitation, and Programming
The prenatal woman	20% of all pregnant women experience pelvic girdle pain, with pain between the iliac crests and gluteal fold, decreased tolerance to prolonged activities or postures ("fidgety"), "catch" in hip Other common pain conditions include muscle overuse conditions, round ligament pain, trochanteric bursitis of the hip TOH is rare but can occur specifically to pregnancy Preterm labor may be misdiagnosed as benign lumbopelvic pain Urinary symptoms may develop	Hormonal changes contribute to increase in lumbopelvic-hip laxity Increase in laxity can lead to poor motor control Postural changes of increase in lumbar lordosis, anterior pelvic tilt, forward head posture Overuse conditions with increase in use of hip abductors, hip external rotators, hip extensors, ankle plantar flexors Round ligament undergoes considerable stretch with growth of uterus and may lead to anterior groin pain, particularly with sit to stand or quick transitional movements Trochanteric bursitis may result from increase mass and side-lying sleep position TOH (rare) may develop from hormonal and biomechanical factors, with sudden and severe pain in hip joint and difficulty bearing weight on affected side Preterm labor may cause "cramping" in low back or abdomen The growing uterus compresses bladder and pelvic diaphragm; pelvic joint laxity creates challenges for pelvic diaphragm muscles; these may contribute to incontinence	Sacroiliac support belt if load transfer tests are positive (e.g., ASLR) Pregnancy abdominal support belt to alleviate round ligament pain Strengthening of transversus abdominis and deep core muscles to improve motor control and reduce pelvic girdle, low back, and round ligament pain Addressing deep stabilizing core muscles (transversus abdominis, multifidus, pelvic diaphragm muscles, breathing diaphragm) with focus on slow, controlled contraction with body awareness Avoiding cues for "bracing" or "drawing in" toward umbilicus (inhibits deep core muscles) Progressing muscle training to functional movement and positions Addressing posture and positions: optimal neutral or "tall" postures promote core muscle function Reassurance that pelvic girdle pain symptoms can be managed with motor control techniques Normalizing posture to reduce strain on hip abductors, adductors, external rotators, extensors Avoiding asymmetrical postures (e.g., cross-legged sitting or stance with weight toward one leg) Manual therapy to address trigger points or pain relief of joints Use of heat or cold therapies (except directly over abdomen) Education in transitional movement patterns or control, sleep positioning, and supports Targeted pelvic diaphragm muscle training as needed for bladder or bowel symptoms
The postpartum woman	At 3 months postpartum, many women report low back pain, hemorrhoids, dyspareunia, urinary and fecal incontinence Low back and pelvic girdle pain persists in nearly half of women 6 months postpartum, more than one third at 18 months Postpartum depression more common in women with low back and pelvic girdle pain DRA (if it occurred) should resolve by 8 weeks postpartum Perineal trauma during delivery increases risk of incontinence, prolapse, and sexual dysfunction	Decrease in muscle control, perineal trauma, and DRA may contribute to persistence of low back and pelvic girdle pain Vaginal delivery in particular may contribute to incontinence, prolapse, pelvic nerve injury, and sexual health symptoms Anal sphincter trauma in particular may contribute to anal incontinence Sacrococcygeal injuries may contribute to coccyx pain Delivery positions prolonged under anesthesia can contribute to neuralgia development Cesarean delivery will involve both postpartum recovery systemically and pelvic-abdominal surgical recovery	It should not be assumed that low back and pelvic girdle pain or DRA arising in pregnancy will resolve on its own; many of these symptoms persist into post-partum period; may address with sacroiliac or abdominal binder supports Instruction in avoiding Valsalva maneuver Incontinence not resolving by 3 months after vaginal delivery should be addressed by pelvic health practitioner Sexual dysfunction or pain that is persisting should be addressed by pelvic health practitioner Postcesarean delivery care should target instruction on infant care and daily activities while healing from surgery, as well as abdominal wall rehabilitation

ASLR, Active straight leg raise; *DRA*, diastasis rectus abdominis; *TOH*, transient osteoporosis of the hip.
*These types of dysfunctions are described throughout the chapter, with brief summaries and highlights for each population given here.

displacement, thus poorer balance) and in continent women.[30] In the same study, electromyographic (EMG) activity of the pelvic diaphragm muscles and erector spinae was greater in women with incontinence; the authors of the study suggested that this EMG difference may contribute to impaired balance as a result of decreased ability of trunk motion to assist with postural correction.[30] The same authors demonstrated in another study that the pelvic diaphragm also plays a role in posture support, with the pelvic diaphragm muscles providing postural muscle responses along with the abdominal muscles.[24] The pelvic diaphragm muscles provide support to the trunk, hip complex, and distal lower extremity.[20] However, this support is likely related more to control and coordination of the pelvic diaphragm and abdominal muscles and less to the power of muscle contraction.[24]

Nonspecific Low Back Pain and Pelvic Diaphragm Muscles

In particular, back pain has been associated with lack of pelvic diaphragm muscle motor control because of the role of pelvic diaphragm muscles in stabilization of the pelvic girdle joints and trunk.[24,28] It serves as a primary core stabilizing muscle with a natural co-contraction of the transversus abdominis muscle. Investigators have demonstrated that the addition of pelvic muscle exercises to a rehabilitation routine for patients with low back pain results in significantly greater improvements in outcome measures and pain reports.[29] Although not specific to pelvic diaphragm muscle involvement, another study[26] showed that people with nonspecific low back pain exhibit a delay in anterior pelvic tilting when transitioning from sitting to standing and also with stand-to-sit movements. Considering that the pelvic diaphragm muscles contract most strongly in a "very tall" and "tall" upright posture,[31,32] with bias toward anterior pelvic tilt, it is possible that a lack of adequate pelvic diaphragm muscle recruitment occurs in these persons.

Hip Pain and Pelvic Diaphragm and Pelvic Wall Muscles

In the differential diagnosis of hip and groin pain, pelvic diaphragm muscle dysfunction or intrapelvic structural involvement is recognized as a possible cause or contributor.[33] Although extensive research does not yet exist, several case reports suggest benefit from addressing intrapelvic structures in patients with hip pain (Table 9-7 summarizes case reports described here). In one report, a 39-year-old woman developed recalcitrant hip pain related to obturator internus muscle tendinitis after 10 minutes of rowing exercises.[34] As an intrapelvic muscle, the obturator internus muscle may receive therapy intervention with intrapelvic interventions (e.g., manual therapy techniques). This patient's pain was reported as being localized to the posterior gluteal region (just medial to the ischial tuberosity),

the anterior groin, and with palpation tenderness along the posterior border of the greater trochanter (all sites of the obturator internus muscle path). Tendinitis was confirmed through both magnetic resonance imaging (MRI) (showing swelling of the obturator internus muscle) and surgical observation of the tendon. Direct surgical intervention to the obturator internus muscle tendon followed by therapy resulted in a 15-month follow-up of full return to function.

Several cases directly implicate pelvic diaphragm muscle retraining to resolve hip pain. In a second case report, a 45-year-old distance (marathon) runner was experiencing deep gluteal and hamstring pain, which was initially diagnosed by the referring physician as a high hamstring strain.[35] This patient presented with pain in the left ischial tuberosity, with ipsilateral diffuse pain extending into the gluteal region and toward the pubic ramus. She reported her injury to occur during a training run in which she "pulled" her hamstring muscle. Over time, this progressed to ischial tuberosity pain with sitting, pain and tingling along the proximal hamstring extending to fibular head, and aching and burning at the ischial tuberosity; symptoms progressed to the point of discontinuing running. Symptoms reduced with rest and shortening her stride length and speed during runs. The patient had no complaints of bowel, bladder, or sexual dysfunction. Physical therapy examination ruled out lumbar, sacroiliac joint, hip joint, or fracture disorders. Based on findings, the initial physical therapy diagnosis was hamstring syndrome, described as gluteal sciatic pain related to recurrent strains of the proximal hamstring, which directed focus of the initial interventions. Because of the lack of full resolution of symptoms, with deep pelvic pain remaining along the inferior pubic ramus and pain remaining at the ischial tuberosity with sitting, the patient went on to receive a physical therapy intravaginal examination of the pelvic diaphragm and pelvic wall structures. This examination revealed reproduction of her "deep pain" with palpation of ipsilateral levator ani muscles along with other findings related to the levator ani muscle overactivity. Physical therapy intervention was added to address the pelvic muscle dysfunction. At 6 months after treatment, the patient's symptoms were resolved, and she returned to full running activities.

A third case report examined the involvement of intrapelvic myofascial involvement in a woman with hip osteoarthritis diagnosed by radiograph.[36] The patient experienced 5 years of symptoms with progressive increase in intensity; symptoms were alleviated but not resolved with trials of nonpelvic physical therapy and massage therapy. Pain complaints were of the left lateral hip, central low back, left lateral knee, and lower leg. Pain was most noticeable with walking and transitional movements. Preference of weight bearing toward her left leg was noted (with the left hip held in an adducted and internally rotated position), along with excessive thoracic kyphosis and lumbar lordosis. The patient confirmed using this stance for more than 20 years in her bank telling job. The patient also demonstrated a preference

TABLE 9-7	Summary of Case Reports Linking Hip Signs and Symptoms to Pelvic Dysfunction	
Demographic Features of Patient	**Hip-Related Signs and Symptoms**	**Pelvic-Related Findings, Interventions, and Outcomes**
39-year-old woman[34]	Recalcitrant hip pain developed after 10 minutes of rowing exercises Pain at posterior gluteal region (just medial to ischial tuberosity), anterior groin, posterior border of greater trochanter (all sites of obturator internus muscle path) MRI and surgical observation confirmed obturator internus tendinitis	Obturator internus muscle may be addressed by intrapelvic techniques (not described in this case) In this case, surgical intervention directed at tendinitis, followed by physical therapy (therapy not described) Full return to function
45-year-old female marathon runner[35]	Deep pain unilateral ischial tuberosity, gluteal region, pubic ramus Patient report of "pulled hamstring" Pain with sitting in proximal hamstring to fibular head Symptoms reduced with rest, shorter stride with running No bowel, bladder, or sexual symptoms reported Initial physical therapy for hip and gluteal region: reduced symptoms, but pain remaining along pubic ramus and deep in hip	Intravaginal palpation of ipsilateral levator ani muscles reproduced usual "deep pain" and revealed muscle overactivity Physical therapy intervention addressed intrapelvic muscle dysfunction At 6 months, symptoms resolved, with full return to running
Woman, bank teller for 20 years[36]	Chronic (5 years) pain in left lateral hip, central low back, left lateral knee, lower leg Pain worse with walking, transitional movements Osteoarthritis of hip diagnosed by radiograph Nonpelvic physical therapy and massage reduced symptoms Postural tendencies persisting from bank telling job (weight bearing toward left leg; left hip held in adducted and internally rotated position; excessive thoracic kyphosis and lumbar lordosis) Preference for cross-legged sitting Reported history of urinary tract infections Musculoskeletal examination findings of trunk, hip, spine dysfunction	Intravaginal examination revealed left obturator internus muscle trigger points and pain, stiffness of ATLA attachment of levator ani muscles Interventions focused on intrapelvic muscle trigger points and stiffness, normalizing postures, lumbopelvic stabilization exercise 70% overall improvement
13-year-old girl[27]	After emergency appendectomy, developed sudden-onset ongoing urinary incontinence and right-sided hip pain Palpation of right lower quadrant surgical scar at 10 months postoperatively caused inhibition of right levator ani, breathing diaphragm, lower trapezius, left gluteus maximus, right abdominal obliques, bilateral psoas, right sternocleidomastoid, and bilateral anterior scalene muscles	Chiropractic intervention to resolve inhibition of affected muscles led to full resolution of urinary incontinence and hip pain (with 6-year follow-up)

ATLA, Arcus tendineus levator ani; *MRI,* magnetic resonance imaging.

for leg crossing. Both these positions place stress on hip rotators if prolonged. A tendency toward leg crossing is also observed clinically as a compensatory mechanism for weakness or poor coordination of deep core muscles. Her history included frequent urinary tract infections, which can contribute to pelvic muscle overactivity. Physical therapy examination testing revealed lumbar spine instability, spine range-of-motion limitations (flexion and extension), hip range-of-motion stiffness and tightness, and overall hip muscle weakness (particularly on the left side). Intravaginal examination revealed left obturator internus trigger points and pain, along with stiffness along the ATLA attachment of the levator ani muscles. In addition, a decrease in

function was noted on multiple outcome measures (eight total, relating to both pelvic symptoms specifically and general function). Interventions focused on addressing the internal obturator internus muscle trigger points and pain, standing and sitting postures (to achieve "neutral" spine, pelvis, and hip positions, including avoiding leg crossing in sitting), and lumbopelvic stabilization exercise progression (with focus on the transversus abdominis and multifidus muscles). At the end of therapy, the patient reported clinically significant differences in outcome measures and a 70% improvement in overall function.

The fourth case involved a 13-year-old girl who developed a sudden onset of ongoing urinary incontinence (occasionally with full bladder loss) and right-sided hip pain following an emergency open appendectomy.[27] The patient presented 10 months postoperatively with incision scars at the umbilicus, just superior to the pubic joint, and the right lower quadrant. The latter scar, when palpated, was associated with inhibition (demonstrated through decreased manual muscle test strength) of the right levator ani, breathing diaphragm, bilateral lower trapezius, left gluteus maximus, right abdominal obliques, bilateral psoas, right sternocleidomastoid, and bilateral anterior scalene muscles. Chiropractic intervention that produced resolution of the inhibition of these muscles led the patient to report that all urinary incontinence and pelvic pain were alleviated, and this improvement continued through a 6-year follow up.

Patient Profile

Because of a lack of high-quality research studies, the demographics and prevalence of persons with underlying pelvic muscle involvement specifically overlapping with lumbar, abdominal, pelvic girdle, hip, and thigh pain are unknown. As discussed previously, findings from smaller studies and case reports demonstrate such overlap of involvement occurring in female patients from their teens to middle age, with obturator internus muscle tendinitis, deep gluteal and proximal hamstring pain, hip osteoarthritis, urinary incontinence, decreased balance abilities, and alterations in postural positions and transitional movements. However, this does not preclude similar involvement in male patients, other age groups, or persons with other symptoms or impairments in the lumbopelvic-hip region or elsewhere in the body. Symptoms of pelvic muscle involvement may or may not be apparent, however, as demonstrated through case report.[35] Thus, lack of bladder, bowel, or sexual symptom reports does not necessarily preclude pelvic muscle involvement. Pelvic muscle symptoms may refer to more distal structures (because of connections into the lower trunk, hip, and thigh) while not affecting function directly at the pelvic outlets. Thus, patients with a plateau in progress of rehabilitation of these areas, or with refractory symptoms in these more distal regions, may have occult underlying pelvic muscle contribution.

Nonetheless, patients who report direct symptoms related to bowel, bladder, or sexual function in addition to lumbopelvic-hip problems should certainly be further screened and evaluated by a well-trained practitioner who has experience in examining the intrapelvic muscles and structures.

Common Mechanisms

Pelvic diaphragm muscles can contribute to lumbopelvic-hip problems, and lumbopelvic-hip impairments may lead to pelvic-related dysfunction and symptoms. Although the cause and effect are not always clearly known, overlap of conditions exists and may be explained by problems in joint structures or in myofascial composition.

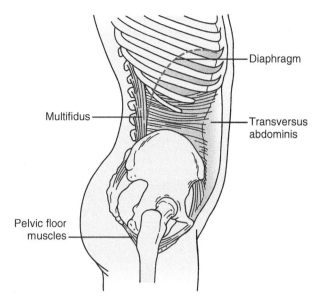

• **Figure 9-9** Deep Core Muscles. (From Magee DJ. *Orthopedic Physical Assessment.* 6th ed. St. Louis: Saunders; 2014.)

With aging, the sacroiliac joint cavity may narrow and experience fibrosis; because of innervation by the lower lumbar and sacral nerves, sacroiliac joint disease may contribute to pain in the pelvis and lower back and along the sciatic nerve distribution.[8]

Tender points or fibrous bands noted with internal palpation of the obturator internus muscle could be peripheral pain generators[37,38] (with pain referral to the anterior groin, thigh, and lateral and posterior hip) and may also contribute to bladder urgency and frequency symptoms.

The pelvic diaphragm muscles play an important role in pelvic girdle joint force closure, by providing support for the sacroiliac and pubic symphysis joints. Investigators have suggested that the most important muscles for stabilizing the sacroiliac joint are the transversus abdominis and pelvic diaphragm muscles (Fig. 9-9).[39] Several examination tests may help identify the cause of pelvic girdle pain or dysfunction; the tests described here are further summarized in Table 9-8.[40-43] Pelvic girdle joint dysfunction may include difficulty in transferring the "load" of the limbs and trunk through the pelvis with walking or other activities.[40] This difficulty in load transfer may be indicated during specific examination tests, including the Stork test (Fig. 9-10), the active straight leg raise (ASLR) test (Fig. 9-11), and pain provocation of the pubic symphysis with a modified Trendelenburg test (Fig. 9-12).[40] Difficulty transferring loads and decreased motor control around the pelvic girdle joints can lead to pain development in the pelvic girdle. Pain provocation of pelvic girdle joints is indicated with the Gaenslen test (Fig. 9-13), the long dorsal sacroiliac ligament (LDL) test (Fig. 9-14), the Patrick test (also known as flexion abduction external rotation (FABER]) (Fig. 9-15), the posterior pelvic pain provocation (P4) test (Fig. 9-16), and the pubic symphysis pain palpation test (Fig. 9-17).[40]

TABLE 9-8	Examination Tests in Pelvic Girdle Pain and Dysfunction		
Examination Test	**Brief Description**		**Statistics**
Active straight leg raise (ASLR)[41]	Test of load transfer through pelvis Patient supine, actively elevates legs (one at a time) off plinth, and asked to rate difficulty of elevating leg; any degree of difficulty indicates problems with load transfer through pelvis		Pain arising in pregnancy or first 3 weeks postpartum: Sensitivity = 0.87 Specificity = 0.94 Correlation with Quebec Back Pain Disability Scale of ≥45: Sensitivity = 1.00
Modified Trendelenburg[42]	Test for pubic symphysis involvement Patient standing and asked to flex one hip and knee to 90 degrees; positive test result indicated by pain in pubic symphysis		Examined in pregnant population (n = 2269): Sensitivity = 0.60-0.62 Specificity = 0.99 Intertester reliability = 0.63
Gaenslen[40]	Test for pelvic girdle pain Patient supine with overpressure of hip flexion and contralateral hip extension; production of usual pain in pelvic girdle joints indicates pelvic girdle pain		Reliability = 0.60-0.72 Sensitivity = 0.71 Specificity = 0.26
Palpation of long dorsal ligament (LDL)[42]	Test for pain provocation with palpation of the posterior sacroiliac ligament, indicating posterior pelvic girdle pain Patient placed prone; sacrum counternutated to increase tension in the LDL; then the LDL is palpated for pain provocation (can be modified to side lying during pregnancy)		Sensitivity = 0.11-0.49 Specificity = 1.00 Intertester reliability = 0.34 Examined in pregnant population (n = 2269) Positive LDL, ASLR, and P4 helps differentiate pelvic girdle from lumbar pain
Patrick (Faber)[42]	Test for pain provocation in hip or in sacroiliac joint Patient positioned in supine figure-4, with overpressure given to the flexed and externally rotated hip; reproduction or provocation of hip pain positive for hip joint involvement; reproduction or provocation of sacroiliac joint pain positive for sacroiliac joint involvement		Sensitivity = 0.40-0.70 Specificity = 0.99 Intertester reliability = 0.54 Examined in pregnant population (n = 2269)
Posterior pelvic pain provocation (P4)[42,43]	Test for pelvic girdle pain Patient supine with test hip in 90 degrees of flexion; clinician places pressure down through femur to stress sacroiliac joint; production of usual pain indicates pelvic girdle pain		Sensitivity = 0.81-0.93 Specificity = 0.80-0.98 Intertester reliability = 0.70 Examined in pregnant populations (range of n = 342 to n = 2269)
Pubic symphysis palpation[42]	Test for pubic symphysis joint pain Patient supine; clinician firmly palpates anterior pubic symphysis		Examined in pregnant population (n = 2269): Sensitivity = 0.60-0.81 Specificity = 0.99 Intertester reliability = 0.89

What has been demonstrated clearly is that objectively measured[44] and palpatory findings of pelvic girdle landmark asymmetry are not associated with low back pain. Thus, palpation should not be used for diagnosis in low back or pelvic girdle pain, but rather as a contribution to the gestalt of the overall examination.

Because of the theory that levator ani support prevents stretching of ligaments and fascia in the pelvis, injury or damage to these muscles may eventually compromise the supportive role of connective tissues in the pelvis.[8,45,46] Given that some of these ligaments connect directly or indirectly into lumbosacral structures, stretch and strain on these ligaments may contribute to low back ache. Without adequate instruction, many women may actually worsen levator ani support by attempting to perform pelvic muscle exercises. It is reported that 42% to 49% of women perform pelvic diaphragm muscle contractions incorrectly on verbal or written instruction,[46] including use of the Valsalva maneuver. The Valsalva maneuver results in an ineffective pelvic muscle contraction, significant substitution with the abdominal and chest wall muscles, increase in intraabdominal pressure, and increase in pelvic diaphragm descent. Use of the Valsalva maneuver to substitute for a pelvic diaphragm muscle contraction may lead to incontinence resulting from ineffective contractions to provide support and closure of the urethra. Additionally, the Valsalva maneuver may lead to poor pelvic stabilization and supportive dysfunction of intrapelvic ligaments (from increased intraabdominal pressure), which may contribute to pelvic girdle pain and CPP symptoms.[46]

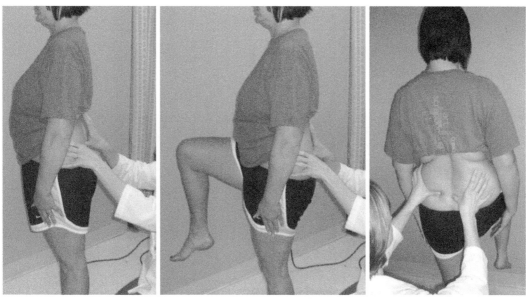

• **Figure 9-10** Stork Test. (Courtesy Section on Women's Health of the American Physical Therapy Association.)

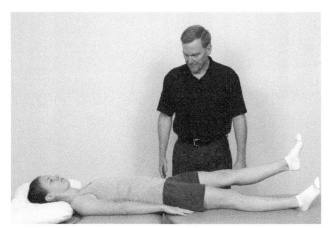

• **Figure 9-11** Active Straight Leg Raise Test. (From Olson KA. *Manual Physical Therapy of the Spine*. 2nd ed. St. Louis: Elsevier; 2016.)

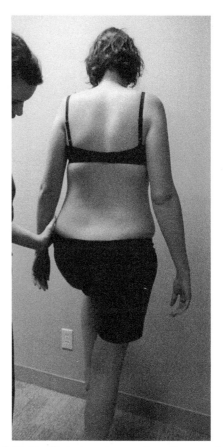

• **Figure 9-12** Modified Trendelenburg Test. (Courtesy Section on Women's Health of the American Physical Therapy Association.)

Postinjury Considerations

The previously described studies and case reports demonstrate that short-term or long-term involvement of intrapelvic musculoskeletal structures may result in lumbopelvic-hip symptoms. The challenge for the orthopedic therapist in the postinjury phase is accurately screening for and determining potential sources of pelvic diaphragm and pelvic wall muscle involvement. However, many of these conditions could also require physical therapy to address extrapelvic structures. Thus, initially, when involvement of intrapelvic structures is uncertain, rehabilitation would appropriately be focused toward an outpatient orthopedic approach that targets the explicit symptoms such as low back pain, hip pain, or impaired balance. In these cases, if the patient is not responding to therapy or the progression of rehabilitation plateaus, then additional examination of the intrapelvic structures may be needed. When specific symptoms implicate pelvic diaphragm muscle dysfunction, such as bladder leakage or urinary frequency and urgency, then early referral to or collaboration with a pelvic health physical therapist is warranted. Other types of health care providers may also

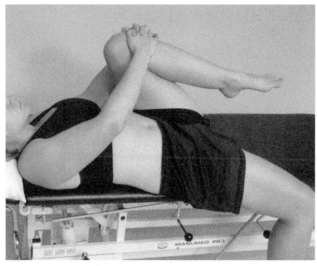

• **Figure 9-13** Gaenslen Test. (From Magee DJ. *Orthopedic Physical Assessment.* 6th ed. St. Louis: Saunders; 2014.)

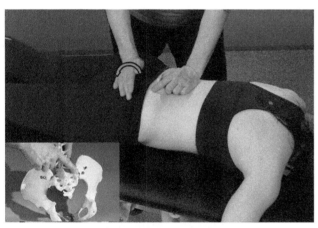

• **Figure 9-14** Long Dorsal Ligament (LDL) Pain Provocation Testing. (From Lee D, Lee L, Vleeming A. *The Pelvic Girdle: An Integration of Clinical Expertise and Research.* 4th ed. Edinburgh: Churchill Livingstone; 2011.)

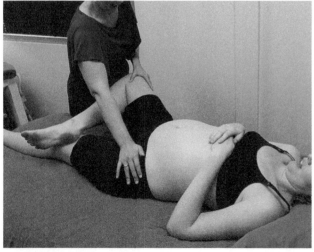

• **Figure 9-15** Patrick Test. (Courtesy Section on Women's Health of the American Physical Therapy Association.)

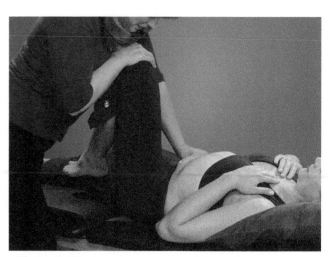

• **Figure 9-16** Posterior Pelvic Pain Provocation (P4) Test. (From Lee D, Lee L, Vleeming A. *The Pelvic Girdle: An Integration of Clinical Expertise and Research.* 4th ed. Edinburgh: Churchill Livingstone; 2011.)

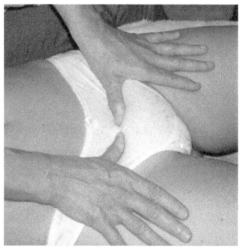

• **Figure 9-17** Pubic Symphysis Pain Palpation Test. (From Grimaldi M. Le périnée douloureux sous toutes ses formes: apport de la médecine manuelle et ostéopathie. Étude clinique. *J Gynecol Obstet Biol Reprod (Paris).* 2008;37:449-456.)

participate in pelvic rehabilitation. Considering their extensive neuromusculoskeletal education, physical therapists may be first-line practitioners when addressing signs and symptoms of a musculoskeletal nature.

Of benefit may be to include specific pelvic screening questions in the examination of every patient who presents with lumbopelvic-hip symptoms. The habit of asking every patient a few questions related to pelvic health may lead to increased likelihood of discovering these potential underlying problems, as well as facilitate earlier intervention for them. Be aware that early screening questions will not identify persons who do not have overt pelvic health symptoms or persons who are uncomfortable sharing and do not report these symptoms. One specific screening tool allows

Three Incontinence Questions

1. During the last 3 months, have you leaked urine (even a small amount)?
   ___YES (continue to question 2) ___NO (you are done with the survey)
2. During the last 3 months, did you leak urine (check all that apply):
   ___ When you were performing some physical activity such as coughing, sneezing, lifting, or exercise?
   ___ When you had the urge or the feeling that you needed to empty your bladder but could not get to the toilet fast enough?
   ___ Without physical activity and without a sense of urgency?
3. During the last 3 months, did you leak urine most often (check only one):
   ___ When you were performing some physical activity such as coughing, sneezing, lifting, or exercise?
   ___ When you had the urge or the feeling that you needed to empty your bladder but could not get to the toilet fast enough?
   ___ Without physical activity and without a sense of urgency?
   ___ About equally as often with physical activity as with a sense of urgency?

Interpretation of Answers

1. YES: UI exists; NO: no UI is identified
2. Identifies urinary symptoms present
3. Determines the type of UI:
   With physical activity: stress UI or mostly stress UI
   With urge: urge UI or mostly urge UI
   Without activity or urge: another cause of UI exists
   Equally as often with physical activity and urge: mixed UI

Sensitivity and Specificity

For urge UI: sensitivity of 0.75; specificity of 0.77
For stress UI: sensitivity of 0.86; specificity of 0.60

From Brown JS, Bradley CS, Subak LL, et al. The sensitivity and specificity of a simple test to distinguish between urge and stress urinary incontinence. *Ann Intern Med.* 2006;144:715-723.
UI, Urinary incontinence.

identification of stress, urge, or mixed urinary incontinence. This tool, called the Three Incontinence Questions (3IQ)[47] is easily and quickly administered (Box 9-1). The three questions ask whether leakage occurs and what preceded the leakage (physical stress to bladder or strong urge). The screen has been demonstrated to have a high sensitivity and specificity of determining urge or stress incontinence.[47]

Early Intervention

With nonspecific low back pain, the deep stabilizing core muscles of the trunk (transversus abdominis, deep segmental fibers of the lumbar multifidus, pelvic diaphragm muscles, and breathing diaphragm) have altered motor control.[48] Thus, initial focus in rehabilitation related to low back pain should center on regaining awareness, control, and normalized motor patterns of these muscles. In particular, precontraction of the transversus abdominis and pelvic diaphragm muscles naturally precedes arm and trunk movements.[49,50] The transversus abdominis provides optimal neuromuscular efficiency to the entire lumbopelvic-hip complex.[50,51]

Early retraining of the transversus abdominis and pelvic diaphragm muscles should be focused on controlled, submaximal contractions.[52] These two muscle groups naturally co-contract,[31,53] although they should be trained individually first to improve conscious awareness of their control. Lee[52] suggested the following goals with initial retraining of the deep core muscles (transversus abdominis, pelvic diaphragm, and deep multifidus fibers): maintain "normal" breathing patterns, with cues for inhalation followed by cues for exhalation with the muscle contraction; cue a performance of a minimal contraction (5% to 10% effort) to avoid recruitment of accessory and global muscles; maintain a neutral pelvis and spine position; keep contraction slow and controlled during concentric and eccentric phases (contraction and release of contraction); position the patient to promote relaxation of global muscles; and, finally, cue the patient to establish a conscious connection between the brain and the muscles being used.

As discussed previously, underactivity of pelvic diaphragm muscles may result in a decreased ability to maintain stabilizing control of the pelvic joints during transfers of trunk or lower extremity loads through the pelvis, such as with single limb stance during walking. Initial management of decreased load transfer ability may include use of a pelvic girdle support belt (or sacroiliac support belt).[54] Simultaneously, the patient is being instructed in increasing supportive motor control of the deep core muscles during potentially exacerbating activities and positions and avoiding excessive stressors to the pelvic girdle joints (e.g., avoiding extreme hip ranges of motion, crossing legs, or bicycle riding). Use of the belt for up to 6 months assists in reducing symptoms while motor control is restored with a specific exercise program.[20]

Rehabilitation Considerations and Programming

Rehabilitation that involves the pelvic diaphragm muscles in conjunction with the lumbopelvic and hip region is likely to center on core muscle awareness and control as described previously, followed by progressive strengthening and functional retraining. For the orthopedic therapist without training in intrapelvic muscle examination, use of real-time ultrasound has been recommended as an option for ensuring appropriate isolation of the transversus abdominis and levator ani muscles in particular (Figs. 9-18 and 9-19).[25]

Because of the role of the pelvic diaphragm muscles in providing pelvic girdle joint support, training of these muscles is valuable and likely necessary for patients with

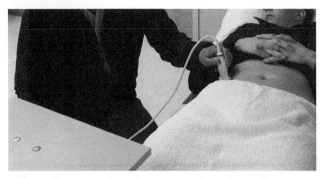

• **Figure 9-18** Real-time Ultrasound Performed With Transversus Abdominis Exercise.

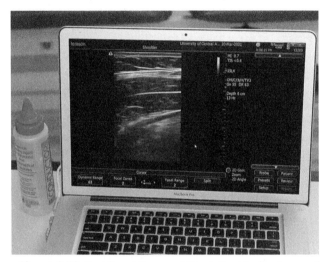

• **Figure 9-19** Real-time Ultrasound Computer Monitor Image of Lower Abdomen and Abdominal Muscles.

inadequate motor control support of the pelvic girdle that is causing pelvic girdle pain.[20]

Transversus Abdominis Muscle Cueing

Considerations should be given to avoiding instructions to use abdominal bracing (with co-contraction of all abdominals) or drawing in of the umbilicus toward spine because these maneuvers can lead to inhibition of the pelvic diaphragm muscles and increase in intraabdominal pressure, which in turn contribute to pelvic health conditions.[31] As described earlier, Lee[52] recommended submaximal cueing for slow, controlled contractions, that will result in a very small amount of movement occurring below the umbilicus and approximately 2 inches medial to the ASIS. Cues that may produce this controlled contraction include "slowly and gently draw the lowest part of the abdomen up and in" (while palpating medial to the ASIS), or "slowly say 'haaaa' as if fogging a mirror." Cues that promote an optimal contraction vary from person to person. Progression of coordination and functional strengthening will lead to submaximal contraction of the transversus abdominis during any movements or activities that require stability of the trunk and pelvis.

Pelvic Diaphragm Muscle Contractions

A correct contraction produces a tightening around the vaginal canal with an inward and upward movement of the perineum. It elevates the bladder anterosuperiorly and moves the urethra anteriorly[55] (to provide closing pressure against the pubic arch). Simultaneous with the bladder and urethral movements, the contraction does not increase bladder pressure.[56] Dynamic MRI has confirmed these components of a correct pelvic muscle diaphragm contraction.[57]

Considering the contribution of pelvic diaphragm muscle function to posture and support of the trunk, pelvis, hip, and lower extremities, intervention for these areas that includes pelvic diaphragm muscle assessment and appropriate training leads to a more thorough and complete rehabilitation process. Pelvic diaphragm muscle retraining involves the following: specific assessment (described later); 8 to 12 submaximal pelvic diaphragm endurance contractions (up to 10-second holds, depending on the patient's abilities) followed by 5 fast contractions (quick "squeeze" and full release of contraction each repetition) twice daily; and approximately 12 weekly clinical therapy visits with a pelvic health therapist who focuses on neuromuscular training and progression.[58,59] This progression should eventually lead to assessment and incorporation of pelvic diaphragm muscle activation with functional activities that typically cause symptoms (e.g., coughing, bending, lifting).[31,32] Instruction of pelvic diaphragm muscle contraction may be best promoted by encouraging the patient to draw in the muscles that "hold back gas," as opposed to asking patients to "hold back urine," because such cues may lead to disruption of normal bladder emptying.[20] Training may initially be enhanced with palpatory and surface (EMG) biofeedback.

Just as pelvic diaphragm muscles contribute to postural control, lumbopelvic posture also affects pelvic diaphragm muscle function. As mentioned earlier, investigators have demonstrated that muscle activity of the pelvic diaphragm muscles is greater in "very tall" and "tall" upright, unsupported sitting. Muscle activity is the least in supported slump sitting. Additionally, subjects report a sensation of stronger pelvic diaphragm muscle activation in the very tall and tall unsupported postures as opposed to slumped supported sitting.[31,32] In theory, the very tall and tall postures may contribute to stronger and more coordinated contractions because of optimal length-tension relationship development of the pelvic diaphragm muscles with a neutral to anterior tilt position of the pelvis. Expiration also promotes pelvic diaphragm muscle activation, and it may be used as a tool to help a patient initially locate and isolate these muscles.[20]

Chronic Pelvic Pain

Table 9-6 summarizes key findings related to various types of pelvic health conditions that may be experienced, including those described here related to pelvic pain.

Definition of Chronic Pelvic Pain and General Information

Pelvic pain is a very general term for pain in the pelvis that may extend to umbilicus, low back, and thighs.[46] Pelvic pain may involve visceral or somatic structures. Pain may be acute or chronic. Acute pelvic pain may arise from the joints of the lumbopelvic region (pubic symphysis, sacroiliac joints, lumbosacral junction, sacrococcygeal joint, and femoral-acetabular joints), ligaments of the lumbosacral and hip region, muscles and tendons in the pelvic region (levator ani, pelvic wall muscles, or surrounding hip, thigh, abdominal, and low back musculature), pelvic viscera, or nervous structures of the tenth thoracic spinal level and below. Acute pelvic pain is frequently diagnosed correctly and is assigned effective interventions.[46] However, some acute conditions may develop into CPP, which is typically of greatest concern clinically because of the challenge in identifying the cause and the significant morbidity associated with this condition. Thus, the center of discussion here is related to CPP.

CPP is nonmalignant[46] and noncyclic pain (meaning that it does not fluctuate with menstrual cycles or hormonal changes) lasting longer than 6 months in the pelvis and possibly extending to the lower abdomen, lower back, or thighs.[60] CPP pain accounts for 40% to 50% of gynecologic laparoscopic operations, 10% of gynecologic office visits, and 12% of hysterectomies.[20,46] Up to 40% of women having hysterectomy for CPP management will have no change in symptoms postoperatively.[46]

Patient Profile

The prevalence of female CPP is reported at 4% to 20% of women, or up to 9 million women, between 15 and 50 years of age.[46] Women older than 50 years of age may also experience pelvic pain, but the prevalence is not reported for this age group. Of women experiencing CPP, up to 60% have not been given a specific diagnosis, and up to 20% have not had diagnostic testing.[46]

Risk factors for CPP development include psychosocial issues, miscarriage, long menstrual cycles, clinical symptoms of pelvic inflammatory disease (PID), and sexual, psychological, or physical abuse during childhood.[46,60] Symptoms may include a variety of neuropathic sensory changes (Table 9-9), inflammation, and skin changes in the affected areas.[60] PID results from sexually transmitted diseases (STDs) and bacteria crossing the cervix; it is diagnosed most frequently in women 15 to 25 years old. PID is the most common cause of female infertility.[20] The most common causes of PID are *Chlamydia* infection and gonorrhea,[20] with worsening of the infection if an intrauterine device or douching is used.[46] Symptoms of STDs include vaginal discharge with foul odor, urinary frequency or burning, painful intercourse, and abnormal vaginal bleeding or spotting.[20]

Musculoskeletal changes typically associated with CPP may contribute to pain symptoms or result from "guarding"

TABLE 9-9	Neuropathic Sensory Changes Associated With Chronic Pelvic Pain	
Sensory Change	**Description**
Allodynia	Pain produced in response to a stimulus that is typically not pain producing (e.g., as light touch)
Dysesthesia	Unexpected or "wrong" sensation produced from a stimulus
Formication	Sensation of an insect crawling on the skin
Hyperalgesia	Exaggerated response to a pain-producing stimulus
Hypoalgesia	Diminished response to stimuli
Metesthesia	Protracted response to stimuli
Paresthesia	Abnormal sensation such as burning, tickling, or tingling

Data from Apte G, Nelson P, Brismee J-M, et al. Chronic female pelvic pain. Part 1. Clinical pathoanatomy and examination of the pelvic region. *Pain Pract.* 2012;12:88-110.

positions in response to the pain. Patients with CPP may exhibit the following: excessive thoracic kyphosis; poor breathing patterns; loss of flexibility in iliopsoas, piriformis, and obturator internus muscles; loss of hip capsule extensibility; apparent asymmetry of pelvic girdle landmarks; hypermobility of the thoracolumbar spine; excessive anterior pelvic tilt with "swayback" posture; and a tendency for unilateral standing patterns.[46]

Common Mechanisms

Several mechanisms may contribute to the development of CPP. However, in 33% to 35% of women undergoing diagnostic laparoscopic procedures to investigate pelvic pain origins, no pathologic condition is found.[46] Because of the potential for pain to arise from musculoskeletal, gynecologic, urologic, gastrointestinal, or neurologic conditions, a differential diagnosis is difficult to develop, thus leading to frustration with management of symptoms for both patient and health care provider.[46] Investigators have even proposed that nonspecific CPP may be a type of complex regional pain syndrome, with possible increased central sensitization of the nervous system.[46] Pain being referred to the pelvic region from a nonpelvic structure or system should also be considered.[46]

Musculoskeletal and neural structures may be a cause of or relate to CPP development. Potential sources of symptoms include the following: pelvic diaphragm muscle and fascial dysfunction[37,46]; compression or irritation of the pudendal, levator ani, iliohypogastric, genitofemoral, ilioinguinal, and lateral femoral nerves; and sacrococcygeal joint mobility disorders.[46]

<table>
<tr><td rowspan="2">TABLE
9-10</td><td colspan="4">**Nerves That May Be Involved in Chronic Pelvic Pain Development**</td></tr>
</table>

Nerve	Structures Innervated	Symptoms of Disorder	Potential Cause of Disorder
Lateral femoral cutaneous nerve	Sensation of lateral thigh	Paresthesia of lateral thigh	Compression between the inguinal ligament and abdomen (pregnancy, obesity) Compression from tight clothing
Iliohypogastric nerve	Skin and muscle of inferior anterior abdominal wall; skin over inguinal and pubic regions	Lateral pelvic pain Suprapubic pain Abdominal muscle weakness	Compression psoas muscle Trauma or surgical insults (cesarean section)
Ilioinguinal and genitofemoral nerves	Skin and muscles of inferior anterior abdominal wall; skin over inguinal and pubic regions; labial skin	Inguinal paresthesia Lower abdominal pain Labia pain	Compression from psoas muscle Compression along inguinal canal
Obturator nerve	Obturator externus, adductors, gracilis, and pectineus muscles; sensation of medial thigh and knee	Hip adductor weakness Medial thigh and knee sensory changes	Compression in obturator foramen (pregnancy, masses, hernia) Compression from psoas muscle Pelvic surgery trauma
Pudendal nerve	Inferior rectal branch: external anal sphincter Perineal branch: labia and muscles of deep and superficial pelvis Anterior clitoral branch: sensory to clitoris	Pain and burning in perineum Pain worsening with sitting Pain lessening with standing	Bicycle riding Surgical injury Vaginal delivery Pelvic ligament hypertrophy
Sciatic nerve	Tibial branch: hip extensors, knee flexors, ankle plantar flexors, everters, and inverters; sensation to posterolateral leg and foot Common fibular branch: foot everters, ankle dorsiflexors, sensation to lateral leg and dorsum of foot	Sensory changes (pain, burning) in posterolateral thigh, leg, foot and dorsum of foot Weakness in supplied muscles Shuffling gait or foot drop	Compression from piriformis muscle Misplaced gluteal injections Pelvic fracture

Data from references 11, 18, and 20.

Pelvic diaphragm muscle underactivity or overactivity, or fascial conditions creating loss of support or excessive tightness, may contribute to CPP. With muscle underactivity and loss of fascial support, the patient has weakness and decreased ability of the muscles to contract when needed. This weakness can result in loss of pelvic diaphragm muscle support to the pelvic girdle joints, thus leading to ineffective motor control and pain development around the sacroiliac and pubic symphysis joints. Pelvic muscle overactivity would involve muscles that do not relax when needed, thus resulting in features of muscle spasm, trigger points, and soft tissue tightness. This overactivity can lead to vaginismus (pain with tampon or sexual entry into the vagina), dyspareunia (pain with sexual activity), coccydynia, proctalgia fugax (sharp rectal pain, possibly related to irritable bowel syndrome),[20] constriction of neurovascular structures (e.g., pudendal nerve), and other pelvic pain conditions and symptoms. Both underactivity and overactivity can lead to bowel and bladder symptoms because of the effects on the correlating pelvic outlets.

Involvement of the nerves that supply the pelvic, hip, and thigh region may be involved (Table 9-10). Injury or trauma to the iliohypogastric nerve may lead to lateral pelvic and suprapubic pain and abdominal muscle weakness.[46] The ilioinguinal and genitofemoral nerves may be affected if inguinal paresthesia and lower abdominal and labia pain are present.[20] Weakness of the hip adductors with sensory changes to the medial thigh and knee may indicate obturator nerve involvement.[20] The obturator nerve is at risk for injury because of its path through the pelvis and the fibroosseous tunnel; thus, pregnancy, pelvic masses, pelvic surgical procedures, orthopedic injuries, hernias, and obturator tunnel narrowing may result in compression and affectation of this nerve.[46] The path and supply of the pudendal nerve are described earlier. The pudendal nerve traverses a winding path from S2 to S4 near bony and ligamentous structures of the pelvis and may contribute to perineal pelvic pain through its sensory and motor supply to the levator ani nerve, the perineal branch, and the dorsal nerve to the clitoris. Involvement of the inferior rectal branch may also lead to symptoms in the anal region. The pudendal nerve may be compressed or experience trauma with anal surgical procedures, vaginal delivery, prolonged bicycle riding, and hypertrophy of the sacrospinous or sacrotuberous ligaments.[46] Pain and burning sensations in the perineal area that worsen with sitting or eliciting activities and improve with standing or abstaining from these activities are typical of pudendal nerve involvement. Nonrecumbent bicycling in particular is an activity that can cause pudendal nerve compression within the pudendal canal[20] (Alcock canal; see Fig. 9-8).

Sacrococcygeal joint dysfunction, or coccydynia, involves pain in and around the coccyx. Coccydynia occurs most often in women and most commonly involves pain with sitting and during transition from sitting to standing.[20] Histories and conditions of patients with coccydynia may include trauma to the coccyx (e.g., a fall directly onto the coccyx), obesity (including a formerly obese state), lumbosacral disk disease, dyspareunia, pelvic diaphragm muscle tension or overactivity, or local neurologic problems (e.g., compression of the sympathetic ganglia just anterior to the sacrococcygeal joint [ganglion impar], sacral nerve root irritation, cauda equina, or meningeal cysts).[20]

Visceral structures may contribute to CPP. An association of symptoms of the urinary viscera with CPP has been well established in the literature, suggestive of the overlap of conditions (but not necessarily that of a causal relationship between the two).[46] Painful bladder conditions, such as interstitial cystitis (IC) and painful bladder syndrome are potential causes of CPP. Pelvic diaphragm muscle dysfunction is present in 87%[20] and bladder storage or emptying symptoms are present in 94%[46] of women diagnosed with IC. Urinary frequency, urgency, nocturia, and burning with urination are reported by women with IC.[20] Pain related to IC often refers to the suprapubic region, but it can also refer to the low back, buttock, and perineal areas. If cultures are not performed, IC is often misdiagnosed as a urinary tract infection,[20] and thus it is mistreated.

Gynecologic viscera may also contribute to CPP. Endometriosis is noted as a diagnosis for 33% of CPP cases, whereas CPP is attributed to "other" gynecologic conditions in another 33%.[46] Endometriosis is a condition in which endometrial tissues are growing outside the endometrial cavity,[20] such as in the pelvic or abdominal cavity. In addition to endometriosis, gynecologic conditions associated with CPP include PID, ovarian cysts, leiomyomas (benign tumors of the muscular wall of the uterus), or adenomyosis (growth of endometrium into the adjacent myometrium of the uterus).[20] CPP and vulvar pain can develop in relation to STDs, including syphilis, *Chlamydia* infection, gonorrhea, human immunodeficiency virus infection and acquired immunodeficiency syndrome, trichomoniasis, vaginitis, and genital herpes.[20] Unfortunately, some of these diseases may initially be asymptomatic, thus leading to development of PID before treatment is initiated.[20]

The genitalia and vagina may also be involved in CPP. Vulvodynia is chronic discomfort of the vulvar structures. Women with vulvodynia may report pain, burning, itching, dyspareunia, stinging, rawness, or "irritation."[20] Vulvar vestibulitis syndrome is a subset of vulvodynia.[20] Patients with vulvar vestibulitis syndrome report introital dyspareunia in particular. The origin of vulvodynia and vulvar vestibulitis syndrome is unclear.[20] Clitorodynia is a form of vulvodynia in which the clitoral branch of the pudendal nerve is affected.[20] Clitoral pain may result from metabolic causes (e.g., diabetic neuropathy), tight clothing, or vigorous stimulation of the clitoris, or it may be idiopathic.[20] Dyspareunia is pain with intercourse at the introitus or the midvaginal or deep vaginal areas,[20] and it may result from other pelvic conditions such as endometriosis, PID, or postsurgical scarring.

CPP development may involve the gastrointestinal system. Bowel conditions that contribute to CPP include diverticulitis, Crohn disease, ulcerative colitis, and chronic appendicitis.[20] Functional gastrointestinal disorders manifest as abdominal pain that is worsened with food intake or bowel movements; irritable bowel syndrome is one type.[20] This syndrome additionally involves intestinal gas, bloating, and cyclic constipation and diarrhea. Irritable bowel syndrome is particularly associated with pelvic pain, with 60% of patients having dysmenorrhea (painful menstrual cycles) as a comorbidity. Up to 50% of physician visits for gastrointestinal issues are related to irritable bowel syndrome.[20]

Vascular structures have also been proposed as a cause of CPP. Pelvic veins may become dilated and result in "pelvic congestion syndrome."[46] Thus, blood flow becomes impaired and may contribute to ischemic factors in CPP.[46]

Pelvic and abdominal surgical procedures may contribute to pain and dysfunction developing in the pelvis. Sutures placed in the sacrospinous ligament (just medial to the ischial spine) can result in compression of the levator ani nerve and can potentially lead to pain or atrophy of the levator ani muscles.[8] Because of the location of a suture in the sacrospinous ligament, the surgical recipient may also complain of point-tender buttock pain on the suture side; often, this is the right side, given the surgeon's dominant handedness. The sacrospinous and anterior longitudinal ligaments of the sacrum serve as suture sites when repairing pelvic organ prolapse.[1] For the Burch retropubic bladder neck suspension (a procedure intended to address urinary incontinence), sutures may be anchored into the iliopectineal ligament along the pubic bone.[1] Scarring, healing abnormalities, infection, inflammation, or other problems at these suture sites may lead to pain and other dysfunction of the soft tissues. Additionally, as noted, these sutures may contribute to nerve irritation or muscle inhibition or atrophy.

Other surgical considerations are complications that have arisen in recent years related to placement of mesh materials for addressing prolapse symptoms. Surgical removal of the mesh is difficult and is typically avoided by many surgeons. Pelvic health providers may address pain symptoms and dysfunction resulting from mesh that has led to tissue erosion or compression or that has caused a reaction from the body.

Early Intervention

In patients with neuralgia symptoms, early intervention may be aimed at reducing stressors to the neural structures to allow healing and regeneration. Thus, initial intervention may include abstaining from or modifying activities that exacerbate symptoms. For instance, with pudendal neuralgia in a cyclist, early intervention may include a brief period of no riding; for the same patient, sitting may need to be performed on a cushion with a perineal cutout to reduce pressure on the pudendal canal.

By the time a patient with CPP participates in physical therapy, symptoms have likely been experienced for a considerable amount of time. Early management should begin with thoroughly educating the patient in the development and mechanisms of chronic pain. Understanding how pain develops and its purpose assists the patient in assuming some control over symptoms (Box 9-2). The following is a brief overview of pain and chronic pain development: Pain does not necessarily indicate that tissues are in a damaged or injured state, but rather it gives the perception that the tissue is in danger.[61] The relationship between tissue damage and pain experienced becomes less predictable the more chronic pain becomes. As pain persists, neurons that bring nociceptive input to the brain become more sensitized even though the input is unchanged, with resulting hyperalgesia or allodynia.[61] As a patient begins to understand that pain is not necessarily a direct indication of tissue damage, she can begin to engage in strategies to reduce pain production without limitations from anxiety and fear of causing or worsening the underlying problems. When tissues are injured, the nociceptive system functions to protect the body. Nociceptive fibers send signals to the brain that mechanical changes have or are occurring in the tissues. The brain then determines whether pain is produced and to what degree pain occurs.[62] Thus, pain is an "output" rather than an "input,"[63] with very individualized influences of cultural, familial, psychological, geographic, and experiential input into the ultimate production of pain.[61] Anxiety and expectation affect pain production as well.[61]

Patients with chronic pain anticipate that movement will cause more pain and thus avoid active motion of the affected body part. Over time, this approach results in altered body schemas, and altered movement patterns.[64,65] Early strategies to facilitate for a patient with CPP should thus include enhancing self-efficacy, learning positive coping strategies, and developing methods and patterns of thinking and movement that will enhance functional recovery.[20] Along these lines, therapy interventions should provide the central nervous system and brain with a representation of the body part that is nonthreatening.[66] Thus, exercise progressing with motions that either are not painful or produce low-level pain is beneficial. Initial motions may simply involve imagining a motion (which can also cause pain production[61]) to submaximal contractions that are isometric or in a small range of motion, to

active movement with stronger contraction and in larger ranges of motion. Individual tailoring of a program is key.[61] Graded exposure to movements and positions can reduce fear and anxiety associated with movement and thus with associated pain production.[64,65] One example is progression in length of sitting time or from softer to firmer sitting surfaces. Another example is progressing from vaginal insertion of a small dilator to larger sizes, with eventual progression to return to intercourse. With graded exposure, care should be taken not to exacerbate symptoms. Additionally, patients should be guided in how to maintain a feeling of control to help decrease anxiety with the progression of graded exposure. For instance, teaching patients positions that allow them more control during intercourse is one way to reduce fear and associated pain symptoms with resuming sexual activity.

• BOX 9-2 Key Features of Chronic Pain Educational Intervention

Providing education to patients with chronic pain on the development and management of chronic pain may empower patients in the rehabilitation process. Listed here are key features to be included in chronic pain education:
- Pain does not always indicate that tissue damage or injury is present.
- Pain can create the perception that tissue is in danger.
- The more chronic pain is, the less predictable is the relationship between actual tissue damage or injury and the degree or type of pain experienced.
- Persisting pain causes nociceptive neurons to become more sensitized, even if the input to the neurons remains the same (hyperalgesia or allodynia develops).
- When tissues are injured, the nociceptive system protects the body by signaling to the brain that mechanical change is occurring in the tissues.
- The brain determines whether pain is produced, with pain being an "output" based on the individual's cultural, familial, psychological, geographic, and experiential inputs.
- Anxiety and expectation can worsen or heighten pain production.
- Patients with chronic pain may anticipate that movement causes more pain and will avoid moving.
- Over time, avoiding movement causes altered body schemas and movement patterns.

Interventional instruction to correlate with chronic pain education is as follows:
- Enhance self-efficacy of the patient; encourage that improvements in pain symptoms, strength, and movement patterns can all occur (even if these take time).
- Teach positive coping strategies for when pain occurs.
- Help develop thinking and movement patterns that will improve functional recovery.
- Progress through movements, postures, and positions that produce either no pain or low-level pain with graded exposure (to reduce anxiety and nonthreatening brain representations of body parts and movements).
- Progress from simple exercises to functional movements with the graded exposure progression.

Data from references 61 to 66.

Rehabilitation Considerations

Because CPP causes are often undiagnosed, intervention and plan of care are often aimed at managing pain and other symptoms.[46] Common methods for addressing CPP currently include counseling or psychotherapy, hormone therapy, provision of reassurance, laparoscopy to rule out serious disease (e.g., malignancy), and surgical interventions. A biopsychosocial approach to intervention is necessary and should include addressing structural disorders in addition to emotional, psychological, motivational, and cognitive factors. These factors contribute to ongoing pain resulting from the peripheral and central sensory sensitization and central processing mechanisms.[48] Pharmaceutical treatments, nerve blocks, neural ablation procedures, or neuromodulation may be offered for pain.[46] Musculoskeletal causes of pain may be successfully managed with conservative measures,[46] including physical therapy.

Physical therapy should incorporate the whole person and take into account the patient's psychosocial status and ability to engage in change.[20] Physical therapy interventions may include education on movement and patient-directed pain management techniques, reestablishment of motor control and postural awareness, stress management techniques, sleep hygiene education, relaxation techniques, physical agents, and manual therapy techniques.[20] Additionally, some dietary modifications may help with some CPP conditions.

Of considerable interest are accurate and specific muscle training and reeducation to address motor control problems, with an initial focus on the patient's ability to identify, isolate, and activate the transversus abdominis and pelvic diaphragm muscles while maintaining a neutral spine and pelvis position,[20] with optimal posture and lordosis.[31,32] Once the patient has consistent control and awareness of the transversus abdominis and pelvic diaphragm muscles, the ability to maintain a normal breathing pattern while contracting and relaxing these muscles should be learned. Many patients use altered breathing patterns to compensate for inadequate core muscle control, such as breath-holding during contraction, shallow breathing, and excessive use of upper trapezius muscles or oblique muscles with inhalation. These altered patterns should be identified and retrained. Once transversus abdominis and pelvic diaphragm muscle contractions are coordinated with correct breathing patterns, multifidus retraining may be added to complete core muscle retraining, particularly when the patient lacks normal sacral nutation.[20] Once the patient has adequate control of the deep core muscles in a static position with neutral spine and pelvis, progression can be made to include secondary stabilizing muscles (latissimus dorsi, gluteus maximus, abdominals [obliques and rectus abdominis], and hamstrings[67]). Further progression would then include dynamic and nonneutral positions as needed for function. A focus on using the muscles in functional movements through the day is beneficial.

Physical agents may include transcutaneous electrical neuromuscular stimulation (TENS), with both high and low frequencies warranting trial to determine what will work for each individual patient.[20,68] As with other areas of the body, TENS may be arranged directly on or near external regions of pain. TENS may also be placed to surround the perineal and vulvar region, although not placed directly on these tissues. Targeting of related spinal nerve roots may also be helpful.

Manual therapy is commonly used to address CPP. Painful ligaments, muscles, or trigger points may be addressed with massage, myofascial release, or friction massage performed either externally or internally through the vagina or rectum. Joint mobilization may also be performed to restore motion or provide pain relief.[20] For instance, a patient with pubic symphysis, lumbosacral, sacroiliac joint, or sacrococcygeal joint contributions to symptoms may benefit from manual mobilization techniques to address pain and stiffness at these joints.

Beneficial relaxation techniques may incorporate diaphragmatic breathing, muscle biofeedback, gentle movements, and postural education to reduce muscle tension.[20] Additionally, activities such as progressive relaxation can increase the patient's awareness of areas of tension holding. These techniques can be used proactively, scheduled as part of the regular home program; they can also be used to address acute pain onset.

For CPP of a visceral nature, the reasonable expectations of physical therapy are to provide pain reduction and increase participation in daily functional activities, rather than to resolve pain symptoms fully.[20] Reduction of pain may result from physical therapy interventions and modalities at the thoracolumbar and lower abdominal region,[20] as well as the pelvic, hip, and thigh region.

Neuralgia-related symptoms may be addressed with a variety of techniques. Neural mobilization may be performed to improve circulation to reduce swelling and improve cellular transport by moving the nerve along its path, with the key to success being that the patient's symptoms are not exacerbated during the mobilizing treatment.[20] Mobilization of iliohypogastric, ilioinguinal, and genitofemoral nerves can be performed with a patient position of ipsilateral hip flexion and contralateral trunk side bending[66]; this may be accomplished with the patient standing with the ipsilateral side next to an adjustable ("hi-lo") table. The foot of the flexed hip and knee is planted on the hi-lo table, which is elevated to a point to support the desired position. The obturator nerve may be mobilized through positioning the patient in supine hook lying or in standing. In supine hook lying, the trunk is first positioned into side bending toward the side being mobilized; next the ipsilateral flexed knee is dropped toward the table (hip external rotation).[20] Alternatively, from the same supine hook-lying start position, the lower extremity of the side being mobilized is repositioned into hip and knee extension and is then moved into a position of hip abduction and external rotation.[20] For standing mobilization of the obturator nerve, a position of stride stance with partial lunging toward the contralateral side is assumed. The patient then moves in and out of hip extension and abduction and hip and knee flexion and extension on the ipsilateral (mobilization) side.[20]

Addressing pudendal neuralgia may involve addressing any overactivity in the pelvic diaphragm muscles that is contributing to compression of the nerve; thus, manual therapy or other interventions may be used to address surrounding muscle tension, trigger points, or areas of tightness. A perineal cutout sitting cushion may be used to reduce tension on the nerve. Avoiding deep squat positions or prolonged sitting (especially with greater hip flexion, such as in a very soft, deep couch) may reduce irritation at the site of the sacrospinous ligament.[20] As discussed previously, incorporating appropriate use of graded exposure and restoring of normal movement patterns should be included. However, for many patients emphasis is needed on decreasing ongoing physical and mechanical stressors to these tissues.

The Prenatal Woman

In Table 9-6, key components of the prenatal female patient are summarized along with the other patient types described in this chapter.

Pregnancy introduces specific musculoskeletal changes that, although often typical, can cause pain and discomfort. During pregnancy, women are frequently told that these ailments will simply resolve after the pregnancy. Evidence indicates that many musculoskeletal problems that develop in pregnancy persist into the postpartum period and beyond. Support for intervening during the pregnancy to alleviate these symptoms and their underlying problems also exists.

Anatomic and physiologic changes with pregnancy involve changes in all body systems, including the pelvic viscera, the pelvic joints, and the entire musculoskeletal system. In the typical nonpregnant woman, all pelvic organs are located within the true pelvis (portion of pelvis below the iliopectineal line, sacral promontory, and upper margin of the symphysis pubis).[8,9] During pregnancy, the uterus eventually outgrows the true pelvis and moves up into the false pelvis and abdomen, with its superior border eventually resting against the inferior border of the breathing diaphragm. The symphysis pubis, sacroiliac, and sacrococcygeal joints soften during pregnancy to allow increased mobility and size of the pelvis for delivery.[8] Estrogen, progesterone, and relaxin are hormones that may be responsible for this softening.[8]

Prenatal Patient Profile

Related to the lumbopelvic-hip region, the pregnant patient may experience a variety of conditions that are discussed throughout this section. Pain conditions commonly include pelvic girdle pain, muscle overuse conditions, round ligament pain, and trochanteric bursitis of the hip. A rarer condition that is specific to late pregnancy and that can

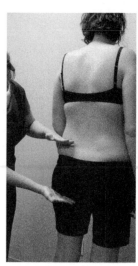

• **Figure 9-20** Pelvic Girdle Pain Region. (Courtesy Section on Women's Health of the American Physical Therapy Association.)

cause pain is transient osteoporosis of the hip (TOH). Specific to obstetric concerns, preterm labor pains can lead to lumbopelvic pain. Finally, urinary incontinence may occur in pregnancy and be related to pelvic muscle underactivity, overactivity, or poor coordination.

Pregnant women most commonly seen in outpatient therapy clinics are those with lumbopelvic-hip discomforts. Pelvic girdle pain is reported in up to 20% of all pregnant women.[40] Pelvic girdle pain is defined as pain between the posterior iliac crests and gluteal fold, particularly in the sacroiliac joint region (Fig. 9-20).[40,69] Pain generally arises in pregnancy sometime between the first trimester and first month postpartum.[40] The onset may be insidious or sudden. Women with pelvic girdle pain likely report decreased tolerance or endurance resulting from pain with prolonged standing, walking, or sitting; the woman feels the need to change positions or activities frequently to alleviate the discomfort. Thus, she is observed as "fidgety" in the waiting or treatment room. In addition, gait may be affected with "catching" or "clicking" of the hip, along with a decrease in gait speed and an increase in horizontal pelvic rotation (to avoid stress on the sacroiliac joints).[40]

Common Mechanisms

It is well accepted and reported, although not thoroughly understood, that contributions to nonpathologic increases in lumbopelvic-hip laxity during pregnancy are likely a result of hormonal changes (increase in estrogen, progesterone, and relaxin).[8] The increase in joint laxity can contribute to poor motor control around the pelvic and hip joints and lead to pelvic girdle pain. Significant postural changes occur during pregnancy, including increases in lumbar lordosis, anterior pelvic tilt, and forward head posture, all of which may contribute to musculoskeletal complaints during pregnancy. However, these postural changes have not been shown to correlate significantly with low back pain intensity.[70] Typical gait pattern changes occurring in pregnancy may contribute to overuse conditions in the hip and lower extremity. These changes include the following: an increase in hip moment and power in coronal and sagittal planes; increase in ankle moment and power in the sagittal plane; and an increase in use of hip abductors, hip extensors, and ankle plantar flexors.[71] Walking velocity also decreases to maintain ground reaction forces with the growing body mass, to allow for more reaction time with perturbations, and to reduce the need for increased coordination that is needed with the changing maternal body.[72] Smaller rotations occur between the trunk and pelvis to allow for increased control of the body. In addition, women increase the front plane of stability by adapting a wider base of support, either through wider foot stance (hip abduction) or through external rotation of the hips and lower extremities.[72] Thus, women may develop muscle overuse conditions in the gluteus medius, piriformis, and other hip abductor and external rotator structures.

The round ligament experiences stretching as the growing uterus moves superiorly into the trunk. The round ligament extends laterally from the uterus and travels into the inguinal canal and mons pubis. Stretching of this ligament may contribute to anterior groin pain in the region of the inguinal canal and pubis, particularly with moving from positions of hip flexion to hip extension, as in going from sitting to standing. This pain is exacerbated with quicker movements.

Trochanteric bursitis is common during pregnancy because of the increased loads on the pelvis, hips, and lower extremities in pregnancy. Additionally, increased forces in side lying while sleeping can cause irritation of the trochanteric bursa. Women with trochanteric bursitis during pregnancy report pain with weight bearing (from iliotibial band compression against the trochanteric bursa), pain with adduction and internal rotation of the hip (for the same reason), and pain with palpation over the greater trochanter.

TOH is another condition that occurs specifically in pregnant women.[73] This condition is theorized to result from hormonal and biomechanical compressive forces in the hip joint in the later stages of pregnancy. TOH has a sudden onset of severe pain in the hip joint with no apparent cause. Pain may refer to the gluteal and groin region. Other symptoms include difficulty with bearing weight through the affected lower extremity; some women find it impossible to bear weight through this joint at all. Hip range of motion is be normal, but pain occurs at the end ranges.[73]

A specific obstetric cause of lower abdominal, hip, and low back pain can include labor contractions. These may be Braxton Hicks contractions, which are "warm-up" exercises of the uterus and do not result in changes in the cervix that lead to imminent labor and delivery. These contractions may occur for several months before delivery, and they come and go with no specific pattern. However, signs of true labor onset involve intense contractions lasting 1 minute or longer and occurring at regular intervals (e.g.,

every 5 minutes or more frequently). These contractions are likely to be described as "cramping" and "menstrual-like." Any progressive labor contractions (which result in changes in the cervix) before 35 weeks of gestation are considered preterm labor and should be regarded as a need for immediate medical attention. Early labor contractions can be triggered by a variety of causes, including maternal or fetal conditions, physical trauma, infections (e.g., urinary tract infections, which are common in pregnancy), dehydration, or overexertion.

Urinary incontinence may also arise during pregnancy. Urinary incontinence is not a normal condition during pregnancy, but several pregnancy-related factors can contribute to its development. As early as the first trimester, the growing uterus begins to add pressure on the underlying urinary bladder. As the uterus and fetus continue to grow, the increase in mass adds pressure on the pelvic diaphragm muscles and continence support structures. As the pelvic joints become more lax, the pelvic diaphragm muscles can be more challenged in providing motor control to the pelvic girdle, support to the trunk, and continence. Women who had suboptimal coordination, control, and strength of the pelvic diaphragm muscles before pregnancy may find that the resultant anatomic and physiologic changes lead to a greater chance of developing incontinence symptoms.

Postinjury Considerations

Pregnancy-related musculoskeletal and gross systemic changes begin as soon as a woman becomes pregnant. Changes continue throughout the pregnancy in rapid spurts, resulting in ongoing postural, gait, center of gravity, and balance changes. Systemic changes, such as increase in blood volume and interstitial fluid levels, also affect the woman's overall musculoskeletal system. For instance, increases in bodily fluids may lead to progressive edema symptoms later in pregnancy, which may affect lower extremity proprioception and cause discomfort. The pregnant woman may have difficulty adapting to her rapidly changing body shape and mass. For some women, these changes may result in a need for encouragement that the challenges she faces with her changing body are typical.

Early Intervention

Early intervention of the musculoskeletal discomforts associated with pregnancy should include reducing compressive forces and providing support for strained tissues as much as possible. For instance, pregnant women with pelvic girdle pain may benefit from use of a sacroiliac support belt (Fig. 9-21), to provide external compressive support to the pelvic girdle joints. Women experiencing round ligament pain may benefit from a pregnancy abdominal support belt that is worn along the underside of and provides an upward lift of the pregnant abdomen. In lifting the abdomen, compressive forces to the round ligament within the inguinal canal may be alleviated. Other early interventions to provide

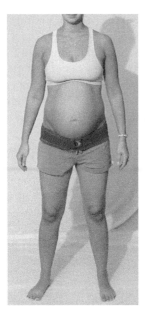

• **Figure 9-21** Pregnant Woman Wearing Sacroiliac Support Belt. (Courtesy Section on Women's Health of the American Physical Therapy Association.)

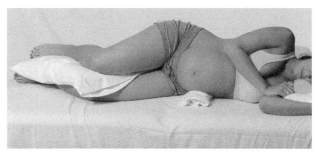

• **Figure 9-22** Supportive Positioning for the Pregnant Woman in Side-lying. (Courtesy Section on Women's Health of the American Physical Therapy Association.)

support for strained tissues may involve strengthening of weakened muscles, such as strengthening the transversus abdominis muscle to elevate the lower abdomen and reduce strain on the pelvic girdle joints and to alleviate pressure on the round ligament during daily activities. Additionally, early instruction (first visit) in sleeping position with adequate pillow support is of immense benefit to the pregnant woman with musculoskeletal discomforts (Fig. 9-22). As shown in Figure 9-22, a woman in side lying is likely to experience relief of pelvic girdle and other lower back symptoms with pillow support under her abdomen (to reduce trunk rotational strain), adequate pillows between the knees (to prevent the top leg from adducting and rotating), and appropriate support for the cervical spine and upper extremities. A small rolled wash cloth or hand towel placed under the waist can also reduce lateral curving of the spine to provide further relief.

Of note are initial interventions related to rehabilitation of pelvic girdle pain that are similar to interventions in nonpregnant patients. Rehabilitation begins with submaximal retraining of the transversus abdominis, pelvic diaphragm, and multifidus, as described previously. Of great value for the pregnant woman experiencing pelvic girdle pain is offering reassurance that her musculoskeletal condition does not indicate structural damage of her pelvic joints and that by improving motor control, her symptoms can be controlled.

Rehabilitation Considerations and Programming

Pelvic Girdle Pain

Systematic review indicates that individually tailored rehabilitation programs with specific therapeutic exercise to improve motor control of the pelvic girdle joints are most beneficial for pregnant women with pelvic girdle pain.[40] In performing examination and developing a program, care should be given to avoid contraindicated positions or movements during pregnancy (Table 9-11). Positions or movements that should be avoided are those that create abdominal compression in middle to late-pregnancy, positions of inversion, and any activities that involve rapid, uncontrolled bouncing, swinging, or sharp twists of the body.[74] Positions or movements to be cautious with include the following: having the buttocks higher than the chest (because of cardiovascular changes and the potential for vaginal air embolus); the supine position 3 minutes or longer after the first trimester (because of the potential to occlude the inferior vena cava); positions that strain the pelvic diaphragm and abdominal muscles; and positions that cause intense stretching of the hip adductors, extreme asymmetrical lower extremity positions, and extreme hip end range of motion positions (because of increased laxity of the pubic symphysis and sacroiliac joints).[74]

As described earlier in the discussion of pelvic pain rehabilitation, training of the deep core muscles is usually necessary for women with pelvic girdle pain in pregnancy. Women who performed pelvic diaphragm muscle training during pregnancy are less likely to report lumbopelvic pain in the last trimester of pregnancy and at 3 months postpartum; this finding indicates that the pelvic diaphragm muscles should not be overlooked in core muscle programming.[75]

Muscle Overuse Conditions

As noted, the gluteus medius, piriformis, hip adductors, and other hip external rotators can become sources of trigger points and muscle tension as a result of postural and gait changes in pregnancy. Education is important for teaching women neutral postures and positions to reduce shortening or strain on these structures and muscles. For instance, avoiding sitting with the legs held in an externally rotated position, as is common with the ankles crossed, prevents increased tension in the external rotators with prolonged sitting. Avoiding crossing the legs reduces strain on the same muscles. Manual therapy can be used to address trigger points and spasm in these muscles. Use of thermotherapy

TABLE 9-11	Contraindicated or Cautionary Positions and Movements During Pregnancy	
Avoid the Following Contraindicated Positions or Movements During Pregnancy		
Position or Movement	**Reasoning**	**Examples**
Abdominal compression in middle to late pregnancy	Places too much pressure onto linea alba and abdominal wall, which are already in overstretched state; compression of deep abdominal vasculature	Crunches or sit-ups; toe touch stretching that causes strain of abdominal wall; prone lying position; plow position in yoga
Inverted positions	Significant hemodynamic changes in pregnancy can affect blood flow; weight of growing uterus on breathing diaphragm in middle to late pregnancy	Headstands, handstands, shoulder stands, or downward dog in yoga
Rapid, uncontrolled bouncing, swinging, or sharp twisting movements	Risk of musculoskeletal injury with rapidly changing body shape and mass affecting motor control and balance and with hormonal changes increasing joint laxity; risk of falls that could cause maternal or fetal injury	Jumping or flipping on trampoline; excessive twisting with trunk rotational sports (e.g., softball, golf, tennis)
Practice Caution With the Following Positions or Movements During Pregnancy		
Position or Movement	**Reasoning**	**Examples**
Buttocks elevated higher than the chest	Cardiovascular and hemodynamic changes in pregnancy can affect blood return; potential for vaginal air embolus (although greater risk in postpartum period)	Bridging exercises with shoulders on floor; plow position or head, hand, or shoulder stands in yoga
Supine for >3 minutes after first trimester	Potential for compression of inferior vena cava and reduction of blood return from lower extremities	Lying flat on back for examination, exercise, or interventions
Positions that strain pelvic diaphragm or abdominal muscles	Pelvic diaphragm is under strain to support the mass of the growing uterus; abdominals are under strain from ongoing stretch with growing uterus; being under strain creates a greater risk for injury	Valsalva or excessive bearing down, causing pelvic diaphragm muscles to bulge outward; plank position can strain abdominals, particularly if the woman is not experienced with performing
Intense stretching of the hip adductors, asymmetrical positions of hips, extreme end range of motion of hips	Increase in laxity of the pelvic girdle joints (pubic symphysis, sacroiliac joints), and thus placing strain on muscles attaching into the pelvis or on the pelvic and hip joints can create a higher risk of injury	Splits; deep asymmetrical lunges or squats; Eve's lunge with Pilates Reformer; pigeon pose in yoga; cross-legged sitting

Data from Stephenson RG, O'Connor LJ. *Obstetric and Gynecologic Care in Physical Therapy.* 2nd ed. Thorofare, NJ: Slack; 2000.

(heat or cold packs) directly over these muscles may also provide relief and reduce muscle spasm. However, pregnant women should not place heat modalities directly over the abdomen or be immersed in hot water as a form of thermotherapy. Some obstetrician-gynecologists also do not allow hot packs to be placed on the low back of a pregnant woman. After manual therapy, cold may be of greatest benefit for also addressing inflammation and swelling in the area. Deep core muscle rehabilitation, as described previously, provides great benefit by promoting the primary stabilizing muscles to support the pelvis and trunk. Thus, the larger hip-moving muscles may be alleviated from overworking and compensating for lack of deep core muscle control. Along these lines, external support (e.g., sacroiliac [see Fig. 9-21] and pregnancy abdominal belts) may also provide relief to these overworked muscles.

Round Ligament Pain

Reducing stretching forces on the round ligament can reduce associated pain. Several interventions may provide relief of this strain. Women can be taught to perform a transversus abdominis muscle contraction before standing to intrinsically support the abdomen and decrease stretching of the round ligament. Instructions for external support of the abdomen (e.g., using the hands to lift under the abdomen or wearing a pregnancy abdominal support belt) with movements that typically cause discomfort can also reduce pain. Encouraging slow movements can also alleviate this ligamentous pain. For instance, if a woman has round ligament pain with transitioning from sitting to standing, or with rolling over in bed, encouraging slow, controlled movements prevents a quick stretch of the ligament and decreases the risk of pain. Addressing any biomechanical, postural, or positional contributions to compression or strain of the anterior pelvic structures may also reduce round ligament discomfort. For instance, addressing and correcting excessive anterior pelvic tilt may reduce pressure through the inguinal region and lessen strain on the overall path of the ligament. Performing manual therapy to address any constriction of the inguinal canal or associated soft tissues may also provide a less constricting path in which the ligament travels.

Trochanteric Bursitis

Typical measures to address bursitis may be used, with consideration to the postural and gait changes of pregnancy that may be adding pressure to the bursa through shortening of the hip external rotations, hip abductors, and iliotibial band. Assessment of these structural contributions may guide education needed for altering posture, biomechanics, and gait to alleviate pressure on the bursa. Women with trochanteric bursitis during pregnancy may need instructions in sleep positions to reduce pressure on the greater trochanter. For instance, if sleeping in side lying, care should be given to not lie directly on the hip by positioning in a quarter-turn position (side lying, but rolled slightly forward or slightly backward to roll the weight off the trochanter). Additionally, if sleeping in side-lying, enough pillow support should extend from between the knees all the way to between the feet such that lower extremities are equidistant apart from the thighs to the ankle. If the top foot is allowed to drop down toward the bottom foot, excessive stress may occur in the hip and sacroiliac joint and iliotibial band and subsequently on the upper trochanter and bursa. Women are often advised to lie on the left side to reduce compressive forces to the inferior vena cava and abdominal aorta because these structures pass directly anterior to the L3 vertebral body (and just slightly to the right side of the vertebral body).

Transient Osteoporosis of the Hip

TOH typically resolves on its own in the postpartum period. Women with TOH during the latter portion of pregnancy benefit from pain relief measures and interventions to prevent muscle atrophy and strength loss. Because of pain with weight-bearing, women with TOH may require a rolling walker or other appropriate assistive device for functional ambulation. Non–weight-bearing exercise may be beneficial in promoting muscle activity surrounding the affected hip joint; in prescribing exercises, pain should be the guide. Women with TOH should perform range-of-motion and isometric exercises without pain. Aquatic exercise may be especially beneficial because it allows the woman to ambulate and perform a variety of stretching, strengthening, and aerobic exercises with gravity reduced on the affected joint. Exercise in water may also provide pain relief and enhance the woman's sense of health by offering greater participation in physical activity.

Urinary Incontinence

Evidence is reported to support performing pelvic diaphragm muscle exercises during pregnancy to reduce urinary incontinence during pregnancy and the postpartum period. Prenatal pelvic muscle exercise is demonstrated to be especially beneficial with the first pregnancy.[76-79] Women who train their pelvic diaphragm muscles report less urinary incontinence at 35 weeks of pregnancy, 6 weeks postpartum, and 6 months postpartum.[78] Pelvic muscle exercises do not appear to adversely "tighten" the muscles because no negative effect has been demonstrated on labor and delivery for women training these muscles during pregnancy.[80] In fact, women performing pelvic diaphragm muscle training prenatally do not have any significant difference in perineal lacerations or tears, nor do they have any difference in need for episiotomy, assisted delivery, or emergency cesarean delivery.[80]

The Postpartum Woman

Key concepts related to the postpartum female patient are given in Table 9-6, along with summaries of the other types of patients described in this chapter.

Women in the postpartum period may experience ongoing musculoskeletal conditions that arose during pregnancy, such as low back and pelvic girdle pain or DRA. Postnatal women may also have problems arising from labor and delivery itself, such as a new onset of urinary incontinence, pelvic organ prolapse, sexual dysfunction, or coccyx injuries. Postpartum recovery may be from vaginal labor and delivery or cesarean delivery. Regardless of delivery method, the reproductive organs and maternal physiologic factors require approximately 6 weeks to return to the pre-pregnancy state.[81] Thus, the postpartum period is a time in which continued physiologic and anatomic changes are occurring.

Patient Profile

Women surveyed in a study at 3 months postpartum reported the following lumbopelvic-related problems: 51%, low back pain; 43%, hemorrhoids; 27%, dyspareunia; 21%, urinary incontinence; and 14%, fecal incontinence.[82]

Reports of low back and pelvic girdle pain persist in up to 43.2% of women at 6 months postpartum,[83,84] as well as in 37% of women at 18 months postpartum.[85] By 2 years postpartum, 8.6% of women will still experience pelvic girdle pain that arose during the pregnancy.[86] Postpartum depressive symptoms are three times more likely in women who experience low back and pelvic girdle pain than in those without.[87] Thus, screening for postpartum depression is valuable when examining a patient with postpartum lumbopelvic pain.

Diastasis rectus abdominis (DRA) (separation of two halves of the rectus abdominis muscle by stretching or separation of the linea alba) is a condition that may arise in

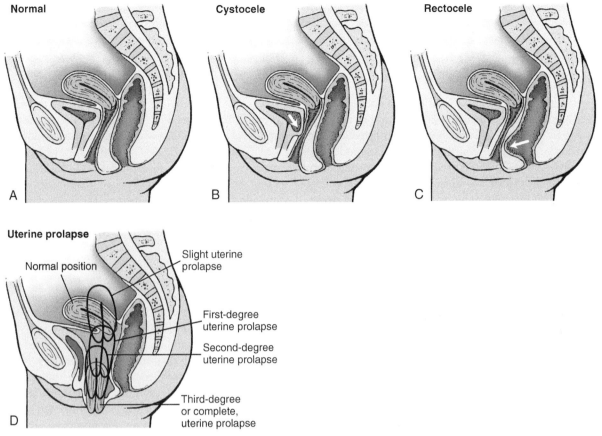

Figure 9-23 Pelvic Organ Prolapse. (From Monahan FD, Neighbors M. *Medical-Surgical Nursing: Foundations for Clinical Practice.* 2nd ed. Philadelphia: W.B. Saunders; 1998.)

pregnancy and persist into the postpartum period. DRA is present in 27% of women during the second trimester of pregnancy; the incidence increases to 66% of women in the third trimester of pregnancy and decreases to 30% of women by 8 weeks postpartum.[18] The separation is considered significant if the distance between the two halves of the rectus abdominis muscles is greater than 2.0 cm.[88] Although the site of the DRA itself is typically painless, women with DRA tend to have higher degrees of abdominal or pelvic region pain.[88] DRA results in a lack of adequate abdominal wall support and thus may contribute to ongoing lumbar and pelvic girdle pain. Along these lines, in theory DRA may also contribute to urinary incontinence by its effect on the core muscles functioning as a unit.

Approximately 60% of postmenopausal women report urinary incontinence,[89] indicating that bladder leakage in women after childbirth does not resolve spontaneously. Postpartum urinary incontinence is reported at 45%,[90] thus indicating the need for pelvic health rehabilitation in nearly half of women who have had a vaginal delivery. Women who have experienced perineal trauma during delivery (e.g., with episiotomy or significant tearing) are at higher risk for also developing fecal incontinence later in life (in middle and old age).[90] Pelvic organ prolapse also is more likely to develop after vaginal delivery (an independent risk factor), with each delivery increasing the risk

(Fig. 9-23). Women with three or more vaginal deliveries have an 8 to 10 times increased risk of prolapse. Other postpartum risk factors for developing prolapse include having had an instrumental delivery (forceps or vacuum), having trauma to the levator ani muscles during delivery, and having had prolapse symptoms during pregnancy.[90-93] Elective cesarean delivery is only partially effective in preventing pelvic organ prolapse.[94]

In addition to incontinence and prolapse symptoms, many women experience sexual dysfunction in the postpartum period. Many women report perineal pain or other pain limiting desired sexual activity after vaginal delivery: 42% immediately after delivery, and 10% reporting persisting sexual pain symptoms at 12 weeks postpartum.[95,96]

Common Mechanisms

Postpartum Pelvic Girdle Pain

As noted previously, lumbopelvic pain may persist into the postpartum period. The mechanisms that contribute to this ongoing pain are not fully understood. It is reasonable that the changes in either the pelvic diaphragm muscles after vaginal delivery or the abdominal muscles after cesarean delivery would affect motor control around the lumbopelvic and hip joints. Persistent DRA may also contribute to continued back and pelvic pain in the postpartum period. The genetic composition of fascia may affect the ability of a

DRA to resolve spontaneously. Chronically increased intraabdominal pressures with poor deep core muscle control and Valsalva maneuver may also contribute to non-resolving DRA.

Vaginal Delivery

Both nerve injuries and muscle injuries in the pelvic region can lead to symptoms of stress urinary incontinence and pelvic organ prolapse.[97] Stress urinary incontinence can arise years after vaginal childbirth. In these cases, pudendal nerve latency has been demonstrated.[46] Women may lose 25% to 35% of levator ani muscle strength after childbirth.[45] Strength loss may result from the stretch and strain trauma on the nervous and muscular structures or from tearing within the levator ani muscles during delivery. Pelvic diaphragm muscle tearing and avulsions in women with stress urinary incontinence have been reported in several studies.[98] In particular, it appears that tearing at the attachments of the pelvic diaphragm muscles has a greater impact than tearing in the muscle belly. With three or more vaginal deliveries, women have significantly thinner pelvic diaphragm muscles than do women who have never given birth.[98] The thinning of the muscles indicates atrophy in the muscles after multiple births.

Pelvic diaphragm nerve injuries are a possibility with vaginal labor and delivery. The levator ani nerve (S3 to S5) provides somatic innervation for conscious control of voiding.[98] This nerve is susceptible to childbirth-related damage because it runs along the cranial surface of the pelvic diaphragm muscles.[98] Denervation of the pelvic diaphragm muscles is reported to occur commonly after childbirth and in women with stress urinary incontinence.[99] The degree of damage typically relates to the degree of trauma occurring during delivery and not to having had multiple deliveries.[100,101] A prolonged active phase of the second stage of labor and having heavier babies leads to greater injury.[101] The pudendal nerve can be stretched up to 20% of its length during the second stage of labor (with 12% stretch being a sufficient amount to cause nerve damage).[46,102] Typically, the denervation worsens in the postpartum years,[46]

likely because of the lack of a strong neuroregenerative response of the pudendal nerve after delivery.[103]

Intrapelvic fascial injuries may also contribute to pelvic symptoms. The ATLA and ATFP are described previously in this chapter. The ATLA provides anterior attachment for the pubococcygeus and puborectalis muscles of the levator ani. The ATFP provides lateral support to the vagina and prevents the vagina and urethra from moving into inferior and posterior positions with increased intraabdominal pressure.[98] Tearing of the ATLA results in an inability of the connective tissues to absorb elevated intraabdominal pressures, thus requiring the pelvic diaphragm muscles to provide greater force than normal. Therefore, damage occurring also to the levator ani muscles increases the risk of incontinence. Apparent genetic contribution to connective tissue consistency (weaker collagen) also seems to affect the development of incontinence and prolapse.[98]

Anal sphincter trauma (grade 3 or 4 perineal laceration) is known to occur in up to 5% of vaginal deliveries (Fig. 9-24), and it is an independent risk factor for developing bladder and anal incontinence. Anal sphincter trauma risk factors include first-time delivery, a large infant, and use of an instrument for delivery (vacuum or forceps, with forceps more likely to cause trauma).[45] However, ultrasound examination demonstrates external anal sphincter defects in up to 38% of women after vaginal delivery, a finding suggesting a high rate of occult trauma to the anal sphincters.[45]

Coccyx fractures and sacrococcygeal joint trauma have been reported to occur during vaginal delivery.[20] Dorsal lithotomy position (supine with hips flexed) in particular may increase the risk because of compression of the sacrum and coccyx between the lying surface and the delivering fetus. This effect is compounded when the fetus is in an occiput posterior position, in which the occiput of the fetal head is positioned against the mother's sacrum and coccyx during delivery (normal position is occiput anterior, or the fetal occiput positioned toward the mother's pubic symphysis). Such injuries can lead to postpartum coccydynia or coccyx injuries.

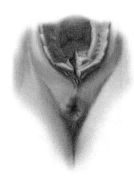
First-degree

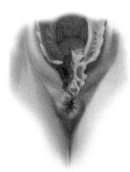
Second-degree

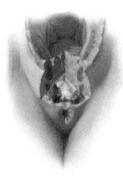
Third-degree

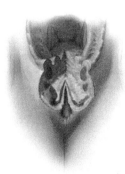
Fourth-degree

• **Figure 9-24** Degrees of Perineal Lacerations Occurring With Childbirth. (From Corton MM, Lankford JC, Ames R, et al. A randomized trial of birthing with and without stirrups. *Am J Obstet Gynecol.* 2012;207:133.e1-133.e5.)

Delivery positioning may also contribute to pelvic or lower extremity neuralgia. In particular, women who have epidural analgesia for labor and delivery may lack protective sensation that communicates a need to move out of a position that may be compromising or compressing a neuromuscular or vascular structure, thereby leading to a compression injury. Overstretch or compression injury could affect any of the nerves or vasculature in the pelvis and lower extremities, depending on the woman's positioning. For instance, clinically (and described in some case reports), postdelivery anesthesia-related neuralgia has been noted to develop specifically in the femoral nerve (with prolonged dorsal lithotomy) or the obturator nerve (with prolonged hip hyperabduction in side lying).

Perineal trauma with vaginal delivery affects sexual health. Risk factors for developing postpartum perineal pain and pain with intercourse include requiring sutures to repair the perineum after delivery and experiencing the first vaginal delivery. Instrumental delivery results in a two and a half times increase in reporting of painful intercourse at 6 months postpartum.[104] Breastfeeding and postpartum depression also appear to have a negative effect on return to sexual function.[105,106]

Cesarean Delivery

Cesarean delivery results in surgical incisions to the abdominal wall and uterus. Of consideration is whether the cesarean delivery was planned or an emergency surgical procedure. In emergency cases, the potential for surgical-related trauma is greater. Nerve irritation or entrapment from abdominal incisions or surgical retractors can result in abdominopelvic pain.[46] After cesarean delivery, women are unlikely to have pelvic diaphragm trauma[45] unless they labored before an unplanned cesarean delivery. A few small randomized controlled trials have demonstrated no difference in isokinetic strength in the abdominal muscles with different types of incisions (Pfannenstiel versus Maylard) after cesarean section.[107] Otherwise, research on the effects of abdominal or cesarean surgical procedures on muscular performance is lacking.

Postpartum Considerations

Pelvic Girdle Pain and Diastasis Rectus Abdominis

As noted previously, assumptions should not be made that low back and pelvic girdle pain or DRA arising in pregnancy will resolve on its own in the postpartum period. Any of these conditions that are persisting should be addressed.

After Vaginal Delivery

Urinary incontinence should resolve within 6 weeks to 3 months after vaginal delivery.[105,108] For women in whom incontinence has not resolved by 3 months postpartum, symptoms tend to persist up to a year and beyond and potentially become a lifetime problem.[90] Thus, women who are reporting leakage after 3 months postpartum should be referred for pelvic rehabilitation.

Sexual Dysfunction

In general, women are instructed to refrain from sexual activity until 6 weeks postpartum to allow recovery of reproductive and sexual structures. Sexual dysfunction related to perineal trauma can be rehabilitated with pelvic health physical therapy. Thus, persistent perineal pain or pain with intercourse may be resolved with referral to a pelvic health therapist.

After Cesarean Delivery

Because cesarean delivery is an abdominopelvic operation, with the mother's abdominal wall and uterus incised, precautions and considerations are similar to those of other abdominopelvic surgical procedures. The special consideration after cesarean delivery is that the mother now has an infant (or infants) to care for in addition to her postsurgical recovery. Thus, it becomes important to assess social and family support and assistance for women right after a postcesarean delivery: is anyone helping her on a daily basis, how much help she is receiving, does she feel she is able to allow others to help, and so on. This information will tell the clinician a great deal about how her physical activities may be affecting her healing and recovery in the postpartum period. Additionally, emergency cesarean deliveries may have a greater negative impact on the health of the mother and infant or infants, and this information is valuable to gather.

Early Intervention

Pelvic Girdle Pain and Diastasis Rectus Abdominis

Early interventions for these musculoskeletal conditions would most likely involve early retraining of the deep core muscles, as described previously, to provide support to the trunk and pelvis. With pelvic girdle pain, a sacroiliac support belt may alleviate acute symptoms until motor control has been reestablished. A postpartum abdominal binder may be a beneficial support in addressing DRA initially. In particular with DRA, focus should be given early on avoiding Valsalva maneuvers with bending, lifting, and childcare to prevent increased strain on the linea alba.

After Vaginal Delivery

Six weeks is generally recommended for initial recovery of reproductive organs from delivery. For a woman who had significant perineal trauma (tearing or lacerations), additional considerations may be needed for perineal healing. Early intervention may still include isometric contractions of the pelvic diaphragm muscles and transversus abdominis at an intensity that does not produce pain. Early contractions promote circulation and begin to reestablish motor control of these deep core muscles.

After Cesarean Delivery

In the acute phases of rehabilitation after cesarean delivery, the concerns are similar to those of any abdominal or pelvic surgical procedure. Initially, diaphragmatic breathing is valuable to begin to provide a source of mobilization to the abdominal wall and promote good breathing patterns. Incision care is important, and use of an abdominal binder with a folded towel directly over the incision gives support.[109] Isometric transversus abdominis and pelvic diaphragm muscle contractions may begin the first day postpartum.[110] After cesarean delivery, the woman may require instruction in appropriate bed mobility and transfers, as well as promotion of early ambulation within tolerance after the first 24 hours postpartum.[111] Additionally, women may need support for breastfeeding, such as pillows to bring the baby to the breast (as opposed to the woman's leaning forward through the trunk toward the infant). The new mother may also require training to perform infant care with body mechanics that prevent stress on the healing abdomen. Pain management may include use of TENS and ice or cold packs around the surgical incision. Postural reeducation should begin early because women are likely to slouch to place slack on the postsurgical abdominal wall.

Rehabilitation Considerations and Programming

Pelvic Girdle Pain

As described previously, pelvic girdle pain is addressed similar to that in pelvic pain conditions and during pregnancy. In the postpartum period, greater attention is needed on body mechanics related to childcare. For instance, ensuring appropriate body mechanics with breastfeeding or bottle feeding, use of infant carriers and strollers, and diaper changing. Discouraging use of infant car seat carriers for mobilizing the baby, in which the mother holds the carrier handle over one arm, is valuable for reducing strain to the spine, trunk, and pelvis.

Diastasis Rectus Abdominis

DRA is important to address because the resultant decreased abdominal support can impair load transfer through the pelvis and trunk with vertical loading tasks such as bending and lifting.[112,113] Thus, DRA may contribute to postpartum lumbopelvic-hip pain and symptoms. DRA is addressed with attention to core muscle retraining in conjunction with exercise of the rectus abdominis while support is given to maintain approximation of the two halves. Precontraction of the transversus abdominis and pelvic diaphragm muscles should occur before and throughout the rectus abdominis exercises (initially and with ongoing progression). A hand is placed on either side of the abdomen to press the two halves of the muscle together physically (Fig. 9-25). Palpation and observation should be performed to ensure that the two halves remain approximated throughout the exercise, with no separation. Initial rectus abdominis exercises in this fashion may simply involve isometric contractions, over time progressing to concentric and eccentric contractions. Progression should occur only as the two halves of the muscle are able to maintain approximation.

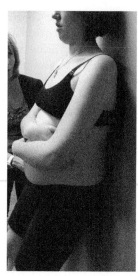

• **Figure 9-25** Diastasis Rectus Abdominis–Reducing Exercise. (Courtesy Section on Women's Health of the American Physical Therapy Association.)

To expound on the need for eccentric contraction ability of the rectus abdominis, a patient may need to learn to maintain appropriate engagement of the rectus abdominis during an activity with reaching overhead, such as placing a heavy item on a high shelf. This motion would require that the patient is able to maintain appropriate supportive muscle contraction, thus preventing excessive anterior force through the abdominal wall, while reaching upward and thus lengthening the muscle at the same time.

Postpartum Urinary Incontinence and Pelvic Organ Prolapse

Because incontinence and prolapse both involve underactivity of the pelvic diaphragm muscles, rehabilitation in the two conditions is quite similar. Although this has not yet been studied, it has been suggested that postpartum perineal pain causes pelvic diaphragm muscle inhibition, with the result that some women do not redevelop appropriate function of the muscles spontaneously. Additionally, although it has not been studied specifically in pelvic muscle retraining, general exercise physiology knowledge supports that after denervation of muscle, the remaining innervated fibers can be beneficially trained.[98] What has been demonstrated is that women with stress urinary incontinence exhibit decreases in coordination (voluntarily and reflexively), force generation, endurance, and ability to perform a quick recruitment of the pelvic diaphragm muscles (recruitment of fast twitch fibers).[98] The literature repeatedly supports pelvic diaphragm muscle training to decrease volume and frequency of urine leakage, improve strength, and increase muscle thickness.[98,113] Specifically, postpartum rehabilitative pelvic diaphragm muscle exercise has been reported to prevent stress urinary incontinence effectively.[114] Successful pelvic muscle diaphragm muscle training to reduce stress urinary incontinence requires that: (1) women can precontract the muscles before leakage-causing events; (2) exercise cause muscle hypertrophy to allow resistance of intraabdominal pressure increases; and (3) automatic firing of the motor units can be improved with motor learning.[115] The optimal number of repetitions, length of hold times, variety of hold times (endurance versus quick contractions), and frequency of pelvic diaphragm muscle contractions has not been established through research. However, investigators have demonstrated that performing 8 to 12 maximal contractions 3 times daily in addition to weekly 45-minute physical therapy sessions may result in improvements; the same benefits do not occur with home exercises alone.[116] Adhering to a pelvic diaphragm muscle exercise program has been found to be the most important predictor of successful incontinence rehabilitation.[117] These reports demonstrate the value of a skilled pelvic health physical therapist for providing adequate instruction, feedback, and accountability to ensure effective training. The need for individualized instruction has been further confirmed in studies demonstrating that few women (even continent women) are able to perform voluntary pelvic diaphragm muscle contractions correctly.[55,118]

A component of pelvic diaphragm muscle rehabilitation may include abdominal muscle training. Multiple studies have demonstrated a co-contraction of the levator ani and transversus abdominis and lower portion of the other abdominal muscles in women who are continent. Submaximal, well-controlled pelvic diaphragm muscle contractions occur with a submaximal transversus abdominis contraction. Maximal pelvic muscle contractions also result in rectus abdominis and oblique muscle contractions.[98] Retraining of the transversus abdominis in particular assists pelvic diaphragm muscle contraction, with attention to submaximal muscle recruitment to avoid excessive simultaneous increase in intraabdominal pressure. However, systematic review does not support the use of transversus abdominis muscle training alone to replace pelvic diaphragm muscle training.[80] Abdominal muscle training should be added only after intrapelvic muscle training has resulted in adequate coordination and initial retraining of the pelvic diaphragm muscles.[80]

In both incontinence and prolapse, sudden increases in intraabdominal pressure are of concern. In asymptomatic women, the pelvic diaphragm muscles should naturally and reflexively contract just milliseconds before coughing,[119] referred to as the cough reflex. In women with stress urinary incontinence, this reflex is diminished or absent.[98] However, the habit of contracting the pelvic diaphragm muscles just before coughing or other activities in which intraabdominal pressure suddenly increases (e.g., sneezing) can reduce incontinence. This technique in Europe was coined "the knack," and some still refer to it as such. In a study of 27 women, 1 week of practicing a precontraction of the pelvic diaphragm muscles reduced urine lost with a moderate cough by 98.2%, and with a deep cough by 73.3%.[120]

In prolapse, fascial and connective tissue damage requires surgical intervention for correction. However, rehabilitating the pelvic diaphragm muscles is highly beneficial.

Improving the coordination, endurance, and strength of these muscles may be a key component to providing long-term support and success for surgical prolapse repairs. Additionally, some women may not be eligible for surgical treatment or may desire trial of less invasive interventions first. One small study found that contraction of the pelvic diaphragm muscles in the supine position could completely reduce the prolapse.[121]

Collaboration With Pelvic Health Therapists

Considering the context for this chapter within this text, it is valuable for the orthopedic practicing therapist to understand the potential for referring to or working alongside a pelvic health physical therapist. The desire of pelvic health therapists is to "put the pelvis back in the body" because it is the base of the trunk, the attachment site of the lower extremities, and the site of convergence for the urologic, gastrointestinal, and reproductive systems. The pelvis is a key part of the body to address with many core muscle function problems, which may span from upper extremity and cervical dysfunction, to thoracolumbar problems, to hip, knee, and ankle dysfunction. Thus, learning about symptoms related to pelvic diaphragm muscle dysfunction may assist in identifying core muscle deficits that may affect rehabilitation throughout the musculoskeletal system. Many history-taking questions related to pelvic health address sensitive topics, thus often limiting gathering of essential information that may lead to accurate diagnosis and intervention. Pelvic health therapists can assist others with the wording and approach for posing these necessary questions.

Most pelvic health therapists practice in outpatient orthopedic settings. Additionally, many pelvic health therapists with board certification in Women's Health (WCS) also have board certification in Orthopedics (OCS), both through the American Board of Physical Therapy Specialties (ABPTS). The WCS encompasses pelvic health (pelvic pain, prolapse and supportive dysfunction, bladder and bowel health, reproductive health); pregnancy and postpartum (musculoskeletal complaints, high-risk pregnancy interventions, postpartum rehabilitation); osteoporosis intervention and fracture rehabilitation; and breast and gynecologic oncology rehabilitation and lymphedema therapy. By 2015, 224 physical therapists had earned the WCS credentials.[122] Many pelvic health practitioners may not have the WCS, but have received formal training or some degree of mentoring to develop their subspecialized skills. Training and education typically come through participation in a Women's Health Physical Therapy Residency (of which there are currently one developing and eight credentialed programs in the country),[123] successful completion of continuing education (typically a course series) in pelvic health or pregnancy and postpartum rehabilitation, or closely working with one or more experienced pelvic health therapists who offer formal or informal mentoring.

Considerations for Collaboration With a Pelvic Health Therapist

The orthopedic therapist may consider referral to or collaboration with a pelvic health therapist when a patient's impairments indicate that possible pelvic health conditions are involved. As noted previously, in some conditions, pelvic health symptoms and conditions overlap with symptoms of the low back, hip, and pelvic ring. The pelvic health therapist could assist in identifying potential neuromusculoskeletal findings that may be addressed with pelvic health therapeutic interventions. The pelvic health therapist may also be helpful in referral to an appropriate health care provider (e.g., a gynecologist, urologist, gastrointestinal practitioner, colon and rectal practitioner, or urogynecologist).

Signs and symptoms that indicate need for consultation with a pelvic health therapist include those related to pelvic diaphragm and pelvic wall myofascial dysfunction and bladder and bowel symptoms. Patient with underactive pelvic diaphragm musculature may report the following: symptoms of urinary leakage; solid or liquid fecal, mucus, or gas leakage from the anus; and symptoms of pelvic organ prolapse (e.g., heaviness or sensation of a lump in the vagina). Patients with overactive pelvic diaphragm musculature may experience pain with intercourse or other sexual activity, pain with urination or defecation, difficulty starting the stream of urine, slow or altered urine flow, urinary frequency or urgency, constipation, and coccydynia. Symptoms of both underactive and overactive pelvic diaphragm muscles can occur in the same person.

However, as noted previously, in some cases patients may not report direct symptoms of intrapelvic neuromusculoskeletal problems. Thus, considerations for pelvic health physical therapy may also include lumbopelvic or hip pain or symptoms that are not resolving with other therapy interventions.

Pelvic Health Therapist Patient Management

Box 9-3 outlines the basic components that may be included in a pelvic health therapist examination and evaluation. Based on patients' reports, patients' goals, and examination findings, this examination may be less or more inclusive of the items described here and in Table 9-5. The history and examination performed by a pelvic health therapist certainly target impairments and functional or activity limitations related to pelvic structures and pelvic health. Additionally, the therapist also provides a thorough external musculoskeletal examination, a lower quarter screening, and, if warranted, an upper quarter screening. More detail on these components is described here.

The patient's history is often key to providing an evaluation of the examination findings. For patients experiencing

---

• BOX 9-3 Pelvic Health Therapy Components

Patient or Client History

- Pain descriptions
- Symptoms related to incontinence (bowel or bladder) and prolapse
- Activities associated with symptoms
- Obstetric and gynecologic history
- Urinary, gastrointestinal, and colorectal-anal history
- Psychosocial screening and history

Outcome Measures and Screening Tools

- May include tools related to affective or depressive states, more global musculoskeletal complaints, and urinary, colorectal, pelvic organ prolapse, and sexual symptoms

Regional Musculoskeletal Examination

- Upper and lower quarter screening
- Assessment of extra-pelvic contributions to pelvic-related symptoms, such as posture, functional movements, gait, and biomechanics
- Screening to differentiate organic from musculoskeletal contributions to abdominal quadrant pain

External Screening of Pelvic Diaphragm Muscles

- Palpation of pelvic diaphragm muscles (under clothing, or over underwear or thin clothing)
  - Screening for tenderness or trigger points
  - Screening for ability of muscle to contract and relax voluntarily
- Step may be excluded if internal muscle examination planned

External Examination of the Perineum

- Visual assessment of vulvar tissues and external genitalia
- Observation of external tissues with voluntary pelvic diaphragm muscle contraction, voluntary relaxation, and voluntary bearing down
- Observation of presence or absence of involuntary contraction (cough reflex)
- Cotton swab test for mapping areas of allodynia
- Anal reflex testing
- External palpation of superficial external pelvic diaphragm muscles

Internal Palpation and Examination of Pelvic Diaphragm Muscles

- Palpation of levator ani, coccygeus, obturator internus, and piriformis muscles for muscle tone and tenderness or trigger points
- Manual muscle testing of the levator ani muscles (strength, endurance, and coordination)
- Assessment of ability to relax and bear down voluntarily
- Assessment of involuntary contraction of levator ani with cough
- Assessment of pelvic organ prolapse (location and degree)

Additional Examination Components That May be Used

- Observation of pelvic muscle activity with surface electromyography biofeedback
- Visualization of muscle activity in abdominopelvic region with real-time ultrasound
- Observation of anal and rectal muscles with anal manometry

pain, history taking should include character, intensity, radiation, and daily chronologic patter of the patient's pain.[46] The patient's reports of the pain patterns help determine somatic versus viscerally related pain. Well-defined, sharp, and localized pain is often somatic.[46] However, if the pain is in a chronic state, peripheral and central sensitization may cause pain symptoms to be diffuse and difficult to provoke or reduce with mechanical tests or interventions. Visceral pain is often described as difficult to localize, vague, achy, cramping, or squeezing; the pain comes in waves and likely refers to other areas.[46] For patients reporting voiding, defecatory, or prolapse symptoms, information should be gathered on frequency and intensity of symptoms and activities associated with the symptoms. For example, does bladder leakage occur in small amounts or large amounts? Does leakage occur with coughing and sneezing, or with sensations of urgency? Do prolapse symptoms worsen toward the end of the day or with certain activities? How does diet affect symptoms of constipation? These descriptions help the therapist to determine what musculoskeletal dysfunction may be contributing to or causing symptoms, such as overactive versus underactive pelvic diaphragm muscles.

For all patients with pelvic health conditions, general information about urologic, gastrointestinal, colorectal and anal, obstetric, and gynecologic history and surgical procedures should be gathered. For instance, information about birth history or injuries, or gynecologic operations, may offer explanations of development of symptoms related to bladder, bowel, or sexual dysfunction. In addition, a patient may not voluntarily report history or symptoms in other pelvic organ systems that are not perceived as being significant or important by the patient. However, asking direct questions about the other organ systems may reveal a constellation of information contributing to the main complaint. For instance, a patient with primary complaints of sexual pain may also have symptoms of urinary urgency and frequency, with all symptoms (pain and urinary) relating to overactive pelvic diaphragm muscles. Knowing the array of symptoms assists the therapist in directing the physical examination.

Psychosocial information is also helpful in understanding potential impact on symptoms and rehabilitation potential. Such information may include depression and anxiety screening, questions related to social or familial support, and pertinent history (e.g., history of physical or sexual abuse) that may contribute to current symptoms.

Outcome measures and screening tools vary based on the patient's complaints. In the pelvic health setting, these measures and tools may replicate those used in other outpatient clinics that relate to overall activity participation and function and more global symptom and pain complaints. Beyond these broader measures are also questionnaires and instruments that focus on specific conditions of pelvic health, such as urinary, colorectal and anal, and sexual problems. Many tools commonly used in pelvic health physical therapy are summarized in Table 9-12, although this list is not exhaustive. These instruments and others, along with their supporting evidence, are also located on the website

of the Section on Women's Health of the American Physical Therapy Association (http://www.womenshealthapta.org/research/functional-outcome-measures).

Screening tools may be used to assess affective or depressive states. Some examples include the *Beck Depression inventory*, the *Edinburgh Postnatal Depression Scale* (EPDS),[124] and the *Depression, Anxiety, Stress Scale* (DASS21). In particular, the EPDS is validated for women who are up to 12 weeks postpartum and was developed to be easily accessible and user friendly for any practitioner.[124] Screening for postpartum depression is pertinent because, as discussed previously, low back pain in the postpartum period is reported to be three times more common in women who also have depressive symptoms.[87] For women who have positive postpartum depression screening results (as indicated by an EPDS score of 10 or greater), referral to the primary care provider or other appropriate health care practitioner is needed for a full examination and evaluation of mental health status.

As noted previously, many patients with pelvic muscle diaphragm dysfunction and conditions often also experience trunk, hip, and lower extremity symptoms. The *Patient-Specific Functional Scale* (PSFS), the *Oswestry Disability Index*, and the *Lower Extremity Functional Scale* (LEFS) are examples of scales commonly used with patients experiencing musculoskeletal complaints outside the pelvis in addition to pelvic-specific conditions. In particular, PSFS is very clinically useful because it allows the patient to identify the specific activities that relate to pain symptoms, with minimally detectable changes identified for follow-up assessments[125] (see Table 9-12). The *Fear Avoidance Beliefs Questionnaire* (FABQ)[126] and the *Pelvic Girdle Questionnaire* (PGQ)[127] are both valid and reliable specifically for patients with pelvic girdle pain, particularly during pregnancy and postpartum.

The majority of Table 9-12 provides information on pelvic-specific condition scales and instruments. Two of the scales listed address pelvic health conditions that encompass multiple systems and functions, including combinations of urinary, colorectal and anal, sexual function, and pelvic organ prolapse symptoms. Examples of these pelvic health encompassing scales include the *Pelvic Floor Impact Questionnaire-7* (PFIQ-7)[128] and the *Pelvic Floor Distress Inventory-20* (PFDI-20).[128]

Other pelvic-specific condition scales either solely address one pelvic organ system or address multiple systems as they affect one specific functional area. The *Geriatric Self-Efficacy Scale for Urinary Incontinence* (GSE-UI)[129] assesses and detects meaningful improvements in the confidence of adults 65 years of age and older to control bladder leakage. Several scales assess colorectal-anal function of incontinence, constipation, or both. Such scales include the *Incontinence Symptoms and Impact on Quality of Life* (ICIQ-B),[130] the *Constipation Scoring System* (CSS),[131] and the *Colorectal Functional Outcome Questionnaire* (COREFO).[132] Sexual function is examined in relation to other pelvic systems in the *Pelvic Organ Prolapse/Urinary Incontinence/Sexual Function Questionnaire*

| TABLE 9-12 | Outcome Measures and Screening Tools Commonly Used in Pelvic Health Settings* |

Outcome Measure or Screening Tools	Description
Edinburgh Postnatal Depression Scale (EPDS)[124]	Screening tool for detecting women at risk for postnatal depression (does *not* diagnose depression; diagnosis requires appropriate examination from qualified practitioner for diagnosing mental health conditions) 10-question scale with maximum score of 30; possible depression score of 10 or greater indicates need for referral to primary care provider or appropriate mental health practitioner for assessment and diagnosis
Patient-Specific Functional Scale (PSFS)[125]	Questionnaire for assessing and detecting changes in patient self-identified activities that are impossible or difficult to perform because of symptoms Patients asked to identify up to 3 important activities and rate difficulty on a scale of 0 (unable to perform) to 10 (able to perform) Minimal detectable change (90% CI) for average score = 2 points Minimal detectable change (90% CI) for a single activity score = 3 points
Fear Avoidance Beliefs Questionnaire (FABQ)[126]	Valid and reliable self-report questionnaire for patients with pelvic girdle pain (tested specifically in pregnant and postpartum population) 2 domains: physical activity (5 questions); work (11 questions)
Pelvic Girdle Questionnaire (PGQ)[127]	Reliable and valid for PGP in pregnancy and postpartum 25 questions in areas of activities of daily living, functional movements, pain, leg symptoms, sleep
Pelvic Floor Impact Questionnaire-7 (PFIQ-7)[128]	Valid and reliable for condition-specific quality of life for women with pelvic floor disorders 7 questions on 3 scales (urinary distress, pelvic organ prolapse, colorectal-anal distress)
Pelvic Floor Distress Inventory-20 (PFDI-20)[128]	Valid and reliable for condition-specific quality of life for women with pelvic floor disorders 20 questions on 3 scales (urinary distress, pelvic organ prolapse, colorectal-anal distress)
Geriatric Self-Efficacy Scale for Urinary Incontinence (GSE-UI)[129]	Responsive and clinically useful for measuring older adults' (≥65 yr) level of confidence for preventing urine loss Improvement of 14 points had a sensitivity of 75.1% and specificity of 78.2% for detecting clinically meaningful changes in urinary incontinence status
Incontinence Symptoms and Impact on Quality of Life (ICIQ-B)[130]	Valid and reliable for evaluation of anal incontinence of varying causes and impact on quality of life 17-item questionnaire in 3 domains: bowel pattern, bowel control, quality of life
Constipation Scoring System (CSS)[131]	Subjective constipation score Score range of 0 to 30 (0 = normal, 30 = severe constipation) Score >15 correlated with objective obstruction causes
Colorectal Functional Outcome Questionnaire (COREFO)[132]	Reliable and valid for evaluating colorectal function after colorectal surgical procedures 5 multi-item scales (number of questions: 9 incontinence, 9 social impact, 2 frequency, 3 stool-related aspects, 3 need for medications)
Pelvic Organ Prolapse/Urinary Incontinence/Sexual Function Questionnaire (PISQ)[131]	Valid and reliable to evaluate sexual functioning in women with urinary incontinence or pelvic organ prolapse 31 questions in 3 domains (behavioral/emotive, physical, partner-related)
Female Sexual Functional Index (FSFI)[133]	Scale of female sexual function with 19-item questionnaire Reliable and valid for assessing domains of subjective arousal, lubrication, orgasm, satisfaction, and pain

CI, Confidence interval.

*This list is not exhaustive, but it provides a summary of many of the global and condition-specific measures that may be used in a pelvic health setting. The evidence for and the actual tools listed here (along with other scales and questionnaires) may be found at http://www.womenshealthapta.org/research/functional-outcome-measures/.

(PISQ).[131] Focus on specific domains of sexual function occurs in the *Female Sexual Functional Index* (FSFI),[133] and in particular this is a sexual function scale that addresses pain with sexual activity and intercourse.

A regional musculoskeletal examination is performed to determine extrapelvic contributions to pelvic-related symptoms, involving lower quarter (and upper quarter as needed) screening along with further examination in implicated areas. Examination also includes adequate examination of the trunk, spine, pelvis, and hips, and it extends to the lower extremities as needed. This may also include screening tests such as the Carnett test, which is used to attempt to differentiate between musculoskeletal and organically originating pain symptoms in the abdominal quadrants. Observation and measurements related to posture (in a variety of positions), transitional movements, gait, and balance may also be performed.

External screening of pelvic diaphragm muscles can be performed by skilled palpation just medial to the ischial tuberosity, over the patient's underwear or thin clothing. Although this screening does not allow the therapist to measure strength or perform a thorough palpation of the muscles, it does allow a screen of the ability of the muscles to contract and voluntarily relax and for pain or discomfort with palpation. External screening described here is typically used only when an internal pelvic diaphragm muscle examination is not performed. For instance, a patient with recalcitrant hip pain that is not responding to nonpelvic therapy may be referred to a pelvic health physical therapist to assess for possible referral or contribution of pelvic diaphragm muscles to the hip symptoms. The therapist may choose to perform this type of screening before deciding that an internal examination is needed. The external assessment also allows the therapist to provide preliminary education to the patient on potential conditions that may be arising from intrapelvic structures. Thus, the therapist is able to build rapport with the patient and help the patient understand why an internal examination may be needed for symptoms that, to the patient, seem to be originating from outside the pelvis.

Perineal observation and internal pelvic examination are performed only after informed consent of the patient. The therapist uses anatomic models or pictures to educate the patient on the anatomy and physiology of the pelvic structures to be examined and explains thoroughly what the examination entails from start to finish before the patient disrobes.

External examination of the perineum includes visual assessment of the vulva, perineal body, clitoris, vestibule, vagina, and anus for apparent presence of infection, inflammation, skin abnormalities, lichen planus, fissures, cysts, or any other visible abnormality. Sensory testing is performed of the external pelvic structures (genitofemoral, ilioinguinal, and branches of the pudendal nerves). Pelvic diaphragm and perineal body movement are observed with instruction to contract and relax the muscles. Additionally, with instruction to cough, observation occurs for reflexive pelvic diaphragm muscle contraction (present or absent) and any urinary or anal leakage. Observation for any visible pelvic organ prolapse is also noted. A cotton swab test may be performed to map areas of allodynia (this test may also be referred to as the Q-Tip test). The anal reflex may be assessed (also called anal wink). The anal reflex involves a quick stroke across the anus; the normal response is a "winking" motion of the anus (afferent pudendal nerve and efferent S2 to S4). External palpation of superficial external pelvic diaphragm muscles (ischiocavernosus, bulbocavernosus, and superficial transverse perineal) is performed to assess for muscle tone and tenderness.

Internal palpation and examination of pelvic diaphragm muscles are necessary for manual muscle test grading and for thorough examination of the pelvic diaphragm structures. Internal digital examination is performed by the therapist either vaginally or rectally. Palpation of the levator ani, coccygeus, obturator internus, and piriformis muscles allows assessment of muscle tone and any tender or trigger points. Additionally, palpation is performed to assess gross intravaginal or intrarectal sensation. Manual muscle testing is performed of the levator ani to assess strength, endurance, and coordination with fast and slow twitch fiber activity; several different pelvic diaphragm manual muscle strength scales have been described in the literature. Assessment of a patient's ability to relax or bear down with the pelvic diaphragm muscles voluntarily is also performed, along with involuntary contraction of the levator ani with a cough. Cough and bearing down are also used to assess pelvic organ or pelvic tissue descent; location and degree of descent are noted.

Additional tools that complement the pelvic examination may include surface EMG biofeedback to assess electrical activity of the pelvic diaphragm muscles during contraction and relaxation, real-time ultrasound to visualize muscle activity during contraction and relaxation (may be performed transabdominally or transperineally) (see Fig. 9-18), and anal manometry to assess the activity of the anal and rectal muscles. These tools can also be used for biofeedback, by allowing the patient to visualize timing and activity of the muscles. Thus, they can be used to "uptrain" or increase activity of a muscle (addressing muscle underactivity) or "downtrain" or decrease unwanted activity of a muscle and improve relaxation (addressing muscle overactivity). Although these tools are helpful for examination and intervention, they should ideally be used in conjunction with the manual intrapelvic examination, which allows the clinician to determine muscle tone, bulk, and atrophy and to assess other qualitative components of the muscle fibers. Internal manual assessment also ensures the accuracy of adjunctive tool findings, such as EMG or pressure readings.

Case Studies

Case Study 9-1 describes the management of a prenatal patient with pelvic girdle pain, and Case Study 9-2 describes a patient with poststroke chronic urinary incontinence.

CASE STUDY 9-1

Management of a Prenatal Patient With Pelvic Girdle Pain

Patient History

A 32-year-old woman at 31 weeks of gestation presented to physical therapy in an outpatient clinic with a complaint of gradual onset of lower back and hip pain, with radiation to the pubic area. She reported that pain began during the eleventh week of gestation and gradually worsened. She described pain as being sharp and starting in the upper gluteal and sacroiliac joint region on the left side, with spread of diffuse achy pain into the midgluteal and lateral hip region as symptoms worsened. Pain occurred "75% of the day" with prolonged positions or activities that involved sitting, standing, or walking. Pain also awakened her sometimes at night (4 nights a week), and it required change of positions or getting out of bed and moving around. Pubic pain occurred less frequently (a few times a day) and was typically sharp and brief, lasting only with an exacerbating activity. Pubic pain occurred with rolling over in bed, crossing the legs or ankles, and stepping up or down on a step or curb. The patient reported that her physician encouraged taking acetaminophen and using freezer gel packs from her local pharmacy to apply over painful areas. The patient was an elementary school teacher who spent most of her day standing or sitting on a tall stool to teach. She rated her pain on numeric rating scale as a 2 out of 10 at the least, worsening to a sharp 8 out of 10 with exacerbating activities. She reported requesting further health care management from her obstetrician when the pain caused her to miss 2 days at work. She reported that before pregnancy she participated in a combination of running, light weight lifting, and kickboxing-style aerobics classes 3 to 5 days per week. After becoming pregnant, she continued running at a slower pace and lesser distances and continued weight lifting. Since her pain had exacerbated the last few weeks, she had discontinued exercise because of decreased tolerance to activity. On questioning, the patient denied any bowel symptoms, but she reported occasional leakage of a few drops of urine with cough or sneeze since becoming pregnant. She reported sexual activity to be affected by pain of the low back and left hip.

The patient reported her goals to include (1) a reduction of pain that would allow sleep without disturbance from pain, (2) participation in some recreational exercise, and (3) the ability to complete workdays to the end of her pregnancy without being limited by pain.

Systems Review

General observations: The patient was initially observed as being "fidgety," having difficulty finding a comfortable position in her waiting room chair. The patient did not use an assistive device. Gait appeared slowed with shortened step length. Gait also occurred with visualization of decrease in normal lower trunk and pelvis rotation, with lack of separation between upper and lower trunk rotation. Her static standing posture showed a posterior pelvic tilt from a lateral view and maintenance of slightly excessive hip abduction and external rotation in anterior and posterior views (occurring more on the left side). She also appeared to bear more weight toward her right lower extremity. She did not exhibit any other remarkable deviations of the trunk, spine, or lower extremities.

Cardiovascular and pulmonary: Blood pressure after 5 minutes of sitting (taken in seated position) was 132/72 mm Hg. Resting heart rate was 68 beats per minute. Respiratory rate was 15 breaths per minute.

Integumentary: A linea nigra (darkened line of skin along linea alba, common and normal in pregnancy) was noted. Mild bilateral swelling was noted in the feet and ankles, although it was nonpitting. No other discolorations, swelling, or skin abnormalities were noted in the trunk (abdomen or back), hips, or lower extremities.

Neuromuscular: Patellar and Achilles reflexes were equal and normal (2+) bilaterally. Sensation to light touch was equal and intact bilaterally to dermatomes L2 to L5, S1, and S2.

Musculoskeletal: Bilateral hip and knee active range of motion was found to be in normal limits. Trunk flexion was in the functional range. Deficits were noted in the several tests and measures, as described next.

Tests and Measures

The patient completed the Pelvic Girdle Questionnaire (PGQ)[127] which has been found to be valid and reliable for assessing the effect of pelvic girdle pain on activities of daily living, functional movements, pain, leg symptoms, and sleep in pregnant and postpartum women. The patient's PGQ demonstrated a raw score of 52, or a 69% score. (A score of 0% indicates no problems at all; a score of 100% indicates symptoms affect to a large extent.)

Next the physical examination was performed. Trunk extension was measured as follows: A tape measure was used to measure the distance between C7 spinous process and S1 spinous process, both in static neutral standing and again at end range of standing extension. The difference noted was 3.5 cm, with patient reporting pain and stiffness in the left side of her low back at end range. This motion was visibly limited.

Results of manual muscle testing for both lower extremities and spine were normal, except for the following: left hip abduction was 4 out of 5 with pain limitation. In addition, the patient demonstrated poor ability to recruit her transversus abdominis muscle in a seated position; she substituted with breath-holding and performed a slight bulging of the abdomen (instead of a controlled drawing up and in of the lower abdomen).

Palpation revealed pain rated at 7 out of 10 over the pubic symphysis joint, and on the left side grossly over the gluteus medius along its attachment to the iliac crest, the gluteus maximus from its superior overlap with the gluteus medius extending down to midbuttock, and the piriformis. Palpation of the gluteus medius also revealed muscle knotting and produced pain referred into the lateral hip, the lower back, and the left sacroiliac joint and sacrum.

Special testing began with the seated slump test and the straight leg raise test to assess for lumbar spine contribution to symptoms. Results of these two tests were negative and ruled out primary spine involvement.

The additional special tests performed were to assess for pelvic girdle and pubic symphysis involvement. The patient demonstrated a positive active straight leg raise test result bilaterally (although most involved when lifting the right leg), indicating difficulty with functional load transfer from the lower extremities to the pelvis. The results of a modified Trendelenburg test was positive for pubic symphysis pain reproduction, a finding also indicating poor load transfer through the pelvic ring. The posterior pelvic pain provocation (P4) test result was positive with reproduction of pain in the left

CASE STUDY 9-1

Management of a Prenatal Patient With Pelvic Girdle Pain—cont'd

gluteus medius and sacroiliac joint region, indicating pelvic girdle pain dysfunction.

External screening of the patient's levator ani function was performed over the patient's underwear and yoga pants. She was positioned in side lying, and the therapist (with gloved hand) palpated the levator ani in the space just inferior and medial to the ischial tuberosity. The patient was asked to contract, relax, and gently bear down through her levator ani. The patient had difficulty contracting the muscle initially, but was able to improve with verbal and manual cues.

Finally, the patient was asked to demonstrate her usual sleeping position. She placed one pillow between her knees, and one under her head in a side-lying position. She reported rolling from one side to the other throughout the night.

Evaluation, Diagnosis, and Prognosis

Based on the patient's history, observation, and physical examination, it was determined that she had pregnancy-related pelvic girdle pain. The patient's reports of pain in the sacroiliac region (with unilateral dominance) and intolerance to prolonged positions or activities or to asymmetrical leg position are typical of posterior pelvic girdle and pubic symphysis pain. The patient demonstrated the following: strength deficits of her left gluteus medius; poor transversus abdominis and levator ani muscle recruitment and coordination (which would lead to decreased muscle support of the pelvic ring and trunk); muscle tenderness, knotting, and pain referral of the gluteals and piriformis; and limited spine extension consistent with this population. Additionally, special testing for pelvic girdle pain and reduced load transfer through the pelvis were demonstrated. The sleeping position she demonstrated would contribute to pain. The onset of symptoms in early pregnancy with progression of symptoms as the pregnancy advanced also indicated this diagnosis.

Intervention

Initially, the patient was reassured that her symptoms were common in pregnancy and were typically able to be managed with conservative treatments. The patient was educated on the role of the deep primary core muscles (transversus abdominis, levator ani, and multifidus) in coordination with the breathing diaphragm for providing stability to her pelvic joints with the progression of pregnancy and with the increase in laxity that normally and necessarily occurred in these joints to prepare for labor and delivery. The patient then learned that her secondary stabilizing muscles in the hips (gluteals and piriformis) were experiencing excessive workloads to compensate for the poor coordination of some of her deeper core muscles, thus leading to the pain in the lumbar-hip region.

Once the patient was reassured about the ability to manage her condition conservatively, both passive and active therapies were introduced. The patient received soft tissue massage and trigger point release along the gluteals and piriformis, with focus on the left gluteus medius to reduce their inhibiting effect on the primary core muscles. This was followed by ice and compression in a side-lying position to reduce inflammation. Thorough instruction and practice of transversus abdominis and levator ani contractions were given, in isolation and in conjunction with one another, with focus on coordinating with

normal breathing patterns. This instruction was performed initially in side lying, where the patient could allow her global secondary stabilizing muscles (namely, the gluteals) to stay at rest. Over subsequent visits, these exercises were progressed to seated and standing positions. By the third visit, the patient was asked to identify three activities throughout the day with which she would functionally activate these muscles (with a submaximal 20% effort contraction to promote control).

The first visit also included instruction and practice set-up of a side-lying sleep positioning. The patient was instructed to purchase long body pillows to place between the legs, extending from the thigh all the way to the feet. She was instructed to keep the two lower extremities "mirroring" one another, such that the uppermost extremity was not allowed to drop into external rotation (with the upper foot dropping down against the bottom one). The patient also practiced placing pillow support under her abdomen to eliminate rotational forces on her spine and hips. She also placed a small rolled towel under her waist to support a neutral spine position in the frontal plane. On practicing in the clinic, the patient reported immediate improvements in comfort levels in a side-lying position. Additionally, the patient was instructed in choosing symmetrical positions of the legs throughout the day (thus, no leg or ankle crossing, and keeping weight distributed evenly on both legs in standing). She was also instructed in log rolling, keeping the legs symmetrical, to get in and out of bed.

Gentle isometrics of seated hip abduction (with a stiff belt positioned around the thighs just above knee level) and hip adduction (with a pillow folded between the knees) were performed to provide gentle distraction forces through the pelvic girdle joints and pain relief.

Additionally, the patient was instructed in the purchase of a sacroiliac support belt. She brought the belt to her second visit, at which time she was instructed in positioning it firmly around the greater trochanters below the abdomen. She was instructed that the belt could be worn under the clothes over underwear, and that it should feel comfortable and reduce discomfort if positioned properly.

The foregoing program was used for a total of 3 weeks, with the patient attending visits once per week. She performed the home exercise program daily and used cold packs as needed. She also changed her sleeping position and reduced asymmetrical leg positions as described.

Reexamination and Termination of Physical Therapy

After 3 weeks of the initial program, the patient was reevaluated. Her PGQ score had reduced to 18%, indicating improvement in function (this questionnaire does not yet have a minimal clinical difference score change defined). She reported a pain to be occasionally at 0 out of 10, averaging a 2 out of 10, and getting up to 4 out of 10 at the worst. She reported feeling more "stable and in control" with use of the transversus abdominis and levator ani during functional movements. She also reported a resolution of the urinary leakage she had been experiencing. She was able to complete workdays with minimal discomfort. She also began walking for exercise and had resumed light weight lifting. She still experienced occasional sharp pubic symphysis pain with rolling over in bed, but with less severity than initially.

Continued

CASE STUDY 9-1

Management of a Prenatal Patient With Pelvic Girdle Pain—cont'd

Tenderness with palpation was now reduced to a small area of the superior portion of the gluteus medius, with resolution of referred pain. Manual muscle test revealed a 5/5 of left hip abduction with no pain. Results of special tests of the pelvic girdle were now negative, with the exception of the active straight leg raise (although performance on this test improved).

Because the patient was now at 34 weeks of gestation and had time restraints on her schedule, she reported feeling confident of being able to continue to manage the symptoms on her own. She agreed to a weekly telephone follow-up for 2 weeks. At the second telephone follow-up, the patient stated that she was satisfied with her progress and ready for discharge from physical therapy.

CASE STUDY 9-2

Chronic Urinary Incontinence in a Woman After Cerebrovascular Accident

Patient History

A 68-year-old woman presented to physical therapy in an outpatient pelvic health clinic with a primary complaint of urinary incontinence that had worsened over the last 6 months after experiencing a cerebrovascular accident (CVA) affecting her right side. She reported experiencing mild leakage with coughing or jogging (stress incontinence) during the year after the birth of her first child 45 years ago, with on and off leakage through the years that she has managed by decreasing fluid intake and using panty liners. The patient was being seen by a physical therapist in an outpatient rehabilitation clinic to address residual trunk and lower extremity weakness on her right side after the CVA. During this time, the patient expressed concern to her therapist about participating in treadmill exercise because of her worsening bladder leakage. At this time, the therapist performed the Three Incontinence Questions (3IQ) with the patient and determined that the patient likely had mixed urinary incontinence (MUI), with a predominance of urge urinary incontinence (UUI). The therapist then referred the patient to the pelvic health clinic for focused pelvic health physical therapy examination and evaluation.

The patient was asked to complete a bladder diary, which revealed that leakage occurred primarily in amounts that were small (few drops) to moderate (dampening of underwear, but not outerwear) in a frequency of two to five times daily. Although not revealed on the diary, the patient reported occasional (once per month) leakage episodes that would result in a need to change outerwear. The diary revealed that leakage occurred most often with sensation of moderate to strong bladder urges and less frequently with coughing, sneezing, and walking. The diary also showed that the patient consumed two six-ounce cups of regular coffee every morning, one "large" glass of tea at lunch, and little else for fluid intake. No significant findings in food intake choices were noted.

The patient reported that leakage had caused her to be fearful of drinking much during the day, of participating in exercise, or in performing activities such as grocery shopping or social outings. She expressed that her goals were the following: (1) feel in control of her bladder urges, (2) return to walking for exercise, and (3) feel that she can grocery shop or go out to dinner or the movies without fear of leaking or having overwhelming strong bladder urges.

Systems Review

General observations: The patient presented as a 68-year-old woman of average build and weight. She ambulated modified independently with use of a straight cane in her right hand. Her gait was observed to occur with a mild trunk lean toward the left. Static sitting and standing posture revealed slight trunk lean toward left, mild increase in thoracic kyphosis and posterior pelvic tilt, and mild forward head posture.

Medications: The patient reports taking irbesartan (Avapro) for blood pressure and an over-the-counter daily vitamin. She also reports having tried a medication to address bladder urgency, but discontinued it because it was not helping and it was causing her to have a dry mouth. She reported that she could not remember the name of this medicine.

Cardiovascular and pulmonary: Taken in sitting position after 5 minutes of rest, blood pressure was 128/80 mm Hg. Resting heart rate was 72 beats per minute. Respiratory rate was 13 breaths per minute.

Integumentary: No remarkable findings with skin or swelling noted of the trunk or extremities.

Neuromuscular: Examination of reflexes deferred because of recent CVA and because the patient is followed by a neurologic physical therapist. Sensation to light touch was intact bilaterally to dermatomes L2 to L5, S1, and S2 (although reported as diminished on the right side).

Musculoskeletal: Gross myotome muscle testing revealed general weakness on the right side. Pelvic health–specific deficits were noted in the following examination.

Tests and Measures

The patient completed and scored 15 (score of 0 = not confident at all, score of 120 = fully confident) on the Geriatric Self-Efficacy Scale for Urinary Incontinence (GSE-UI), indicating relatively low confidence in her ability to control her bladder. The GSE-UI is a scale that is reliable and valid for persons 65 years old and older to assess for confidence in bladder control.

Next, a physical examination of the patient was completed. The patient was educated on the pelvic diaphragm muscle with use a three-dimensional pelvis model with muscles, including location and function of the muscles. The patient was also instructed on physical therapy examination of these muscles and other pelvic structures that provide continence.

Chronic Urinary Incontinence in a Woman After Cerebrovascular Accident—cont'd

The patient was given the opportunity to ask questions about the examination. The patient provided informed consent to participating in an intrapelvic physical therapy examination (vaginal). She disrobed from the waist down and was positioned in supine with knees bent and feet supported on the examination table.

External observation of the perineum revealed mild atrophy of vulvar tissues and visible descent of her perineal body. When asked to contract her levator ani muscle ("squeeze as if you are holding back urine or gas"), the patient gave a slight contraction followed by an outward bulge of the perineum, indicating poor recruitment and poor coordination of the levator ani muscles. The patient was then asked to provide active relaxation of the muscles ("gently bear down as if trying to release gas"), revealing a mild paradoxical contraction of the levator ani muscles. No visible prolapse was noted externally. Sensation to light touch revealed intact and bilateral equal sensation in S2 to S5 dermatomes and throughout the perineum. Cotton swab testing did not reveal any areas of allodynia. The anal reflex (anal wink) testing revealed a present reflex.

Single digit (gloved) internal examination was then performed. This examination revealed reports of tenderness and "burning" pain with palpation grossly at the posterior portion of the levator ani (pressing into the muscles in a direction downward toward the treatment table). Reproduction of urgency occurred with this posterior levator ani pressure and also of the levator ani just adjacent to the urethra bilaterally. No other areas of tenderness or muscle tension were noted. The right levator ani muscles and obturator internus felt atrophied compared with the left side. Strength testing revealed 1/5 on the right (a "trace" contraction), and a 2/5 on the left (a contraction but no "lift" of the palpating digit occurred). The patient was asked to contract again and was given further manual and verbal cues to elicit a contraction without the patient's bearing down; the patient was able to perform a contraction with this assistance.

Endurance testing revealed the patient's ability to hold a levator ani muscle contraction for 3 seconds and to repeat this contraction three times before fatiguing. The patient was unable to perform "quick flicks" (quick contractions occurring in 1 second or less), thus indicating poor coordination of these muscles. When asked to bear down, the patient again performed a paradoxical levator ani contraction, with the patient unable to perform correctly during the initial visit. No pelvic organ prolapse was noted in a resting position of the levator ani; because of paradoxical contractions, the presence of prolapse was not assessed with bearing down. Finally, the patient was instructed in performing a transversus abdominis contraction (because the levator ani and transversus abdominis naturally co-contract); this resulted in an outward bulging of the lower abdomen, thereby indicating poor coordination of the transversus abdominis muscle.

After instruction in a home exercise program for the levator ani, the patient was then instructed to dress.

Evaluation, Diagnosis, and Prognosis

Based on the patient's history, observation, and physical examination, she was diagnosed with MUI, being predominated by UUI. The patient demonstrated strength, coordination, and palpation deficits consistent with this patient population. The early onset after childbirth, with a gradual worsening over time, followed by acute worsening after a CVA affected gross body neuromuscular function are also potential symptom contributors for older women experiencing incontinence. The patient's tenderness to palpation of the levator ani muscles contributes to poor coordination of the levator ani and UUI symptoms. The weakness and poor coordination both contribute greatly to the stress urinary incontinence (leakage with physical activity or coughing and sneezing).

Intervention

First, the patient received gentle passive stretching (digital and intravaginal) of the posterior portion of the levator ani, along with gentle friction massage to the periurethral musculature. The improvement in muscle flexibility and reduction in pain with soft tissue manual therapy were intended to reduce inhibition of muscle contraction. After 10 minutes of treatment, the patient reported a decrease in tenderness in these areas and demonstrated improved control with levator ani muscle contraction. This treatment was repeated at subsequent visits as needed, with gradual resolution of tenderness and muscle tension as the muscle coordination and strength improved.

The patient was initially instructed in levator ani muscle contractions, with a focus on controlled contractions at a submaximal recruitment effort to reduce compensatory muscle contractions of the hip or abdomen. The patient started with 5 repetitions of 3-second holds, to be performed 6 times a day (thus a total of 30 repetitions a day). Over time, these exercises were increased in hold-time as the patient demonstrated improvements in endurance, until she was able to hold a submaximal contraction for 8 seconds times 10 repetitions.

The patient was also educated the first day on fluid intake. She expressed understanding that a decrease in fluid intake could lead to less dilute (more concentrated) urine, which can contribute to bladder urgency. She also learned about potential bladder irritants, such as the caffeine in her coffee and tea. She agreed to reduce her caffeinated beverages by half the amount and to replace those amounts with water. Over subsequent visits, the patient reduced her caffeine intake to two 8-ounce cups or less per day and increased her plain water intake to six 8-ounce cups to dilute her urine and thus decrease intravesical irritation and urgency.

At her second visit a week later, the patient demonstrated that she was able to contract her levator ani muscles consistently and correctly, but she still demonstrated difficulty in coordinating these contractions with a normal breathing pattern. On this visit, focus was given to teaching the patient how to coordinate breathing with levator ani muscle contractions: while the muscles were at rest, the patient was asked to take in a "normal" breath, then exhale and contract the muscles at the same time. After much practice in clinic this day, she was able to perform this correctly. No increase in endurance hold times was given for the home program yet. She was also instructed in a side-lying transversus abdominis contraction with similar coordination of breathing and a submaximal recruitment to prevent substitution from more

Continued

global trunk or hip muscles. The patient was able to perform these exercises correctly by the end of the visit.

At her third visit a week later, the patient now demonstrated the ability to coordinate endurance levator ani contractions with normal breathing patterns and to perform them without substitution from global muscles. Endurance hold times and repetitions for home program were increased. Quick flicks were added to target fast twitch muscle fibers of the levator ani and to begin to train the muscles for contracting quickly with activities such as coughing or sneezing.

Reexamination

After 4 weeks of physical therapy and adherence to home exercise program and instructions, the patient was formally reevaluated. The patient's score on the GSE-UI had improved from a score of 15 to a score of 40, indicating an increase in confidence in her ability to control bladder symptoms. An improvement of 14 points or more is reported to have good specificity (78.2%) and sensitivity (75.1%) for detecting clinically meaningful changes. The patient reported less leakage with coughing or sneezing. She still experienced strong urges, but they were occurring less frequently. She was still concerned about participating in exercise or in being away from her home for long periods.

Her strength had improved to 3/5 (lift of the palpating digit) to manual muscle test on her left side, and to 2/5 on the right. Endurance had now increased to 5-second holds for six repetitions. She was now able to perform five quick contractions in a 10-second period. She now had no tenderness in the paraurethral musculature and reported a reduction in the tenderness of the posterior levator ani (intensity and area of tenderness). She reported that leaking had reduced to only once or twice daily, and intensity of urges was moderate or less. The amount of leakage that occurred had not changed (still ranging from small to moderate amounts). She also demonstrated good control with transversus abdominis muscle contractions and was able to coordinate these with normal breathing patterns.

Treatment Progression and Advancing of Functional Training

Levator ani and transversus abdominis muscle exercises for the home program, along with gradual changes in fluid intake instructions, continued to be progressed. Additionally, the patient was introduced to urge suppression techniques. These techniques involved the following: when the patient felt a strong urge come on, she was to attempt to remain calm with normal breathing patterns. Ideally she would remain or become stationary, and sit in a chair if one were available. These first steps promote a calming of any sympathetic nervous system inputs. Additionally, sitting would place pressure on the perineum, which would provide inhibitory input to the bladder. The patient was then instructed to perform submaximal effort quick flicks, which would further provide inhibition to the

bladder. Once the urge had passed, she could then either walk to a restroom to empty her bladder if she still had a sensation of bladder fullness. Or if she no longer had a sensation of bladder urge or fullness, she could then continue with her usual activity. She was encouraged that this technique would take practice and that with time would assist in increasing her bladder control.

Additionally, the patient was instructed in performing levator ani contractions in a functional manner to reduce leakage. She was instructed initially to contract these muscles just before and to maintain the contraction with a cough or sneeze ("squeeze before you sneeze"). Over time, this was progressed to contracting the muscles during transitional movements and then with more prolonged activities such as walking. With increase in length of the activity, the patient was instructed to decrease the intensity of the contraction and focus on being able to maintain a prolonged controlled contraction at a low level. She was given the analogy that her levator ani muscles were on a "dimmer switch," and that the intensity needed to be greater for short bursts of intense stress to the bladder, such as with cough or sneeze ("turn the dimmer on high"). The intensity needed to be less for long periods of bladder control, such as during walking for exercise ("turn the dimmer down low" to conserve energy).

Termination of Physical Therapy

At 7 weeks of physical therapy, the patient expressed satisfaction with her progress and believed that she was ready to continue to manage symptoms independently. Her GSE-UI score had improved to 105/120, indicating significant improvements in her confidence to control her urinary symptoms. She was asked to complete a final bladder diary and return the following week.

At 8 weeks, her bladder diary revealed the following: Bladder leakage now occurred in only small amounts (a few drops that did not dampen her underwear) and at a frequency of twice per week total. Strong urges had resolved, and normal bladder urgency now occurred with a full bladder. The patient now drank one 8-ounce cup of coffee in the morning, followed by water the rest of the day. Bladder emptying frequency was normal (averaging five to eight times in each 24-hour period).

Intrapelvic examination revealed that levator ani muscle coordination with contraction, relaxation, and gentle bearing down were all normal. No tenderness was noted in the levator ani. Manual muscle strength testing revealed a bilateral 3/5 of the levator ani. Endurance of the levator ani had increased to 8 seconds for 10 repetitions. She was able to perform 7 quick flicks in a 10-second period. Instruction to cough and elicit an involuntary muscle contraction also demonstrated normalized coordination of the levator ani. The patient was discharged from therapy with instruction in an ongoing home exercise program to maintain levator ani and transversus abdominis coordination, strength, and endurance.

References

1. AAPC. *ICD-10 code translator.* <https://www.aapc.com/icd-10/codes/>; Accessed January 30, 2015.

2. Shamliyan TA, Wyman JF, Pink R, et al. Male urinary incontinence: prevalence, risk factors, and preventive interventions. *Rev Urol.* 2009;11:145-165.

3. Kim JC, Cho KJ. Current trends in management of post-prostatectomy incontinence. *Korean J Urol.* 2012;53:511-518.

4. Matthew AG, Goldman A, Trachtenberg J, et al. Sexual dysfunction after radical prostatectomy: prevalence, treatments, restricted use of treatments and distress. *J Urol.* 2005;174:2105-2110.

5. Shamloul R, Ghanem H. Erectile dysfunction. *Lancet.* 2013;381:153-165.

6. Hao Z-Y, Li H-J, Wang Z-P, et al. The prevalence of erectile dysfunction and its relation to chronic prostatitis in Chinese men. *J Androl.* 2011;32:496-501.

7. Anothaisintawee T, Attia J, Nickel JC, et al. Management of chronic prostatitis/chronic pelvic pain syndrome: a systematic review and network meta-analysis. *JAMA.* 2011;305:78-86.

8. Corton MM. Anatomy of the pelvis: how the pelvis is built for support. *Clin Obstet Gynecol.* 2005;48:611-626.

9. Dietrick CS III, Gehrich A, Bakaya S. Surgical exposure and anatomy of the female pelvis. *Surg Clin North Am.* 2008;88:223-243.

10. Hobel CJ, Chang AB. Normal labor, delivery, and postpartum care: anatomic considerations, obstetric analgesia and anesthesia, and resuscitation of the newborn. In: Hacker NF, Moore JG, Gambone JC, eds. *Essentials of Obstetrics and Gynecology.* 4th ed. Philadelphia: Saunders; 2004.

11. Gilroy AM. *Anatomy: An Essential Textbook.* New York: Thieme; 2013:107, 319, 324-326.

12. Brody LT, Irion J. The female athlete. In: Irion JM, Irion GL, eds. *Women's Health in Physical Therapy.* Philadelphia: Lippincott Williams & Wilkins; 2010.

13. Miller A, MacDougall J, Tarnopolsky M, et al. Gender differences in strength and muscle fiber characteristics. *Eur J Physiol.* 1993;66:254-262.

14. Huston L, Wojtys E. Neuromuscular performance characteristics in elite female athletes. *Am J Sports Med.* 1996;24:427-436.

15. Wojtys EM, Huston LJ, Schock HJ, et al. Gender differences in muscular protection of the knee in torsion in size-matched athletes. *J Bone Joint Surg Am.* 2003;85:782-789.

16. Granata KP, Wilson SE, Padua DA. Gender differences in active musculoskeletal stiffness. Part I. Quantification in controlled measurements of knee joint dynamics. *J Electromyogr Kinesiol.* 2002;12:119-126.

17. Granata KP, Padua DA, Wilson SE. Gender differences in active musculoskeletal stiffness. Part II. Quantification of leg stiffness during functional hopping tasks. *J Electromyogr Kinesiol.* 2002;12:127-135.

18. Boissonnault J, Stephenson RG. The obstetric patient. In: Boissonnault WG, ed. *Primary Care for the Physical Therapist Examination and Triage.* 2nd ed. St. Louis: Saunders; 2011.

19. Messelink B, Benson T, Berghmans B, et al. Standardization of terminology of pelvic floor muscle function and dysfunction: report from the pelvic floor clinical assessment group of the International Continence Society. *Neurourol Urodyn.* 2005;24:374-380.

20. Nelson P, Apte G, Justiz R III, et al. Chronic female pelvic pain. Part 2. Differential diagnosis and management. *Pain Pract.* 2012;12:111-141.

21. Frank J, Mistretta P, Will J. Diagnosis and treatment of female sexual dysfunction. *Am Fam Physician.* 2008;77:635-642.

22. Berman JR. Physiology of female sexual function and dysfunction. *Int J Impot Res.* 2005;17:544-551.

23. Travell J, Simons G. *Myofascial Pain and Dysfunction: The Trigger Point Manual.* 2nd ed. Philadelphia: Lippincott Williams & Wilkins; 1991.

24. Smith MD, Coppieters MW, Hodges PW. Postural response of the pelvic floor and abdominal muscles in women with and without incontinence. *Neurourol Urodyn.* 2007;26:377-385.

25. Whittaker J. Abdominal ultrasound imaging of pelvic floor muscle function in individuals with low back pain. *J Man Manip Ther.* 2004;12:44-49.

26. Claeys K, Dankaerts W, Janssens L, Brumagne S. Altered preparatory pelvic control during the sit-to-stance-to-sit movement in people with non-specific low back pain. *J Electromyogr Kinesiol.* 2012;22:821-828.

27. Cuthbert SC, Rosner AL. Conservative management of post-surgical urinary incontinence in an adolescent using applied kinesiology: a case report. *Altern Med Rev.* 2011;16:164-171.

28. Smith MD, Russell A, Hodges PW. Disorders of breathing and continence have a stronger association with back pain than obesity and physical activity. *Aust J Physiother.* 2006;52:11-16.

29. Bi X, Zhao J, Zhao L, et al. Pelvic floor muscle exercise for chronic low back pain. *J Int Med Res.* 2013;41:146-152.

30. Smith MD, Coppieters MW, Hodges PW. Is balance different in women with and without stress urinary incontinence? *Neurourol Urodyn.* 2008;27:71-78.

31. Sapsford R. Rehabilitation of pelvic floor muscles utilizing trunk stabilization. *Man Ther.* 2004;9:3-12.

32. Sapsford R, Richardson C, Stanton W. Sitting posture affects pelvic floor muscle activity in parous women: an observational study. *Aust J Physiother.* 2006;52:219-222.

33. Enseki KR, Kohlrieser D. Rehabilitation following hip arthroscopy: an evolving process. *Int J Sports Phys Ther.* 2014;9:765-773.

34. Rohde RS, Ziran BH. Obturator internus tendinitis as a source of chronic hip pain. *Orthopedics.* 2003;26:425-426.

35. Podshun L, Hanney WJ, Kolber MJ, et al. Differential diagnosis of deep gluteal pain in a female runner with pelvic involvement: a case report. *Int J Sports Phys Ther.* 2013;8:462-471.

36. Buss ML, Clinton SC. Pelvic floor functional and impairment limitations in a female with hip osteoarthritis. *Top Geriatr Rehabil.* 2013;29:239-245.

37. Weiss JM. Pelvic floor myofascial trigger points: manual therapy for interstitial cystitis and the urgency-frequency syndrome. *J Urol.* 2001;166:2226-2231.

38. Dommerholt J, Bron C, Franssen J. Myofascial trigger points: an evidence-informed review. *J Man Manip Ther.* 2006;14:203-221.

39. Pel JJM, Spoor CW, Pool-Goudzwaard AL, et al. Biomechanical analysis of reducing sacroiliac joint shear load by optimization of pelvic muscle and ligament forces. *Ann Biomed Eng.* 2008;36:415-424.

40. Vleeming A, Albert HB, Ostegaard HC, et al. European guidelines for the diagnosis and treatment of pelvic girdle pain. *Eur Spine J.* 2008;17:794-819.

41. Mens JM, Vleeming A, Snijders CJ, et al. Reliability and validity of the active straight leg raise test in posterior pelvic pain since pregnancy. *Spine (Phila Pa 1976)*. 2001;26:1167-1171.

42. Albert H, Godskesen M, Westergaard J. Evaluation of clinical tests used in classification procedures in pregnancy-related pelvic joint pain. *Eur Spine J*. 2000;9:161-166.

43. Ostgaard HC, Zetherstrom G, Roos-Hansen E, Svanberg G. The posterior pelvic pain provocation test in pregnant women. *Eur Spine J*. 1994;3:258-260.

44. Levangie PK. The association between static pelvic asymmetry and low back pain. *Spine (Phila Pa 1976)*. 1999;24:1234-1242.

45. Dietz HP, Lanzarone V. Vaginal delivery results in significant trauma to the levator ani muscle. *Obstet Gynecol*. 2005;106(4):707-712.

46. Apte G, Nelson P, Brismee J-M, et al. Chronic female pelvic pain. Part 1. Clinical pathoanatomy and examination of the pelvic region. *Pain Pract*. 2012;12:88-110.

47. Brown JS, Bradley CS, Subak LL, et al. The sensitivity and specificity of a simple test to distinguish between urge and stress urinary incontinence. *Ann Intern Med*. 2006;144:715-723.

48. Jull GA, Richardson CA. Motor control problems in patients with spinal pain: a new direction for therapeutic exercises. *J Manipulative Physiol Ther*. 2000;23:115-117.

49. Cresswell AG, Oddson L, Thorstensson A. The influence of sudden perturbations on trunk muscle activity and intra-abdominal pressure while standing. *Exp Brain Res*. 1994;98:336-341.

50. Hodges PW, Richardson AC. Contraction of the abdominal muscles associated with movement of the lower limb. *Phys Ther*. 1997;77:132.

51. Hodges PW, Richardson AC, Jull G. Evaluation of the relationship between laboratory and clinical tests of transversus abdominis function. *Physiother Res Int*. 1996;1:30-40.

52. Lee D. *The Pelvic Girdle*. 3rd ed. Edinburgh: Churchill Livingstone; 2004.

53. Critchley D. Instructing pelvic floor contraction facilitates transversus abdominis thickness increase during low-abdominal hollowing. *Physiother Res Int*. 2002;7:65-75.

54. Mens JM, Damen L, Snijders CJ, Stam HJ. The mechanical effect of a pelvic belt in patients with pregnancy-related pelvic pain. *Clin Biomech (Bristol, Avon)*. 2006;21:122-127.

55. Christensen LL, Djurhuus JC, Constantinou CE. Imaging of pelvic floor contractions using MRI. *Neurourol Urodyn*. 1995;14:209-216.

56. Kiesswetter H. EMG-patterns of pelvic floor muscles with surface electrodes. *Urol Int*. 1976;31:60-69.

57. Bo K, Lilleas F, Talseth T, et al. Dynamic MRI of the pelvic floor muscles in an upright sitting position. *Neurourol Urodyn*. 2001;20:167-174.

58. Tsao H, Hodges PW. Immediate changes in feedforward postural adjustments following voluntary motor training. *Exp Brain Res*. 2007;181:537-546.

59. Beith ID, Synnott RE, Newman SA. Abdominal muscle activity during the abdominal hollowing maneuver in the four point kneeling and prone positions. *Man Ther*. 2001;6:82-87.

60. American College of Obstetricians and Gynecologists Committee on Practice Bulletins (ACOGCPB-G). Chronic pelvic pain: clinical management guidelines for obstetricians-gynecologists. ACOG Practice Bulletin number 51. *Obstet Gynecol*. 2004;103:589-605.

61. Moseley L. Using visual illusion to reduce at-level neuropathic pain in paraplegia. *Pain*. 2007;130:294-298.

62. Hilton S, Vandyken C. The puzzle of pelvic pain: a rehabilitative framework for balancing tissue dysfunction and central sensitization. I. Pain physiology and evaluation for the physical therapist. *J Womens Health Phys Ther*. 2011;35:103-111.

63. Melzack R. Evolution of the neuromatrix theory of pain. *Pain Pract*. 2005;5:85-94.

64. Moseley L, Zalucki N, Birklein F, et al. Thinking about movement hurts: the effect of motor imagery on pain and swelling in people with chronic arm pain. *Arthritis Rheum*. 2008;59:623-631.

65. Moseley L. A pain neuromatrix approach to patients with chronic pain. *Man Ther*. 2003;8:130-140.

66. Butler D. *The Sensitive Nervous System*. Australia: Noigroup; 2000.

67. Hungerford B, Gilleard W, Hodges P. Evidence of altered lumbopelvic muscle recruitment in the presence of sacroiliac joint pain. *Spine (Phila Pa 1976)*. 2003;28:1593-1600.

68. De Andres J, Chaves S. Coccygodynia: a proposal for an algorithm for treatment. *J Pain*. 2003;4:257-266.

69. Kanakaris NK, Roberts CS, Giannoudis PV. Pregnancy-related pelvic girdle pain: an update. *BMC Med*. 2011;9:1-15.

70. Franklin ME, Conner-Kerr T. An analysis of posture and back pain in the first and third trimesters of pregnancy. *J Orthop Sports Phys Ther*. 1998;28:133-138.

71. Foti T. A biomechanical analysis of gait during pregnancy. *J Bone Joint Surg Am*. 2000;82:625-632.

72. Wu W. Gait coordination in pregnancy: transverse pelvic and thoracic rotations and their relative phase. *Clin Biomech (Bristol, Avon)*. 2004;19:480-488.

73. Spinarelli V. Hip fracture in a patient affected by transient osteoporosis of the femoral head during the last trimester of pregnancy. *Orthopedics*. 2009;32:385.

74. Stephenson RG, O'Connor LJ. *Obstetric and Gynecologic Care in Physical Therapy*. 2nd ed. Thorofare, NJ: Slack; 2000.

75. Morkved S. Evidence for pelvic floor physical therapy for urinary incontinence during pregnancy and after childbirth. In: Bo K, Berghmans B, Morkved S, Van Kampen M, eds. *Evidence-Based Physical Therapy for the Pelvic Floor*. Philadelphia: Elsevier; 2007.

76. Morkved S. Pelvic floor muscle strength and thickness in continent and incontinent nulliparous pregnant women. *Int Urogynecol J Pelvic Floor Dysfunct*. 2003;15:384-390.

77. Reilly ET, Freeman RM, Waterfield MR, et al. Prevention of postpartum stress incontinence in primigravidae with increased bladder neck mobility: a randomized controlled trial of antenatal pelvic floor exercises. *BJOG*. 2002;109:68-76.

78. Sampselle CM. Effect of pelvic muscle exercise on transient incontinence during pregnancy and after birth. *Obstet Gynecol*. 1998;91:406-412.

79. Hay-Smith J, Morkved S, Fairbrother KA, Herbison GP. Pelvic floor muscle training for prevention and treatment of urinary and faecal incontinence in antenatal and postnatal women. *Cochrane Database Syst Rev*. 2009;(4):CD007471.

80. Bo K, Morkved S, Frawley H, Sherburn M. Evidence for benefit of transversus abdominis training alone or in combination with pelvic floor muscle training to treat female urinary incontinence: a systematic review. *Neurourol Urodyn*. 2009;28:368-373.

81. Hacker NF, Moore JG. *Essentials of Obstetrics and Gynecology.* Philadelphia: Saunders; 1986.

82. Figuers C. *A study of postpartum women: description of reported health issues within the first three months post-pregnancy.* Poster presented at: American Physical Therapy Association Combined Sections Meeting; February 7, 2004; Nashville, TN.

83. Ostgaard HC, Anderson GB. Postpartum low-back pain. *Spine (Phila Pa 1976).* 1992;17:53-55.

84. Ostgaard HC. Back pain in relation to pregnancy: a 6-year follow up. *Spine (Phila Pa 1976).* 1997;22:2945-2950.

85. Larsen EC, Wilken-Jensen C, Hansen A, et al. Symptom-giving pelvic girdle relaxation in pregnancy. I. Prevalence and risk factors. *Acta Obstet Gynecol Scand.* 1999;78:105-110.

86. Albert H, Godskesen M, Westergaard J. Prognosis in four syndromes of pregnancy-related pelvic pain. *Acta Obstet Gynecol Scand.* 2001;80:505-510.

87. Gutke A, Josefsson A, Oberg B. Pelvic girdle pain and lumbar pain in relation to postpartum depressive symptoms. *Spine (Phila Pa 1976).* 2007;32:1430-1436.

88. Parker MA, Millar LA, Dugan SA. Diastasis rectus abdominis and lumbo-pelvic pain and dysfunction: are they related? *J Womens Health Phys Ther.* 2009;33:15-22.

89. Brown JS, Grady D, Ouslander JG, et al. Prevalence of urinary incontinence and associated risk factors in postmenopausal women. *Obstet Gynecol.* 1999;94:66-70.

90. Rortveit G, Subak LL, Thom DH, et al. Urinary incontinence, fecal incontinence and pelvic organ prolapse in a population-based, racially diverse cohort: prevalence and risk factors. *Female Pelvic Med Reconstr Surg.* 2010;16:278-283.

91. Rortveit G, Brown J, Thom DH, et al. Symptomatic pelvic organ prolapse: prevalence and risk factors in a population-based, racially diverse cohort. *Obstet Gynecol.* 2007;109:1396-1403.

92. Slieker-ten Hove MC, Pool-Goudzwaard AL, Eijkemans MJ, et al. Symptomatic pelvic organ prolapse and possible risk factors in a general population. *Am J Obstet Gynecol.* 2009;200:184.e1-184.e7.

93. Whitcomb EL, Rortveit G, Brown JS, et al. Racial differences in pelvic organ prolapse. *Obstet Gynecol.* 2009;114:1271-1277.

94. Sze EH, Sherard GB 3rd, Dolezal JM. Pregnancy, labor, delivery, and pelvic organ prolapse. *Obstet Gynecol.* 2002;100:981-986.

95. Glazener CM, Abdalla MI, Russell IT, Templeton AA. Postnatal care: a survey of patients' experiences. *Br J Midwifery.* 1993;1:67-74.

96. Glazener CM, Abdalla MI, Straud P, et al. Postnatal maternal morbidity: extent, causes, prevention, and treatment. *Br J Obstet Gynaecol.* 1995;102:282-287.

97. Smith AR, Hosker GL, Warrell DW. The role of pudendal nerve damage in the aetiology of genuine stress incontinence in women. *Br J Obstet Gynaecol.* 1989;96:29-32.

98. Madill SJ, McLean L. A contextual model of pelvic floor muscle defects in female stress urinary incontinence: a rationale for physiotherapy treatment. *Ann N Y Acad Sci.* 2007;1101:335-360.

99. Agarwal P, Rosenburg ML. Neurological evaluation of urinary incontinence in the female patient. *Neurologist.* 2003;9:110-117.

100. Tunn R, Paris S, Fischer W, et al. Static magnetic resonance imaging of the pelvic floor muscle morphology in women with stress urinary incontinence and pelvic prolapse. *Neurourol Urodyn.* 1998;17:579-589.

101. Allen RE, Hosker GL, Smith AR, et al. Pelvic floor damage and childbirth: a neurophysiological study. *Br J Obstet Gynaecol.* 1990;72:S15-S17.

102. Benson JT. Neurophysiologic control of lower urinary tract. *Obstet Gynecol Clin North Am.* 1989;16:733-752.

103. Washington-Cannon T, Damaser MS. Pathophysiology of the lower urinary tract: continence and incontinence. *Clin Obstet Gynecol.* 2004;47:28-35.

104. Signorello LB, Harlow BL, Chekos AK, Repke JT. Postpartum sexual functioning and its relationship to perineal trauma: a retrospective cohort study of primiparous women. *Am J Obstet Gynecol.* 2001;184:881-888.

105. Rowland M, Foxcroft L, Homman WM, Patel R. Breastfeeding and sexuality immediately postpartum. *Can Fam Physician.* 2005;51:1366-1367.

106. Morof D, Barrett G, Peacock J, et al. Postnatal depression and sexual health after childbirth. *Obstet Gynecol.* 2003;102:1318-1325.

107. Giacalone P-L, Daures J-P, Vignal J, et al. Pfannenstiel versus Maylard incision for Cesarean delivery: a randomized controlled trial. *Obstet Gynecol.* 2002;99:745-750.

108. Burgio K, Zyczynski J, Locher J, et al. Urinary incontinence in the 12-month postpartum period. *Obstet Gynecol.* 2003;102:1291-1298.

109. Noble E. *Essential Exercises for the Childbearing Year.* Boston: Houghton Mifflin; 1988.

110. LaPorta Krum L, del Fin M, Ford R, et al. Effect of conservative physical therapy management status post cesarean section: a randomized control group design. *J Womens Health Phys Ther.* 2006;30:27-28.

111. Mayo Clinic Staff. *C-section: what you can expect.* <www.mayoclinic.org/tests-procedures/c-section/basics/what-you-can-expect/prc-20014571/>; Accessed September 5, 2015.

112. Lee D, Lee LJ, McLaughlin L. Stability, continence and breathing: the role of fascia in both function and dysfunction and the potential consequences following pregnancy and delivery. *J Body Mov Ther.* 2007;12:333-348.

113. Berghmans LC, Hendricks HJ, Bo K, et al. Conservative treatment of stress urinary incontinence in women: a systematic review of randomized clinical trials. *Br J Urol.* 1998;82:181-191.

114. Chiarelli P, Murphy B, Cockburn J. Promoting urinary continence in postpartum women: 12-month follow-up data from a randomized controlled trial. *Int Urogynecol.* 2004;15:99-105.

115. Bo K. Pelvic floor muscle training is effective in treatment of female stress urinary incontinence, but how does it work? *Int Urogynecol.* 2004;15:76-84.

116. Bo K, Hagen R, Kvarstein B, et al. Pelvic floor muscle exercise for the treatment of female stress urinary incontinence. III. Effects of two different degrees of pelvic floor muscle exercises. *Neurourol Urodyn.* 1990;9:489-502.

117. Lagro-Janssen TL, Debruyne FM, Smits AJ, van Weel C. Controlled trial of pelvic floor exercises in the treatment of urinary stress incontinence in general practice. *Br J Gen Pract.* 1991;41:445-449.

118. Bo K, Stien R. Needle EMG registration of striated urethral wall and pelvic floor muscle activity patterns during cough, Valsalva, abdominal, hip adductor, and gluteal muscle contractions in nulliparous healthy females. *Neurourol Urodyn.* 1994;13:35-41.

119. Deindl FM, Vodusek DB, Hesse U, et al. Activity patterns of pubococcygeal muscles in nulliparous continent women. *Br J Urol.* 1993;72:46-51.

120. Miller JM, Ashton-Miller JA, DeLancey JO. A pelvic muscle precontraction can reduce cough-related urine loss in selected women with mild SUI. *J Am Geriatr Soc.* 1998;46:870-874.

121. Yang A, Mostwin JL, Rosenshein NB, et al. Pelvic floor descent in women: dynamic evaluation with fast MR imaging and cinematic display. *Radiology.* 1991;179:25-33.

122. American Board of Physical Therapy Specialties (ABPTS). *ABPTS certified specialists statistics. Updated 8/27/2014.* <http://www.abpts.org/About/Statistics/>; Accessed September 5, 2015.

123. American Board of Physical Therapy Residency and Fellowship Education (ABPTRFE). *Directory of residency programs.* <http://www.abptrfe.org/apta/abptrfe/Directory.aspx?navID=10737432672/>; Accessed September 5, 2015.

124. Cox JL, Holden JM, Sagovsky R. Detection of postnatal depression: development of the 10-item Edinburgh postnatal depression scale. *Br J Psychiatry.* 1987;150:782-786.

125. Stratford P, Gill C, Westaway M, Binkley J. Assessing disability and change on individual patients: a report of a patient specific measure. *Physiother Can.* 1995;47:258-263.

126. Grotle M, Garratt AM, Krogstad Jenssen H, Stuge B. Reliability and construct validity of self-report questionnaires for patients with pelvic girdle pain. *Phys Ther.* 2012;92:111-123.

127. Stuge B, Garratt A, Krogstad Jenssen H, Grotle M. The Pelvic Girdle Questionnaire: a condition-specific instrument for assessing activity limitations and symptoms in people with pelvic girdle pain. *Phys Ther.* 2011;91:1096-1108.

128. Barber MD, Walters MD, Bump RC. Short forms of two condition-specific quality-of-life questionnaires for women with pelvic floor disorders (PFDI-20 and PFIQ-7). *Am J Obstet Gynecol.* 2005;193:103-113.

129. Tannenbaum C, Brouillette J, Michaud J, et al. Responsiveness and clinical utility of the geriatric self-efficacy index for urinary incontinence. *J Am Geriatr Soc.* 2009;57:470-475.

130. Cotterill N, Norton C, Avery KN, et al. Psychometric evaluation of a new patient-completed questionnaire for evaluating anal incontinence symptoms and impact on quality of life: the ICIQ-B. *Dis Colon Rectum.* 2011;54:1235-1250.

131. Agachan F, Chen T, Pfeifer J, et al. A constipation scoring system to simplify evaluation and management of constipated patients. *Dis Colon Rectum.* 1996;39:681-685.

132. Bakx R, Sprangers MA, Oort FJ, et al. Development and validation of a colorectal functional outcome questionnaire. *Int J Colorectal Dis.* 2005;20:126-136.

133. Rosen R, Brown C, Heiman J, et al. The Female Sexual Function Index (FSFI): a multidimensional self-report instrument for the assessment of female sexual function. *J Sex Marital Ther.* 2000;26:191-208.

10

Influence of Lumbosacral Disorders on the Differential Diagnosis of Hip Pain

WILLIAM J. HANNEY AND MOREY J. KOLBER

CHAPTER OUTLINE

Anatomy and Pain

Up to 84% of adults will experience an episode of low back pain (LBP) at some point in their lifetime.[1] Clinically, the term low back pain is often a misnomer because disorders arising from the lumbosacral region may manifest with a wide array of pain referral patterns, inclusive of both somatic and radicular presentations. From a pain referral perspective and integral to this chapter's purpose is the understanding that lumbosacral disorders may manifest as hip or pelvic pain. In addition, evidence suggests that hip and lumbosacral disorders may coexist, further confounding the diagnostic process.[2,3] Thus, clinicians and researchers alike must be cognizant of the multifactorial etiology of pain when evaluating a patient with a presumed hip disorder.

The potential for lumbosacral disorders to masquerade as hip pain along with the prevalence of coexisting hip and spine disorders may lead to diagnostic uncertainty and omissions of care in certain instances. Although most clinicians would surmise that a diagnostically elusive hip examination should steer the assessment process toward potential referral sources such as the lumbosacral spine, the precise cause of the pain may be clinically occult to clinicians without a sound diagnostic acumen. Thus, a clear model for the differential diagnosis of hip pain would seemingly be a valuable tool for both the beginning and advancing clinician's armamentarium.

The goal of steering the examination toward a valid pathoanatomic etiology has implications for quality of care, prognosis, treatment emphasis, and wiser allocation of scarce health care resources. With rising health care costs and the realization of visit restrictions, the clinician's diagnostic acumen will undoubtedly be the requisite skill set for promptly identifying the problem at hand and steering care. The consequence of misdiagnosis can lead to delayed care, which has both economic (e.g., unnecessary tests and interventions) and clinical consequences (e.g., persistent symptoms). Inarguably, a clinical methodology for discerning referred lumbosacral symptoms from hip disease should facilitate a more accurate diagnosis and timely recovery by directing appropriate treatment and evaluative measures.

Accordingly, this chapter presents a reductionist approach to the differential diagnosis of hip pain among patients with suspected lumbosacral disorders. A primer for signs and symptoms suggestive of the need for evaluating neighboring lumbosacral disease is first introduced. Subsequently, evidence-based symptom referral patterns and clinical predictors are presented for the more common lumbosacral disorders that may manifest as hip pain. Finally, case studies are used at the chapter conclusion to provide the reader an opportunity to synthesize the information into clinically relevant scenarios. On conclusion of this chapter, the reader will have a broader understanding of the multifaceted considerations to be made when evaluating patients with presumed hip disorders of uncertain etiology.

Anatomy and Pain Patterns

The neuromuscular and skeletal anatomy of the lumbosacral spine is intricate, and a baseline level of knowledge is necessary to understand the pain patterns and referral sources discussed in this chapter. Although this chapter introduces basic anatomic concepts associated with more common pathoanatomic conditions stemming from the lumbosacral spine, a more detailed review of lumbosacral anatomy is presented in Chapter 1. Recognizing relevant anatomic structures and their contribution to the clinical presentation (e.g., potential for pain and associated referral patterns) serves as a requisite cognitive attribute for the clinical differentiation of pain. Although limitations may be ascribed to using a rigid pathoanatomic model for treatment (e.g., pain is a multidimensional impairment), a substantial body of evidence exists to highlight the diagnostic utility of this approach. Thus, considerable efforts were undertaken in this chapter to connect pain patterns with their associated pathoanatomic tissues.

Pain Behavior

The topic of pain behavior may refer to the multiple dimensions of pain including, but not limited to, quantity, quality, location, and response to the examination. Variability exists among different anatomic tissues with regard to pain prevalence, location, referral patterns, and response to the examination. This variability aids the assessment process and, when combined with a familiarity of evidence-based diagnostic testing clusters, may lend insight into the underlying cause of the clinical presentation. Most clinicians would agree that an understanding of the potential sources of lumbosacral disorders and their associated behaviors (e.g., referral patterns) may be useful in steering the clinician toward an accurate diagnosis. Thus, the primary focus of this section is to present an overview of pain behaviors in the context of recognizing a lumbosacral disorder manifesting as hip pain.

Pain emanating from the lumbosacral spine and referred to a neighboring or distal location is often classified as either somatic or radicular, depending on the pathoanatomic origin. Somatic sources of pain can be divided into superficial and deep components. These sources include structures such as the skin, superficial fascia, tendon sheaths, and periosteum.[4] Deep somatic pain stems from pathologic conditions and may include structures such as the periosteum, cancellous bone, disk, nerves, muscles, tendons, ligaments, and blood vessels.[4] Somatic referred pain is created by stimulation of nerve endings within the superficial and deep somatic structures.[4] Somatic structures tend to have a consistent clinical presentation and are generally described as dull, aching, gnawing, or diffuse. Patients with somatic pain generally have an absence of neurologic signs and symptoms (e.g., paresthesia, focal weakness, hypoactive deep tendon reflexes, loss of sensation) because the symptoms are generated from the nerve endings, rather than from compression of individual spinal nerves or nerve roots. Deep somatic pain tends to cause unique clinical presentations in that it is poorly localized and may be referred superficially or distally. Unique to deep somatic pain is the possibility of associated autonomic phenomenon such as sweating, pallor, or even changes in pulse and blood pressure.[4]

Neuropathic pain stems from chemical or mechanical stimuli to the peripheral or central nervous system. Neuropathic pain can occur from injury to peripheral nerves, dorsal root ganglia, pathways in the spinal cord, or neurons located in the brain. Symptoms stemming from the neurologic system are unique because pain is not caused by stimulation of nociceptors, but instead results from malfunction or mechanical trauma of the nervous system itself. Disturbances in afferent and efferent transmission of nervous signals may produce changes in sensory and motor function. Neuropathic pain or symptoms that stem from mechanical or chemical irritation of the spinal nerve or nerve root often have a distinct presentation and are considered to be radicular (e.g., radiculopathy).

Radicular symptoms generally have a consistent qualitative (e.g., sharp, shooting, burning, paresthetic) and physiologic (e.g., location) pattern. Compression, aberrant traction, or chemical irritation of a particular nerve root often manifests in a symptom referral pattern (e.g., dermatome) consistent with the nerve's sensory distribution (see Fig. 10-2) that may, in some cases, refer to a region of the hip (e.g., L1 nerve root compression referred to groin and anterior proximal thigh). Qualitative descriptors that are pathognomonic of a neural origin include tingling (e.g., paresthesia) or an electric shock type of sensation. Moreover, compression of spinal nerve roots may, in some cases, lead to focal myotomal weakness and other neurologic signs such as hypoactive deep tendon reflexes and sensory anesthesia. Neuropathic pain may not respond to medications typically used for somatic disorders such as opiates or narcotics.

The diagnostic challenge to the clinician resides in the intimate association between both somatic and neurogenic (radicular) sources of pain in the hip and lumbosacral complex. To complicate the situation further, it is not uncommon for patients to present with symptoms stemming from both the somatic and neurologic systems concurrently or, in many cases, simultaneous hip and lumbar disorders. For example, a lumbar disk herniation compressing the L2 nerve root would produce focal somatic pain in the right lower back in an oblique pattern from the lower back to the groin or proximal medial thigh. The somatic pain may be described as dull, whereas the nerve root compression may be described as shooting and could be associated with paresthesias. Concurrent pathologic conditions and the potential for pain pattern overlap from lumbosacral referral, and hip disorders may confound the diagnostic process when the clinician is unfamiliar with pain behavior. Fortunately, a substantial body of evidence exists on lumbosacral pain behavior to help steer clinicians toward a more precise diagnosis.[5-9]

Pain Location

The location of a patient's pain may provide insight into the pathoanatomic cause of the problem. Evidence suggests that structures from the hip and lumbosacral spine have recognizable pain patterns with regard to location and response to the examination.[7-10] Supplementary to pain location, symptom response to testing may provide greater insight into the underlying origin. Symptom response to the examination may be classified into the following three categories: concordant reproduction (e.g., test or activity reproduces specific symptoms that parallel patient report), an absent response, or a change in location. From a simplistic perspective, one could, with reasonable certainty, recognize that pain reproduced with hip or lumbosacral movements originates from the hip or lumbosacral spine, respectively. However, a shortcoming to this approach resides in concurrent movements at the hip and lumbosacral spine. Nevertheless, this simplistic logic should not be overlooked because it should prove useful when combined with an understanding of pain behavior and evidence-based testing clusters known to support the diagnostic process.

> The presence of paresthesias or pain described as shooting or burning that follows a dermatomal path is pathognomonic of a neuropathic etiology. Sources of lumbosacral radiculopathy should be investigated in such cases. More common sources of lumbosacral radiculopathy include foraminal stenosis and disk disorders.

The evidence showing that anatomic structures have a defined pain location and referral pattern stems from studies of a descriptive nature of inquiry as well as those comparing clinical patterns of lumbosacral pain by using advanced evaluative measures. In regard to the lumbosacral spine, a substantial body of evidence has been gleaned from investigations comparing clinical patterns (e.g., pain behavior and physical testing) with the results of advanced evaluative measures such as diagnostic injections or provocative

TABLE 10-1	Tissue Origin of Low Back Pain	
Tissue	**Anatomic Site of Pain**
Lumbar fascia*	Low back pain along the central region or site of vessel-nerve perforation
Paravertebral muscle*	Localized low back pain only, primarily at the site of bone attachment or vessel-nerve perforation
Posterior longitudinal ligament	Central low back pain
Facet capsule*	Localized low back pain with occasional buttock referral
Posterior dura	Buttock and leg
Anterior dura	Back and buttock
Compressed nerve root	Buttock, leg, and foot
Central annulus	Central low back
Central lateral annulus	Ipsilateral low back
Vertebral end plate	Back

Modified from Kuslich SD, Ulstrom CL, Michael CJ. The tissue origin of low back pain and sciatica: a report of pain response to tissue stimulation during operations on the lumbar spine using local anesthesia. *Orthop Clin North Am.* 1991;22(2):181-187.
*Rarely produced pain.

diskography.[6-8,11-13] Additional insight into pain location and referral patterns has been recognized from investigations performed during the course of surgical procedures in which structures are noxiously stimulated or mechanically provoked.[5]

Kuslich and colleagues[5] evaluated the tissue origin of LBP and sciatica in 193 consecutive patients undergoing surgical procedures. In the aforementioned investigation, the investigators sought to evaluate potential sources of pain, pain patterns, and location. The most common sources of pain included the outer portion of the annulus fibrosis, nerve roots, vertebral end plate, and dura matter. Table 10-1 summarizes the sources of pain, as well as the more common pain location and referral patterns for each of the tested tissues. In summary, the investigators reported that the annulus fibrosis, when stimulated, produced local LBP on the ipsilateral side. Thus, noxious chemical or mechanical stimulation of the annulus, as seen in diskogenic disorders, would lead to ipsilateral pain. Moreover, central annulus stimulation induced central pain. The posterior dura matter, which may be noxiously engaged with degenerative changes, produced LBP, as well as referred pain into the lower extremity excluding the foot. The anterior dura matter, a potential site of compression from disk disease, produced local lumbar and buttock pain only. The facet joints were a less common source of pain; however, when present, they produced local LBP at the region of stimulation (e.g., focal and ipsilateral), which occasionally referred into the buttock region as a result of capsular stimulation. Nerve roots, when noxiously compressed, produced lower extremity symptoms that referred into the foot. Muscular, facet, or diskogenic tissues would not be expected to produce thigh, leg, or foot symptoms unless contact with the dura or nerve root is present. Of particular clinical importance to the differential diagnosis process is that in the aforementioned study only the nerve root produced symptoms into the foot; thus, a radicular pattern or pain pattern that traveled into the leg and foot would invariably imply nerve root compression or irritation.

In addition to the data provided by Kuslich and associates, several studies investigated pain patterns associated with the more common lumbosacral disorders using diagnostic gold standards (e.g., diskography and diagnostic anesthetic blocks).[6-8,11-13] Specifically, pain patterns arising from the facet and sacroiliac joints, intervertebral disk, and nerve root compression syndromes were reported.

Facet joint disease, independent of the stenosis sequela (degenerated facet joints causing stenosis), is thought to produce pain from the capsule, with symptoms commonly reported as ipsilateral or asymmetrical LBP that may radiate into the gluteal (buttock) region and that could be mistaken for sacroiliac or proximal hamstring disorders.[7,8,14] Pain from the facet joint rarely refers into the lower extremity; however, in cases of referral, the pattern is somatic and does not follow a particular dermatomal path or refer into the foot.[5,7] Moreover, facet joint pain would not be expected to be associated with nerve root symptoms such as paresthesia or neurologic signs such as motor weakness or sensory anesthesia.

Pain arising from the sacroiliac joint is often located in the buttock region (below L5) with a majority of patients pointing to a region within 2 cm of the posterior superior iliac spine (Fig. 10-1).[7,8,15] Sacroiliac joint pain is primarily unilateral and is rarely an independent source of pain below the knee.[5-9]

Diskogenic pain from the lumbar spine, unlike the facet and sacroiliac joint, is highly variable and depends on whether the disk itself has intimate contact with neighboring tissues. Diskogenic pain is predominantly reported in the lower back, focal to the site of involvement. Evidence suggests that central disk disorders would produce central LBP, with right-sided disk disease producing focal right LBP.[5,8] Sources of referred pain from diskogenic disorders seem interdependent on the affected tissue, whereas disk protrusion compressing a nerve root would be expected to cause back and buttock pain, as well as symptoms in the leg and foot, representative of the particular nerve root pattern of innervation. Unique to diskogenic disorders is the concept of variable pain patterns often referred to as centralization and peripheralization.[7,8] Centralization occurs when symptoms move from distal to a more proximal location,[16] and it tends to be a positive prognostic indicator because it implies a clinical presentation amena-

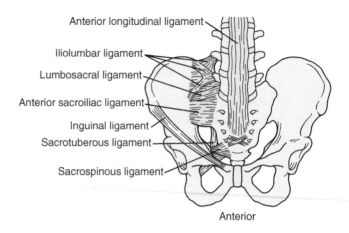

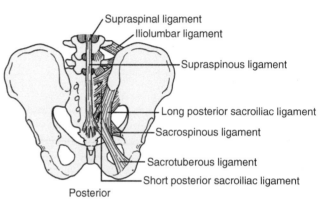

• **Figure 10-1** Sacroiliac Joint Pain Location. (From Magee DJ. *Orthopedic Physical Assessment.* 6th ed. St. Louis: Saunders; 2014.)

ble to treatment.[17] Peripheralization, conversely, occurs when symptoms extend or move in a distal manner[16] and is generally a poor prognostic indicator.[17] More serious disk disease, such as extrusions or large protrusions compressing a nerve root, are more likely to peripheralize in response to interventions. From a clinical perspective, it would seem logical that right-sided diskogenically induced LBP pain that peripheralizes into the foot with movement or over time is suggestive of a morphologic change (e.g., progression from a bulge to a protrusion or extrusion) suggestive of nerve root irritation. Conversely, centralization may imply resolution of intimate contact between the disk and neighboring tissue or a more anatomic relocation of a displaced nucleus.[11,18,19]

Although nerve root or dorsal root ganglia irritation from a chemical or mechanical means is indeed a source of pain, each nerve root generally manifests with a unique symptom location that allows clinicians to discern the location of the disorder (Table 10-2). Other than symptom patterns, the presence of neurologic signs such as hypoactive deep tendon reflexes, diminished sensation, and motor impairments alludes to a nerve root disorder.[20] The etiology of nerve root–related pain is multifactorial, and in the case of pain referring into the hip, this pain is often the result of a lumbar disk herniation or foraminal stenosis present at the upper lumbar spine. The following

TABLE 10-2	Physical Examination Findings for Lumbar Segmental Nerve Root Lesions		
Level	**Myotome**	**Dermatome**	**Reflexes**
T12	None	Lower abdominal and inguinal area	None
L1	None	Back, anterior thigh, as well as medial upper thigh	None
L2	Psoas and hip adductors	Back to anterolateral to proximal medial thigh	None
L3	Psoas and quadriceps	Back, upper buttock to anterior and medial thigh to knee	Diminished or absent patellar reflex
L4	Tibialis anterior and extensor hallucis	Medial buttock, lateral thigh to medial lower leg and medial aspect of foot	Diminished or absent patellar reflex
L5	Extensor hallucis, peroneals, gluteus medius, and dorsiflexors	Buttock, posterior and lateral thigh to anterolateral aspect of leg to the dorsum of foot	None
S1	Ankle plantar flexors, hamstrings, and peroneals	Buttock, thigh, and posterior leg and lateral foot	Diminished or absent Achilles reflex
S2 to S4	Diminished control of the pelvic floor muscles contributing to inhibited control of bowel and bladder control	Perineum, genitals, and lower sacrum	Absent or diminished anal wink

section outlines the expected clinical presentation of the various nerve roots that may be affected in patients with lumbosacral disorders.

Nerve Root Lesions

Nerve root lesions of the lower thoracic and lumbar spine typically refer pain distally into the hip, thigh, lower leg, and foot[5] (Fig. 10-2). Symptoms distributed in these regions may give the impression of hip pain in some cases; however, a clear description of referral patterns for each nerve root may provide the clinician with insight into potential sources of pain. Moreover, nerve root lesions produce a host of signs and symptoms (paresthesia, myotomal weakness, sensory disturbance) not commonly encountered in hip disorders. When a nerve root is chemically irritated or mechanically compressed in the absence of neurapraxia or axonotmesis (temporary or more permanent loss of conduction with degeneration), only nerve root symptoms would be expected during the clinical examination.

T12 Nerve Root Lesion

The twelfth thoracic nerve root exits between the twelfth thoracic and first lumbar vertebrae. Nerve lesions at this level often refer symptoms from the midback coursing around the torso to the lower abdominal region. Ventrally, the symptoms would manifest proximal to the iliac crest to the region just superior to the public symphysis (see Fig. 10-2, A). Generally, no myotomes or deep tendon reflexes are attributed to this level. A key differentiating factor here is the pain pattern. Symptoms associated with thoracic nerve root disorders manifest around the thorax at the approximate level of the lesion.

L1 Lumbar Nerve Root Lesion

The first lumbar nerve root exits between the first and second lumbar vertebrae. A lesion of the first lumbar nerve root would refer symptoms from the midback, around the torso to the lower abdominal region and proximal medial thigh. Ventral symptoms would reside over the pubic symphysis (see Fig. 10-2, B). Generally, no myotomes or deep tendon reflexes are attributed to this level.

L2 Lumbar Nerve Root Lesion

The second nerve root exits between the second and third lumbar vertebrae. A lesion at this level would refer symptoms from the midback, around the torso to the proximal anterior and medial thigh (see Fig. 10-2, C). Examination may reveal weakness of the psoas and hip adductors.

L3 Lumbar Nerve Root Lesion

A third lumbar nerve root lesion often refers symptoms along the midlumbar spine that extend to the upper buttock, coursing in an oblique pattern to anterior and medial thigh, ending at the knee medial to the patella (see Fig. 10-2, D). Examination findings may include a weakness of the psoas and quadriceps, as well as diminished patellar tendon reflexes.

L4 Lumbar Nerve Root Lesion

The L4 nerve root exits between the fourth and fifth vertebrae. Patients with a fourth lumbar nerve root lesion may describe pain located in the midlumbar spine, outer thigh, and leg extending to the medial foot and great toe (see Fig. 10-2, E). They may also demonstrate weakness of the tibialis anterior and possibly great toe extension. Furthermore, the patellar tendon reflex may be diminished or absent.

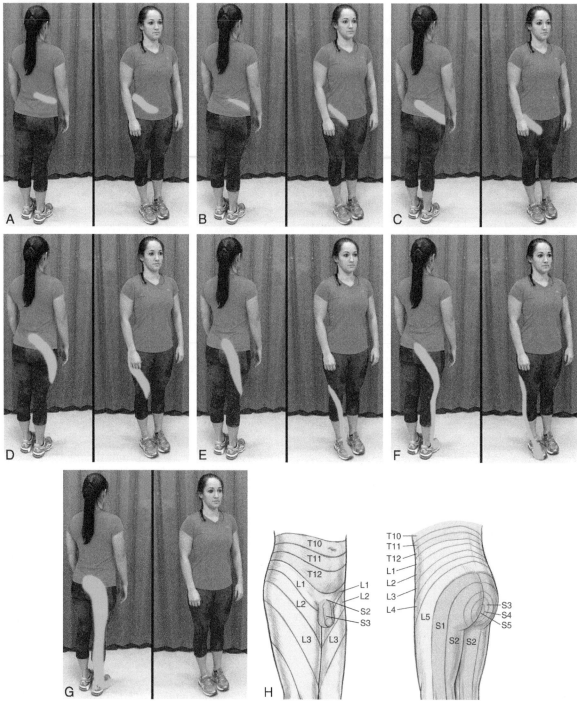

• **Figure 10-2** Referred Pain Patterns for Lumbar Nerve Root Lesions. **A,** T12. **B,** L1. **C,** L2. **D,** L3. **E,** L4. **F,** L5. **G,** S1. **H,** S2 to S4. (**H,** From Brown DL. *Atlas of Regional Anesthesia.* 4th ed. Philadelphia: Saunders; 2010.)

L5 Lumbar Nerve Root Lesion

The L5 nerve root lies between L5 and the first sacral vertebra. Patients with a fifth lumbar nerve root lesion generally describe pain in the sacroiliac region, as well as the lower buttock, lateral thigh, down to the anterolateral leg and dorsum of foot excluding the first and fifth toes (see Fig. 10-2, *F*). Weakness of the extensor hallucis longus, peroneals, gluteus medius, and dorsiflexor muscles may be present.

S1 Nerve Root Lesion

First sacral nerve root lesions refer symptoms, which may be described as low back and buttock pain that extends to the plantar aspect of the foot and heel (see Fig. 10-2, *G*). On examination, myotomal weakness of the gastrocnemius-soleus complex, peroneals, and hamstring muscles may be identified. On further examination, the patient may also have atrophy of the gluteal and intrinsic foot muscles, as well as hypoesthesia of the calf and lateral foot. The Achilles deep tendon reflex may be diminished or absent.

S2 to S4 Nerve Root Lesion

Although a lesion of the second, third, or fourth sacral nerve root is rare, it may be present as a result of disk herniations, cyst formation, malignant disease, or trauma. These lesions are often described as pain in the lower sacral or peritoneal and genital area (see Fig. 10-2, *H*). In addition, patients may describe saddle paresthesia and demonstrate a diminished or absent anal wink. Irrespective of the specific diagnosis, neuropathic pain manifests as radiculopathy, and each nerve root has a relatively consistent clinical presentation, as outlined in Table 10-2.

Changes in bowel or bladder function, as well as saddle region sensory changes, are pathognomonic for cauda equina syndrome. Cauda equina syndrome, when suspected, is a medical emergency because of the potential for incomplete neurologic recovery. Patients suspected of having cauda equina syndrome should be referred for emergency medical care immediately. Depending on the cause of symptoms, patients may benefit from surgical intervention to relieve pressure on the involved nerve root. Ahn and colleagues[21] published a metaanalysis of surgical outcomes after cauda equina syndrome secondary to lumbar disk herniation. When disk herniation was involved, the most common levels were L1 to L2 (27%), L3 to L4 (26%), and L5 to S1 (22%), whereas levels least often involved were L4 to L5 (16%) and L2 to L3 (9%). The findings of this study reinforce the importance of immediate medical care. A significant difference was found when comparing patients receiving surgical decompression before and after the 48-hour mark. Patients who underwent surgical treatment within 48 hours demonstrated greater resolution of sensory and motor deficits, as well as better urinary and rectal function.

Further to pain location, changes in response to testing may assist in the clinical evaluation and decision-making process. As stated previously, activity isolated to a particular region that provokes concordant symptom reproduction adds to the diagnostic process from a face validity perspective. Moreover, symptoms originating from the lumbar spine that change in response to movement may provide insight into the cause. Primary reference to a change in symptoms in response to testing involves the concepts of centralization and peripheralization, which are invariably linked to diskogenic disorders.[11] Patients with spinal stenosis are more likely to peripheralize with extension or ipsilateral lumbar flexion and to report symptom resolution with lumbar flexion or contralateral lateral flexion. More importantly, when a patient's symptoms centralize or peripheralize in response to lumbar movements, the clinician may eliminate hip disease as the source of symptoms. Furthermore, evidence suggests that symptoms arising from the sacroiliac joint and facet disorders neither peripheralize nor centralize in response to movements.[7]

Although pain sources and associated referral patterns have been defined in the literature, clinicians should not solely rely on location (in lieu of a prudent clinical examination) as their source for diagnosis because overlap exists. The next section of this chapter presents clinical characteristics for the more common sources of lumbosacral disorders that may refer pain to the hip and pelvis. Although a baseline discussion of pathologic features for each condition is given, the objectives reside in providing content imperative to the differential diagnosis. A discussion of interventions for treating lumbosacral conditions is beyond the scope of this chapter.

Lumbosacral Conditions

The differential diagnosis of pelvic and hip disorders is often complicated by competing pathologic conditions with a similar pain referral location, as well the prevalence of concurrent disease. This section discusses selected lumbosacral disorders that should be considered when a patient presents with hip pain and the underlying cause is not clear. Information is provided in the context of the differential diagnosis of lumbosacral disorders from an evidence-based perspective using studies that are inclusive of diagnostic reference standards where applicable. In cases where there is a paucity of evidence, a pragmatic approach grounded in biologic plausibility is presented.

Trigger Points and Myofascial Pain

Although evidence from pain pattern and diagnostic studies rarely implicate muscle or fascia as a source of chronic pain, muscle or fascia is nevertheless an established source of clinical symptoms. Some reports suggest (based on the clinical examination) that approximately 85% of the population will report myofascial pain during their lifetime.[22] Myofascial pain syndrome (MPS) is characterized by the presence of a myofascial trigger point, which has been defined as a tender point in a taut band of muscle.[23] Trigger points typically are characterized by an area of muscle tenderness that can be provoked by palpation or mechanical stimulation.[24] This stimulation also produces referred pain that is perceived at a location distal from the trigger point.[25] Two primary types of trigger points are active and latent trigger points.[24] Active trigger points contribute to symptoms at rest, and the familiar symptoms are reproduced when pressure is placed on them. Latent trigger points generally are not symptomatic at rest and cause symptoms only when pressure is placed over the offending area.[24]

The pathogenesis of myofascial pain is not fully understood. Mechanical stress, metabolic deficiencies, and psychological influences have all been found to interact with myofascial pain.[26] Several contributing factors to the pathophysiology of myofascial tenderness have been suggested, including trauma, overuse, poor posture, psychological stress, mechanical overload, growth hormone deficiency, inflammatory diseases, alcohol toxicity, and constrictive clothing.[27,28] Maintaining prolonged postures and repetitive activities with light loads may be mechanisms of injury that a patient would not recognize as readily as he or she would a specific traumatic event.[29]

Patient Profile

Patients with myofascial pain and trigger points in the lumbopelvic region generally report pain without a specific mechanism of injury. Symptoms are often provoked with prolonged static positions and are generally referred to distal locations.[25] Patients describe muscular pain as being steady, aching, and deep, whereas examination findings reveal specific tenderness that provokes familiar symptoms with focal pressure. Patients also may have a taut band and "twitch response" to palpation. Referral patterns vary; however, those muscles with the most common referral patterns in the lumbopelvic hip complex are the iliopsoas, gluteus medius, quadratus lumborum, piriformis, erector spinae, and hamstring muscles (Fig. 10-3). Although some of the trigger points and structures responsible for myofascial pain may indeed be anatomically classified with the hip itself, myofascial disorders can be differentiated from other competing disorders such as extraarticular strains or nerve root disorders based on both symptom location and areas of tenderness. Moreover, an absence of macrotrauma or microtrauma may help steer the clinician away from extraarticular pathologic conditions.

> Patients with myofascial pain syndrome may present with pain patterns similar to those of contractile tissue lesions of the hip. Contractile lesions of the hip may be differentiated by a known mechanism of injury and pain with weakness during manual muscle testing. Patients with myofascial pain syndrome often experience exacerbations in the absence of a mechanism of injury and present with palpable tenderness as a primary finding.

Diskogenic Disorders

Diskogenic disorders are significant contributors to LBP and are the primary source of pathologic conditions in many studies investigating sources of lumbosacral disorders.[5-8] Descriptions of diskogenic disorders range from internal disk derangements to annular tears and extrusions. Diskogenic disorders with external morphologic changes such as protrusions, extrusions, and sequestrations may produce symptoms stemming from the annulus itself or from contact with structures such as the dura matter and nerve roots.

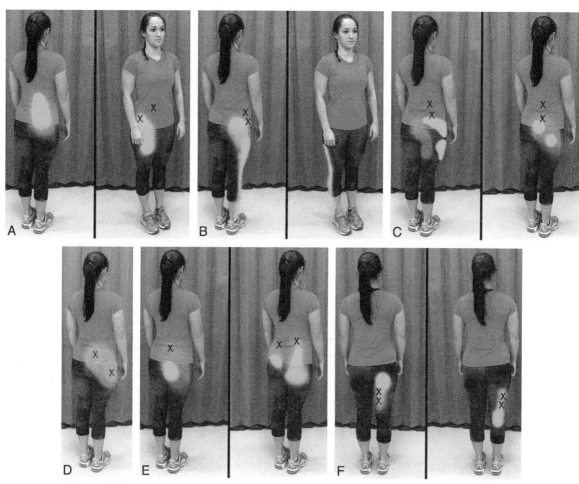

• **Figure 10-3** Myofascial Pain Referral Patterns. **A,** Iliopsoas. **B,** Gluteus medius. **C,** Quadratus lumborum. **D,** Piriformis. **E,** Erector spinae. **F,** Hamstring. Note that *x* indicates the primary location from which the symptoms originate.

The mechanism of injury is variable, ranging from no apparent reason to activities such as combined flexion with rotation or lifting. During rotation, a majority of force is accommodated or resisted by the contralateral facet joint, as well as by the supraspinous ligament. Therefore, the disk alone provides a minority of resistive force during rotation. However, when rotation is coupled with other movements, such as flexion and rotation, the disk may be at greater risk for injury. The annulus is most susceptible in the posterior or posterolateral fibers.[30] This again is another reason that specific combined movements such as flexion and rotation may be caustic to disk function.

The degenerative process can contribute to diskogenic disorders as well. Normally, the intervertebral disk is a closed system, and compressive forces expand the nuclear material outward, thereby placing greater internal pressure on the annulus. During the degenerative process, the annular fibers degrade and become unable to accommodate these forces. This desiccation of the disk leads to narrowing disk height and the potential for encroachment of key spaces in the spinal column. In time, the degenerative sequelae of the disk itself may lead to spondylosis or degenerative changes in the spine.

Patient Profile

Box 10-1 provides an overview of characteristics of diskogenic disorders. Patients with diskogenic symptoms may report pain that is isolated to the lower back or may describe referred or radicular symptoms. Diskogenic symptoms may manifest in the midline, bilaterally or unilaterally, and referral depends on structures mechanically compressed. In the early stages or in less complex cases of diskogenic disorders, patients often report central or unilateral LBP. Diskogenic lesions on the right side of disk tend to produce right-sided symptoms, whereas central disease tends to produce central or bilateral LBP.[5] Pain referral is often from the posterior annulus and posterior longitudinal ligament and in some cases may refer to the buttock region. If the diskogenic lesion contacts the dura, symptoms may be referred to the thigh; however, pain that follows a specific nerve root pattern (as described in the pain referral section of this chapter) suggests nerve root compression. Nonetheless, as the degenerative condition progresses, key spaces in the spine may be compromised, and patients may have a clinical presentation of foraminal stenosis (discussed in next section). If the lateral foraminal canal is occupied by disk herniation, patients may present with unilateral symptoms in a distribution consistent with the involved nerve root level.[31]

Generally, patients with diskogenic disorders describe some positions or movements that decrease symptoms and others that provoke them, a situation that indicates a directional preference. A directional preference is present when movements or positions in a particular direction decrease or abolish pain or cause referred pain emanating from the spine to centralize or retreat in a proximal direction.[32] The previous section on centralization and peripheralization provides insight into more common symptom responses to movement. In particular, evidence suggests that these patients will have pain with sitting to standing or with prolonged sitting and generally can walk off their symptoms (see Box 10-1).

On examination, these patients often have positive neural tension signs assessed by the straight leg raise (Fig. 10-4), crossover sign (Fig. 10-5), or Slump sit test (Fig. 10-6) if compression of lower lumbosacral nerve roots (or dura matter) exists, whereas a prone knee flexion test

---

• BOX 10-1   Diskogenic Pathologic Features

Pain location midline, unilateral or bilateral
Somatic or radicular, or both
Centralization or peripheralization
Directional preference favoring extension
Pain provoked on rising from sitting
Loss of lumbar extension following flexion
Positive neural tension testing (straight leg raise or Well) with a
    radiculopathy presentation

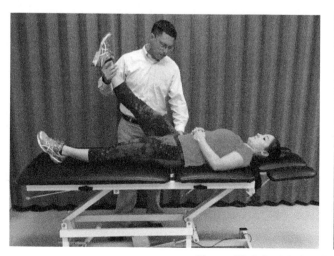

Description:
The patient is in the supine position. The examiner passively elevates the involved leg. A positive test result occurs when concordant lower extremity pain is produced. A positive test for nerve root compression or irritation would be confirmed by symptoms that are increased with added dorsiflexion and decreased with plantarflexion.

Reference Standard:
Lumbosacral nerve root compression identified with magnetic resonance imaging.

Diagnostic Utility:
Sensitivity: 97%; Specificity: 57%; +LR: 2.23; −LR: 0.05.[70]

• **Figure 10-4** Straight Leg Raise Test. *LR,* Likelihood ratio.

(Fig. 10-7) would predict upper lumbar dura or root compression.[33] In particular, a positive straight leg raise result has an odds ratio of 3.7 for disk herniation, whereas a positive crossover sign demonstrates an odds ratio exceeding 4.0. Reduced deep tendon reflexes and motor or sensory loss may exist in cases of prolonged compression when a neurapraxia has developed. Additionally, patients with a loss of extension during the physical examination are thought to have a presentation associated with diskogenic symptoms.[12] Patients with diskogenic disorders who centralize in

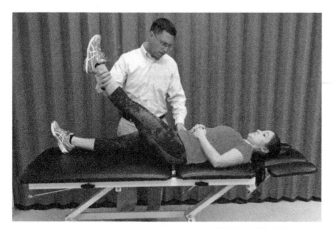

Description:
The patient lies in a supine position. The examiner passively raises the asymptomatic leg. A positive finding occurs if there is a reproduction of the concordant leg symptoms in the contralateral leg.

Reference Standard:
Surgical visualization of protruded lumbar intervertebral disks.

Diagnostic Utility:
Sensitivity: 43%; Specificity: 97%; +LR: 14.3; –LR: 0.59.[71]

• **Figure 10-5** Crossover Sign. *LR,* Likelihood ratio.

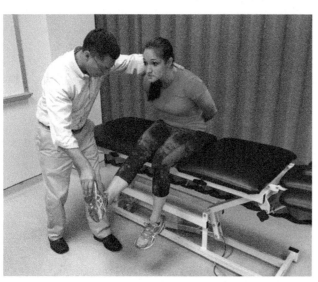

Description:
The patient sits and slumps forward while the examiner passively extends the patient's knee while maintaining dorsiflexion and evaluates for reproduction of concordant symptoms. The patient then extends the neck and symptoms are again evaluated. A positive test result occurs when the concordant symptoms are provoked in the slump position and eased when neck flexion is released.

Reference Standard:
Herniated nucleus pulposus identified on computed tomography and/or magnetic resonance imaging.

Diagnostic Utility:
Sensitivity: 83%; Specificity: 55%; +LR: 1.82; –LR: 0.32.[72]

• **Figure 10-6** Slump Sit Test. *LR,* Likelihood ratio.

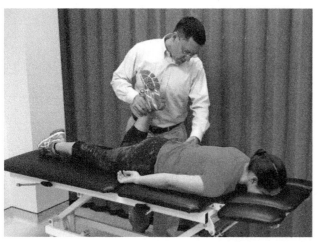

Description:
The patient lies prone. The examiner passively flexes the patient's knee, moving the foot toward the buttock. A positive test result occurs if a reproduction of the concordant symptoms presents.

Reference Standard:
Operative visualization of herniation.

Diagnostic Utility:
Sensitivity: 84%; Specificity: NT; +LR: NA; –LR: NA.[73]

• **Figure 10-7** Prone Knee Flexion Test. *LR,* Likelihood ratio; *NA,* not applicable; *NT,* not tested.

response to lumbar movements in a particular direction (e.g., directional preference) are thought to have a good prognosis, whereas those who peripheralize in response to movements in all directions are more likely to have a poor prognosis. In particular, patients with diskogenic disorders often experience centralization with lumbar extension with or without laterally directed movements of positioning.

A study by Donelson and colleagues[11] compared the clinical examination with the diagnostic gold standard for disk disease (i.e., diskography) and found that patients with diskogenic disorders were likely to centralize, with the exception of those patients with a disk extrusion or incompetent annulus, who were likely to peripheralize in response to both flexion and extension.

> Patients with diskogenic pain often experience a symptom change in response to lumbar movements. Similar to femoral acetabular impingement, hip-trunk flexion and sitting are reported sources of aggravation. However, unlike disk disorders, femoral acetabular impingement is associated with pain reproduction during hip adduction and internal rotation.

Degenerative Disorders

Spondylosis refers to spinal degenerative osteoarthritis that begins at the disk and progresses along the articulation between the neural foramina or zygapophysial joints.[34] If the condition is advanced, it may compromise the central or lateral foraminal canal and contribute to motor or sensory disturbances, which include muscle weakness, pain, or paresthesia.[35] The end progression of spondylosis is spinal stenosis. Spinal stenosis is a narrowing of specific spaces in the spine that include the lateral foraminal or central canal. Narrowing of these spaces often contributes to LBP and leg pain, which are exacerbated with activities such as standing or walking. It is most common in patients older than 48 years of age and is one of the primary reasons for surgical treatment in patients older than the age of 65 years.[30,36]

Activities that compromise the posterior spinal elements include standing or walking and may contribute to exacerbation of symptoms. Conversely, flexion-biased activities such as sitting or leaning forward generally ease symptoms.[37] Two primary types of foraminal canal narrowing are recognized. Central canal narrowing is often associated with conditions such as facet arthrosis, thickening of the ligamentum flavum, or a central intervertebral disk bulge,[38] whereas lateral foraminal canal stenosis may compromise the spinal nerve roots as they exit the lateral space between adjacent vertebrae. A loss of intervertebral disk height may contribute to narrowing of this space.

Patient Profile

Box 10-2 lists common characteristics associated with degenerative disorders. Because of the degenerative and progressive nature of spondylosis, the condition often has no specific mechanism of injury, and symptoms manifest insidiously.[39] Patients with spondylosis generally describe symptoms that include a deep ache and morning stiffness. Depending on the severity, symptoms may ease with activity throughout the course of the day. However, in advanced cases, compromise of the central or lateral foraminal canal may result in neurologic symptoms or signs.[40] Symptoms include referred pain and paresthesia into the lower extremity and are exacerbated with activities that further compromise the neural canal such as prolonged standing or walking.[35] Moreover, activities such as slouched sitting and bending are likely to relieve symptoms.[6,30,41]

Changes in pain location are based on morphologic changes to the lateral foramen with movements.[42] Specifically, evidence suggests that extension and ipsilateral lateral flexion narrow the foramen by 12% and 8%, respectively.[42] Conversely, flexion and contralateral lateral flexion increase the foraminal space by 11% and 8%, respectively.[42] Examination findings for spondylosis consist of localized pain in the early stages. In advanced cases (because of the compressive origin), however, neurologic findings may be present including altered deep tendon reflexes, sensory anesthesia, ataxia, and motor weakness.

On examination, the patient may present with a positive treadmill test result, which requires the patient to walk on a level treadmill at a comfortable pace until symptoms manifest. The amount of time to onset of symptoms is recorded. The patient then sits down, the time until symptoms return to baseline is recorded, and the test is then repeated with the patient walking on the treadmill at a 15-degree incline. Again, the time to onset of symptoms and the time to resolution of symptoms while sitting are recorded. Researchers found that earlier onset of symptoms with level walking to be consistent with a clinical diagnosis of lumbar spinal stenosis (sensitivity, 68%; specificity, 83%).[43] In addition, a longer total treadmill walking time during incline when compared with level walking was indicative of lumbar spinal stenosis (sensitivity, 50%; specificity, 92%). Finally, prolonged recovery after level walking was also consistent with the clinical diagnosis of stenosis (sensitivity, 82%; specificity, 68%).

● BOX **10-2** **Common Characteristics Associated With Degenerative Disorders**

Age >48 years
Pain location midline, unilateral or bilateral
Somatic or radicular, or both, with leg pain most
    dominant
Peripheralization with lumbar extension
Symptom production with walking or standing, or both
Directional preference favoring flexion

Nerve root compression from intervertebral stenosis and meralgia paresthetica are both likely to produce paresthesias. The pattern of paresthesias from meralgia paresthetica follows a vertical pathway to the anterolateral thigh, whereas nerve root compression travels in an oblique pattern. The pelvic compression test may reduce symptoms from meralgia paresthetica and does not affect nerve root compression. Furthermore, symptoms of intervertebral stenosis are abolished with lumbar flexion, whereas meralgia paresthetica is unaffected by lumbar spine positioning.

Spondylolysis

Spondylolysis is a condition associated with dissolution of or a defect in the lumbar pars interarticularis.[44,45] The most common level for this condition is L5, with L4 the second most common.[46] This condition generally has various causes, ranging from trauma to overuse injuries. Although spondylolysis is commonly asymptomatic, some patients may report sharp pain with specific movements such as extension or rotation; however, this finding alone is not a conclusive clinical test result.[46,47] Patients at risk for spondylolysis include those who participate in athletic activities requiring repeated and forceful extension or loading such as gymnastics, wrestling, American football, weight lifting, or competitive cheerleading.[46,48,49] Some evidence suggests that younger male athletes are at particular risk.[46] In addition, a sedentary lifestyle in adolescence with low tone and poor postural control may place undue stress on the posterior elements of the spine that may manifest with a pars interarticularis defect over time.[50] If a pars interarticularis defect is suspected, plain radiography with an oblique view should be considered, although evidence suggests that up to 49% of pars defects are radiographically occult.[46] Further imaging studies may be considered if plain film radiographs are inconclusive.

Patient Profile

Symptoms are often reported as a dull ache in the lower back, and men are generally more symptomatic than women.[44,46] If symptoms are present, often no mechanism of injury has been identified, and patients report an insidious onset of pain. Movements that close the posterior elements, such as extension, or functional activities, such as standing or walking, may exacerbate symptoms,[51] although this is not always the case. On physical examination, patients may demonstrate localized tenderness with a posteroanterior spring test over the involved segment; however, these results alone are not conclusive.[46,52]

Spondylolisthesis

Spondylolisthesis is a slippage of one vertebra on another. Normally, the posterior facets resist this forward motion, although several circumstances can create a predisposition for slippage.[53] Five different types of spondylolisthesis have been identified: dysplastic, isthmic, degenerative, traumatic, and pathologic.[54] The isthmic variety involves a lesion of the pars interarticularis, whereas translation permitted by the facet joint is referred to as dysplastic.[55] The dysplastic and isthmic types account for the majority of cases in children. Degenerative spondylolisthesis is secondary to facet incompetence and degenerative changes in the disk, which permit translation of one vertebra on another.[44] Traumatic spondylolisthesis is attributed to a fracture of the posterior elements other than the pars interarticularis. Other cases of spondylolisthesis result from a primary disease such as tumor and are referred to as pathologic spondylolisthesis. The dysplastic and isthmic types are considered congenital, whereas the degenerative, traumatic, and pathologic types are categorized as acquired.[56]

Spondylolisthesis is typically graded based on the percentage of slip and is measured from a line along the posterior cortex of the S1 body to the posteroinferior corner of the L5 vertebra. Grading is then performed using the following classification: grade I, 1% to 25%; grade II, 26% to 50%; grade III, 51% to 75%; grade IV, 76% to 100%; and grade V, more than 100%.[56,57] If conservative measures do not provide relief or if neurologic signs and symptoms appear, surgical treatment may be indicated. Degenerative spondylolisthesis is often associated with a diagnosis of spinal stenosis and results from the aging process, in which the osseous and articular structures become weak and unable to maintain relative spinal column alignment. This disorder is more common in persons who are older than 50 years of age and typically occurs at the L3 to L4 or L4 to L5 segmental levels.[56]

Patient Profile

The most common period for slipping associated with spondylolisthesis is between 10 and 15 years of age.[58] Symptoms generally occur in a patient's second or third decade of life and may or may not be related to the degree of slippage. Pain is generally mechanical and located along the midline, as well as the lumbosacral junction. In addition, symptoms may manifest as unilateral or bilateral leg pain, which is often consistent with neurogenic claudication.[59] A lateral radiographic study would confirm the presence and degree of slippage, whereas an oblique view or magnetic resonance image would help determine the cause.

Spinal Instability

Generally, instability suggests excessive movement in a given lumbar motion segment that contributes to pain.[59] Box 10-3 outlines a summary of clinical characteristics associated with radiographic instability of the lumbar spine. Instability can be a contentious diagnosis depending on how the condition is defined. Attempts have been made to quantify spinal instability with flexion-extension radiographs, with increased movement of one vertebrae beyond a predefined criteria (e.g., 15% or >3 mm) constituting instability.[52] Fritz and associates[60] found variables such as age, lumbar flexion range of motion, total extension range of motion, the Beighton scale for general ligamentous laxity, and segmental intervertebral motion testing to be associated with radiographic identification of spinal instability. This study suggests that the clinical examination may be helpful in developing a course of treatment to address spinal instability. Clinical instability is a less well-defined condition, and this suggests that a patient may benefit from a stabilization-based treatment program. Regardless of how instability is defined, evidence suggests that an exercise-based trunk stabilization program may help with some of these patients.

Patient Profile

Patients with lumbar instability often complain of recurrent episodes of LBP that occur over time.[61] Physical activity or a static posture tends to be provocative for patients with instability, and individuals may describe a sense of being unstable. A minor ache is often described; however, symptoms are generally inconsistent. On examination, a patient may present with a positive prone instability test result (Fig. 10-8) and a positive passive lumbar extension test result (Fig. 10-9).[61,62] Abbott and associates[52] studied the accuracy of manual palpation of segmental mobility when compared with radiography (Fig. 10-10). These investigators found a high level of specificity for translation lumbar spinal instability but showed poor sensitivity (specificity, 0.89; sensitivity, 0.29). Essentially, the investigators reported that if instability is identified, then it is likely present; however, a negative test result is often inconclusive because of the number of false-negative results (approaching 70%).

• BOX 10-3 Clinical Findings Associated With Radiographic Lumbar Instability

Age <37 years
Pain location variable
Somatic or radicular, or both
Isolated lumbar flexion >53 degrees
Beighton scale >2
Lack of hypomobility or hypermobility, or both, during segmental mobility testing

---

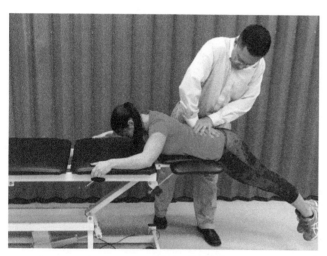

Description:
The patient lies prone over the end of a treatment plinth. The examiner applies a PA spring over a spinous process to identify a provocative segment. The patient is then asked to lift the legs while holding onto the plinth. The examiner applies a PA spring over the identified tender segment. A pain decrease with the legs lifted constitutes a positive test.

Reference Standard:
Success deemed with a stabilization program.

Diagnostic Utility:
Sensitivity: 72%; Specificity: 58%; +LR: 1.7; −LR: 0.48.[61]

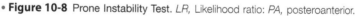

• **Figure 10-8** Prone Instability Test. *LR,* Likelihood ratio: *PA,* posteroanterior.

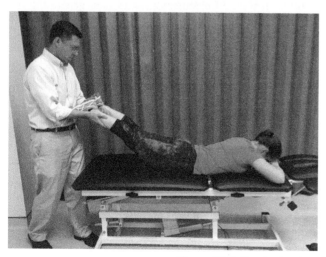

Description:
The patient lies prone while the examiner elevates both lower extremities approximately 30 cm and gently pulls while maintaining the knees extended. A positive test result occurs if the patient reports pain or abnormal sensation in the lumbar region.

Reference Standard:
Radiologic evaluation of instability.

Diagnostic Utility:
Sensitivity: 84%; Specificity: 90%; +LR: 8.84.[62]

• **Figure 10-9** Passive Lumbar Extension Test. *LR,* Likelihood ratio.

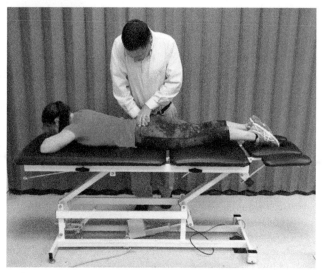

Description:
The patient lies prone while the clinician applies a posteroanterior central pressure to the spinous processes.

Reference Standard:
Radiologic evaluation of translational instability.

Diagnostic Utility:
Sensitivity: 29%; Specificity: 89%; +LR: 2.63; –LR: 0.79.[52]

• **Figure 10-10** Posterior-Anterior Mobility Assessment. *LR,* Likelihood ratio.

• **BOX 10-4** **Clinical Characteristics Associated With Sacroiliac Joint Pain**

Somatic pain primarily within 2 cm of the posterior superior iliac spine
Unilateral pain below L5 with referral to thigh
Pain provoked rising from sitting
Absence of centralization and peripheralization
No directional preference
Three or more positive sacroiliac joint provocation test results

---

Patients with spinal instability may report audible sounds such as popping or cracking similar to patients with hip conditions such as labral tears or osteoarthritis (OA). Clinical examination should elucidate the cause of symptoms because spinal instability is associated with hypermobility and pain during segmental mobility testing of the spine, which would not affect hip OA or labral disorders. Hip OA and labral disorders would be provoked by hip movements that would not affect spinal instability. Special tests such as Faber (Patrick) and Scour maneuvers would help to differentiate spinal instability from hip disease more clearly.

Sacroiliac Joint Pain

Sacroiliac joint pain describes symptoms that originate at the sacroiliac joint.[63] Pain generated from the sacroiliac joint can refer pain to other parts of the hip and pelvis and rarely to the leg (nonradicular).[7,8,64] The mechanical features associated with sacroiliac pain are controversial. Some evidence appears to suggest a small amount of movement, which occurs at the sacroiliac joint.[65] However, it is not clear how movement influences symptoms. Mechanisms that may contribute to sacroiliac pain include trauma, overuse, or pregnancy. Unfortunately, a myriad of ligamentous, fascial,

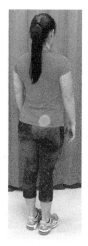

• **Figure 10-11** Sacroiliac Pain Symptom Distribution.

and muscular structures is present in the lumbopelvic complex, with an extensive array of pain-generating nociceptors. This can make isolation of the pain-generating structures difficult with the clinical examination alone. Nevertheless, sufficient evidence exists to support a valid diagnostic testing cluster. This section focuses on signs and symptoms identified based on research using the diagnostic gold standard of a double block injection.

Patient Profile

Box 10-4 presents clinical characteristics associated with sacroiliac joint pain. Patients with sacroiliac pain may describe a specific mechanism of injury, or in certain cases the pain may occur for no apparent reason. Symptoms generally manifest in the posterior and superior aspect of the hip at a region within 2 cm of the posterior superior iliac spine (Fig. 10-11). Unlike with facet or diskogenic pain, the location of symptoms is rarely above L5.[7] Moreover, pain is primarily unilateral, and although symptoms

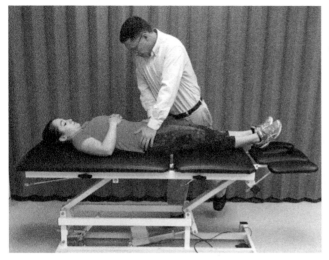

Description:
The patient lies supine while the examiner places firm downward pressure over the anterior superior iliac spines. A positive result occurs if concordant symptoms are reproduced.

Reference Standard:
80% pain relief with injection of local anesthetics into sacroiliac joint

Diagnostic Utility:
Sensitivity: 60%; Specificity: 81%; +LR: 3.20; –LR: 0.49.[13]

• **Figure 10-12** Distraction Sacroiliac Provocation Test. *LR,* Likelihood ratio.

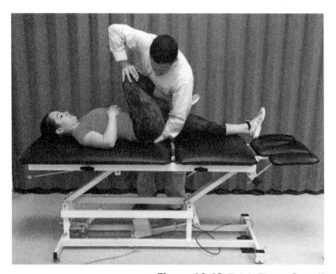

Description:
The patient lies supine while the ipsilateral hip flexed. The examiner places one hand under the sacrum and supports the patient's ipsilateral hip with their other hand. A downward force is imparted along the long axis of the femur toward the plinth. A positive result is reproduction of concordant symptoms.

Reference Standard:
80% pain relief with injection of local anesthetics into the sacroiliac joint

Diagnostic Utility:
Sensitivity: 88%; Specificity: 69%; +LR: 2.80; –LR: 0.18.[13]

• **Figure 10-13** Thigh Thrust Sacroiliac Provocation Test. *LR,* Likelihood ratio.

are predominately located over the sacroiliac joint, referral of symptoms may extend into the gluteal region.[9,66] Activities such as walking or standing may be provocative, but no consistency of activity provocation has been observed in these patients, with the exception of pain during sitting to standing transitions.[7,8] A patient's history often identifies symptoms associated with sit to stand; however, these symptoms are generally unaffected by walking or sitting.[8] On examination, results of the following provocation tests may be positive: distraction sacroiliac provocation test (Fig. 10-12); thigh thrust sacroiliac provocation test (Fig. 10-13), Gaenslen sacroiliac provocation test, right and left sides (Fig. 10-14); compression sacroiliac provocation test (Fig. 10-15); and sacral thrust sacroiliac provocation test (Fig. 10-16). Laslett and colleagues[13] evaluated a battery of provocation tests and found them to be more accurate than individual tests. This study found stronger predictive ability when results of three of the five provocation tests were

positive. A caveat to the results of the aforementioned tests is that their validity depends on the patient's not having a directional preference and exhibiting no evidence of centralization or peripheralization with lumbar movements.[67] When hip disease is suspected and the patient primarily has gluteal pain, sacroiliac joint involvement can be ruled out by using the five aforementioned tests.

Sacroiliac joint disorders may manifest with hip weakness and focal pain, similar to extraarticular sources of hip pain. Key diagnostic criteria to differentiate extraarticular contractile disorders from sacroiliac pain include the five special tests described by Laslett and associates, as well as pain location. Sacroiliac joint pain is often located at the S2 region (frequently referred to as the Fortin area) and refers inferiorly. Extraarticular hip disorders manifest with focal pain and tenderness over the affected muscle, along with a specific pattern of weakness.

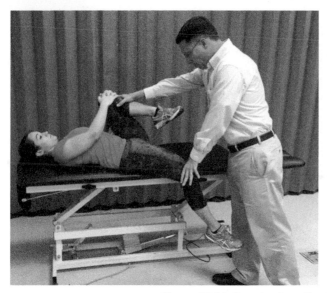

Description:
The patient lies supine with the ipsilateral hip flexed and the contralateral leg hanging off the edge of a plinth. The examiner places a downward force, moving the ipsilateral innominate into posterior rotation while stabilizing the contralateral leg. A positive test occurs if concordant symptoms are reproduced.

Reference Standard:
80% pain relief with injection of local anesthetics into the sacroiliac joint

Diagnostic Utility:
RIGHT: Sensitivity: 53%; Specificity: 71%; +LR: 1.84; –LR: 0.66.[13]

LEFT: Sensitivity: 50%; Specificity: 77%; +LR: 2.21; –LR: 0.65.[13]

• **Figure 10-14** Gaenslen Sacroiliac Provocation Test. *LR,* Likelihood ratio.

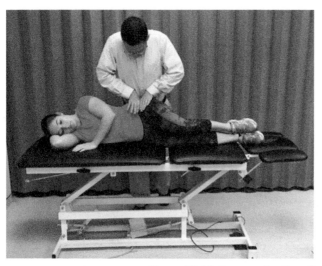

Description:
The patient is in a side-lying position with hips and knees comfortably flexed. The examiner stands behind the patient and applies a downward force over the iliac crest. A positive result occurs if concordant symptoms are reproduced.

Reference Standard:
80% pain relief with injection of local anesthetics into the sacroiliac joint

Diagnostic Utility:
Sensitivity: 69%; Specificity: 69%; +LR: 2.20; –LR: 0.46[13]

• **Figure 10-15** Compression Sacroiliac Provocation Test. *LR,* Likelihood ratio.

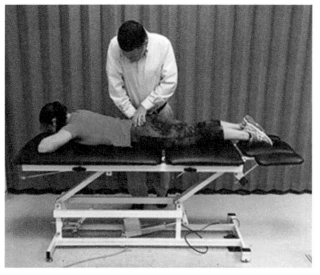

Description:
The patient is in a prone position. The examiner places a firm downward pressure over the sacral base. A positive test result occurs if concordant symptoms are reproduced.

Reference Standard:
80% pain relief with injection of local anesthetics into the sacroiliac joint

Diagnostic Utility:
Sensitivity: 63%; Specificity: 75%; +LR: 2.50; –LR: 0.49[13]

• **Figure 10-16** Sacral Thrust Sacroiliac Provocation Test. *LR,* Likelihood ratio.

Coccydynia

The coccyx articulates along the most inferior position of the sacrum, and movement occurs in either an anterior or a posterior direction. Many ligamentous structures surround this articulation, and substantial pain can therefore be generated from the coccyx joint. The most common mechanism for a coccyx injury is a slip and fall onto the buttock. Although pain predominately manifests over the coccyx, severe symptoms may extend into the posteromedial aspect of the hip.

Patient Profile

The coccyx consists of three to five fused vertebrae, which form a curvature with an anterior concavity. This conformation, in combination with its relative position to the sacrum, makes it susceptible to be forced into a flexed position. This is particularly the case with a slip and fall onto the buttocks, the most common mechanism. The condition can be difficult to diagnose, depending on how diffusely the pain manifests. Patients with a true coccyx injury have exquisite point tenderness over the sacrococcygeal joint. Depending on how diffusely the symptoms manifest, clinicians should consider ruling out both intraarticular and extraarticular hip disorders.

Facet Joint Disorders

Facet joint pain is thought to result from capsular irritation or the degenerative sequelae. Although the prevalence of facet joint pain has been reported, conditions emanating from this area remain less common than diskogenic or sacroiliac disorders.

Patient Profile

Box 10-5 presents common clinical characteristics associated with facet joint disorders. Pain from the facet joint is typically unilateral and somatic. Referral past the knee is rare unless the condition is degenerative, which has a clinical presentation more closely aligned with that of foraminal stenosis. The historical presentation for facet joint disorders is often inconclusive; however, the recumbent position tends to provide the greatest symptom relief.[68] Unlike in diskogenic and sacroiliac disorders, pain is not provoked when rising from sitting.[7,8,69] Although spinal movements may be limited as expected with a joint disorder, no consistent directional preference is observed, and centralization and peripheralization are absent.[7,8,14] From a face validity perspective, one could surmise the presence of hypomobility or pain with segmental mobility testing of the affected region. Box 10-6 provides a sample differential diagnosis of hip pain.

• BOX 10-5   Clinical Characteristics Associated With Facet Joint Pain

Somatic pain
Unilateral with primary referral to gluteal and rarely distal
Pain not provoked by rising from sitting
Absence of centralization and peripheralization
No directional preference
No symptoms with coughing or sneezing

• BOX 10-6   Differential Diagnosis

Patient Examination

A 45-year-old woman presents with right gluteal pain that travels toward her lateral hip. The primary pain location is the posterior superior iliac spine (PSIS). Onset was insidious. The pain has progressively worsened over the past year, and last month it worsened for no apparent reason. Symptoms have been relieved with ibuprofen and heat. The chief complaint is pain when transitioning from sitting to standing. Walking is generally pain free as required for daily function; however, symptoms increase on running. The patient denies audible sounds and does not report a change in symptoms with sitting or standing. Radiographs were not obtained.

Physical examination reveals normal posture in standing with a mild loss of lumbar lordosis in sitting. Hip active range of motion is within normal limits and pain free, with the exception of right hip extension, which is normal albeit painful at end-range. Muscle performance testing of the hip is symmetrical, with no focal weakness. Results of log roll and impingement testing are negative. The Faber-Patrick test result is positive on the right. Palpation of the hip reveals tenderness at the greater trochanter bilaterally; otherwise, it is normal, with no temperature changes or atrophy. Thoracolumbar active range of motion is normal and pain free, with no change in pain pattern during motion.

Disposition

The patient's history does not suggest hip disease. Given the patient's age, it is unlikely that hip osteoarthritis or lumbar stenosis is present. Moreover, the patient's age potentially may help rule out spinal instability. The absence of audible sounds helps support the exclusion of osteoarthritis and instability as potential sources of the pain at the hip and spine. Pain primarily in the gluteal region with a focal point of the PSIS is strongly associated with a sacroiliac joint disorder. Pain during transitioning from sitting to standing suggests either diskogenic or sacroiliac joint pain. Given that the pain has no apparent directional preference and does not change location, it seems unlikely that diskogenic disease or foraminal stenosis would be the source. Moreover, the absence of focal low back pain helps rule out a facet joint disorder. The absence of a mechanism of injury helps exclude a muscle strain (hip, pelvic, and lumbar) and subacute trauma such as spondylolysis.

Continued

• BOX 10-6 | Differential Diagnosis—cont'd

The physical examination reveals normal hip active range of motion, with pain only during end range hip extension; this finding, when combined with symmetrical muscle testing of the hip, helps to rule out hip disease. Finding an absence of a directional preference and normal thoracolumbar mobility helps to exclude a premise of lumbar disease (e.g., facet, disk, stenosis) more definitively. Although tenderness is present at the greater trochanter, it is bilateral and thus would seem irrelevant; with no other areas of tenderness, no pain with muscle testing, and an insidious onset, muscle disease can be excluded. This patient has an essentially unremarkable hip examination aside from pain with unilateral hip extension.

Given the pain location of the ipsilateral gluteal region with focal PSIS tenderness and pain on sitting to standing,

the sacroiliac joint seems a plausible cause of the condition. This premise can be further supported with an absence of centralization and peripheralization with lumbar mobility testing and no directional preference. Pain with end-range hip extension may not be unusual with sacroiliac disease because the position closely resembles the Gaenslen test. Further investigation could include additional special tests for focal hip disorders, as well as the testing cluster (sacral spring, thigh thrust, compression, distraction, and Gaenslen) used for the sacroiliac joint. Should symptoms remain elusive to the clinical examination, radiographs could aid in detection of minor structural changes or morphologic abnormalities of the hip or lumbosacral spine.

Summary

This chapter presents a pragmatic approach for differentiating symptoms of pain reported at the hip region. As established early in this chapter, hip pain has a multifactorial etiology, and conditions from the lumbosacral spine may indeed masquerade as a hip disorder. It is imperative that clinicians possess the diagnostic acumen to evaluate lumbopelvic and hip pain differentially. To that end, this chapter presents signs and symptoms of value for appropriate classification of patients. Information stemming from pain behavior and clinical testing, when combined, often provides a clear depiction of a patient's complaint. Finally, specific lumbosacral conditions are discussed with an emphasis on clinical characteristics vindicated from investigative studies. A theoretical framework is created within which the clinician can evaluate the patient's signs and symptoms and gain insight into the diagnosis. The chapter concludes with case studies in which it is not clear whether the symptoms are stemming from the hip or the lumbosa-

cral complex. The reader has an opportunity to evaluate the examination finding and subsequent plan of care. A discussion section is also provided in the case study so the reader can better understand the decision-making process in determining the ultimate plan of care.

Case Studies

Patient care can be a challenge, and rarely are clinical presentations exactly the same as described in texts. Multiple factors must be considered beyond diagnosis and treatment. Case Studies 10-1 to 10-3 are hypothetical; however, they are based on the authors' clinical experiences. The cases presented may not fit into a clear diagnostic category, but the process is clearly described to provide the reader with examples of how the text material may be applied to clinical practice.

CASE STUDY 10-1

Hip Pain

Patient History

Mr. Smith is a 48-year-old man who presents to the clinic with a primary complaint of right hip pain with no specific mechanism of injury. Currently, he is employed as an accountant and sits for a majority of the day in front of a computer. It is the end of tax season, and therefore he recently finished several months of 12-hour workdays. The symptoms seem to have progressed during this time. Initially, the pain was described as a dull ache "deep" in the hip joint. However, as the symptoms have progressed, he describes pain that radiates from the midback, around the torso to the proximal anterior and medial thigh. The pain seems to increase with prolonged sitting and eases as he walks around. His past medical history is significant for controlled hypertension. Mr. Smith's primary goal is to return to work pain free.

Examination Findings

Observation: On observation, Mr. Smith stands approximately 5 feet 9 inches tall and weighs approximately 220 pounds.

Range of motion: His lumbar range of motion is limited in all directions but most significantly in flexion. Repeated extension seemed to ease his symptoms, which became less prominent in his thigh after several repetitions. Moreover, assessment of his hip range of motion revealed general limitations of hip flexion on the right as well as internal rotation.

Strength: On examination, all hip strength on the right is weak, with particular weakness noted of the hip flexors. Strength on the contralateral side is within normal limits.

CASE STUDY 10-1

Hip Pain—cont'd

Muscle length tests: Muscle length tests reveal restrictions of the iliotibial band bilaterally and a positive Ober test result bilaterally. A Thomas test reveals tight hip flexors on the right and normal on the left.

Special tests: Special tests reveal a negative straight leg raise test result and a negative well leg raise test result; however, the femoral nerve tension test result is positive. In addition, the scour test result is negative, as are all sacroiliac provocation tests.

Patient outcome measures: He reports a numeric pain rating score to be 5 out of 10 at the moment, 8 out of 10 at its worst, and 3 out of 10 at its best (an average numeric pain rating score of 5.33).

Assessment

On examination, the patient presents with right-sided hip pain with weakness, as well as muscle length restrictions of select muscles on that side. Hip range of motion demonstrates a lack of internal rotation on the right, a finding is consisted with osteoarthritis (OA); he also presents with positive neural tension for an upper lumbar plexus injury. However, the scour test is negative and therefore would assist in ruling out intraarticular hip disorders. Therefore, the working diagnosis is an L2 nerve root lesion.

Plan of Care

The plan of care focuses primarily on the symptoms that seem to stem from the upper lumbar region. Therefore, treatment will consist of working within the patient's movement direction of preference, to centralize the symptoms. A trial of mechanical traction will be considered if symptoms cannot be centralized by traditional repeated movements. Although the patient seems to have no intraarticular pathologic condition, the hip

has significant limitation of hip internal rotation, which has been associated with hip OA and low back pain. Therefore, range of motion and mobilization techniques will be imparted to target the decreased range of motion and improve mobility. Finally, a strengthening program will be initiated, targeting the hip musculature as well as the superficial core muscles. The plan of care will consist of eight visits (twice weekly week for 4 weeks).

Outcome

After eight visits, the patient reported significant improvement in symptoms, with an average numeric pain rating score of 1.33 out of 10. He reports an ability to sit for 2 to 3 hours at a time with no increase in symptoms. Currently, he does report some mild symptoms in the upper lumbar spine; however, this is only with certain movements and is not constant.

Discussion

This case highlights two conditions that have a similar referral pattern. Hip OA and an L2 nerve root lesion both refer pain to the hip and anterior thigh. The examination findings did present some contradictory findings. For example, the limitation of hip internal rotation is often associated with OA; however, this condition was ruled out with the scour test, which is generally more sensitive. The femoral nerve tension test result was positive, although it tends to be more sensitive, and a positive finding is not as accurate. Therefore, the primary diagnosis of an upper lumber plexus lesion could not be assigned with confidence. The outcome of this case was positive. However, if the patient had failed to improve after two to four visits, the clinician should have considered reevaluating the conditions to determine whether the correct diagnosis was applied.

CASE STUDY 10-2

Spondylolisthesis

Patient History

Jordan is a 16-year-old competitive female gymnast with a complaint of low back pain. She has had back pain on and off for several years, although she recently reports a significant increase in the pain after a fall from the balance beam. When not injured, she trains 2 to 3 hours a day and is competing at a national level. She describes her pain as centrally located in the mid-low back, with no significant radiating pain into her legs. However, if her pain is really severe, she does report some pain into her thighs. She indicates that her pain is worse when extending backward. This is particularly the case when she performs a back flip or presents her arms in the air after a dismount. Currently, her pain is rated at 5 out of 10. It is reported to be 1 to 2 out of 10 when she rests, although it can be as high as 8 out of 10 if she is performing an activity that requires forceful extension. Other than the back pain, her past medical history is not significant.

Examination Findings

Observation: On observation, the patient appears to be an athletic girl with a slightly exaggerated lordosis. She stands 5 foot 2 inches tall and weighs 105 pounds.

Range of motion: Range of motion is within normal limits in all directions, with the exception of extension, which is limited by pain. During forward bending, she reports some muscle tightness and pulling at end-range.

Strength: The patient has no myotomal deficits and no significant muscle strength deficits, with the exception of trunk extension. She was able to hold the Biering-Sorensen test position for lumbar extensor endurance for approximately 100 seconds, which is appropriate for the general population; however, the expectation is higher for an athlete at her level. She reports that her inability to hold the trunk extensor position longer was caused by pain.

Muscle length tests: The patient is exceedingly flexible and demonstrates no significant muscle length restrictions, with the exception of some relative tightness of the hip flexors bilaterally.

Palpation: On palpation, the paravertebral muscles appear guarded, with a palpable step at L4.

Special tests: Results are as follows: straight leg raise, negative; well leg raise, negative; prone instability test, positive; and passive lumbar extension test, positive.

Imaging studies: Plain film radiography consisting of anteroposterior, lateral, and oblique views was performed.

Continued

CASE STUDY 10-2

Spondylolisthesis—cont'd

The oblique (right and left posterior oblique) and lateral views of the lumbar spine reveal a defect in the right and left pars interarticularis with grade 2 spondylolisthesis, respectively.

Assessment

On assessment, the patient appears to have a hyperlordotic posture and some muscle length restrictions, which may place pressure on the posterior column of the spine. She has some muscle guarding on palpation of the lumbar erector spinae that may suggest a muscle strain. However, the positive results of the prone instability test and the quadrant test suggest a possible structural defect in the posterior element of the spine. Plain film radiography confirms this with grade 2 spondylolisthesis present.

Plan of Care

The plan of care includes education of the athlete and her parents about avoidance of extension movements, as well as the potential for a progression of the condition. Treatment will also consist of flexibility training for the hip flexors as well as core training targeting the local muscle system. Furthermore, the patient will also be instructed to avoid hyperlordotic postures.

Outcome

After much consultation with the athlete's sports medicine team, it was decided that she would retire from competition. Her coach offered her a position as an assistant to keep her active in gymnastics. She still has discomfort on occasion, although she reports overall pain to be approximately 1 out of 10 and quite often she is pain free.

Discussion

On initial presentation, this patient may appear to have a simple muscle strain after falling from the balance beam. The muscle pulling sensation in forward bending and the increased tone of the para spinal muscles are consistent with the mechanism of injury. However, on further examination, the positive quadrant test result implicated a structural defect in the posterior element. This finding, along with the positive prone instability test result, warranted further examination. Plain radiography confirmed the diagnosis; however, in cases of spondylolysis without spondylolisthesis, magnetic resonance imaging may be required to identify the pars defect.

CASE STUDY 10-3

Bilateral Lower Extremity Symptoms

Patient History

Mr. Johnson is a 68-year-old retired man. He is relatively active and attempts to golf two times a week, as well as walk 3 miles each morning. Lately he has been complaining of leg pain, which has progressed and limited his walking abilities. Currently, he has to use the golf cart and is able to walk only about a half mile before his leg pain increases. There was no specific accident to which he can attribute to the pain; however, his walking distances have progressively become shorter because of the symptoms. The symptoms are described as a pain or numbness in both legs that gives the lower extremities the sensation of being heavy. The symptoms start in the buttocks and gradually extend down his legs. These symptoms progress during standing or walking for any amount of time. When the symptoms are really severe, they extend all the way down to his calf muscles. His goal is to return to playing 18 holes of golf two to three times a week without a cart and walk his normal 3 miles per day. His past medical history is positive for medically controlled high blood pressure. He also has coronary artery disease and osteoarthritis in the lower lumbar spine.

Examination Findings

Observation: On observation, it is noted that the patient is a well-developed man of medium stature. He stands approximately 5 foot 8 inches tall and weighs approximately 195 pounds. In closer observation of his posture, it is noted that he stands with his center of gravity displaced slightly forward.

Range of motion: Lumbar range of motion is limited to approximately 75% of the expected normal in all directions, with the exception of extension. Lumbar extension active range of motion is limited to approximately 50% of the expected normal, with slight pain on end-range. A significant loss of hip range of motion is noted, with approximately 5 degrees of internal rotation, 20 degrees of external rotation, –5 degrees of hip extension, and 120 degrees of hip flexion bilaterally.

Strength: Trunk strength demonstrated marked weakness, and he is unable to maintain any standard trunk strength testing positions. In addition, his hip strength is generally reduced, with particular weakness of hip abduction.

Muscle length tests: Muscle length restrictions are noted. The Thomas test result is positive for muscle length restriction of the hip flexors bilaterally, and the Ober test result is positive for iliotibial band and tensor fasciae latae restrictions.

Special tests: Results are as follows: straight leg raise test, negative; crossed leg raise test, negative; and posteroanterior joint mobility, significant for a general decrease in mobility. In addition, the patient has a positive graded treadmill test result in which he reports a reproduction of calf pain at a 3 mph pace within 4 minutes of walking with no incline. Symptoms manifest at approximately 8 minutes while walking at the same pace and on a 15% incline.

Outcome measures: The patient's numeric pain rating scale is 5 out of currently, 2 out of 10 at its best, and 8 out of 10 at its worst.

CASE STUDY 10-3

Bilateral Lower Extremity Symptoms—cont'd

Assessment

On assessment, the patient appeared to be in moderate discomfort as he forced himself to walk 2 miles this morning. On examination, he appears to have a forward flexed posture and complains of pain, primarily in his calf muscles. The examination is consisted with neurogenic claudication; however, the presence of vascular claudication is considered.

Plan of Care

The plan includes referral to physical therapy two times per week for 6 weeks. Treatment will include instruction to avoid standing or walking for any extended length of time. Further rehabilitation will consist of stretching of the muscle length restriction, general strengthening of the trunk and lower extremity musculature, and a graded conditioning program on a recumbent bicycle.

Outcome

On discharge, the patient's numeric pain rating scale was 0 out of 10 currently, 4 out of 10 at its worst, and 0 out of 10 at its best. In addition, the patient was able to walk for normal daily activities such as grocery shopping and general mobility around his home; however, he was unable to walk a round of golf without a significant increase in his symptoms. He also elected to use a recumbent stationary bicycle for exercise rather than walking.

Discussion

This case highlights a situation in which the patient describes little back pain but significant bilateral leg pain extending into the calf muscles. Although direct hip disease is unlikely, considering the bilateral symptoms, he does have a past medical history of arthritis in the lower lumbar spine that may inhibit mobility of the lower lumbopelvic complex. In addition, the patient describes symptoms consistent with vascular or neurogenic claudication. This is a particularly important finding considering his past medical history of high blood pressure and coronary artery disease. However, the treadmill test result was positive for neurogenic claudication, and therefore the plan of care progressed addressing that primary diagnosis. Treatment appeared to have a positive outcome; however, it is important for patients who present with neurogenic claudication to understand that adaptation of normal activities is generally necessary. The patient in this case was able to continue golfing, although he had to use a cart to complete the entire round without significant pain. He also adapted his normal fitness routine of walking to include a recumbent bicycle. The seated position on a recumbent bicycle would open the posterior element of the spine and avoid provocative extension positions. In the end, a combination of physical therapy and adaptation of normal activities significantly affected this patient's pain, perceived disability, and function.

References

1. Cassidy JD, Carroll LJ, Cote P. The Saskatchewan health and back pain survey: the prevalence of low back pain and related disability in Saskatchewan adults. *Spine (Phila Pa 1976)*. 1998;23(17):1860-1866, discussion 1867.
2. Horvath G, Koroknai G, Acs B, et al. Prevalence of low back pain and lumbar spine degenerative disorders: questionnaire survey and clinical-radiological analysis of a representative Hungarian population. *Int Orthop*. 2010;34(8):1245-1249.
3. Hoogeboom TJ, den Broeder AA, Swierstra BA, et al. Joint-pain comorbidity, health status, and medication use in hip and knee osteoarthritis a cross-sectional study. *Arthritis Care Res*. 2012; 64(1):54-58.
4. Goodman CC, Snyder TK. *Differential Diagnosis for Physical Therapists Screening for Referral*. 5th ed. St. Louis: Saunders; 2012.
5. Kuslich SD, Ulstrom CL, Michael CJ. The tissue origin of low back pain and sciatica: a report of pain response to tissue stimulation during operations on the lumbar spine using local anesthesia. *Orthop Clin North Am*. 1991;22(2):181-187.
6. Laslett M, McDonald B, Tropp H, et al. Agreement between diagnoses reached by clinical examination and available reference standards: a prospective study of 216 patients with lumbopelvic pain. *BMC Musculoskelet Disord*. 2005;6:28.
7. Young S, Aprill C. Characteristics of a mechanical assessment for chronic lumbar facet joint pain. *J Man Manip Ther*. 2000;8(2): 78-84.

8. Young S, Aprill C, Laslett M. Correlation of clinical examination characteristics with three sources of chronic low back pain. *Spine J*. 2003;3(6):460-465.
9. Fortin JD, Falco FJ. The Fortin finger test an indicator of sacroiliac pain. *Am J Orthop*. 1997;26(7):477-480.
10. Khan AM, McLoughlin E, Giannakas K, et al. Hip osteoarthritis: where is the pain? *Ann R Coll Surg Engl*. 2004;86(2): 119-121.
11. Donelson R, Aprill C, Medcalf R, Grant W. A prospective study of centralization of lumbar and referred pain: a predictor of symptomatic discs and anular competence. *Spine (Phila Pa 1976)*. 1997;22(10):1115-1122.
12. Laslett M, Aprill CN, McDonald B, Oberg B. Clinical predictors of lumbar provocation discography: a study of clinical predictors of lumbar provocation discography. *Eur Spine J*. 2006;15(10): 1473-1484.
13. Laslett M, Aprill CN, McDonald B, Young SB. Diagnosis of sacroiliac joint pain validity of individual provocation tests and composites of tests. *Man Ther*. 2005;10(3):207-218.
14. Laslett M, McDonald B, Aprill CN, et al. Clinical predictors of screening lumbar zygapophyseal joint blocks: development of clinical prediction rules. *Spine J*. 2006;6(4):370-379.
15. Murakami E, Aizawa T, Noguchi K, et al. Diagram specific to sacroiliac joint pain site indicated by one-finger test. *J Orthop Sci*. 2008;13(6):492-497.
16. Werneke M, Hart DL, Cook D. A descriptive study of the centralization phenomenon: a prospective analysis. *Spine*. 1999; 24(7):676-683.

17. Werneke M, Hart DL. Centralization phenomenon as a prognostic factor for chronic low back pain and disability. *Spine.* 2001;26(7):758-764, discussion 765.

18. Kolber MJ, Hanney WJ. The dynamic disc model: a systematic review of the literature. *Phs Ther Rev.* 2009;14(3):181-187.

19. Takasaki H, May S, Fazey PJ, Hall T. Nucleus pulposus deformation following application of mechanical diagnosis and therapy: a single case report with magnetic resonance imaging. *J Man Manip Ther.* 2010;18(3):153-158.

20. Tokuhashi Y, Satoh K, Funami S. A quantitative evaluation of sensory dysfunction in lumbosacral radiculopathy. *Spine (Phila Pa 1976).* 1991;16(11):1321-1328.

21. Ahn UM, Ahn NU, Buchowski JM, et al. Cauda equina syndrome secondary to lumbar disc herniation: a meta-analysis of surgical outcomes. *Spine (Phila Pa 1976).* 2000;25(12): 1515-1522.

22. Fleckenstein J, Zaps D, Rüger LJ, et al. Discrepancy between prevalence and perceived effectiveness of treatment methods in myofascial pain syndrome: results of a cross-sectional, nationwide survey. *BMC Musculoskelet Disord.* 2010;11:32.

23. Gerwin RD, Shannon S, Hong CZ, et al. Interrater reliability in myofascial trigger point examination. *Pain.* 1997;69(1–2): 65-73.

24. Gerwin RD, Dommerholt J, Shah JP. An expansion of Simons' integrated hypothesis of trigger point formation. *Curr Pain Headache Rep.* 2004;8(6):468-475.

25. Harden RN, Bruehl SP, Gass S, et al. Signs and symptoms of the myofascial pain syndrome: a national survey of pain management providers. *Clin J Pain.* 2000;16(1):64-72.

26. Hong CZ, Simons DG. Pathophysiologic and electrophysiologic mechanisms of myofascial trigger points. *Arch Phys Med Rehabil.* 1998;79(7):863-872.

27. Hanten WP, Olson SL, Butts NL, Nowicki AL. Effectiveness of a home program of ischemic pressure followed by sustained stretch for treatment of myofascial trigger points. *Phys Ther.* 2000;80(10):997-1003.

28. Kannan P. Management of myofascial pain of upper trapezius: a three group comparison study. *Glob J Health Sci.* 2012;4(5): 46-52.

29. Aguilera FJM, Martín DP, Masanet RA, et al. Immediate effect of ultrasound and ischemic compression techniques for the treatment of trapezius latent myofascial trigger points in healthy subjects: a randomized controlled study. *J Manipulative Physiol Ther.* 2009;32(7):515-520.

30. Cook C, Brown C, Michael K, et al. The clinical value of a cluster of patient history and observational findings as a diagnostic support tool for lumbar spine stenosis. *Physiother Res Int.* 2011;16(3):170-178.

31. Albeck MJ. A critical assessment of clinical diagnosis of disc herniation in patients with monoradicular sciatica. *Acta Neurochir (Wien).* 1996;138(1):40-44.

32. Long A, Donelson R, Fung T. Does it matter which exercise? A randomized control trial of exercise for low back pain. *Spine (Phila Pa 1976).* 2004;29(23):2593-2602.

33. Suri P, Rainville J, Katz JN, et al. The accuracy of the physical examination for the diagnosis of midlumbar and low lumbar nerve root impingement. *Spine (Phila Pa 1976).* 2011;36(1): 63-73.

34. Bernard TN Jr, Kirkaldy-Willis WH. Recognizing specific characteristics of nonspecific low back pain. *Clin Orthop Relat Res.* 1987;217:266-280.

35. Arnoldi CC, Brodsky AE, Cauchoix J, et al. Lumbar spinal stenosis and nerve root entrapment syndromes: definition and classification. *Clin Orthop Relat Res.* 1976;115:4-5.

36. Amundsen T, Weber H, Nordal HJ, et al. Lumbar spinal stenosis conservative or surgical management? A prospective 10-year study. *Spine (Phila Pa 1976).* 2000;25(11):1424-1435, discussion 1435-1436.

37. Wiltse LL, Kirkaldy-Willis WH, McIvor GW. The treatment of spinal stenosis. *Clin Orthop Relat Res.* 1976;115:83-91.

38. Bridwell KH. Lumbar spinal stenosis: diagnosis, management, and treatment. *Clin Geriatr Med.* 1994;10(4):677-701.

39. Katz JN, Harris MB. Clinical practice: lumbar spinal stenosis. *N Engl J Med.* 2008;358(8):818-825.

40. Amundsen T, Weber H, Lilleas F, et al. Lumbar spinal stenosis: clinical and radiologic features. *Spine (Phila Pa 1976).* 1995; 20(10):1178-1186.

41. Fritz JM, Delitto A, Welch WC, Erhard RE. Lumbar spinal stenosis: a review of current concepts in evaluation, management, and outcome measurements. *Arch Phys Med Rehabil.* 1998; 79(6):700-708.

42. Fujiwara A, An HS, Lim TH, Haughton VM. Morphologic changes in the lumbar intervertebral foramen due to flexion-extension, lateral bending, and axial rotation: an in vitro anatomic and biomechanical study. *Spine (Phila Pa 1976).* 2001; 26(8):876-882.

43. Fritz JM, Erhard RE, Delitto A, et al. Preliminary results of the use of a two-stage treadmill test as a clinical diagnostic tool in the differential diagnosis of lumbar spinal stenosis. *J Spinal Disord.* 1997;10(5):410-416.

44. Ko SB, Lee SW. Prevalence of spondylolysis and its relationship with low back pain in selected population. *Clin Orthop Surg.* 2011;3(1):34-38.

45. Petersen T, Laslett M, Thorsen H, et al. Diagnostic classification of non-specific low back pain: a new system integrating patho-anatomic and clinical categories. *Physiother Theory Pract.* 2003; 19(4):213-237.

46. Kobayashi A, Kobayashi T, Kato K, et al. Diagnosis of radiographically occult lumbar spondylolysis in young athletes by magnetic resonance imaging. *Am J Sports Med.* 2013;41(1): 169-176.

47. Thein-Nissenbaum J, Boissonnault WG. Differential diagnosis of spondylolysis in a patient with chronic low back pain. *J Orthop Sports Phys Ther.* 2005;35(5):319-326.

48. Nau E, Hanney WJ, Kolber MJ. Spinal conditioning for athletes with lumbar spondylolysis and spondylolisthesis. *Strength Cond J.* 2008;30(2):43-52.

49. Heck JF, Sparano JM. A Classification system for the assessment of lumbar pain in athletes. *J Athl Train.* 2000;35(2): 204-211.

50. Smeets RJ, Wade D, Hidding A, et al. The association of physical deconditioning and chronic low back pain: a hypothesis-oriented systematic review. *Disabil Rehabil.* 2006;28(11):673-693.

51. Hanney WJ, Pabian PS, Smith MT, Patel CK. Low back pain: movement considerations for exercise and training. *Strength Cond J.* 2013;35(4):99-106.

52. Abbott JH, McCane B, Herbison P, et al. Lumbar segmental instability: a criterion-related validity study of manual therapy assessment. *BMC Musculoskelet Disord.* 2005;6:56.

53. Fritz JM, Cleland JA, Childs JD. Subgrouping patients with low back pain: evolution of a classification approach to physical therapy. *J Orthop Sports Phys Ther.* 2007;37(6):290-302.

54. Wiltse LL, Newman PH, Macnab I. Classification of spondylolisis and spondylolisthesis. *Clin Orthop Relat Res.* 1976;117:23-29.

55. Borkow SE, Kleiger B. Spondylolisthesis in the newborn: a case report. *Clin Orthop Relat Res.* 1971;81:73-76.

56. Hu SS, Tribus CB, Diab M, Ghanayem AJ. Spondylolisthesis and spondylolysis. *J Bone Joint Surg Am.* 2008;90(3):656-671.

57. Meyerding H. Spondylolisthesis. *Surg Gynecol Obstet.* 1932;54:371-377.

58. Manchikanti L. Epidemiology of low back pain. *Pain Physician.* 2000;3(2):167-192.

59. O'Sullivan PB. Lumbar segmental "instability": clinical presentation and specific stabilizing exercise management. *Man Ther.* 2000;5(1):2-12.

60. Fritz JM, Piva SR, Childs JD. Accuracy of the clinical examination to predict radiographic instability of the lumbar spine. *Eur Spine J.* 2005;14(8):743-750.

61. Hicks GE, Fritz JM, Delitto A, McGill SM. Preliminary development of a clinical prediction rule for determining which patients with low back pain will respond to a stabilization exercise program. *Arch Phys Med Rehabil.* 2005;86(9):1753-1762.

62. Kasai Y, Morishita K, Kawakita E, et al. A new evaluation method for lumbar spinal instability: passive lumbar extension test. *Phys Ther.* 2006;86(12):1661-1667.

63. Broadhurst NA, Bond MJ. Pain provocation tests for the assessment of sacroiliac joint dysfunction. *J Spinal Disord.* 1998;11(4):341-345.

64. Berthelot JM, Labat JJ, Le Goff B, et al. Provocative sacroiliac joint maneuvers and sacroiliac joint block are unreliable for diagnosing sacroiliac joint pain. *Joint Bone Spine.* 2006;73(1):17-23.

65. Buyruk HM, Snijders CJ, Vleeming A, et al. The measurements of sacroiliac joint stiffness with colour Doppler imaging: a study on healthy subjects. *Eur J Radiol.* 1995;21(2):117-121.

66. Slipman CW, Jackson HB, Lipetz JS, et al. Sacroiliac joint pain referral zones. *Arch Phys Med Rehabil.* 2000;81(3):334-338.

67. Laslett M, Young SB, Aprill CN, McDonald B. Diagnosing painful sacroiliac joints: a validity study of a McKenzie evaluation and sacroiliac provocation tests. *Aust J Physiother.* 2003;49(2):89-97.

68. Revel M, Poiraudeau S, Auleley GR, et al. Capacity of the clinical picture to characterize low back pain relieved by facet joint anesthesia: proposed criteria to identify patients with painful facet joints. *Spine (Phila Pa 1976).* 1998;23(18):1972-1976, discussion 1977.

69. Laslett M, Oberg B, Aprill CN, McDonald B. Zygapophysial joint blocks in chronic low back pain a test of Revel's model as a screening test. *BMC Musculoskelet Disord.* 2004;5:43.

70. Vroomen PC, de Krom MC, Wilmink JT, et al. Diagnostic value of history and physical examination in patients suspected of lumboscral nerve root compression. *J Neurol Neurosurg Psychiatry.* 2002;72(5):630-634.

71. Kerr RSC, Cadoux-Hudson TA, Adams CBT. The value of accurate clinical assessment in the surgical management of the lumbar disc protrusion. *J Neurol Seurosurg Psychiatry.* 1988;51:169-173.

72. Stankovic R, Johnell O, Maly P, Willner S. Use of lumbar extension, slump test, physical and neurological examination in the valuation of patients with suspected herniated nucleus pulposus: a prospective clinical study. *Man Ther.* 1999;4(1):25-32.

73. Porchet F, Fankhauser H, De Tribolet N. Extreme lateral lumbar disc herniation: clinical presentation in 178 patients. *Acta Neurochir (Wien).* 1994;127(3-4):203-209.

11

Hip and Pelvic Injuries

PETER AARON SPRAGUE

CHAPTER OUTLINE

Hip and pelvic injuries comprise a wide-ranging group of injuries that can affect diverse patient populations. The incidence of hip fractures has been reported to be 957 in 100,000 in women and 414 in 100,000 in men.[1] Pelvic trauma has a lower incidence, comprising only 3% of all skeletal injuries, but it is among the most devastating of all skeletal injuries because of the significant comorbidities and high mortality rates associated with these injuries.[2] The causes of these injuries range from high-energy traumatic events, such as from motor vehicle accidents, sports injuries, and high falls, which are associated with younger populations, to low-energy events, such as falls from standing height, which are responsible for these fractures in geriatric individuals with compromised bone mass and for pathologic fractures in younger patients.[3] The treatments of these injuries are varied and depend on the characteristics of the fracture itself, surgeon-based idiosyncrasies, the presence of comorbidities, and the age of the individual patient.

Regardless of the type of injury, successful management of patients with these injuries depends on a thorough understanding of the patient's goals, expectations, lifestyle, and premorbid functional status and on the presence of any disease or condition that affects the health of the individual. The ultimate goals for the individual are to restore optimal function from a whole body standpoint and reduce the morbidity sequelae. The identification and correction of specific predisposing factors responsible for the original injury and the identification of current variables that may lead to a subsequent injury are crucial to positive long-term outcomes. To accomplish these objectives, it is necessary to address the patient's physical, environmental, and psychological factors. For this reason, an interprofessional team approach to the medical management and rehabilitation of the patient yields superior outcomes.[4] Depending on the severity of injury and additional medical complexities of the patient, the team can include professionals in the fields of nursing, occupational therapy, physical medicine and rehabilitation, physical therapy, social work, interventional radiology, and surgery.

Trauma to the hip and pelvis can include fracture-dislocation of the femoral head, fractures of the femoral neck and acetabulum, fractures of the pelvis, ligamentous disruption of the pelvis, proximal femur fractures, and stress reactions. Accordingly, this chapter explores the variety of traumatic injuries found throughout the hip and pelvis. The chapter begins with a description of the various types of hip fractures, and pelvic trauma is discussed later in the chapter. Classification schemes for the various injuries are described, as well as associated causes, complexities, and issues with management.

Hip Fractures

Fractures of the hip can be intracapsular (fracture occurring within the joint capsule) or extracapsular (fracture occurring outside of the hip joint capsule). The capsule of the hip joint attaches to the acetabulum around the labrum, surrounds the femoral head, and extends down the femoral neck. Union and function in intracapsular fractures depend on vascular integrity of the femoral head and bone density within the femoral neck. Extracapsular fractures are at risk from mechanical loads because these fractures are found in regions of tendon insertions for the large hip and pelvis muscles.

Hip fractures can consist of proximal femur fractures, femoral neck fractures, intertrochanteric fractures, and acetabular fractures. The site of a hip fracture is associated with the type of trauma causing the injury as well as specific medical complications of the patient.

Proximal Femur Fractures

The three types of proximal femur fractures are femoral head fractures, femoral neck fractures, and intertrochanteric fractures. Femoral head and femoral neck fractures are considered intracapsular injuries, or injuries that are found within the joint capsule, whereas intertrochanteric fractures are extracapsular. For reference, the capsule of the hip joint has longitudinal fibers that are anchored by transverse fibers around the base of the femoral neck, running over the femoral head, and attaching to the labrum by the arcuate fibers. Femoral head fractures may also be associated with hip dislocation and acetabular fractures, thereby posing significance when considering emergence of management,

prognosis, and long-term management. The causes, presentation, and management of each of these types of proximal femur fractures are unique and are explained in more detail in the following sections.

Femoral Head Fractures, Acetabular Fractures, and Posterior Dislocation

Femoral head and acetabular fractures are rare, serious injuries that are associated with a posterior hip dislocation from a high-energy traumatic event.[5] These injuries typically occur when an axial force is applied to the shaft of the femur while the hip is in a position of flexion, adduction, and internal rotation. Fracture-dislocations of the hip are most common in motor vehicle accidents, motor vehicle versus pedestrian accidents, high falls, and, more rarely, injuries related to sport. Given the nature of injury, the population most commonly injured consists of men between the ages of 20 and 30 years.[6] Because of the large forces at play during the injury, hip dislocations are seen with concomitant injuries up to 95% of the time. Most of these other injuries are nonorthopedic, most commonly head, thoracic, or abdominal injuries. The orthopedic injuries associated with posterior hip dislocation include, in order of prevalence, acetabular fractures, other fractures of the lower and upper extremities, and femoral head fractures[7] (Fig. 11-1).

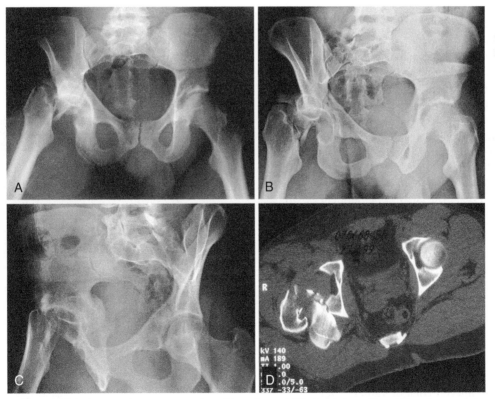

• **Figure 11-1** Preoperative anteroposterior pelvic radiograph **(A)**, Judet views **(B** and **C)** and computed tomography **(D)** show a severely displaced lateral femoral neck fracture with posterior dislocation of the femoral head in combination with a transverse acetabular fracture. (From Tannast M, Mack PW, Klaeser B, Siebenrock KA. Hip dislocation and femoral neck fracture: decision-making for head preservation. *Injury.* 2009;40:1118-1124.)

Comorbidities

Careful examination and evaluation of the patient with a hip fracture-dislocation must be made to identify all other injuries sustained during the traumatic event, including the head, spine, abdomen, and extremities. Rectal, perineal, and vaginal examinations should be made to rule out open fractures. Neurovascular considerations directly related to the dislocation warrant immediate and emergency consideration. The superior gluteal artery may be lacerated during this injury, and examination for sciatic, obturator, and femoral nerve injury should be made. Hip dislocations are considered a medical emergency, and after ruling out contraindications such as femoral neck fractures, closed reduction with the patient under anesthesia should be performed as soon as possible to diminish the risk of avascular necrosis (AVN) of the femoral head, as well as sciatic nerve injury. AVN is more likely to occur in hips that are not relocated within 6 hours of injury.[7] Evaluation and documentation of the sciatic nerve before and after reduction are recommended because of the common injuries of the sciatic nerve during dislocation. As many as 30% of posterior hip dislocations are associated with sciatic nerve injuries, typically involving the peroneal branch of the sciatic nerve, which could result in foot drop.[8] Another postsurgical complication that may arise is heterotopic ossification (HO), with a reported incidence as high as 64%. A higher incidence of HO has been associated with an anterior surgical approach.[9]

Acetabular Fractures

Acetabular fractures are serious albeit rare injuries, with a reported incidence of approximately 3 in 100,000 annually.[10] In younger populations, these injuries are associated with high-energy traumatic events, such as motor vehicle accidents. Fractures of the acetabulum in older populations are generally caused by lower-energy trauma associated with falls from a standing height. The incidence of these fractures in the older population is increasing.[11]

The acetabulum has been described as being supported between the anterior and posterior columns of the innominate bone (Fig. 11-2). The anterior column consists of the anterior wall of the acetabulum, the anterior ilium, the superior pubic ramus, and the iliopectineal ramus. The posterior column is made up of the posterior wall and dome of the acetabulum, the ischial tuberosity, and the quadrilateral plate of the ilium. Classification and treatment of these injuries are based on an understanding of these columns.

The Letournel classification of acetabular fractures classifies the injury relative to the anatomic features of the fracture (Fig. 11-3). These fractures are divided into two types of fractures: elementary types and associated types. The elementary types consist of isolated fractures found in the anterior wall, anterior column, posterior wall, and posterior column of the ischium, as well as transverse fractures. The associated types of fractures cover combined regions and are subclassified as follows: posterior column and posterior wall fractures, posterior wall and transverse fractures,

T-shaped fractures, anterior column and hemitransverse fractures, and fractures involving both columns.

Plain radiographs, specifically anteroposterior pelvis and Judet views, are recommended for identifying the presence of these fractures, whereas computed tomography (CT) scans provide accurate assessment of fracture anatomy and character.[5] An understanding of the type of trauma that caused the injury can provide valuable information on the possibility of other potential comorbidities associated with the trauma, as well as any preexisting comorbidities that may influence management choices. If the patient has no associated hip dislocation, treatment of acetabular fractures is not considered an emergency; however, surgical treatment should be performed within the first 7 days after injury.[5] This approach affords the trauma team time to make the patient physiologically stable and ready for surgery. Traction, a common practice following hip dislocation, may be applied through a pin in the distal femur with approximately 5 kg of weight. Traction may also be used during the surgical procedure.

Acetabular fractures with less than 2 mm of displacement may be treated nonoperatively if joint congruency remains good and the joint is stable. Displaced acetabular fractures are treated by internal fixation. The goal of surgical treatment is to provide good stability in the acetabulum to allow for early range of motion and good congruency between the femoral head and acetabulum. Internal fixation is preferred to percutaneous fixation because of the difficulties in achieving accurate reduction and estimating the appropriate depth of screw penetration to avoid intraarticular insult with external fixation. The choice of surgical approach varies with the characteristics of the fracture, other

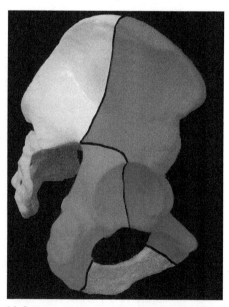

• **Figure 11-2** Pelvic Osteology Showing Anterior and Posterior Columns of the Innominate Bone. (From Stevenson AJ, McArthur JR, Acharya, MR, et al. Principles of acetabular fractures. *Orthop Trauma.* 2014;28:141-150.)

comorbidities, and the experience of the surgeon, although these fractures are typically reduced with lag screws and held in place with neutralization plates (Fig. 11-4).

If the hip joint is considered stable after the surgical procedure, rehabilitation following acetabular fracture involves early restoration of hip joint range of motion. Because of weight-bearing strain on the acetabulum, the patient should be non–weight bearing for 6 weeks and partially weight bearing for an additional 6 weeks. During this time, rehabilitation should also consider any comorbidities, such as head injury, spinal injuries, and other orthopedic trauma.[5] Weight-bearing considerations in nonoperative management should be based on the location of fracture site, assessment of fracture site healing, bone mass, and other comorbidities associated with the individual patient. HO should be considered if the patient is complaining of hip pain during the postoperative period, because a relatively high incidence of HO is reported in these populations.

Acetabular fractures in older adults occur from low-energy trauma and are usually complicated by comorbidities that may have predisposed the patient to this injury initially. A common example of this is the presence of osteoporosis when combined with a more active lifestyle. Acetabular fractures in patients older than 60 years of age typically display anterior column displacement and roof impaction along with comminution of the quadrilateral surface of the ilium.[11] Management of these injuries in older adults considers the status of all the body's systems as much as the

fracture site itself. Figure 11-5 contains more detailed information.

Femoral Head Fractures

Femoral head fractures are rare, with an incidence between 5% and 15% of all posterior hip dislocations.[12] Several classifications have been described for a femoral head fracture, and the Pipkin classification is the most widely used. The Pipkin classification considers the location of the fracture within the femoral head, as well as any other fractures that may be present in a different portion of the femur or involvement of the acetabulum (Fig. 11-6). The diagnosis is made initially by radiographs, and fracture-dislocation of the hip can be viewed on a trauma anteroposterior pelvis radiograph.

A hip fracture-dislocation is considered an orthopedic emergency and should be managed initially by closed reduction. Reduction that is delayed longer than 6 hours after injury is associated with an increased risk for AVN of the hip. CT scan should be obtained after closed reduction to assess the reduction and evaluate for intraarticular comminution. If fracture fragments are found, they can be managed by either surgical excision or fixation. A fragment that is large enough to allow for internal fixation should be fixed. Smaller fragments found on the non–weight-bearing portions of the femoral head can be excised without consequence to outcome. If the hip is unable to be reduced, or if a femoral neck fracture is also present, an emergency open reduction is performed.

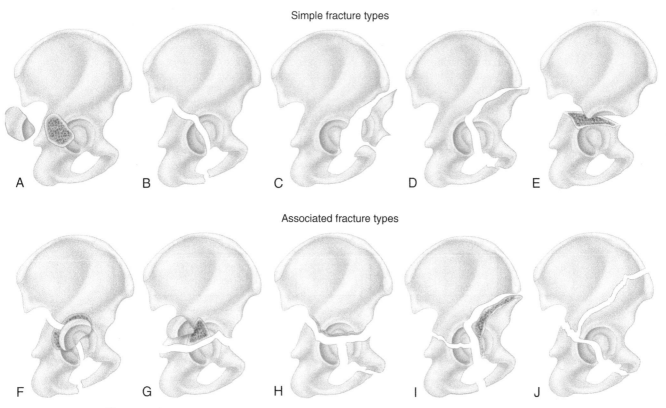

• **Figure 11-3** Letournel Classification of Acetabular Fractures. (From Canale ST, Beaty JH. Campbell's *Operative Orthopaedics*. 12th ed. Philadelphia: Mosby; 2013.)

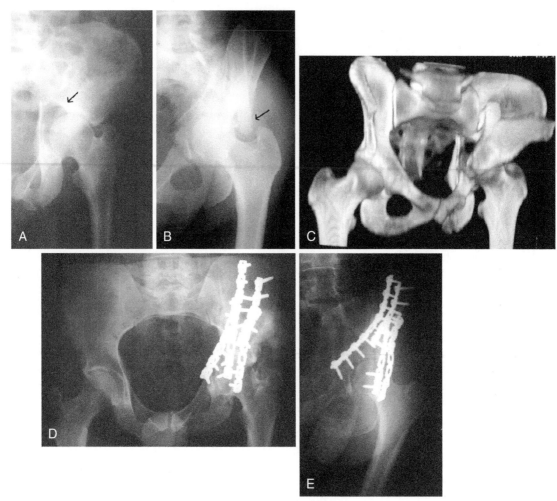

• **Figure 11-4** Type II Both-Column Fracture, With Split of the Second Fragment on the Origin of the Iliopubic Branch. Surgical treatment with posterior step first (double plate) and delayed anterior step (iliac and iliopubic plate). **A,** Preoperative anteroposterior view (*arrow* points to fracture). **B,** Preoperative obturator view (*arrow* points to fracture). **C,** Three-dimensional computed tomography reconstruction that clearly shows the fragments and their displacement, **D** and **E,** Anteroposterior and obturator radiographs 3 years after surgical treatment. (From Pierannunzii L, Fischer F, Tagliabue L, et al. Acetabular both-column fractures: essentials of operative management. *Injury.* 2010;41:1145-1149.)

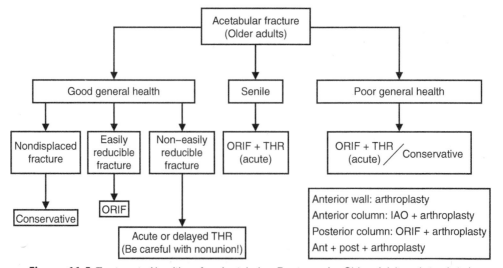

• **Figure 11-5** Treatment Algorithm for Acetabular Fractures in Older Adults. *Ant.,* Anterior; *IAO,* intraacetabular osteosynthesis; *ORIF,* open reduction and internal fixation; *Post.,* posterior; *THR,* total hip replacement. (From Guerado E, Cano JR, Cruz E. Fractures of the acetabulum in elderly patients: an update. *Injury.* 2012;43[suppl 2]:S33-S41.)

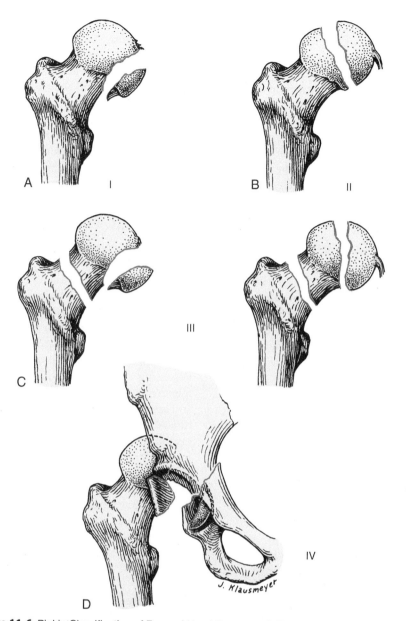

• **Figure 11-6** Pipkin Classification of Femoral Head Fractures. **A,** Type I, femoral head fracture distal to the fovea **B,** Type II, femoral head fracture extending through the fovea centralis **C,** Type III, femoral head fracture with femoral neck fracture **D,** Type IV, femoral head fracture with acetabular fracture. (From Browner BD, Jupiter JB, Levine AM, et al. *Skeletal Trauma: Basic Science, Management and Reconstruction.* 4th ed. Philadelphia: Saunders; 2009.)

The goals of the definitive management of a femoral head fracture are to reduce the femoral head, thus leaving good alignment of the hip joint, and clear any bony fragments from the joint. Most femoral head fractures are managed surgically; however, a Pipkin type I fracture may be managed nonsurgically if good alignment with closed reduction is achieved and the CT scan confirms that no other bone fragments are interposed within the joint. The risk of osteonecrosis with delayed surgical treatment warrants open reduction in the absence of a CT scan or delay of imaging greater than 6 hours.

For Pipkin type III fractures, the femoral neck must be surgically reduced and fixed first. Then the femoral head fracture can be managed according to the reduction achieved by fixation of the femoral neck. If the femoral head fragment is still displaced, surgical reduction or excision will be performed based on the location and size of the fragment. Pipkin type IV fractures are managed by fixation of the acetabulum and the femoral head. The approach is determined by the location of the acetabular fracture.

Postoperative Management

Typically, it is recommended that the patient bear partial weight (equal to the weight of the limb) on the involved side for 8 weeks. After 8 weeks, a progression toward full weight bearing should begin. Decisions on weight-bearing progression should be made according to healing, as evidenced by imaging (CT-directed pelvic oblique radiograph) and the overall medical status and function of the patient. If all fragments are removed and no other surgical fixation is performed, the patient may be managed as weight bearing as tolerated immediately. If a posterior surgical approach is used, initial postoperative precautions for range of motion of the hip include no hip flexion greater than 90 degrees and no hip adduction or internal rotation.

Rehabilitation should begin immediately, to assist the patient in gaining mobility and function to allow for an expedient and safe transition home. If, during the course of rehabilitation, hip pain worsens and joint mobility becomes more limited, AVN of the femoral head may be suspected. The incidence of osteonecrosis of the femoral head at 2 years has been reported at 11%.[13]

Femoral Neck Fractures

Fractures of the femoral neck account for almost half of all hip fractures and are most commonly found in older populations in association with falls.[14] Femoral neck fractures do occur in younger populations (>50 years of age) and may be divided into two groups, with different mechanisms of injury. Femoral neck fractures in patients younger than 40 years of age are typically caused by high-energy trauma, such as motor vehicle accidents. Another group of younger patients between the ages of 40 and 50 years may sustain these fractures after lower-energy traumatic events, typically a fall. Fractures in younger populations associated with low-energy trauma typically are associated with significant medical comorbidities and a higher rate of alcohol dependency.[15] Femoral neck fractures are considered intracapsular injuries because the joint capsule encompasses the femoral head and neck and anchors to the distal end of the femoral neck. Three ways to manage these fractures are recommended: closed reduction with internal fixation, open reduction with internal fixation, or hip arthroplasty. The choice of definitive treatment depends on the characteristics of the individual patient. Physiologically young patients who demonstrate high levels of activity, good bone health, and few comorbidities are managed differently from physiologically old patients, who are physically inactive and have poor bone health and multiple comorbidities. Differences in fracture patterns and the expected level of activity after injury pose very different implications for proper choice of definitive care.

Femoral Neck Fractures in Younger Patients

Initial management of these fractures in younger populations is considered an emergency, to reestablish blood supply to the femoral head, thus minimizing the risk of AVN. However, when reviewing the literature comparing AVN incidence with the timing of surgery, no associations can be made. In addition, timing of surgical treatment has no relationship with the incidence of nonunion.

In one report of hip fractures, populations younger than 65 years of age had a relatively higher incidence of pathologic fractures (11%) than did populations older than 65 years of age (1.4%).[3] Of the younger population, 18% of

the fractures were associated with patients who had a history of alcohol abuse. AVN is a concern in the younger patient with a femoral neck fracture. A metaanalysis investigating displaced femoral neck fractures in younger patients (aged 15 to 50 years) found the overall incidence of AVN to be 22.5%. No differences in the incidence of AVN were observed between groups undergoing surgical treatment within 12 hours of injury and groups receiving treatment more than 12 hours following injury. Prospective data demonstrate, at the 2-year mark, no differences in incidence of AVN in these populations when surgical treatment was performed before or after a 48-hour period after injury.

The relationship of different fixation devices and the presence of AVN or nonunion and overall outcome have not been investigated in younger populations. The choices of hardware for femoral neck fractures vary and may include compression screws, dynamic fixed angle devices, static fixed angle devices, and locked plates.

The Pauwels classification is the most commonly used classification system to describe femoral neck fractures (Fig. 11-7). Classification is based on the angle of the fracture line relative to a horizontal line drawn from the iliac crest. Possessing a more vertical orientation, a Pauwels type III fracture has an increased risk for nonunion as well as AVN, and careful consideration of the forces placed on these fractures during rehabilitation activities is required. Although justification for the use of fixed-angle implants can be made from a biomechanical perspective in treatment of these shear force–type fractures, no advantage has been shown over the use of multiple compression screws.[16] Nonunion has been associated with poor screw fixation placement and with the presence of a posterior comminution.[17,18] Although an increase in intracapsular pressure is associated with femoral neck fractures, no benefit has been demonstrated when capsular decompression has been performed.[19]

Femoral Neck Fractures in Older Patients

Outcomes using nonoperative management of femoral neck fractures in older adults show significantly higher incidence of comorbidities (e.g., pneumonia, thromboembolic events, decubitus ulcers) and nonunion than in patients who underwent surgical fixation.[20,21] The timing of surgery is important for the management of hip fractures in older adults. Delay of surgical treatment for more than 24 hours is associated with significantly higher mortality rates at the 30-day and 1-year postoperative marks (Table 11-1). No differences in mortality rates were found with delayed versus nondelayed surgery in patients who had significant medical comorbidities requiring preoperative treatment. This evidence supports the preoperative management of these comorbidities, even if it delays the surgical procedure.[22]

The Garden classification system is most commonly used for femoral neck fracture classification in older patients (Fig. 11-8). Treatment options include internal fixation, hemiarthroplasty, and total hip arthroplasty (THA). Internal fixation has higher risk of nonunion (>30%) in patients with osteoporosis.[23] Even if union is successfully achieved by

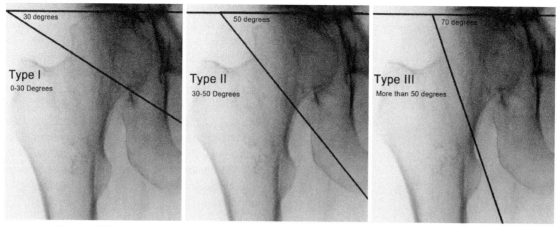

• **Figure 11-7** Pauwels Classification of Femoral Neck Fractures. **Left,** Type I. The fracture angle is greater than 30 degrees. **Middle,** Type II. The fracture angle is between 30 and 70 degrees. **Right,** Type III. The fracture angle is greater than 70 degrees. (From Van Embden D, Roukema GR, Rhemrev SJ, et al. The Pauwels classification for intracapsular hip fractures: is it reliable? *Injury.* 2011;42:1238-1240.)

TABLE 11-1	**Surgical Timing in Hip Fractures in Older Adults**			
Author	**Study Design**	**Level of Evidence**	**Number**	**Summary**
Zukerman et al, 1995*	Prospective observation	B	367	Surgical delay >48 hr doubled 1-year mortality (hazard ratio, 1.76)
Moran et al, 2005†	Prospective observation	B	2,660	Fit for surgery patients at presentation and surgical delay >4 days demonstrated increased 90-day (hazard ratio of 2.25; 95% CI: 1.2-4.3) and 1-yr mortality rates (hazard ratio, 2.4; 95% CI: 1.45-3.99)
Bottle and Aylin, 2006‡	Prospective observation	B	129,522	Delay in surgery >24 hr associated with increased in-hospital death odds ratio 1.39 (95% CI: 1.34-1.44), and when comorbidities were controlled, odds ratio fell to 1.27 (95% CI: 1.23-1.32)
Radcliff et al, 2008§	Prospective observation	B	5,683	Surgical delay of >4 days after admission associated with an increased risk of death within the first 30 days (odds ratio, 1.29; 95% CI: 1.02 to 1.61)
Shiga et al, 2008¶	Metaanalysis	B	257,367	Surgical delay of >48 hr increased 30-day and 1-year mortality rates by 41% (odds ratio, 1.41; 95% CI: 1.29-1.54) and 32% (odds ratio, 1.32; 95% CI: 1.21-1.43)

From Lowe JA, Crist BD, Bhandari M, Ferguson TA. Optimal treatment of femoral neck fractures according to patient's physiologic age: an evidence-based review. *Orthop Clin N Am.* 2010; 41:157-166.
CI, Confidence interval.
*Zuckerman JD, Skovron ML, Koval KJ, et al. Postoperative complications and mortality associated with operative delay in older patients who have a fracture of the hip. *J Bone Joint Surg Am.* 1995;77:1551-1556.
†Moran CG, Wenn RT, Sikand M, Taylor AM. Early mortality after hip fracture: is delay before surgery important? *J Bone Joint Surg Am.* 2005;87:483-489.
‡Bottle A, Aylin P. Mortality associated with delay in operation after hip fracture: observational study. *BMJ.* 2006;332:947-951.
§Radcliff TA., Henderson WG, Stoner TJ, et al. Patient risk factors, operative care, and outcomes among older community-dwelling male veterans with hip fracture. *J Bone Joint Surg Am.* 2008;90:34-42.
¶Shiga T, Wajima Z, Ohe Y. Is operative delay associated with increased mortality of hip fracture patients? Systematic review, meta-analysis, and meta-regression. *Can J Anaesth.* 2008;55:146-154.

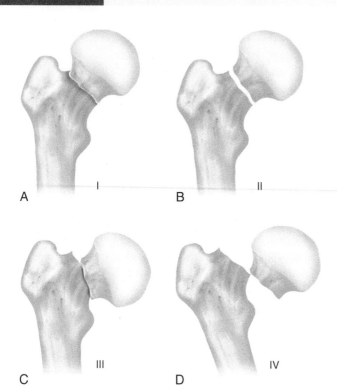

• **Figure 11-8** Garden Classification System for Femoral Neck Fractures. **A,** Garden type I, incomplete fracture line through the femoral neck. It may have some impaction. **B,** Garden type II, fracture line extending completely through the femoral neck with no displacement. **C,** Garden type III, femoral neck fracture with partial displacement. **D,** Garden type IV, femoral neck fracture with complete displacement. (From Waddell JP. *Fractures of the Proximal Femur: Improving Outcomes.* Philadelphia: Saunders; 2011.)

fixation, varus collapse and impaction of the neck have been found in 64% and 39% of patients, respectfully.[20,24] The presence of both impaction and varus collapse of the femoral neck is associated with poorer outcomes and predicts the need for an assistive device to assist with ambulation. THA is associated with higher blood loss and infection rates, and the incidences of surgical revision and progressive increase in pain are higher in patients undergoing internal fixation than with arthroplasty; higher costs are associated with internal fixation than with arthroplasty.[25,26] Because of these concerns, internal fixation is considered only for patients who are young, have good bony integrity, and have a Garden type I fracture.

Callaghan and associates[21] proposed a patient-related algorithmic approach to treatment. Their algorithm suggests that nondisplaced fractures should be managed with closed reduction and surgical fixation with screws. A displaced fracture in a younger patient is managed with open reduction and internal fixation. A displaced fracture in a physiologically older patient with good cognitive functioning can be managed with THA. Blomfeldt and colleagues[27] compared outcomes between hemiarthroplasty and THA in the management of femoral neck fractures and found superior outcomes in the THA group that continued to strengthen at the 4-year mark. Keating and associates[23]

found superior outcomes in the THA group when comparing THA with hemiarthroplasty and internal fixation. These investigators also investigated the cost associated with each procedure and found that, although cost was initially the least in the fixation group, overall cost was much less in the THA group after all associated complications were managed in the internal fixation group. A patient demonstrating cognitive impairments would be managed with a hemiarthroplasty because of the concerns of a high incidence of hip joint dislocation (32%) following THA in cognitively impaired older populations, which is a much higher incidence than THA performed in cognitively intact populations.[25,26,28-32]

Intertrochanteric Fractures

The intertrochanteric region is the extracapsular portion of the proximal femur between the femoral neck and the lesser trochanter (Fig. 11-9). Intertrochanteric fractures comprise approximately one third of all hip fractures occurring from low-energy falls and are commonly seen in older, female, osteoporotic populations.[33] Fractures in this region in younger populations are rare and typically are associated with high-energy blunt trauma. Absence of high-energy trauma in young populations, a history of malignant disease, hip pain just before a fall, or incidental findings of lesions on radiographs are all causes for suspicion of a pathologic fracture in this region. If falls are not associated with tripping, concern for a syncopal episode and its various causes is warranted. In addition, the patient may demonstrate poor balance in standing and with gait that predisposes him or her to a fall. All risk factors, from medical to functional, should be addressed during the course of care.

Classification of these fractures can be defined as one of five types. Type I is a nondisplaced, stable intertrochanteric fracture without comminution. Type II is a stable, minimally comminuted, but displaced fracture. Type III has a large posteromedial comminuted area and is unstable. Type IV consists of an intertrochanteric fracture with a subtrochanteric component and is considered unstable. A type V intertrochanteric fracture is a reverse obliquity fracture; the fracture line in this type of fracture extends laterally, and this fracture is also considered unstable.

Treatment of these injuries is with internal fixation. The method of fixation is determined by the fracture pattern. Dynamic hip screws may be used; these devices allow some impaction to occur along the barrel of the screw that is thought to enhance healing. A plate may be used to ensure that too much shortening does not occur because that may decrease muscular forces on the hip and result in gait abnormalities.[33]

Medical Complications Following Hip Fracture

More than 90% of hip fractures occur in older populations and are associated with medical comorbidities. This may be a primary reason that 1-year mortality rates have been reported to be higher than 20%.[34-36] Frequently cited medical complexities associated with hip fracture operations

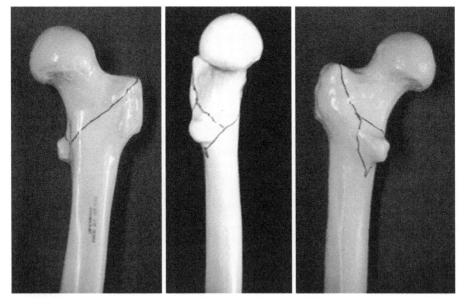

• **Figure 11-9** Intertrochanteric Fracture Sites. (From Park SY, Park J, Rhee DJ, et al. Anterior or posterior obliquity of the lag screw in the lateral view: does it affect the sliding characteristics on unstable trochanteric fractures? *Injury.* 2007;38:785-789.)

include the development of cardiac complications and anemia. Cardiac complications typically occur in patients with a premorbid cardiac condition and are usually related to myocardial ischemia. Patients who experienced early postoperative, clinically verified myocardial ischemia have a higher mortality rate at 1 year (35%).[36] Another cardiovascular complexity is deep vein thrombosis, which is always a risk in any postoperative population. The risk of this complication is greatly diminished with the prophylactic use of thrombolytic agents.[37]

Pulmonary complications can occur in as much as 4% of the population undergoing hip fracture surgery. Older adults are more prone to contract pulmonary infections and develop pneumonia because of changes in immune responses,[38] as well as lung epithelium,[39] associated with age. Pulmonary complications are associated with increased length of hospitalization. Early and frequent mobilization of the patient and the thoracorespiratory complex should assist in diminishing the risk of developing these complications.

Older patients exhibit a high incidence of mortality related to cognitive changes termed postoperative delirium; this condition has also been identified in 13.5% to 33% of the postsurgical population.[40] Observing for changes in mentation and careful consideration of cognition during the early postoperative period should be emphasized. The rehabilitation professional should ensure that the patient is able to respond to commands and to understand the precautions and orders regarding his or her functional status. Any observed changes in cognition should be reported to the health care team. Speech and occupational therapists may assist in improving cognitive processing and restoring function around any changes in mentation.

Pelvic Rim Trauma

Pelvic rim injuries range from lower-energy pubic ramus fractures to high-energy trauma with multiple fracture sites, ligamentous failure, and significant hemorrhage. If injury of the pelvis is suspected, initial anteroposterior radiographs of the pelvis are performed. If abnormal findings are present, then CT scan and radiographs of the pelvic inlet and outlet should be performed. These findings guide classification and subsequent treatment.

Several classification systems for pelvic fractures have been described. The Young-Burgess classification (Fig. 11-10) and the Tile classification are the most commonly used and referenced classification systems. Each of these systems offers a different conceptualization of traumatic injuries to the pelvis and provides important information on the stability of the pelvic rim, as well as the magnitude and vectors of force causing the injury, that may identify the need to rule out other possible comorbidities (see Table 11-1; Figs. 11-11 and 11-12).

Classification

Understanding the mechanisms behind the injury to the pelvis is important because it will provide information on the magnitude of forces and, subsequently, the extent of the trauma endured by the body. The Young-Burgess classification system classifies pelvic injury based on the mechanism of injury. Three types of injury are identified; anteriorposterior compression (APC), lateral compression (LC), and vertical shear (VS).

APC injuries occur as a result of compressive forces placed on the pelvis in an anterior to posterior or posterior

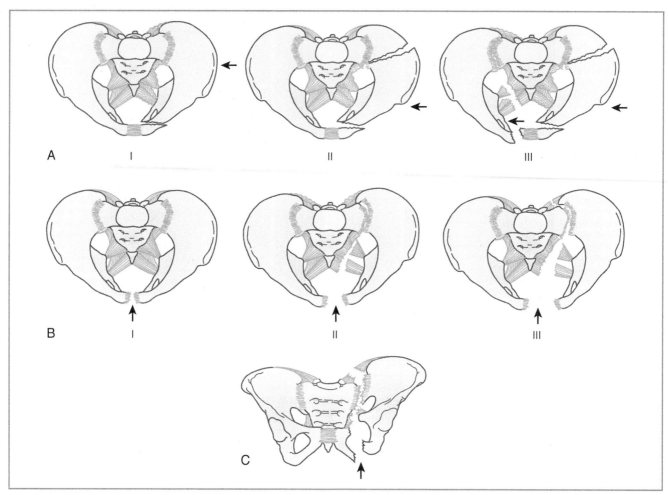

• **Figure 11-10 A** to **C,** Young-Burgess classification of pelvic trauma. (Redrawn from Young JWR, Burgess AR: *Radiologic Management of Pelvic Ring Fractures.* Baltimore: Urban & Schwarzenberg; 1987.)

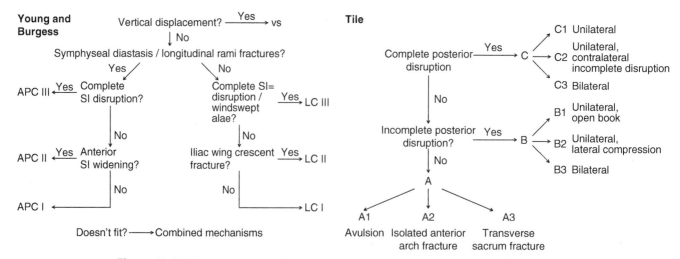

• **Figure 11-11** Comparison of Pelvic Trauma Classifications. *APC,* Anterior-posterior compression; *LC,* lateral compression; *SI,* sacroiliac. (From Osterhoff G, Scheyerer MJ, Fritz Y, et al. Comparing the predictive value of the pelvic ring injury classifications systems by Young and Burgess and by Tile. *Injury.* 2014;45:742-747.)

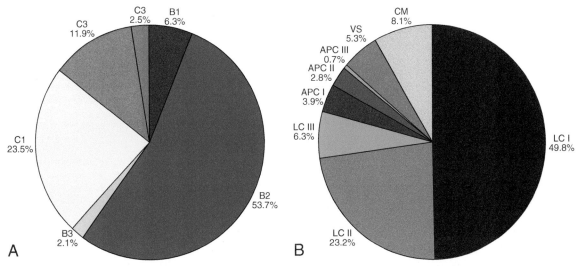

• **Figure 11-12** Fracture Types. Distribution of pelvic ring fracture types according to the classifications by Tile (**A**) and Young-Burgess (**B**). *APC,* Anterior-posterior compression; *CM,* combined mechanisms; *LC,* lateral compression; *VS,* vertical shear. (From Osterhoff G, Scheyerer MJ, Fritz Y, et al. Comparing the predictive value of the pelvic ring injury classifications systems by Tile and by Young and Burgess. *Injury.* 2014;45:742-747.)

to anterior direction. To identify the magnitude of force and define the extent of injury, APC injuries are subclassified into three different types of injuries. APC I injuries have less than 2.5 cm of pubic symphysis separation without affecting the integrity of the posterior elements of the pelvis. APC II injuries are characterized by pubic symphysis widening greater than 2.5 cm. For the pubic symphysis to widen this amount, disruption of the anterior sacroiliac ligaments, the sacrotuberous ligament, and the sacrospinous ligaments must occur. APC type III injuries include injuries to the posterior ligaments of the sacroiliac joint along with division of all the other structures found in APC II injuries. Fractures are not common in APC injuries, but, when present, they demonstrate a vertical orientation in the ramus. The amount of compressive force placed on the pelvis during injury directly relates to the traumatic changes identified on imaging. Much higher forces yield APC III injuries than APC I injuries. The clinical implications of this concept can be found in the increased need for blood transfusions, higher fluid replacement, and higher mortality rates in APC III injuries versus APC I injuries.[41] Greater forces cause greater injury, as well as an increased likelihood of comorbidity, such as trauma to the head, chest, spine, and abdomen.[41]

APC injuries are difficult to differentiate accurately. Often, radiographs are performed with the patient in a pelvic binder used to help maintain pelvic rim stability against rising hemodynamic pressures associated with bleeding and fluid responses to trauma. The binder may reduce the APC injury as it appears on film. In addition, unstressed radiographs, or radiographs performed under non–weight-bearing load, will not demonstrate the true nature of pelvic rim stability.

Young-Burgess LC injuries are injuries that occur from a compressive load applied laterally across the pelvis. These injuries are associated with bony fractures of the pelvis more than APC injuries, with fractures occurring in more of a horizontal or coronal plane than fractures associated with APC injuries. LC I injuries occur during a force directed onto the posterior and lateral portion of the pelvis. Ramus fractures and sacral fractures are seen with this type of injury. The severity of sacral fractures varies directly with the amount of force applied to the pelvis during injury, ranging from incomplete to complete fractures of the sacrum. LC II injuries are caused by a lateral force from the anterior part of the pelvis that mechanically forces the anterior aspect of the ilium to move medially and the posterior aspect to move laterally. These forces can result in sacral fracture, posterior disruption of the sacroiliac joint, and fractures of the ilium. LC III injuries occur from forces in the same vector as LC II injuries, although with greater energy causing additional damage to the contralateral hemipelvis including anterior sacroiliac injury and sacrotuberous and sacrospinous ligament injuries. VS injuries are a result of an axially applied load onto the pelvis, such as a high fall. These injuries cause a shearing of the hemipelvis relative to the sacrum, with complete tears of the sacrotuberous and sacrospinous ligaments or fractures of the ilium.

Although the Young-Burgess classification scheme provides an understanding of pelvic injuries as they relate to injury mechanism and severity of forces, it does not provide information on pelvic rim stability (see Figs. 11-11 and 11-12). The Tile classification system does classify pelvic injuries according to stability into one of three types (Fig. 11-13). In type A injuries, the pelvic ring is considered stable. Injuries are in isolated areas and do not contribute to instability of the pelvis. Such injuries can include avulsion fractures, sacrococcygeal dislocation, complete fractures of the innominate, and transverse fractures of the sacrum and coccyx. Avulsion fractures are often found in young athletic patients in whom the immature apophysis is

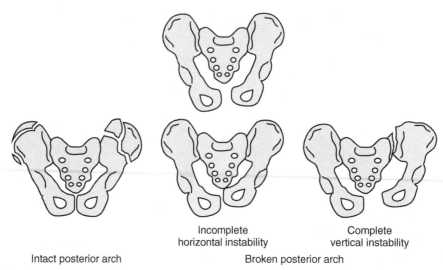

Intact posterior arch

Incomplete
horizontal instability

Broken posterior arch

Complete
vertical instability

• **Figure 11-13** Tile Classification System of Pelvic Injury by Instability. (Redrawn from Ul Haq R, Dhammi IK, Srivastava A. Classification of pelvic fractures and its clinical relevance. *JOTR.* 2014; 7[1]:8-13.)

overcome by strong and repetitive muscular forces. The most common sites of avulsion fractures around the hip and pelvis have been reported to be the ischial tuberosity, the anterior inferior iliac spine, the anterior superior iliac spine, and, to a lesser extent, the pubic symphysis and iliac crest.[42] Avulsion fractures are typically found in active adolescents; soccer and gymnastics are the sports with the highest reported incidences of avulsion fractures.[42] The onset of the pain is sudden, and the pain is provoked by athletic activity and improves with rest. Localized tenderness and swelling are present over the area of avulsion, and ecchymosis may also be seen in the acute phase. Weakness may be present in the involved musculotendinous unit, and stretching of the muscle may produce pain at the attachment sites. Acute fractures may not be seen on radiographs during the acute phases. CT scan and magnetic resonance imaging can be used to identify apophyseal injuries. The use of musculoskeletal ultrasound to diagnose avulsion fractures has also been reported in the literature, and it provides an expedient and cost effective tool for diagnosis.[43] Avulsion fractures can usually be managed successfully by rest and a guided return to normal sport activity by week 8 after injury.[44]

Contusions to the pelvis are most commonly associated with participation in contact sports, particularly at the elite level, where impact forces are higher.[45] Contusions to the iliac crest and associated soft tissues, often called hip pointers, are painful and often very disabling. The exact incidence of these injuries is unreported. However, these contusions occur much less frequently than do injuries to other regions throughout the lower kinetic chain.[45] The pain associated with these injuries results from significant subperiosteal edema and hematoma to the surrounding soft tissues and can be caused by a direct blow to the pelvis from an opposing player or a surface associated with a particular sport (i.e., a check into the boards during hockey or fall directly onto ice during ice skating). Patients present with significant pain and tenderness over the site of injury and may present with an antalgic gait. Initial treatment should focus

on controlling the swelling and bleeding by compression wrapping and cryotherapy. Assistance with gait by using crutches should be provided until the patient can demonstrate a normal gait, and rehabilitation should ensue with an emphasis on the restoration of lumbopelvic-hip mobility, motor control, and strength.

Type B injuries are partially stable. If one of the sacroiliac joints is disrupted and the other is spared, then only part of the pelvic rim is unstable. This can occur in so-called *open book* injuries, in which one innominate is rotated externally, thus gapping the pubic symphysis and one of the sacroiliac joints anteriorly. The opposite can occur, in which an innominate bone is rotated internally as a result of failure of the posterior ligamentous elements of the pelvis and overlap of the pubic symphysis. An injury involving both sides of the pelvis, thus rendering each side partially unstable, would be classified as a type B injury, resulting from the partial stability of each hemipelvis. If complete unilateral or bilateral disruption of hemipelvis is present, a Tile type C classification is used. Type C injuries are characterized by a complete separation of the innominate from the sacrum and the contralateral innominate at the pubis. This can occur on one or both sides. Because of the complete separation, the hemipelvis is rotationally and vertically unstable.

The Orthopaedic Trauma Association/AO (OTA/AO) expanded on the Tile classification and even added the Young-Burgess classification in as a subgrouping. This classification scheme is advantageous because it allows for an understanding of both the effects of mechanistic forces and the stability of the pelvis.

Reliability of these classification systems has been reported to be moderate to good. The Young-Burgess classification system has shown slightly higher reliability than the Tile classification.[46] Use of CT scanning and combining the two systems have been found to enhance reliability.[46] Reliability in classification of severe pelvic injuries is very low for the Young-Burgess and OTA/OA classification systems.

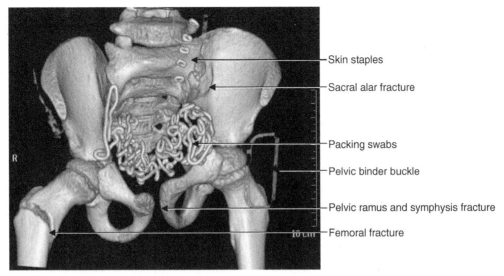

- Skin staples
- Sacral alar fracture
- Packing swabs
- Pelvic binder buckle
- Pelvic ramus and symphysis fracture
- Femoral fracture

• **Figure 11-14** Graphic showing the pelvic and femoral fractures and pelvic packs that clearly protrude from the pelvic brim to impinge on the femoral vessels. (From Cox SG, Westgarth-Taylor CJ, Dix-Peek SI, Millar AJ. Pre-peritoneal pelvic packing in a paediatric unstable pelvic fracture: an undescribed complication of lower limb compartment syndrome. *Injury.* 2013;44:258-260.)

Emergency Care

Multiple considerations are required in the management of pelvic fractures. Initial assessment of the patient should be made to identify the presence and source of hemorrhage. Death within 24 hours of injury is mostly the result of hemorrhage.[47] Bleeding can occur from arterial and venous structures, as well as from the bone at the fracture site itself. Bleeding is in direct relation to the pelvic trauma incurred; pubic ramus fractures can cause obturator vessel damage, and anterior sacroiliac joint injuries can cause damage to the hypogastric and gluteal vascular branches. It is common to have multiple sources of hemorrhage, thereby posing difficulties in the management of these injuries.[48] If the clinician must manage complex patients with hemorrhage and pelvic injuries, it is recommended that specific coordination and planning among the trauma team members should occur to standardize and organize an approach that will optimize patient care.[49]

In APC injuries, initial stabilization of the patient can be achieved through the use of a pelvic binder (Fig. 11-14).[50] This device will assist in providing stability to the pelvic rim through compressive forces around the pelvic rim. The binder can be a sheet or a commercially available device designed specifically for this function. The patient is bound around the level of the trochanters and anchored with clamps versus knots to avoid areas of increased compression. Binding the pelvis should be avoided if LC II injuries are present. The binder may cause further internal rotation of the hemipelvis and accentuate the injury. External fixation may also be used as a method of pelvic stabilization if other emergency surgical procedures are necessary, such as control of intraabdominal bleeding.[51] Iatrogenic injuries to intrapelvic vasculature can easily occur with the use of external

fixation devices. Most trauma centers now use binders and save external fixation for use by experienced surgeons in patients in whom binding may be contraindicated (i.e., degloving injuries to the hip and leg, hemipelvis internally rotated).

Once all sources of extrapelvic bleeding have been controlled or ruled out, attention can be given to bleeding in the pelvic region. Significant arterial bleeding and bleeding from the fracture site are common in pelvic fractures. If the patient is still hemodynamically unstable following binding or external fixation, then the bleeding will be controlled by several methods. Preperitoneal packing may be used to control venous and bony bleeding and may be the initial method used to restore hemodynamic stability and allow other areas of hemorrhage to be addressed (i.e., head, viscera). Preperitoneal packing is an invasive procedure in which laparotomy pads are placed in the retroperitoneal space on each side of the iliac vessels and are inserted through a midline incision above the pubis. The packs are removed again after several days. If patient is still hemodynamically unstable after packing and addressing other sources of bleeding, then angiography may be performed to identify local areas of arterial bleeding. Embolization, a minimally invasive occlusive procedure targeting specific arteries using the introduction of embolic agents, may be used to arrest arterial bleeding. An interventional radiology team performs these procedures.

The goal of surgical fixation is to stabilize the pelvic rim. Considerations of the type of injury assist in the clinical reasoning involved in surgical decision making. APC type I injuries are not managed surgically. APC type II injuries managed with fixation show good outcomes.[52,53] Stabilization for APC type II injuries is performed either with anterior fixation or a combination of anterior and posterior fixation. The choice to use posterior fixation is based on the integrity of the posterior sacroiliac ligaments. If these ligaments are disrupted, fixation is warranted to stabilize the pelvic rim posteriorly. Anterior and posterior fixation is used to stabilize APC type III injuries. LC injuries provide challenges because the stability of the fracture is often difficult to identify. Weight-bearing films are recommended, as is the application of the push-pull test on the hemipelvis to assess for sagittal plane stability. Management can range from conservative to anterior and posterior fixation. VS and combined injuries are always managed with fixation.

Postoperative management promotes early movement and weight bearing when safe. Considerations regarding activity must be communicated throughout the medical team and are in direct accordance with pelvic rim stability. Unstable injuries in the vertical plane, such as APC type III and VS injuries, should be treated as non–weight bearing on the involved side for 8 to 12 weeks. The surgeon should direct the weight-bearing orders. Vertical plane rotational injuries, such as LC type I and stable type II, in which vertical stability is not compromised, may be managed as weight bearing as tolerated, although clear communication with the surgeon regarding weight bearing is paramount.

Coccyx Injuries

The exact incidence of coccyx fractures is unreported; however, a higher incidence of coccygeal pain and injury is associated with female gender and obesity.[54] Causes of coccyx injury and pain can range from trauma (falls backward and landing on coccyx region) to the presence of infection, hypermobility or hypomobility of the sacrococcygeal joint, or tonal changes of the pelvic floor musculature. Prolonged sitting on firm and narrow surfaces can also contribute to coccyx pain. The presence of pain in this region has also been associated with psychological disorders.[55]

Coccyx pain resolves without the need for intervention in most cases. If management is necessary, the use of cushioning or donut hole devices for sitting is often recommended, along with the prescription of nonsteroidal antiinflammatory medications for the management of pain. If these measures do not work, more invasive procedures, such as intrarectal manipulation, can be used.[56] Recalcitrant cases of coccyx pain may be managed with injection to the ganglion impar, which is the sympathetic ganglion located just anterior to the sacrococcygeal junction.[57]

Rehabilitation Considerations Following Hip and Pelvic Trauma

Rehabilitation following hip and pelvic trauma should include an early, intensive, multidisciplinary approach. The goal in the acute setting should focus on early mobility and interventions that are more intensive and frequent. Studies showed that intense early physical therapy and occupational therapy provided subjects with greater level of function at discharge from the hospital and at the 2-week and 1-month postoperative point, as well as a shorter length of hospital stay.[58-62] Early therapeutic interventions should focus on the restoration of functional movement, with the goal of maximizing independence with bed mobility, transfers out of bed, static standing balance, and ambulation. Early range of motion of the hips and lower extremities is important to avoid joint stiffness and to help prevent deep vein thrombosis and pulmonary complications. Progressive strengthening exercises can reverse muscle inhibition and motor control changes associated with injuries and pain in musculature surrounding the pelvis. These changes have been shown to originate from the premotor cortex.[63] A focus on retraining musculature by active muscle contraction has been shown to reverse these aberrant central changes of motor control in the lumbopelvic-hip region. Active retraining of the transversus abdominis muscle, pelvic floor musculature, diaphragm, lumbar multifidus, gluteus, and lower extremity musculature can be taught to the patient to perform throughout the day, during the times when the patient is not in rehabilitation. These improvements in muscle activity and strength should then be worked into functional movement patterns to focus on restoration of the active mobility required to perform self-care tasks.

Ambulatory status should be steadily improved in these patients. Weight-bearing status should be defined by the orthopedic surgeon. Other comorbidities and a premorbid gait and functional status should be ascertained when able to provide a prognosis and frame realistic goals for mobility. Fractures and weight-bearing status of the other extremities create additional considerations when choosing an appropriate assistive device.

Patients discharged from the hospital to an inpatient rehabilitation facility have demonstrated significantly greater functional improvement over subjects discharged to a skilled nursing facility.[61] Patients discharged directly to their home and who received home-based rehabilitation demonstrated significantly greater functional recovery at 12 months after injury and greater community ambulation scores at the 4-, 8-, and 12-month mark than patients who went to an inpatient rehabilitation setting following discharge from the hospital.[64,65]

In the inpatient setting, the focus on improving muscle strength, range of motion, and functional mobility should continue. High-intensity physical therapy and intense strengthening of the quadriceps muscles have been shown to improve patient balance, reduce the length of stay in the rehabilitation setting, and improve general mobility.[66] The rehabilitation team should understand the circumstances surrounding the patient's discharge from the inpatient rehabilitation setting. Considerations of the physical environment of the home (including the presence of stairs, layout of bathrooms for toileting and bathing, family support) allow the team to focus on potential barriers to safety and independence and address functional mobility in a manner that will directly relate to independent function within the home.

If the patient is discharged home, return to independent activity can be performed practically and directly address the circumstances surrounding functional limitations. Intense strengthening should still be employed in the home setting, with an emphasis on integrating strength and mobility gains into functional movement pattern retraining. Strength gains alone have been shown not to result in changes to functional movement patterns. Challenging the patient in functional activities such as rolling in bed and accessing different positions of the developmental sequence are low-load activities that will help to retrain the body's ability to move through space independently by accessing the appropriate of joint mobility, muscle control, and proprioception required to complete a task successfully.

Once the patient has been cleared to return to full weight-bearing status, a determination of safety for ambulation assistance must be made. The higher-functioning patient will likely need to be progressed in a stepwise manner back to independent ambulation by gradually increasing weight bearing on the involved limb or limbs and decreasing the level of assistance offered from assistive devices for gait. Aerobic exercise, strengthening, and con-

tinued progression in functional movement pattern retraining should be emphasized, with patient-specific goals and family and societal expectations acting as the foundation for decisions about activity-specific interventions and eventually discharge. A younger patient with high-energy pelvic trauma needs to return to a higher level of function than does an older patient.

Older patients, or patients compromised functionally by medical complexities, should be carefully assessed for safety and fall risk when returning back to full weight-bearing status. In many cases, the persistent use of an assistive device may be necessary to ensure safety and reduce fall risk. Various fall-risk assessment tools have shown validity in a variety of settings. Decisions regarding functional mobility should be based on an objective measure of fall risk, balance, a comprehensive understanding of all medical and social factors of the involved patient, the patient's and caregivers' goals, and communication with the entire medical team.

Case Study

Case Study 11-1 describes an APC type II pelvic injury and a distal radial fracture in a young man.

CASE STUDY 11-1

Pelvic Injury and Nondisplaced Comminuted Distal Radial Fracture in a Young Patient

A 22-year-old man suffered an anterior-posterior compression type II injury to the pelvis and a nondisplaced comminuted distal radial fracture. Through examination, it was determined that internal fixation would be performed to the anterior and posterior right hemipelvis once the patient was hemodynamically stable and all other comorbidities were excluded. The radial fracture was managed with a long arm cast. Physical therapy (PT) and occupational therapy (OT) were ordered immediately. OT addressed all self-care activities and ruled out cognitive impairments that may have been caused by head trauma not found on computed tomography. PT began to mobilize the patient, by working with OT to optimize independent function with out of bed to chair transfers and toileting. PT also addressed gait by using a walker with a platform attachment for the right upper extremity. Weight-bearing orders from the surgeon were for non–weight bearing at the right wrist and weight bearing as tolerated to partial weight bearing of the right lower extremity. Initial foundational exercises consisted of the following: instruction in and performance of diaphragmatic breathing exercises; active contraction of the transversus abdominis muscle and pelvic floor musculature; active and purposeful contractions of the rectus and oblique abdominal muscles through the "pelvic clock" exercise; gluteal, quadriceps, and hamstring isometric exercises; and passive hip range of motion into flexion.

The patient and the patient's family were able to provide a social history. The patient is employed full time as a motorcycle mechanic and lives with his wife in a single story house that is compliant with the Americans With Disabilities Act. They have no children. On discharge to the home 5 days later, the patient was independent with his transfers and was able to dress and

bathe with the assistance of his wife. Home health PT and OT were ordered. The occupational therapist assessed the patient's function within the home. The patient was deemed safe with all self-care activities with assistance from his wife. A plan was made to restart OT on his hand to assist with reintegration back to the demands of his job once the cast was removed and the fracture of the radius showed sufficient healing. PT continued to work on overall mobility, including rolling from supine to prone, standing balance, and strength and range of motion of the extremities and trunk. Progressive resistive exercises were used to enhance strength of the knee and ankle musculature and all the muscle groups of the noninvolved limbs. Pelvic and modified trunk proprioceptive neuromuscular facilitation exercises were used to improve active muscle control in the lumbopelvic-hip region.

At 4 weeks, the patient was given full weight-bearing orders. The arm cast was cut to below the elbow (but still limited supination and pronation) at 2 weeks, and it was cut to the midforearm at 4 weeks. Progressive resistive exercises were continued. Mobility work was added to include functional movement through developmental sequencing positions to help access and restore the joint mobility and muscle timing required to complete more complex movement patterns. Proprioceptive neuromuscular facilitation was continued for trunk mobility and stability and exercises in quadruped, and bridging sequences were added to help improve posterior trunk muscle functioning. The patient was progressed from a walker to a single crutch under the left arm for ambulation. Gait training was performed with a cane in the left hand to off-weight the right side and assist with balance. The patient was progressed to a cane as soon as he was able to

Continued

CASE STUDY 11-1

Pelvic Injury and Nondisplaced Comminuted Distal Radial Fracture in a Young Patient—cont'd

demonstrate a normal, noncompensated gait using a cane. At that point, gait training would begin without the use of an assistive device, and the cane was discontinued when the patient demonstrated normal, safe, and noncompensated gait on level surfaces, inclines, steps, and stairs.

At 6 weeks, the patient continued rehabilitation in an outpatient clinic. He was independently ambulating in the community at that time but still exhibited pain and movement dysfunctions. The cast was removed from the upper extremity, and OT began to address the upper extremity limitations with the goal of returning the arm to full function to participate in all duties and demands associated with his job. To identify specific residual dysfunctions relating to the patient's overall mobility, a Selective Functional Movement Assessment (SFMA) was performed, revealing residual joint mobility and tissue extensibility dysfunctions in the right hip into extension patterns. A modified Thomas test (see Chapter 2) revealed tissue extensibility limitations in the iliopsoas, tensor fasciae latae, and quadriceps musculature on the right. The SFMA also found dysfunctions in unilateral standing and squatting. The unilateral standing dysfunction resulted from motor control impairments in the lumbopelvic hip region. The patient demonstrated a positive Trendelenburg sign on the right and difficulty maintaining unilateral standing balance on the right. Residual hip flexion limitations on the right and motor control impairments contributed to the inability to squat fully, which is a motion required for his job.

Manual therapy techniques were used to improve hip and lumbar joint mobility and tissue extensibility. The patient was instructed in self-stretching and band-assisted mobilization with movement exercises to improve hip joint and muscle mobility. Proprioceptive neuromuscular facilitation was added for the lower extremities, with manual resistance to be able to maximize muscle activity in different portions of the pattern. Aerobic exercise was performed 5 days per week for a minimum of 20 minutes and included walking and the stationary bicycle.

Foundational motor control correctives were added initially to address the motor control issue in the pelvis during unilateral standing. These included side-lying leg raises with

cues to not flex the hip, roll out of side lying either forward or backward, and no hiking of the pelvis. This was to isolate gluteus medius activity. The patient was asked also to balance in tandem half kneeling in a neutral hip position to isolate and force lumbopelvic stability to maintain his balance. Once stable in this position, the patient was challenged further by maintaining the position with eyes closed, working resisted chops and lifts out of this pattern, and standing from half kneeling. The pattern was progressed through a lunging exercise progression to improve strength and reinforce lumbopelvic stability in a split-stance pattern because he will likely function within this type of movement for his job.

Unilateral standing balance was addressed by having the patient maintain balance in standing without a pelvic drop. Visual feedback in a mirror was used for this maneuver. The patient was progressed to unilateral balancing on compliant surfaces. Once unilateral standing balance was maintained without compensation, unilateral squat patterns were introduced. Using a mirror for feedback, the patient was asked to squat without letting the knee and lower extremity adduct or internally rotate, thus forcing frontal plane control over the femur from the gluteus maximus muscle and control over the pelvis by the gluteus medius muscle. When good control of the unilateral squat pattern was demonstrated, the patient was instructed in a hip hinge pattern in which hip flexion would occur while maintaining stability of the spine. A long dowel was placed along the patient's back contacting the sacrum, midthoracic region, and back of the head to ensure that no flexion occurred anywhere along the spine while dropping into hip flexion patterns. This action was performed in bilateral and unilateral squat patterns. Once both patterns were performed with good lower extremity and trunk control, then the squat patterns were loaded. Kettlebells were used to load single squat patterns. Bilateral goblet squats were added, and deadlifting patterns were trained. These patterns were loaded to help train the patient in safe lifting patterns for his return to work.

The patient returned to full function and work at the 4-month mark.

References

1. Bauer CA, Coca-Perraillon M, Cutler DM, Rosen AB. Incidence and mortality of hip fractures in the United States. *JAMA.* 2009;302:1573-1579.
2. Grotz M, Allami MK, Harwood P, et al. Open pelvis fractures: epidemiology, current concepts of management and outcome. *Injury.* 2005;36:1-13.
3. Karantana A, Boulton C, Bouliotis G, et al. Epidemiology and outcome of fracture of the hip in women aged 65 years and under. *J Bone Joint Surg Br.* 2011;93:658-664.
4. Halbert J, Crotty M, Whitehead C, et al. Multi-disciplinary rehabilitation after hip fracture is associated with improved outcome: a systematic review. *J Rehabil Med.* 2007;39:507-512.
5. Stevenson AJ, McArthur JR, Acharya MR, et al. Principles of acetabular fractures. *Orthop Trauma.* 2014;28:141-150.
6. Dreinhofer KE, Schwarzkopf SR, Haas NP, Tscherne H. Isolated traumatic dislocation of the hip: long-term results in 50 patients. *J Bone Joint Surg Br.* 1994;76:6-12.
7. Hak DJ, Goulet JA. Severity of injuries associated with traumatic hip dislocation as a result of motor vehicle collisions. *J Trauma.* 2009;47:60-63.
8. Issack PS, Helfet DL. Sciatic nerve injury associated with acetabular fractures. *HSS J.* 2009;5:12-18.
9. Swiontkowski MF, Winquist RA, Hansen ST Jr. Fractures of the femoral neck in patients between the ages of twelve and forty-nine years. *J Bone Joint Surg Am.* 1984;66:837-846.
10. Laird A, Keating JF. Acetabular fractures: a 16-year prospective epidemiological study. *J Bone Joint Surg Br.* 2005;87:969-973.
11. Ferguson TA, Patel R, Bhandari M, Matta JM. Fractures of the acetabulum in patients aged 60 years and older: an epidemiological and radiological study. *J Bone Joint Surg Br.* 2010;92:250-257.

12. Hougaard K, Thomsen PB. Coxarthrosis following traumatic posterior dislocation of the hip. *J Bone Joint Surg Am.* 1987;69:679-683.

13. Kumar MN, Belehall P, Ramachandra P. PET/CT study of temporal variations in blood flow to the femoral head following low-energy fracture of the femoral neck. *Orthopedics.* 2014;37:e563-e570.

14. Karagas MR, Lu-Yao GL, Barrett JA, et al. Heterogeneity of hip fracture: age, race, sex, and geographic patterns of femoral neck and trochanteric fractures among the US elderly. *Am J Epidemiol.* 1996;143:677-682.

15. Robinson CM, Court-Brown CM, McQueen MM, Christie J. Hip fractures in adults younger than 50 years of age: epidemiology and results. *Clin Orthop Relat Res.* 1996;312:238-246.

16. Liporace F, Gains R, Collinge C, Haidukewych GJ. Results of internal fixation of Pauwel's type-3 vertical femoral neck fractures. *J Bone Joint Surg Am.* 2008;90:1654-1659.

17. Lindequist S. Cortical screw support in femoral neck fractures: a radiographic analysis of 87 fractures with a new mensuration technique. *Acta Orthop Scand.* 1993;64:289-293.

18. Upadhyay A, Jain P, Mishra P, et al. Delayed internal fixation of fractures of the neck of the femur in young adults: a prospective, randomised study comparing closed and open reduction. *J Bone Joint Surg Br.* 2004;86:1035-1040.

19. Maruenda JI, Barrios C, Gomar-Sancho F. Intracapsular hip pressure after femoral neck fracture. *Clin Orthop Relat Res.* 1997;340:172-180.

20. Zlowodski M, Jonsson A, Paulke R. Shortening after femoral neck fracture fixation: is there a solution? *Clin Orthop Relat Res.* 2007;461:213-218.

21. Callaghan JJ, Liu SS, Haidukewych GJ. Subcapital fractures a changing paradigm. *J Bone Joint Surg Br.* 2012;94(suppl A):19-21.

22. Battle A, Aylin P. Mortality associated with delay in operation after hip fracture. *BMJ.* 2006;332:947-951.

23. Keating JF, Grant A, Masson M, et al. Displaced intracapsular hip fractures in fit, older people: a randomized comparison of reduction and fixation, bipolar hemiarthroplasty and total hip arthroplasty. *Health Technol Assess.* 2006;9:1-65.

24. Zlowodzki M, Brink O, Switzer J, et al. The effect of shortening and varus collapse of the femoral neck on function after fixation of intracapsular fracture of the hip. *J Bone Joint Surg Br.* 2008;11:1487-1494.

25. Lu-Yao GL, Keller RB, Littenberg B, et al. Outcomes after displaced fractures of the femoral neck: a meta-analysis of one hundred and six published reports. *J Bone Joint Surg Am.* 1996;76:15-25.

26. Ravikumar KJ, Marsh G. Internal fixation versus hemiarthroplasty versus total hip arthroplasty for displaced subcapital fractures of femur: 13 year results of a prospective randomized study. *Injury.* 2000;31:793-797.

27. Blomfeldt R, Tornkvist H, Eriksson K, et al. A randomized controlled trial comparing bipolar hemiarthroplasty with total hip replacement for displaced intracapsular fractures of the femoral neck in elderly patients. *J Bone Joint Surg Br.* 2007;89:160-165.

28. Johansson T, Jacobsson SA, Ivarsson I, et al. Internal fixation versus total hip arthroplasty in the treatment of displaced femoral neck fractures: a prospective randomized study of 100 hips. *Acta Orthop Scand.* 2000;71:597-602.

29. Holmberg S, Kale'n R, Thorngren KG. Treatment and outcome of femoral neck fractures: an analysis of 2418 patients admitted from their own homes. *Clin Orthop Relat Res.* 1987;218:42-52.

30. Conn KS, Parker MJ. Undisplaced intracapsular hip fractures: results of internal fixation in 375 patients. *Clin Orthop Relat Res.* 2004;421:249-254.

31. Iorio R, Healy WL, Lemos DW, et al. Displaced femoral neck fractures in the elderly: outcomes and cost effectiveness. *Clin Orthop Relat Res.* 2001;383:229-242.

32. Soderqvist A, Miedel R, Ponzer S, Tidermark J. The influence of cognitive function on outcome after a hip fracture. *J Bone Joint Surg Am.* 2006;88:2115-2123.

33. Grisso JA, Kelsey JL, Strom BL, et al. Risk factors for fall as a cause of hip fracture in women: the Northeast Hip Fracture Study Group. *N Engl J Med.* 1991;324:1326-1331.

34. Mantilla CB, Horlocker TT, Schroeder DR, et al. Frequency of myocardial infarction, pulmonary embolism, deep venous thrombosis, and death following primary hip or knee arthroplasty. *Anesthesiology.* 2002;96:1140-1146.

35. Huddleston JM, Gullerud RE, Smither F, et al. Myocardial infarction after hip fracture repair: a population-based study. *J Am Geriatr Soc.* 2012;60:2020-2026.

36. Beaupre LA, Jones CA, Saunders LD, et al. Best practices for elderly hip fracture patients: a systematic overview of the evidence. *J Gen Intern Med.* 2005;20:1019-1025.

37. Lo IL, Siu CW, Tse HF, et al. Pre-operative pulmonary assessment for patients with hip fracture. *Osteoporos Int.* 2010;21:S579-S586.

38. Busse PJ, Mathur SK. Age-related changes in immune function: effect on airway inflammation. *J Allergy Clin Immunol.* 2010;126:690-699.

39. Dolan MM, Hawkes WG, Zimmerman SI, et al. Delirium on hospital admission in aged hip fracture patients: prediction of mortality and 2-year functional outcomes. *J Gerontol A Biol Sci Med Sci.* 2000;55:M527-M534.

40. Osterhoff G, Ossendorf C, Wanner GA, et al. Posterior screw fixation in rotationally unstable pelvic ring injuries. *Injury.* 2011;42:992-996.

41. Rossi F, Dragoni S. Acute avulsion fractures of the pelvis in adolescent competitive athletes: prevalence, location and sports distribution of 203 cases collected. *Skeletal Radiol.* 2001;3:127-131.

42. Pisacano RM, Miller TT. Comparing sonography with MR imaging of apophyseal injuries of the pelvis in four boys. *AJR Am J Roentgenol.* 2003;181:223-230.

43. Metzmaker JN, Pappas AM. Avulsion fractures of the pelvis. *Am J Sports Med.* 1985;13:349-358.

44. Feeley BT, Powell JW, Muller MS, et al. Hip injuries and labral tears in the national football league. *Am J Sports Med.* 2008;36:2187-2195.

45. Koo H, Leveridge M, Thompson C, et al. Interobserver reliability of the Young-Burgess and Tile classification systems for fractures of the pelvic ring. *J Orthop Trauma.* 2008;22:379-384.

46. Smith W, Williams A, Agudelo J, et al. Early predictors of mortality in hemodynamically unstable pelvis fractures. *J Orthop Trauma.* 2007;21:31-37.

47. Metz CM, Hak DJ, Goulet JA, Williams D. Pelvic fracture patterns and their corresponding angiographic sources of hemorrhage. *Orthop Clin North Am.* 2004;35:431-437.

48. Langford JR, Burgess AR, Liporace FA. Haidekewych GJ. Pelvic fractures. Part 1. Evaluation, classification, and resuscitation. *J Am Acad Orthop Surg.* 2013;21:448-457.

49. Routt ML Jr, Falicov A, Woodhouse E, Schildhauer TA. Circumferential pelvic antishock sheeting: a temporary resuscitation aid. *J Orthop Trauma.* 2006;20(suppl):S3-S6.

50. Miller PR, Moore PS, Mansell E, et al. External fixation or arteriogram in bleeding pelvic fracture: initial therapy guided by markers of arterial hemorrhage. *J Trauma.* 2003;54:437-443.

51. Matta JM. Indications for anterior fixation of pelvic fractures. *Clin Orthop Relat Res.* 1996;329:88-96.

52. Tornetta P III, Dickson K, Matta JM. Outcome of rotationally unstable pelvic ring injuries treated operatively. *Clin Orthop Relat Res.* 1996;329:147-151.

53. Maigne JY, Doursounian L, Chatellier G. Causes and mechanisms of common coccydynia: role of body mass index and coccygeal trauma. *Spine (Phila Pa 1976).* 2000;25:3072-3079.

54. Nathan ST, Fisher BE, Roberts CS. Coccydynia: a review of pathoanatomy, aetiology, treatment and outcome. *J Bone Joint Surg Br.* 2010;12:1622-1627.

55. Maigne JY, Chatellier G. Comparison of three manual coccydynia treatments: a pilot study. *Spine (Phila Pa 1976).* 2001; 26:E479-E483.

56. Foye PM, Buttaci CJ, Stitik TP, Yonclas PP. Successful injection for coccyx pain. *Am J Phys Med Rehabil.* 2006;85:783-784.

57. Sagi HC, Coniglione FM, Stanford JH. Examination under anesthetic for occult pelvic ring instability. *J Orthop Trauma.* 2011;25:529-536.

58. Cameron ID, Lyle DM, Quine S. Accelerated rehabilitation after proximal femoral fracture: a randomised controlled trial. *Disabil Rehabil.* 1993;15:29-34.

59. Swanson CE, Day GA, Yelland CE, et al. The management of elderly patients with femoral fractures: a randomised controlled trial of early intervention vs. standard care. *Med J Aust.* 1998; 169:515-518.

60. Koval KJ, Chen AL, Aharonoff GB, et al. Clinical pathway for hip fractures in the elderly: the Hospital for Joint Diseases experience. *Clin Orthop Relat Res.* 2004;425:72-81.

61. Jette AM, Harris BA, Cleary PD, Campion EW. Functional recovery after hip fracture. *Arch Phys Med Rehabil.* 1987;68: 735-740.

62. Mitchell SL, Stott DJ, Martin BJ, Grant SJ. Randomized controlled trial of quadriceps training after proximal femoral fracture. *Clin Rehabil.* 2001;15:282-290.

63. Kane RL, Chen Q, Finch M, et al. Functional outcomes of posthospital care for stroke and hip fracture patients under Medicare. *J Am Geriatr Soc.* 1998;46:1525-1533.

64. Giusti A, Barone A, Oliveri M, et al. An analysis of the feasibility of home rehabilitation among elderly people with proximal femoral fractures. *Arch Phys Med Rehabil.* 2006;87:826-831.

65. Kuisma R. A randomized, controlled comparison of home versus institutional rehabilitation of patients with hip fracture. *Clin Rehabil.* 2002;16:553-561.

66. Tsao H, Danneels LA, Hodges PW. Smudging the motor brain in young adults with recurrent low back pain. *Spine (Phila Pa 1976).* 2011;36:1721-1727.

Lower Extremity Muscles and Nerve Innervations*

TABLE A-1 — **Spinal Nerve Root Innervations of the Muscles of the Lower Extremity**

Muscle	L¹	L²	L³	L⁴	L⁵	S¹	S²	S³
Psoas minor	**X**							
Psoas major	*X*	**X**	**X**	*X*				
Iliacus		**X**	**X**	*X*				
Pectineus		**X**	**X**	*X*				
Sartorius		**X**	**X**					
Quadriceps		*X*	**X**	*X*				
Adductor brevis		**X**	**X**	*X*				
Adductor longus		**X**	**X**	*X*				
Gracilis		**X**	**X**	*X*				
Obturator externus			**X**	**X**				
Adductor magnus		*X*	**X**	**X**	**X**	*X*		
Gluteus medius				**X**	**X**	**X**		
Gluteus minimus				**X**	**X**	**X**		
Tensor fasciae latae				**X**	**X**	**X**		
Gluteus maximus					**X**	**X**	*X*	
Piriformis						**X**	**X**	
Gemellus superior					**X**	**X**	**X**	
Obturator internus					**X**	**X**	**X**	
Gemellus inferior				**X**	**X**	**X**		
Quadratus femoris				**X**	**X**	**X**		
Biceps (long head)					*X*	**X**	**X**	
Semitendinosus					*X*	**X**	**X**	**X**
Semimembranosus					*X*	**X**	**X**	*X*
Biceps (short head)						**X**	**X**	*X*
Tibialis anterior				**X**	**X**			
Extensor hallucis longus				*X*	**X**	**X**		
Extensor digitorum longus				*X*	**X**	**X**		
Fibularis tertius				*X*	**X**	**X**		
Extensor digitorum brevis				*X*	**X**	**X**		
Fibularis longus				*X*	**X**	**X**		
Fibularis brevis				*X*	**X**	**X**		
Plantaris				*X*	**X**	**X**		
Gastrocnemius						**X**	**X**	
Popliteus				**X**	**X**	**X**		
Soleus					*X*	*X*	**X**	
Tibialis posterior				*X*	**X**	*X*		
Flexor digitorum longus					**X**	**X**	**X**	
Flexor hallucis longus					*X*	**X**	**X**	
Flexor digitorum brevis					*X*	**X**	**X**	
Abductor hallucis					*X*	**X**	**X**	
Flexor hallucis brevis					*X*	**X**	**X**	
Lumbrical I					*X*	**X**	**X**	
Abductor digiti minimi						*X*	**X**	**X**
Quadratus plantae						*X*	**X**	**X**
Flexor digiti minimi						*X*	**X**	**X**
Abductor digiti minimi						*X*	**X**	**X**
Adductor hallucis						*X*	**X**	**X**
Plantar interossei							**X**	**X**
Dorsal interossei							**X**	**X**
Lumbricals II, III, IV						*X*	**X**	**X**

Spinal Nerve Root: L¹–L⁵ = Lumbar; S¹–S³ = Sacral.

X, Major distribution.

*From Neumann DA. Kinesiology of the Musculoskeletal System: Foundations for Rehabilitation. 2nd ed. St. Louis: Mosby; 2010.

Hip and Knee Musculature

Adductor Brevis
Proximal attachment: anterior surface of the inferior pubic ramus
Distal attachment: proximal one third of the linea aspera of the femur
Innervation: obturator nerve

Adductor Longus
Proximal attachment: anterior surface of the body of the pubis
Distal attachment: middle one third of the linea aspera of the femur
Innervation: obturator nerve

Adductor Magnus
Anterior Head
Proximal attachment: ischial ramus
Distal attachment (horizontal fibers): extreme proximal end of linea aspera of femur
Distal attachment (oblique fibers): entire linea aspera of the femur
Innervation: obturator nerve

Posterior (Extensor) Head
Proximal attachment: ischial tuberosity
Distal attachment: adductor tubercle of the femur
Innervation: tibial portion of sciatic nerve

Articularis Genu
Proximal attachment: anterior surface of the distal femoral shaft
Distal attachments: proximal capsule and synovial membrane of the knee
Innervation: femoral nerve

Biceps Femoris
Long Head
Proximal attachments: from a common tendon with the semitendinosus; originating from a medial impression on the posterior surface of the ischial tuberosity and part of the sacrotuberous ligament
Distal attachment: head of the fibula
Innervation: tibial portion of the sciatic nerve

Short Head
Proximal attachment: lateral lip of the linea aspera below the gluteal tuberosity
Distal attachment: head of the fibula
Innervation: common fibular (peroneal) portion of the sciatic nerve

Gemellus Inferior
Proximal attachment: upper part of the ischial tuberosity
Distal attachment: blends with the tendon of the obturator internus
Innervation: nerve to the quadratus femoris and gemellus inferior

Gemellus Superior
Proximal attachment: dorsal surface of the ischial spine
Distal attachment: blends with the tendon of the obturator internus
Innervation: nerve to the obturator internus and gemellus superior

Gluteus Maximus
Proximal attachments: outer ilium, posterior gluteal line, thoracolumbar fascia, posterior side of sacrum and coccyx, and part of sacrotuberous and posterior sacroiliac ligaments
Distal attachments: gluteal tuberosity and iliotibial band
Innervation: inferior gluteal nerve

Gluteus Medius
Proximal attachment: outer surface of the ilium, above the anterior gluteal line
Distal attachment: lateral surface of the greater trochanter
Innervation: superior gluteal nerve

Gluteus Minimus
Proximal attachment: outer surface of the ilium between the anterior and inferior gluteal lines, as far posterior as the greater sciatic notch
Distal attachments: anterior-lateral aspect of the greater trochanter and portion of superior capsule of the joint
Innervation: superior gluteal nerve

Gracilis
Proximal attachments: anterior aspect of lower body of pubis and inferior ramus of pubis
Distal attachment: proximal medial surface of the tibia just posterior to the upper end of the attachment of the sartorius
Innervation: obturator nerve

Iliopsoas
Psoas Major
Proximal attachments: transverse processes and lateral bodies of the last thoracic and all lumbar vertebrae including the intervertebral disks
Distal attachment: lesser trochanter of the femur

Iliacus
Proximal attachments: superior two thirds of the iliac fossa, inner lip of the iliac crest, and small region of the sacrum across the sacroiliac joint
Distal attachment: lesser trochanter of the femur through the lateral side of psoas major tendon
Innervation of Iliopsoas: femoral nerve (psoas major also receives branches from L1)

Obturator Externus
Proximal attachments: external surface of the obturator membrane and surrounding external surfaces of the inferior pubic ramus and ischial ramus
Distal attachment: medial surface of the greater trochanter at the trochanteric fossa
Innervation: obturator nerve

Obturator Internus
Proximal attachments: internal side of the obturator membrane and immediately surrounding surfaces of the inferior pubic ramus and ischial ramus; bony attachments extend superiorly within the pelvis to the greater sciatic notch
Distal attachment: medial surface of the greater trochanter just anterior and superior to the trochanteric fossa
Innervation: nerve to the obturator internus and gemellus superior

Pectineus
Proximal attachment: pectineal line on superior pubic ramus
Distal attachment: pectineal (spiral) line on the posterior surface of the femur
Innervation: femoral nerve and occasionally a branch from the obturator nerve

Piriformis
Proximal attachment: anterior side of the sacrum between the sacral foramina; blends partially with the capsule of the sacroiliac joint
Distal attachment: apex of the greater trochanter
Innervation: nerve to the piriformis

• BOX A-1 Attachments and Innervation of the Muscles of the Lower Extremity—cont'd

Popliteus

Proximal attachment: by an intracapsular tendon that attaches to the lateral aspect of the lateral femoral condyle
Distal attachments: posterior surface of the proximal tibia above the soleal line; also attaches to lateral meniscus
Innervation: tibial nerve

Psoas Minor

Proximal attachments: transverse processes and lateral bodies of the last thoracic and the first lumbar vertebra including the intervertebral disk
Distal attachment: pubis near the pectineal line
Innervation: branches from L1

Quadratus Femoris

Proximal attachment: lateral surface of the ischial tuberosity just anterior to the attachments of the semimembranosus
Distal attachment: quadrate tubercle (middle of intertrochanteric crest)
Innervation: nerve to the quadratus femoris and gemellus inferior

Rectus Femoris

Proximal attachments: straight tendon—anterior inferior iliac spine; reflected tendon—groove around the superior rim of the acetabulum and into the capsule of the hip
Distal attachment: base of the patella and, through the patellar tendon, the tibial tuberosity
Innervation: femoral nerve

Sartorius

Proximal attachment: anterior superior iliac spine
Distal attachment: along a line on the proximal medial surface of the tibia
Innervation: femoral nerve

Semimembranosus

Proximal attachment: lateral impression on the posterior surface of the ischial tuberosity
Distal attachments: posterior aspect of the medial condyle of the tibia; additional attachments include the medial collateral ligament, oblique popliteal ligament, popliteus muscle, and medial meniscus
Innervation: tibial portion of the sciatic nerve

Semitendinosus

Proximal attachments: from a common tendon with the long head of the biceps femoris originating from a medial impression on the posterior surface of the ischial tuberosity and part of the sacrotuberous ligament
Distal attachment: proximal medial surface of the tibia, just posterior to the lower end of the attachment of the sartorius
Innervation: tibial portion of the sciatic nerve

Tensor Fasciae Latae

Proximal attachment: outer surface of the iliac crest just posterior to the anterior superior iliac spine
Distal attachment: proximal one third of the iliotibial band of the fascia lata
Innervation: superior gluteal nerve

Vastus Intermedius

Proximal attachment: anterior-lateral regions of the upper two thirds of the femoral shaft
Distal attachments: lateral base of the patella and, through the patellar tendon, the tibial tuberosity
Innervation: femoral nerve

Vastus Lateralis

Proximal attachments: upper region of intertrochanteric line, anterior and inferior border of the greater trochanter, lateral region of the gluteal tuberosity, lateral lip of the linea aspera
Distal attachments: lateral capsule of the knee, base of the patella, and, through the patellar tendon, the tibial tuberosity
Innervation: femoral nerve

Vastus Medialis

Proximal attachments: lower region of intertrochanteric line, medial lip of linea aspera, proximal medial supracondylar line, fibers from adductor magnus
Distal attachments: medial capsule of the knee, base of the patella, and, through the patellar tendon, the tibial tuberosity
Innervation: femoral nerve

Ankle and Foot Musculature

Extensor Digitorum Longus

Proximal attachments: lateral condyle of tibia, proximal two thirds of the medial surface of the fibula, and adjacent interosseous membrane
Distal attachments: by four tendons that attach to the proximal base of the dorsal surface of the middle and distal phalanges through the dorsal digital expansion
Innervation: deep branch of the fibular (peroneal) nerve

Extensor Hallucis Longus

Proximal attachments: middle section of the medial surface of the fibula and adjacent interosseous membrane
Distal attachments: dorsal base of the distal phalanx of the great toe
Innervation: deep branch of the fibular nerve

Fibularis (Peroneus) Brevis

Proximal attachment: distal two thirds of the lateral surface of the fibula
Distal attachment: styloid process of the fifth metatarsal
Innervation: superficial branch of the fibular nerve

Fibularis (Peroneus) Longus

Proximal attachments: lateral condyle of tibia, head, and proximal two thirds of the lateral surface of the fibula
Distal attachment: lateral surface of the medial cuneiform and lateral side of the base of first metatarsal bone
Innervation: superficial branch of the fibular nerve

Fibularis (Peroneus) Tertius

Proximal attachments: distal one third of the medial surface of the fibula and adjacent interosseous membrane
Distal attachment: dorsal surface of the base of the fifth metatarsal
Innervation: deep branch of the fibular nerve

Flexor Digitorum Longus

Proximal attachments: posterior surface of the middle one third of the tibia just medial to the proximal attachment of the tibialis posterior
Distal attachments: by four separate tendons to the base of the distal phalanx of the four lesser toes
Innervation: tibial nerve

Flexor Hallucis Longus

Proximal attachment: distal two thirds of most of the posterior surface of the fibula
Distal attachment: plantar surface of the base of the distal phalanx of the great toe
Innervation: tibial nerve

Continued

Gastrocnemius

Proximal attachments: by two separate heads from the posterior aspect of the lateral and medial femoral condyle
Distal attachment: calcaneal tuberosity through the Achilles tendon
Innervation: tibial nerve

Plantaris

Proximal attachments: most inferior part of lateral supracondylar line of the femur and oblique popliteal ligament of the knee
Distal attachment: joins the medial aspect of the Achilles tendon to insert on the calcaneal tuberosity
Innervation: tibial nerve

Soleus

Proximal attachments: posterior surface of the fibula head and proximal one third of its shaft and from the posterior side of the tibia near the soleal line
Distal attachment: calcaneal tuberosity through the Achilles tendon
Innervation: tibial nerve

Tibialis Anterior

Proximal attachments: lateral condyle and proximal two thirds of the lateral surface of the tibia and the interosseous membrane
Distal attachment: medial and plantar aspects of the medial cuneiform and the base of the first metatarsal
Innervation: deep branch of the fibular nerve

Tibialis Posterior

Proximal attachments: proximal two thirds of the posterior surface of the tibia and fibula and adjacent interosseous membrane
Distal attachments: tendon attaches to every tarsal bone but the talus, plus the bases of the second through the fourth metatarsal bones; main insertion is on the navicular tuberosity and the medial cuneiform bone
Innervation: tibial nerve

Intrinsic Muscles of the Foot

Extensor Digitorum Brevis

Proximal attachment: lateral-distal aspect of the calcaneus just proximal to the calcaneocuboid joint
Distal attachments: usually by four tendons: one to the dorsal surface of the great toe, and the other three join the tendons of the extensor digitorum longus of the second through the fourth toes
Innervation: deep branch of the fibular nerve

Layer 1
Abductor Digiti Minimi

Proximal attachments: medial and lateral processes of the calcaneal tuberosity, plantar aponeurosis, and plantar surface of the base of the fifth metatarsal bone with flexor digiti minimi
Distal attachment: lateral side of the proximal phalanx of the fifth toe, sharing an attachment with the flexor digiti minimi
Innervation: lateral plantar nerve

Abductor Hallucis

Proximal attachments: flexor retinaculum, medial process of the calcaneus and plantar fascia
Distal attachment: medial side of the base of proximal phalanx of the hallux, sharing an attachment with the medial tendon of the flexor hallucis brevis
Innervation: medial plantar nerve

Flexor Digitorum Brevis

Proximal attachments: medial process of calcaneal tuberosity and central part of the plantar fascia
Distal attachments: each of four tendons splits and inserts on the sides of the plantar aspect of the base of the middle phalanx of the lesser toes
Innervation: medial plantar nerve

Layer 2
Lumbricals

Proximal attachments: from the tendons of the flexor digitorum longus muscle
Distal attachments: each muscle crosses the medial side of each metatarsophalangeal joint to insert into the dorsal digital expansion of the four lesser toes
Innervation: to second toe—medial plantar nerve; to third through fifth toes—lateral plantar nerve

Quadratus Plantae

Proximal attachments: by two heads from the medial and lateral aspect of the plantar surface of the calcaneus, distal to the calcaneal tuberosity
Distal attachment: lateral border of the flexor digitorum longus common tendon
Innervation: lateral plantar nerve

Layer 3
Adductor Hallucis

Proximal attachments
  Oblique head: plantar aspect of the base of the second through fourth metatarsal and the fibrous sheath of the fibularis longus tendon
  Transverse head: plantar aspect of the ligaments that support the metatarsophalangeal joints of the third through fifth toes
Distal attachments: both heads converge to insert on the lateral base of the proximal phalanx of the great toe along with the lateral tendon of the flexor hallucis brevis
Innervation: lateral plantar nerve

Flexor Digiti Minimi

Proximal attachments: plantar surface of the base of the fifth metatarsal bone and fibrous sheath covering the tendon of the fibularis longus
Distal attachment: lateral surface of the base of the proximal phalanx of the fifth toe blending with the tendon of the abductor digiti minimi
Innervation: lateral plantar nerve

Flexor Hallucis Brevis

Proximal attachments: plantar surface of the cuboid and lateral cuneiform bones and on parts of the tendon of the tibialis posterior muscle
Distal attachments: by two tendons in which the lateral tendon attaches to the lateral base of the proximal phalanx of the great toe with the adductor hallucis, and the medial tendon attaches to the medial base of the proximal phalanx of the great toe with the abductor hallucis; a pair of sesamoid bones is located within the tendons of this muscle
Innervation: medial plantar nerve

Layer 4
Dorsal Interossei

Proximal attachments
  First: adjacent sides of the first and second metatarsals
  Second: adjacent sides of the second and third metatarsals
  Third: adjacent sides of the third and fourth metatarsals
  Fourth: adjacent sides of the fourth and fifth metatarsals

• BOX A-1   Attachments and Innervation of the Muscles of the Lower Extremity—cont'd

*Distal attachments**

First: medial side of the base of the proximal phalanx of the second toe

Second: lateral side of the base of the proximal phalanx of the second toe

Third: lateral side of the base of the proximal phalanx of the third toe

Fourth: lateral side of the base of the proximal phalanx of the fourth toe

Innervation: lateral plantar nerve

*Attaches into the dorsal digital expansion of the toes.

Plantar Interossei

Proximal attachments

First: medial side of the third metatarsal

Second: medial side of the fourth metatarsal

Third: medial side of the fifth metatarsal

*Distal attachments**

First: medial side of the proximal phalanx of the third toe

Second: medial side of the proximal phalanx of the fourth toe

Third: medial side of the proximal phalanx of the fifth toe

Innervation: lateral plantar nerve

Appendix B

Hip Functional Performance Tests

TABLE B-1 Summary of Functional Performance Tests with Evidence of Validity to Hip Function

Test	Category	Relationship With Hip Function	Interpretation of Test Results
Deep squat	Movement	Patients with femoroacetabular impingement demonstrate less squat depth and altered lumbopelvic kinematics	Patients with femoroacetabular impingement have mean peak squat depth of 41% of leg length Normal mean peak squat depth is 32% of leg length
Single-leg squat	Movement	Subjects graded as "poor" on the single leg squat test exhibit weaker and slower muscle activation of the hip abductors than those graded as "good"	Subjects were ordinally graded (good, fair, poor) on ability to maintain balance, postural control, and lower body alignment during 5 repetitions of a single leg squat to 60 degrees
Single leg stance	Balance	Provocation of pain during 30-sec single-leg stance has shown sensitivity (100%) and specificity (97.3%) in detecting tendinopathy of the gluteus medius and minimus	Positive test result is an increase of pain within 30 sec of single leg stance Normal function of the hip abductors maintains the pelvis nearly perpendicular to the femur in a single leg stance position Normal is 30 sec of single leg stance without pain
Star excursion balance test (SEBT)	Balance	Hip flexion range of motion explained 86%-92% of SEBT reach distances Hip abduction and extension strength have a moderate correlation ($r = .48-.51$) to posterior-medial and posterior-lateral reach distances Elicits activation of the gluteus medius at 49% of maximal volitional isometric contraction during medial reach	Anterior reach difference ≥ 4 cm is 2.5 times risk for injury A composite score standardized to leg length <94% is 6 times more likely for injury

From Kivlan BR, Martin RL. Functional performance testing of the hip in athletes: a systematic review for reliability and validity. *Int J Sports Phys Ther.* 2012;7(4):402-412.

TABLE B-2 Evidence of Reliability and Normative Values for Functional Performance Tests in Physically Active Subjects

Test	Category	Average Age of Subjects (yr)	Evidence of Reliability	Normative Values for Healthy Subjects
Single leg squat test	Movement	24 ± 5	.61-.80 (intrarater)	"Good" to "excellent" alignment of hip flexion (<65 degrees), hip adduction (<10 degrees), and knee valgus (<10 degrees)
Functional movement screen	Movement	22 ± 4	.97 (interrater)	15-16 composite score
Single leg balance test (Trendelenburg test)	Balance	33 ± 11 (males) 28 ± 8 (females)	.58 (intrarater) MDC >4 degrees of pelvic on femoral angle	Normal pelvic on femoral angle = 83 degrees (range, 76-94 degrees)
Single leg balance (10-sec balance test with eyes closed)	Balance	21 ± 2 (males) 28 ± 8 (females)	.21 (test-retest) 1.00 (interrater)	Maintain postural control and balance on a single limb with eyes closed for 10 sec

TABLE B-2 Evidence of Reliability and Normative Values for Functional Performance Tests in Physically Active Subjects—cont'd

Test	Category	Average Age of Subjects (yr)	Evidence of Reliability	Normative Values for Healthy Subjects
Balance error scoring system	Balance	21 ± 2 (males) 28 ± 8 (females)	.74 (test-retest) SDD = 9.4 errors (intertester) 7.3 errors (intratester)	9.1 errors: female gymnasts 14.1 errors: female basketball players 5-7 errors: male baseball players
Star excursion balance test	Balance	22 ± 4 (males) 23 ± 3 (females)	.84-.92 (test-retest) .35-.93 (interrater) SDD = 6%-8% of the subject's limb length	Anterior reach difference <4 cm >94% of composite score
Single leg hop	Hop/jump	23 ± 3 (males) 22 ± 4 (females) 25 ± 4	.80-.96 (test-retest) SDD = 22% of the subject's limb length	Females = 157% of leg length Males = 189% of leg length
Triple hop	Hop/jump	23 ± 3 (males) 22 ± 4 (females) 25 ± 4	.80-.95 (test-retest) SDD: Females = 48% of leg length Males = 64% of leg length	Females = 505% of leg length Males = 585% of leg length
Timed hop test	Hop/jump	23 ± 3 (males) 22 ± 4 (females) 25 ± 4 years	.60-.84 (test-retest) SDD: Females = .21 sec Males = .23 sec	Females = 2.06 sec Males = 1.76 sec LSI >99%
One-legged hop test (medial and lateral)	Hop/jump	Male hockey players 20 ± 3	.87-.95 (test-retest)	Medial = 157 cm and lateral = 160 cm for male hockey players 2% difference between medial and lateral distances
Side hop test (timed test)	Hop/jump	Female athletes 22 ± 2 College students 20 ± 2	.48-.84 (test-retest) MDC = 5.82 sec	Females = 8.20 sec Males = 7.36 sec
Side hop test (number in 30 sec)	Hop/jump	Male and female 28 ± 4	.87-.93 (test-retest)	50 hops
Figure 8 hop test	Hop/jump	Female athletes 22 ± 2 College students 20 ± 2	.85-.99 (test-retest) MDC = 4.59 sec	Females = 12.47 sec Males = 11.36 sec LSI = 81 sec
Crossover hop test (for time)	Hop/jump	College students 20 ± 2	.96 (test-retest) MDC = 1.03 sec	2.7-2.8 sec
Crossover hop test (for distance)	Hop/jump	23 ± 3 (males) 22 ± 4 (females) 25 ± 4	.86-.96 (test-retest) SDD = 55%-59% of the subject's leg length	Females = 480% of leg length Males = 555% of leg length
Square hop test (for time)	Hop/jump	College students 20 ± 2	.90 (test-retest) MDC = 3.88 sec	15-16 sec
Square hop test (for number of jumps)	Hop/jump	Males and females 28 ± 4	.58-.85 (test-retest)	62 jumps
Agility T-test	Agility	23 ± 3 (males) 22 ± 4 (females)	.82-.96 (test-retest) SDD: Males = .48 sec Females = .58 sec	Males = 10.7 sec Females = 13.0 sec
Modified agility test	Agility	Males and females 21 ± 4	.83 (test-retest)	9.59 sec
Reactive agility test	Agility	Male Australian football players 17 ± 1	.91 (test-retest)	2.42-2.96 sec

Modified from Kivlan BR, Martin RL. Functional performance testing of the hip in athletes: a systematic review for reliability and validity. *Int J Sports Phys Ther.* 2012;7(4):402-412.

LSI, Limb symmetry index; *MDC,* minimal detectable change; *SDD,* smallest detectable difference.

Appendix C

Radiography of the Hip: Lines, Signs, and Patterns of Disease*

The complex anatomy of the pelvis and the often subtle but significant radiographic findings can be challenging to the radiologist. A sound understanding of the standard radiographic techniques, normal anatomy, and patters of disease affecting the pelvis can be helpful in accurate diagnosis. This article will review the common radiographic projections in conventional radiography of the pelvis and hip and will discuss radiographic anatomy, including the various lines used to evaluate the pelvis and hip joint. Specific signs and patterns of disease will be addressed, with the goal of providing a fundamental approach to interpreting hip and pelvis radiographs.

Radiographic Technique

Commonly used radiographic projections of the pelvis and proximal femur include the anteroposterior (AP) view of the pelvis, anterior and posterior oblique (Judet) views of the pelvis, AP view of the hip, and frog-leg lateral (Dan Miller) view of the hip.[1-3] The AP radiograph of the pelvis (Fig. C-1) or hip is taken with the patient supine and both feet in approximately 15 degrees of internal rotation. This reduces the normal 25 to 30 degree femoral anteversion, allowing better visualization of the femoral neck.[2] Judet views are performed with the patient in a 45 degree oblique position.[2,3] When the affected hip is in a posterior oblique position, the posterior column and anterior acetabular rim are well seen (Fig. C-2). Conversely, with the affected hip in the anterior oblique position, the anterior column and posterior acetabular rim are well seen. The frog-leg lateral view (Fig. C-3) is performed with the patient supine, feet together, and thighs maximally abducted and externally rotated.[2] The radiographic tube is angled 10 to 15 degree cephalad, directed just above the pubic symphysis.[2] The anterior and posterior aspects of the femoral neck, as well as the lateral aspect of the femoral head, are seen with this projection.

Additional views that may be helpful include the pelvic outlet (Ferguson) view, the pelvic inlet view, and the groin lateral (Dan Miller) view of the hip. The Ferguson view is performed in the same position as the AP view, with the radiographic tube angled 30 to 35 degrees cephalad, and the central beam directed at the center of the pelvis.[2] This projection allows excellent visualization of the sacroiliac joints, the pubic rami, and the posterior acetabular rim (Fig. C-4). The pelvic inlet view is performed in the same position as the AP view, with 30 to 35 degrees of caudal angulation of the radiographic tube.[2] This view allows visualization of the sacral promontory, the iliopectineal line (anterior column), the ischial spine, and the pubic symphysis (Fig. C-5). The groin-lateral view of the hip is performed with the patient supine, the unaffected leg elevated and abducted, and the affected leg extended.[2] The radiographic tube is directed horizontally toward the medial aspect of the affected hip with 20 degrees of the cephalad angulation (Fig. C-6).

Anatomy

The pelvis is composed of three bones, the ilium, ischium, and pubis, all of which contribute to the structure of the acetabulum.[2-5] The ilium is composed of a body and a large flat portion called the iliac wing.[5] The body forms, with the bodies of the ischium and pubis, the roof of the acetabulum. The arcuate line is a bony ridge projecting from the sacroiliac joint to the pubis, dividing the iliac body from the iliac wing. The superior border of the iliac wing is the iliac crest. Anteriorly, there are two projections from the ilium, the anterior superior and inferior iliac spines. Posteromedially, the ilium articulates with the sacrum via the sacroiliac joint. The distal one-third of the sacroiliac joint is a synovial joint, whereas the proximal two thirds forms a syndesmosis.[5]

The pubis is composed of a body and two rami.[5] The pubic body fuses with the iliac and ischial bodies to form the anterior border of the acetabulum. The superior pubic rami project anteroinferiorly from the acetabuli. A linear body ridge along the superomedial border of the superior pubic ramus is present, called the pectin pubis, or pectineal line. This is continuous with the arcuate line of the ilium, forming the iliopectineal line (Fig. C-7), the anterior border of the "anterior column."[2,3] The iliopectineal line is an important osseous landmark to visualize on every radiograph of the hip or pelvis, as traumatic, metabolic, or neoplastic conditions affecting the anterior column of the pelvis

*Article reprinted with permission from Campbell SE: Radiography of the hip: lines, signs, and patterns of disease. *Semin Roentgenol.* 2005;40(3):290-319.

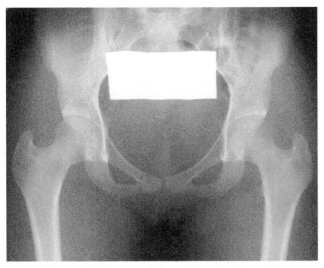

• **Figure C-1** Anteroposterior radiograph of the pelvis.

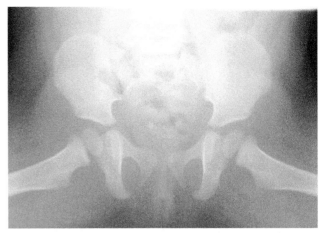

• **Figure C-3** Frog-leg lateral radiograph of the pelvis.

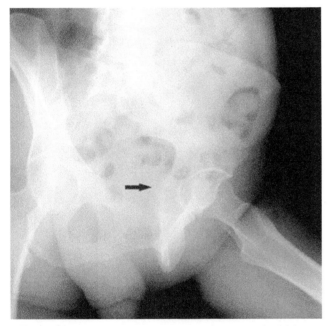

• **Figure C-2** Forty-five-degree posterior oblique view of the left acetabulum reveals a nondisplaced fracture through the posterior column.

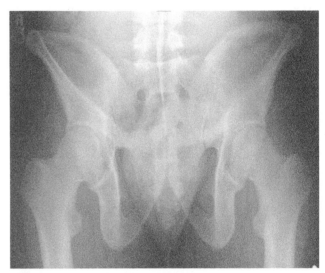

• **Figure C-4** Pelvic outlet view allows good visualization of the sacroiliac joints and pubic rami.

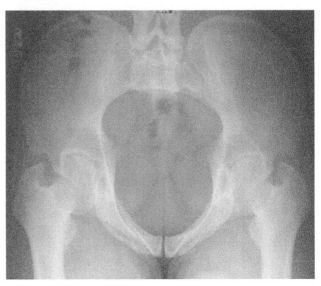

• **Figure C-5** Pelvic inlet view reveals the sacral promontory and iliopectineal line to good advantage.

will cause discontinuity, thickening, or an abnormal course of this line.[3,4] The inferior pubic rami project inferiorly from the medial border of the superior rami and have a symphyseal surface, which articulates with the pubic symphysis. The pubic symphysis may be widened in traumatic symphyseal diastasis or in bladder exstrophy (Fig. C-8).

The ischium is also composed of a body and two rami.[5] The body forms the posterior border of the acetabulum. At birth, the three bones contributing to formation of the acetabulum are not fused and are separated by the triradiate cartilage.[6] A posterior projection from the body of the ischium is called the ischial spine. The curved notch between the posterior inferior iliac spine and the ischial spine is the greater sciatic notch, and the notch between the ischial

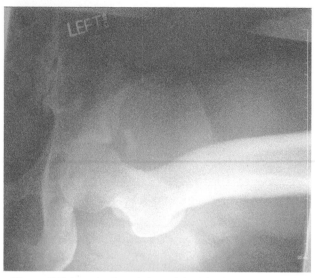

• **Figure C-6** Long-leg lateral view of the left hip shows prominent femoral head–neck junction, narrowing of the anterosuperior joint space, and sclerosis of the anterosuperior acetabulum. Heterotopic bone formation is seen from previous hip arthroscopy for anterior labral débridement in a patient with femoroacetabular impingement.

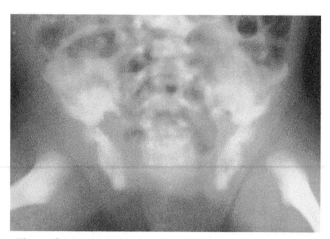

• **Figure C-8** Marked widening of the pubic symphysis is seen in this patient with bladder exstrophy.

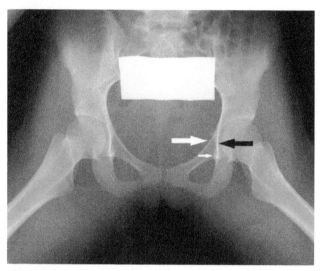

• **Figure C-7** The iliopectineal line is part of the anterior column *(large white arrow)*; ilioischial line is part of the posterior column *(black arrow)*, and has a teardrop appearance *(small white arrow)*.

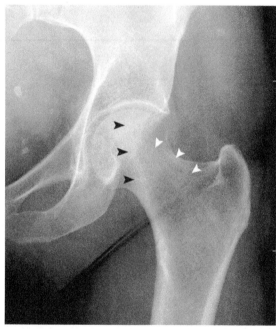

• **Figure C-9** Anteroposterior view of the hip shows the principal compressive *(black arrowheads)* and principal tensile *(white arrowheads)* trabeculae.

spine and the ischial tuberosity is the lesser sciatic notch. The superior ramus of the ischium extends inferiorly from the body to the ischial tuberosity. On the AP radiograph, a line can be drawn from the ilium to the ischial tuberosity and is called the ilioischial line.[3,4] This line is part of the "posterior column" (see Fig. C-7) and is also an important landmark to be visualized on every radiograph of the pelvis. The inferior ischial ramus projects anteriorly to fuse with the inferior pubic ramus, forming the obturator foramen.

The proximal femur can be divided into the femoral head, femoral neck, trochanters, and femoral shaft.[5] The fovea is seen at the medial aspect of the femoral head. The

femoral neck can be divided into subcapital, transcervical, basicervical, intertrochanteric, and subtrochanteric portions.[2] The latter three of these are extracapsular. The femoral head is normally angulated approximately 125 to 135 degrees with respect to the long axis of the femoral shaft, and anteverted approximately 25 to 30 degrees.[2,5] The major trabeculae of the proximal femur are well demonstrated on the AP radiograph.[2] Long, arc-shaped trabeculae extending from the femoral head to the intertrochanteric ridge are the principal tensile trabecular, while the principal compressive trabecular are more vertically oriented, coursing along the medial aspect of the femoral neck (Fig. C-9).

Lines

On the standard AP view of the pelvis, the iliopectineal line (also called the iliopubic line) extends from the medial border of the iliac wing, along the superior border of the superior pubic ramus[2-4] to end at the pubic symphysis (see Fig. C-1). This line is seen as the inner margin of the pelvic ring and defines the anterior column of the pelvis (see Fig. C-7). As mentioned earlier, the anterior column is well demonstrated by a 45-degree anterior oblique radiograph.[3] Fractures extending through the anterior column disrupt the contour of this line (Fig. C-10). In addition, this line may be thickened in patients with Paget disease[7] or in patients with familial idiopathic hyperphosphatasia.[8]

The ilioischial line also begins at the medial border of the iliac wing and extends along the medial border of the ischium[2-4] to end at the ischial tuberosity (see Fig. C-4). This defines the posterior column of the pelvis (see Fig. C-7). As mentioned earlier, the posterior column is well demonstrated by a 45-degree posterior oblique radiograph.[3] Fractures extending through the posterior column of the pelvis disrupt the contour of the ilioischial line (see Fig. C-2).

The anterior rim of the acetabulum is seen as the more medial of two obliquely oriented arc-shaped lines on the AP view[2-4] (Fig. C-11). The anterior acetabular rim is seen well in profile on the 45-degree posterior oblique view[2] (see Fig. C-2). The posterior rim of the acetabulum is the more lateral arc-shaped line on the AP radiograph and is seen well in profile on the 45-degree anterior oblique view.[2] The teardrop represents a summation of shadows of the medial acetabular wall[9] (see Fig. C-7). Teardrop distance is measured from the lateral edge of the teardrop and the femoral head. Side-to-side comparison of the teardrop distance can be useful to evaluate for hip joint effusion or for hip dysplasia.[9]

Line of Kline is a line drawn along the long axis of the superior aspect of the femoral neck, which normally will intersect the epiphysis. The Shenton arc is a smooth curvilinear line connecting the medial aspect of the femoral neck with the undersurface of the superior pubic ramus. A horizontal line connecting the triradiate cartilages (Hilgenreiner line) and a perpendicular line through the lateral edge of the acetabulum (Perkins line) define four quadrants in which, in normal hips, the femoral head should be in the lower inner quadrant.

The sacroiliac joints are seen at an angle on the AP radiograph, resulting in some overlap of structures. The normal sacroiliac joint is a syndesmotic joint in its upper two thirds and a synovial joint in its lower (anterior) one third.[5] The lower sacroiliac joint is well seen on a pelvic outlet view.[2] A normal sacroiliac joint will have a thin white line without erosions or sclerosis (see Fig. C-4).[1,2] Early sacroiliitis may demonstrate erosions and apparent widening of the sacroiliac joint space.[10] Subchondral sclerosis develops due to reactive changes in the bone.[2,10]

The sacral foramina are symmetric foramina with thin, well-defined rims. Disruption or irregularity of the sacral

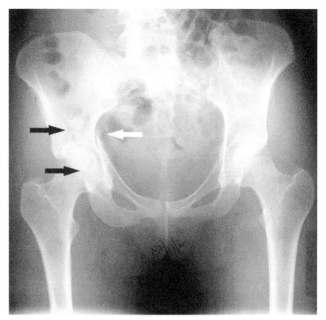

• **Figure C-10** The iliopectineal line is disrupted *(white arrow)* indicating anterior column fracture. There is also a comminuted fracture through the posterior column and posterior acetabular wall *(black arrow).*

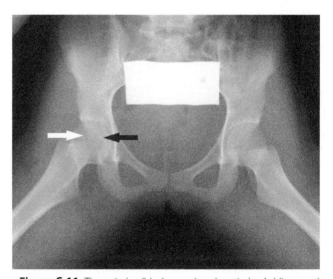

• **Figure C-11** The anterior *(black arrow)* and posterior *(white arrow)* walls of the acetabulum.

foramina may be a subtle clue to traumatic or insufficiency fractures of the sacrum. Inability to visualize the thin rims of the sacral foramina may be a clue to the presence of a lytic mass or erosive process in the sacrum (Fig. C-12).

Several osseous projections of the pelvis and hip serve as tendon attachments and can be avulsed with tendon injuries.[5,11-13] The external abdominal oblique muscles insert on the iliac crest. The anterior superior iliac spine serves as the site of origin of the sartorius muscle. The rectus femoris originates at the anterior inferior iliac spine (Fig. C-13). The hamstrings originate from the ischial tuberosity and inferior pubic ramus (Fig. C-14). The adductor muscles originate from the inferior pubic ramus near the pubic symphysis (Fig. C-15). The gluteus medius and minimus insert on the greater trochanter of the femur. The iliopsoas tendon inserts on the lesser trochanter.

Fat Stripes

Several fat planes can also be seen on the AP radiograph.[5,14] The gluteal fat stripe is seen as a straight line paralleling the superior aspect of the femoral neck on a true AP radiograph and represents normal fat between the gluteus minimus tendon and the ischiofemoral ligament (Fig. C-16). This line bulges superiorly in the presence of a hip joint effusion (Fig. C-17).[14] The iliopsoas fat stripe is seen as a lucent line immediately inferior to the iliopsoas tendon (see Fig. C-16). The obturator fat stripe parallels the iliopectineal line and

is formed by normal pelvic fat adjacent to the obturator internus muscle (see Fig. C-16), which may be displaced by fracture, hematoma, or mass.

Box C-1 summarizes the important anatomic landmarks to be evaluated on every radiograph of the pelvis and hip joint.

Patterns of Disease

Trauma

The various radiographic projections mentioned earlier are used to determine which anatomic structures are disrupted

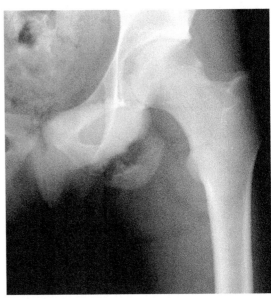

• **Figure C-14** Complete avulsion of the ischial tuberosity, hamstring muscle origin.

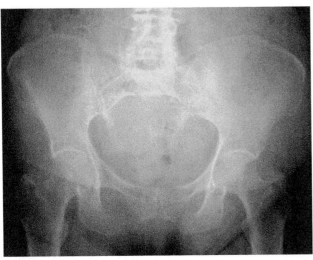

• **Figure C-12** The sacrum is destroyed by a lytic mass (chordoma). Note the absence of the sacral foraminal lines.

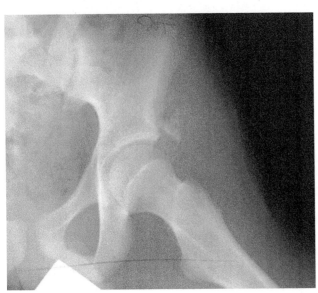

• **Figure C-13** Multiple osseous fragments at the anterior inferior iliac spine are seen from a rectus femoris avulsion.

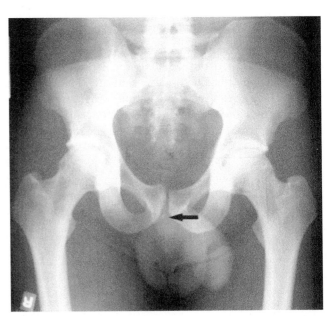

• **Figure C-15** Small bone avulsion at the inferior aspect of the right pubic symphysis (arrow).

in traumatic injuries to the pelvis. Injuries to the pelvis or hip may be fractures, dislocations, stress or insufficiency fractures, or avulsion injuries. In the setting of pelvic trauma, consideration should be given to the status of the nerves, arteries, and veins of the pelvis and proximal thigh, since their proximity to the osseous pelvis places these structures at risk.[15]

Pelvic Fractures

The Young and Burgess classification system divides pelvic fractures into types by mechanism of injury.[16] Anteroposte-

rior compression, lateral compression, vertical shear (Fig. C-18), and combined mechanical injuries are commonly associated with high-energy trauma, such as motor vehicle accidents. Associated injuries are common and can be life-threatening, including pelvic hemorrhage, especially with lateral compression and anteroposterior compression injuries.[15] Stabilization with pelvic compression, though useful in come pelvic fractures, is contraindicated in lateral compression injuries as it may compound the degree of collapse.[17]

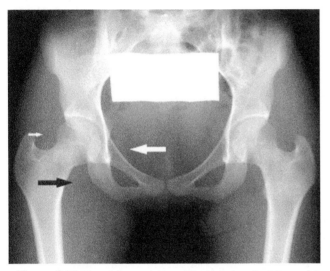

• **Figure C-16** The gluteus minimus fat stripe *(small white arrow)*, obturator internus fat stripe *(large white arrow)*, and iliopsoas fat stripe *(black arrow)*.

> ### • BOX C-1 Radiographic Evaluation of the Pelvis and Hip Joint
>
> Symphysis pubis <5 mm in width
> Sacroiliac joint 2-4 mm in width
> Pelvic ring should have no disruption
> Obturator ring should have no disruption
> Sacral foraminal lines should be visible
> Check transverse processes of lower lumbar vertebrae for fracture
> Check the fat stripes: gluteal, iliopsoas, obturator internus
> Iliopectineal or arcuate line disruption = fracture of anterior column
> Ilioischial line disruption = fracture of posterior column
> Radiographic U or teardrop
> Acetabular roof
> Anterior lip of the acetabulum
> Posterior lip of the acetabulum
> Line of Klein drawn along superior edge of femoral neck should intersect epiphysis
> Shenton line, drawn between medial border of femoral neck and superior border of obturator foramen, should be smooth, continuous arc

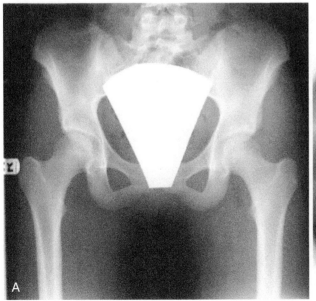
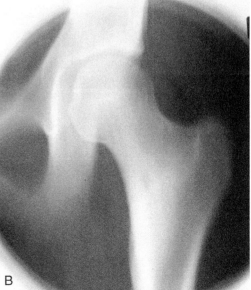

A

B

• **Figure C-17 A,** The left hip joint is distended, as seen by elevation of the gluteus minimus fat stripe. Subtle sclerosis in the medial base of the left femoral neck is almost imperceptible. **B,** Tomographic view demonstrates the nidus of an osteoid osteoma.

Avulsions

Avulsion injuries (see Figs. C-13 to C-15) are most commonly sports-related acute traumatic injuries.[11,12] They can occur from chronic overuse, and in this setting, differentiation from osteomyelitis or neoplasm can be difficult radiographically.[11,12] Special note is made of avulsion injuries in adults with no history of trauma, as this should raise the possibility of an underlying neoplasm.[13]

Acetabular Fractures

The Judet and Letournel classification system divides acetabular fractures into anterior column, anterior acetabular rim, posterior column, posterior acetabular rim, transverse, T-type, posterior column and wall (Fig. C-19), transverse and posterior wall, anterior column and posterior hemitransverse fractures, or both column associated fractures.[18] In 2004, Harris and co-workers described a new computed tomography (CT)-based classification of acetabular fractures.[19]

Femoral Head Fractures

Femoral head fractures are uncommon injuries, occurring typically in the setting of posterior hip dislocation.[20] Risk of avascular necrosis from this injury is high. Interposed

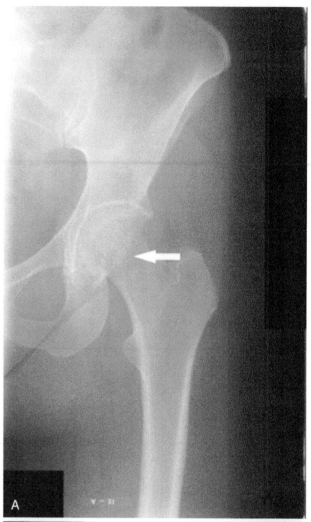

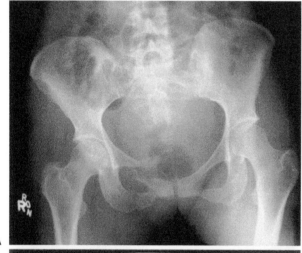

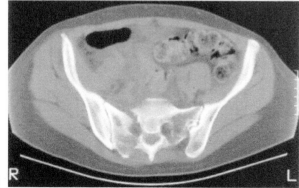

• **Figure C-18 A,** The right superior and inferior pubic rami and right sacral ala are disrupted, rand the right femoral head and acetabulum lie cephalad compared with the left. **B,** The sacral fracture is better seen on computed tomography scan. Vertical shear injury.

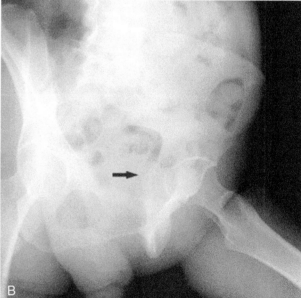

• **Figure C-19 A,** Fracture line through the posterior acetabular wall is seen. Anterior column is intact. **B,** The fracture through the posterior column is better seen on the 45-degree posterior oblique view.

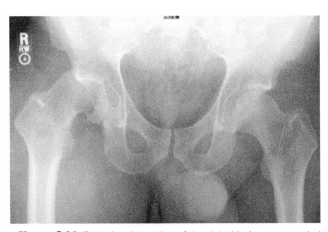

• **Figure C-20** Posterior dislocation of the right hip is accompanied by femoral head fracture and posterior acetabular wall fracture, making this a Pipkin type IV fracture.

fracture fragments may prohibit closed reduction.[20] The Pipkin classification divides these injuries into those with fracture fragment located below the fovea (type I, seen in 35% of cases), fracture fragment above the fovea (type II, 40% of cases), a combined fracture of the femoral head and neck (type III, 10% of cases), and combined fracture of the femoral head and posterior acetabular wall (type IV, 15% of cases; Fig. C-20).[20]

Femoral Neck Fractures

Several different classification systems have been suggested for classification of femoral neck fractures (Fig. C-21). Probably the most widely used is the Garden system, which divides subcapital fractures of the femoral neck into grades I to IV.[21] Grade I is technically an incomplete fracture, though it has become customary to include impacted non-displaced fractures as Grade I, since the treatment is the same.[21] Grade II is a complete fracture, nondisplaced. Grade III is a complete fracture with partial displacement and rotation. Due to the medial rotation of the proximal fragment with respect to the distal fragment, the trabecular lines of the femoral head do not align with those of the acetabulum.[22] Grade IV is completely displaced, so that the femoral head is no longer located in the acetabulum, and the trabeculae are aligned with those of the acetabulum.[22] The Garden system has consistently demonstrated low interobserver reliability in the literature,[21,22] although there is a consistently higher rate of complications, such as avascular necrosis, with the higher grades (Fig. C-22). One report found that the method of treatment was nearly always the same for grade III fractures as grade IV, while another report found that there was insufficient difference in fracture healing between grades III and IV to justify the distinction.[21,23] Thus, several authors have suggested a simplification of the Garden system into nondisplaced fractures and displaced fractures. Among other classifications, the Pauwels system has been reported to have poor ability to predict fracture healing and risk of complications, and the AO system has demonstrated poor interobserver and intraobserver agreement.[21,23]

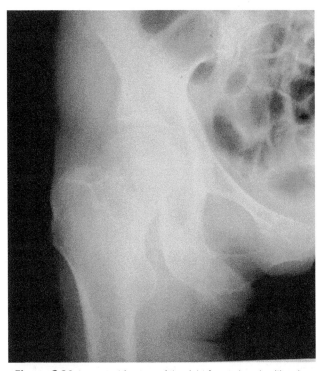

• **Figure C-21** Impacted fracture of the right femoral neck with valgus angulation.

Basicervical fractures of the femoral neck are generally considered separately, since they have much less risk of non-union or avascular necrosis.[23] Intertrochanteric fractures may occur in a slightly older age group than femoral neck fractures, and perhaps as a result of this, appear to have a slightly higher rate of morbidity and mortality.[24]

Stress Fractures

Stress fractures may be defined as either "fatigue" fractures, occurring from abnormal stress on normally mineralized bone, or "insufficiency" fractures, occurring from normal stress on osteoporotic or poorly mineralized bone.[25] The earliest radiographic appearance of stress fracture is graying of the cortex due to bone resorption. Subsequently, a subtle area of scleroses, usually linear and oriented perpendicular to the trabeculae, is seen. The appearance progresses from smooth periosteal elevation to increasing amounts of periosteal new bone formation, as attempted healing takes place (Fig. C-23).[25] Complete healing of the stress fracture is manifested by thick periosteal reaction, with disappearance of the fracture line.[25] If continued stress occurs, however, the fracture may progress, rather than healing (Fig. C-24). Tensile side stress fracture requires longer time to heal than compressive side stress fracture and may need surgical intervention. Occasionally, osteoid osteoma (see Fig. C-17) or infection could appear radiographically similar to a stress fracture. CT or magnetic resonance (MR) imaging can be helpful in this differential diagnosis by demonstrating the fracture line.[25] Radionuclide bone scan and MR imaging are more sensitive than radiography for early detection of stress fractures.

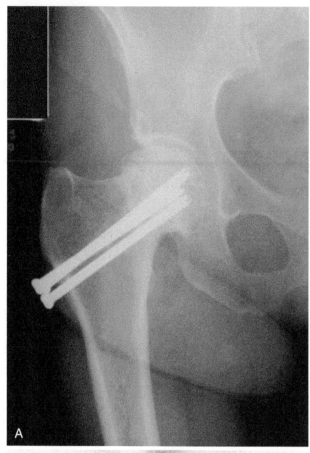

A

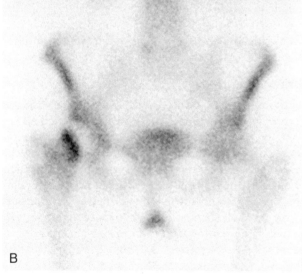

B

• **Figure C-22 A,** Fixation of subcapital femoral neck fracture, with subsequent development of avascular necrosis. **B,** Bone scan from the same patient showing photopenic defect within the right femoral head consistent with avascular necrosis.

Slipped Capital Femoral Epiphysis

Evaluation for slipped capital femoral epiphysis (SCFE) can be assessed using the anteroposterior and frog-leg lateral views of the hip.[2] The condition occurs most commonly in adolescents, around the time of puberty.[26] Boys are affected more commonly than girls, with patients tending to be

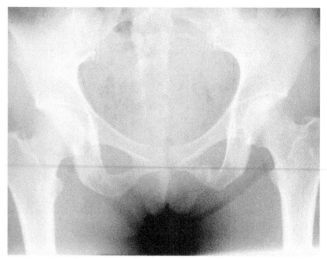

• **Figure C-23** Healing stress fracture of the left inferior pubic ramus.

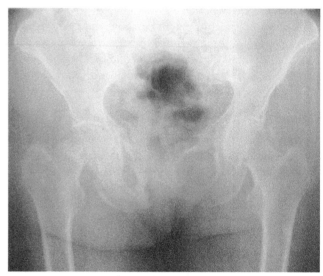

• **Figure C-24** Stress fractures of the right femoral neck and superior and inferior pubic rami. There is varus angulation of the femoral neck fracture.

overweight. SCFE represents a Salter type I fracture, through the physis, resulting in the femoral neck.[26] Radiographically, there may be widening or blurring of the physis or an apparent loss of epiphyseal height on the anteroposterior view.[27] A line drawn along the long axis of the superior aspect of the femoral neck, the line of Kline, normally will intersect the epiphysis, but may not do so in the case of SCFE (Fig. C-25).[2,26] Complications include avascular necrosis and chondrolysis. In the chronic setting, a Herdon hump and secondary osteoarthritis may be seen.[2]

Infection
Septic Joint

Septic joint occurs most commonly from pyogenic infection[28] and may result from hematogenous dissemination, contiguous spread of infection from local tissues, direct

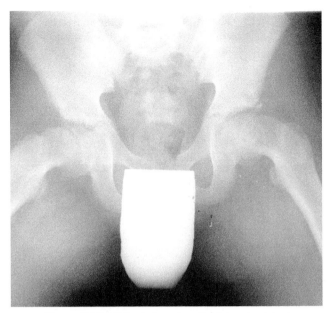

• **Figure C-25** Bilateral slipped capital femoral epiphysis.

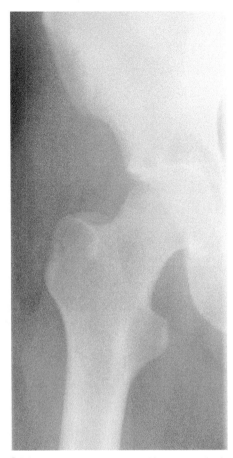

• **Figure C-26** There is complete loss of joint space in the right hip, without appreciable osteophyte formation. Erosions of the superior acetabulum are present. Joint aspiration yielded pus. Arthrogram demonstrates filling defects within the joint (not shown).

inoculation, or contamination at surgery. If an effusion is present, it may manifest radiographically with increased teardrop distance[29] or elevation of the gluteus minimus fat stripe, but these findings can be unreliable.[29] Subacute or chronic infections demonstrate bone erosions, loss of joint space (Fig. C-26), and areas of avascular necrosis.[30] A joint aspiration is typically necessary to confirm the diagnosis.

Septic Sacroiliitis

Septic sacroiliitis is an uncommon infection seen most commonly in pediatric patients and young adults and occasionally in the peripartum period. Due to vague presenting symptoms and difficulty in localization at physical examination, diagnosis is often delayed.[31] The sacroiliac joints may be involved with pyogenic or tuberculous infection, arising most commonly from blood-borne pathogens.[32] Erosions of the sacroiliac joints may be seen (Fig. C-27) and may be associated with osteomyelitis or soft-tissue abscess. Differentiation between infectious and inflammatory sacroiliitis can at times be challenging (Table C-1). Joint aspiration is often necessary for diagnosis.[32]

Tuberculosis

Osseous or articular involvement by tuberculous infection occurs in approximately 1% to 3% of all tuberculous infections (Fig. C-28).[2,33] Slowly progressive monoarticular arthritis involving large joints such as the hip or knee is the most common presentation of tuberculous arthritis, though polyarticular involvement can occur and can be mistaken for inflammatory arthritis.[33,34] A low index of suspicion is indicated, as tuberculous infection is frequently not considered until irreversible damage to the joint has already taken place. Synovial biopsy improves diagnostic yield over aspiration of synovial fluid alone.[33,34]

Osteomyelitis

Osteomyelitis of the pelvis is much rarer than osteomyelitis of tubular bones, occurring most commonly in the ilium from hematogenous dissemination.[35] Symptoms are often nonspecific, and diagnosis is frequently delayed.[35] Radiographically, lytic lesions, sclerosis, smooth periosteal reaction, and/or a soft-tissue mass may be seen (Fig. C-29).[2,35]

Arthritis

Osteoarthritis

The radiographic hallmark of osteoarthritis is joint space narrowing.[36] Most commonly, this narrowing is associated with subchondral sclerosis, marginal osteophytes, cyst formation, and superolateral subluxation of the femoral head (Fig. C-30). An atrophic form of osteoarthritis has been described with joint space narrowing and superolateral subluxation of the femoral head, but with minimal osteophyte formation. The atrophic type is most common in elderly women and is more frequently associated with hip dysplasia than the hypertrophic type of osteoarthritis.[37] Altered weight bearing due to traumatic injury or congenital anomalies may predispose to early development of osteoarthritis.

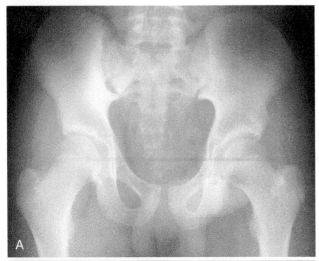

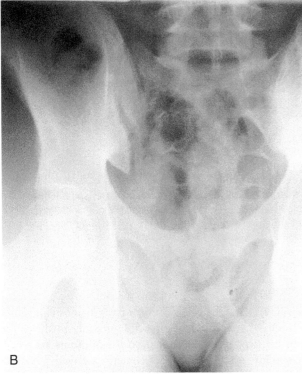

• **Figure C-27 A** and **B,** Erosions and sclerosis of the right sacroiliac joint are seen. Aspiration yielded pyogenic infection.

TABLE C-1	Distinguishing Features Between Septic Sacroiliitis and Spondyloarthropathy	
Radiologic Features	Septic Sacroiliitis	Spondyloarthropathy
Fluid within the sacroiliac joint	+	+
Joint space widening	+	+
Subchondral erosions	+/−	+
Subchondral bone marrow edema	+	+
Subchondral sclerosis	−	+
Transarticular bone bridges	−	+
Shiny corner sign or "Romanus" lesion	−	+
Bilateral involvement	−	+
Muscle infiltration	+	−
Abscess	+	−
Sequestration	+	−
Subperiosteal infiltration or "lava cleft phenomenon"	+	−

Neuropathic Arthropathy

Severe, occasionally rapidly progressive degeneration of the hip joint has been described in the setting of spinal cord injuries or sensory abnormalities (Fig. C-31).[38] The cause is hypothesized to be an absence of the normal protective mechanisms of the neuromuscular structures about the joint.[39]

Rheumatoid Arthritis

Rheumatoid arthritis is an autoimmune disease affecting approximately 1% of the population, characterized by chronic, repeated episodes of synovial inflammation with eventual destruction and deformity of affected joints.[40]

Bilateral, symmetric involvement of the hands and wrists is most common, but any joint may be involved. In the hip, distention of the joint and/or bursae, joint space narrowing, and protrusion acetabuli may be seen (Fig. C-32).[2,40]

Seronegative Spondyloarthropathies

The seronegative spondyloarthropathies include ankylosing spondylitis, enteropathic arthropathy, Reiter's disease, and psoriasis. Radiographs of the pelvis in these disorders may demonstrate "whiskering" of the iliac crests and ischial tuberosity, sacroiliitis, protrusio acetabuli,[41] and/or lower lumbar spine fusions or osteophytes. Involvement of the sacroiliac joints occurs in the synovial portion of the joint, which is the caudal (and anterior) one third of the joint.[42] Bilateral symmetric sacroiliitis is classically present in ankylosing spondylitis or enteropathic arthropathy. Psoriatic arthritis and Reiter's disease classically cause asymmetric sacroiliitis, although it can be bilateral, and can at times appear symmetric.[43] Early inflammatory sacroiliitis may demonstrate erosions, particularly on the iliac side of the joint (Fig. C-33). Later there is sclerosis on both sides of the joint. In the chronic setting, fusion of the sacroiliac joints may occur (Fig. C-34).[43]

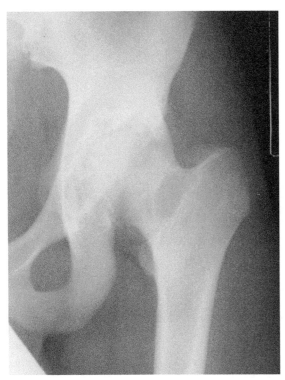

• **Figure C-28** Erosions of the femoral neck, femoral head, and acetabulum, with severe loss of joint space are due to tuberculous arthritis.

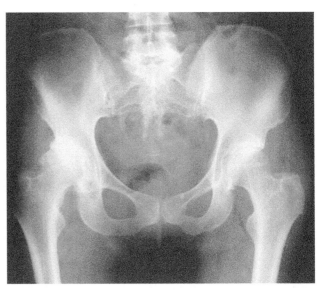

• **Figure C-30** Characteristic findings of osteoarthritis: superior joint space narrowing, subchondral sclerosis, osteophyte formation, and mild superolateral subluxation of the right femoral head.

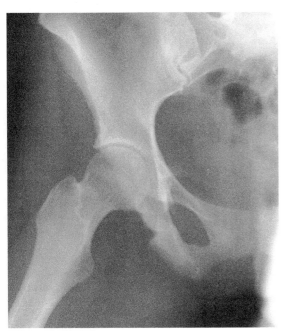

• **Figure C-29** Sclerosis and irregularity of the right ischium are demonstrated, due to chronic osteomyelitis.

Connective Tissue Diseases

Systemic lupus erythematosus patients are particularly at risk for osteonecrosis due to chronic corticosteroid intake and probably due to the auto-inflammatory process itself as well.[43] Evaluation for osteonecrosis can be assessed on

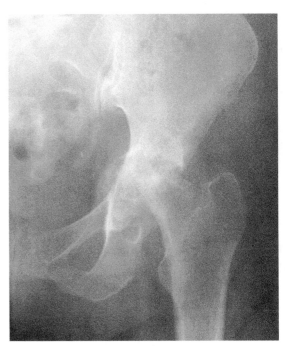

• **Figure C-31** Severe joint space narrowing, destruction, debris within the left hip joint, and protrusio acetabuli are due to neuropathic joint.

standard views of the hip, but a more sensitive evaluation is obtained with MR imaging or radionuclide bone scan. Osteoporosis is also a sequela of this disease and may present clinically as an insufficiency fracture of the sacrum, pubic ramus, acetabulum, or femoral neck.

Dermatomyositis patients often develop soft-tissue calcifications, most commonly in the proximal upper and lower extremities (Fig. C-35), and more often in children than in adults.[44] There is evidence that in juvenile dermatomyositis, up-regulation of genetic markers involved in

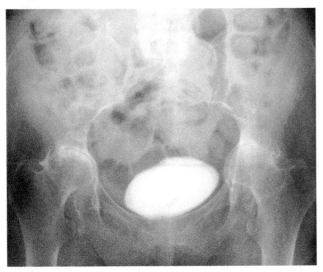

• **Figure C-32** Symmetric joint space loss and erosions of the femoral heads and acetabular protrusio are due to rheumatoid arthritis.

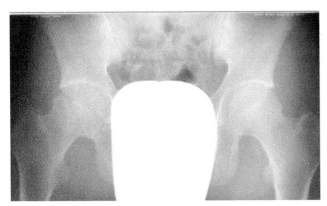

• **Figure C-33** Erosions and sclerosis of the sacroiliac joint bilaterally are seen symmetrically. Ankylosing spondylitis.

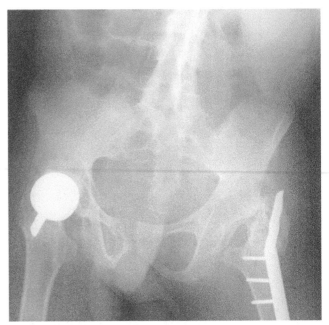

• **Figure C-34** Complete fusion of the left and near complete fusion of the right sacroiliac joints are seen. There is also fusion of the facet joints and spinous processes in the lumbar spine. Deformity and dislocation of the left hip is also noted. Chronic ankylosing spondylitis.

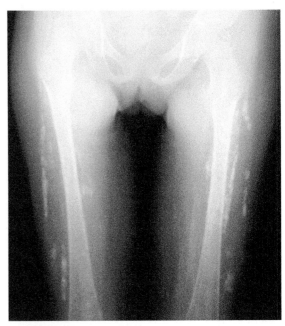

• **Figure C-35** Extensive soft-tissue calcifications are noted bilaterally in the lower extremities of this patient with dermatomyositis.

producing interferon-alpha and interferon-beta occurs, possibly as a result of exposure to a viral antigen.[45]

Scleroderma patients also may develop soft-tissue calcifications but typically have myriad other manifestations of the disease involving the hands and other organs, such as esophagus, small bowel, colon, and lungs.[43]

Metabolic, Synovial, and Crystal Deposition Diseases

Osteonecrosis

Osteonecrosis represents death of bone and may be caused by a wide variety of disease processes including trauma, alcoholism, Gaucher disease, other infiltrative processes, sickle cell disease (Fig. C-36), radiation, and many others.[46] The end result of these processes is decreased blood supply to the bone. In some cases, such as Legg-Calve-Perthes disease, no cause is evident. According to the Ficat staging,[47] the hip may have a normal appearance (stage I), vague increased density in the femoral head (stage II), subchondral collapse of the femoral head often producing a "crescent" appearance (stage III) (Fig. C-37), or secondary osteoarthritis in the chronic setting (stage IV). MR imaging and radionuclide bone scan are much more sensitive than plain film radiography for the detection of early osteonecrosis (see Fig. C-37).[43]

Legg-Calve-Perthes Disease

Legg-Calve-Perthes disease occurs more commonly in males, between the ages of 4 and 8 years.[48] The condition is bilateral

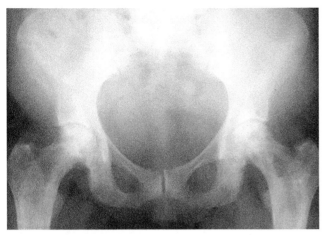

• **Figure C-36** Abnormal appearance of the bones diffusely, with marked, patchy sclerosis in bilateral femoral heads, superior acetabuli, and pubic symphysis, resulting from repeated episodes of avascular necrosis in a patient with sickle cell disease.

in about 10% of cases.[48] The etiology is unknown, leading it to be termed "idiopathic osteonecrosis." Radiographically, Perthes disease presents similarly to other types of osteonecrosis, as described earlier (Fig. C-38). Overgrowth of the articular cartilage as a result of the osteonecrosis results in the eventual development of a large, deformed femoral head, called coxa magna. Associated lateral subluxation of the femoral head and secondary osteoarthritis may be seen. Treatment of Perthes disease varies from conservative to various types of acetabular or femoral osteotomies to maintain the femoral head in the acetabulum.[48]

Osteoporosis

Osteoporosis represents normally mineralized bone but with decreased overall amount of bone mass.[2] This can occur from a wide variety of congenital or acquired causes and manifests radiographically as increased lucency in the bone and cortical thinning. The risk of fracture increases with severity of osteoporosis. Singh and co-workers attempted a radiographic classification based on the theory that there is progressive loss of trabeculae (see Fig. C-9) with increasing severity of osteoporosis.[49] The Singh index divides this process into six grades of trabecular loss. In grade 6, all major trabecular groups are still present. In grade 5, some trabecular in the secondary compressive, secondary tensile, and greater trochanter groups are lost, while the remaining trabeculae in the principal compressive and tensile groups are slightly reduced in number, while the secondary groups are nearly completely absent. In grade 3, there is a break in continuity of the principal tensile trabecular group. In grade 2, only the principal compressive group of trabeculae remains, which are reduced in number. In grade 1, even the principal compressive trabecular group is markedly reduced in number. Reports have varied in the literature concerning the reliability of the Singh index for measuring severity of osteoporosis.[50] Dual energy x-ray

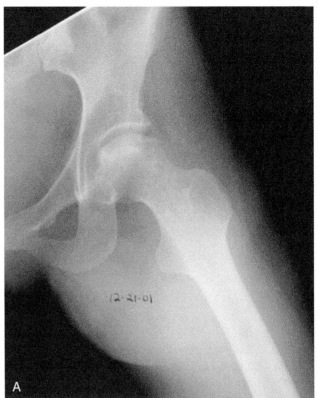

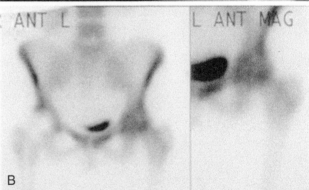

• **Figure C-37** **A,** In this frog-leg lateral view of the left hip, flattening of the femoral head contour and subchondral lucency denote collapse from avascular necrosis. **B,** Bone scan in the same patient with photopenic defect in the superolateral femoral head, where bone is necrotic. The remainder of the femoral head shows increased uptake, due to the reparative response of surrounding bone.

absorptiometry (DEXA) is more sensitive and accurate in quantifying osteoporosis.[50]

Hyperparathyroidism

Primary or secondary forms of hyperparathyroidism may occur.[51] Primary hyperparathyroidism results from excess production of parathyroid hormone by the parathyroid gland. Secondary hyperparathyroidism occurs as a result of phosphate retention by poorly functioning renal tubules, leading to excess excretion of serum calcium and subsequent increase in release of parathyroid hormone.[51] Subperiosteal bone resorption and cortical thinning may be seen, similar to the appearance seen in the phalanges.[51] Brown tumors

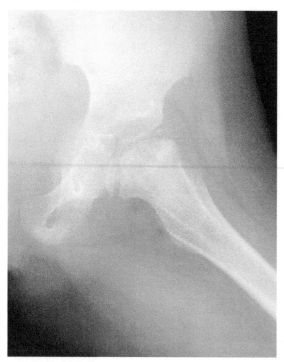

• **Figure C-38** Severe collapse of the left femoral head in a patient with Legg-Calve-Perthes disease.

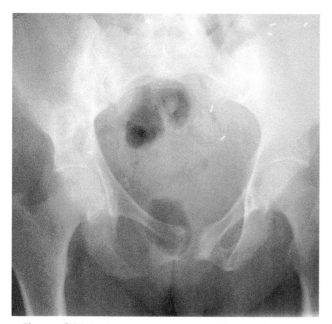

• **Figure C-39** Subperiosteal bone resorption is noted in the pubic symphysis and sacroiliac joint bilaterally, and a lucent lesion is noted in the right superior acetabulum (Brown tumor). Hyperparathyroidism.

may occur (Fig. C-39). A "rugger-jersey" appearance to the vertebral bodies may be noted.[51]

Osteomalacia

Osteomalacia represents abnormally mineralized bone and may be caused by inadequate intake of vitamin D, inadequate absorption of vitamin D due to malabsorptive states

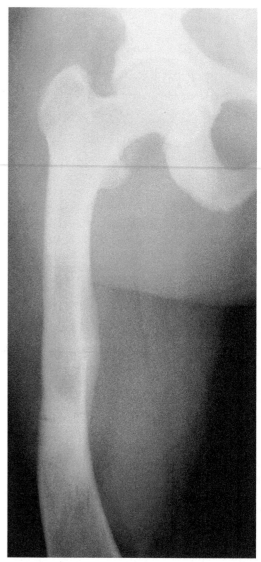

• **Figure C-40** There is bowing of the femur, a lucent line perpendicular to the shaft (Looser zone), and thickening of the medial femoral cortex in this patient with osteomalacia.

or surgical bypass, or inadequate formation of the biologically active form of vitamin D due to renal or hepatic disease.[52] Osteomalacia has also been associated with other underlying disorders including Wilson disease, neurofibromatosis, and some neoplasms.[2] Looser zones, which are essentially poorly healed stress fractures due to inadequate callus formation, may be seen[52] (Fig. C-40). These appear as linear lucencies, perpendicular to the cortex of the bone, occurring typically in the medial cortex of the femoral neck, as well as the pubic rami, ischial rami, ribs, and scapulae. When osteomalacia is due to renal dysfunction, the radiographic manifestations of secondary hyperparathyroidism usually predominate, including subperiosteal bone resorption and cortical thinning.[2]

Rickets

Rickets is the pediatric correlate of osteomalacia, resulting from abnormal mineralization of bone due to inadequate vitamin D intake, absorption, or hydroxylation. Different types of rickets have been described, with infantile rickets typically found in patients between the ages of 6 months and 2 years[53] (Fig. C-41). The various types of vitamin D resistant rickets are typically found in patients older than 3 years of age and are characterized by shortening and bowing of long bones, occasionally with sclerosis and ectopic ossifications[54] (Fig. C-42). It may be seen with glycosuria or with defective renal tubular absorption of amino acids, glucose, and phosphate (Fanconi syndrome).[2]

Paget Disease

Paget disease has a characteristic appearance on radiographs, bone scan, MR, or CT with coarsened trabeculae and thickening of the cortex[55] (Fig. C-43). Paget disease typically occurs in patients older than the age of 50 years and progresses in three phases—predominately lytic, mixed lytic and sclerotic, and finally, sclerotic.[2,55] Increased osteoclastic activity leads to abnormal bone remodeling. The etiology of Paget disease is unknown, although a viral etiology is hypothesized.[55] Similar to osteomalacia, Looser zones may form, representing inadequately healed stress fractures. A small percentage of patients with Paget disease will develop a secondary sarcoma.[56] New development of a lytic lesion or soft-tissue mass associated with Pagetoid bone is evidence of sarcoma formation. These tend to be high-grade lesions with a poor prognosis.[2,56]

A similar radiographic appearance may be seen in familial idiopathic hyperphosphatasia, with abnormalities seen diffusely[53] (Fig. C-44).

Pigmented Villonodular Synovitis

Pigmented villonodular synovitis (PVNS) is a disorder of synovial proliferation characterized by recurrent effusions, with bleeding into the joint, bursa, or tendon sheath affected.[57] The knee is most commonly affected, but the disease can affect any synovial joint. In the hip, erosions may be seen in the femoral head, femoral neck, or acetabulum[57] (Fig. C-45). MR is the imaging modality of choice, demonstrating synovial proliferation, effusion, and the paramagnetic effect of hemosiderin,[57] which may also be seen in patients with hemophilia or rheumatoid arthritis. Recurrence after synovectomy occurs in as many as 50% of cases.[2]

Synovial Osteochondromatosis

Synovial osteochondromatosis is a metaplasia of the synovium, most commonly involving the knee, although any joint may be involved.[58] Radiographs may demonstrate multiple ossified bodies in the joint space, with joint effusion, erosions on one or both sides of the joint, and scalloping of the femoral neck[59] (Fig. C-46). Joint narrowing and osteophyte formation may be absent until late in the course of the disease. The chondroid bodies in the joint may or may not be ossified, but are evident at MR imaging or arthrography.[59] The amount of ossification increases over time. About 5% develop malignant degeneration.[58]

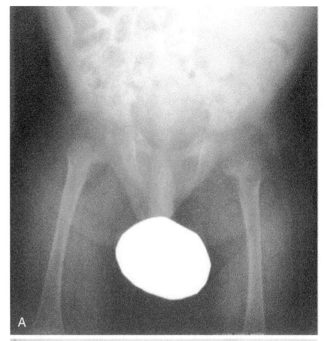
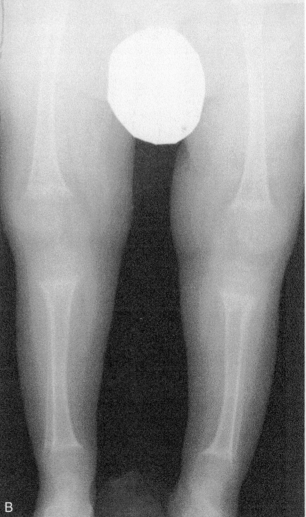

• **Figure C-41** **A** and **B,** Widened, frayed physis, broad metaphysis, and osteopenia are characteristic of infantile rickets.

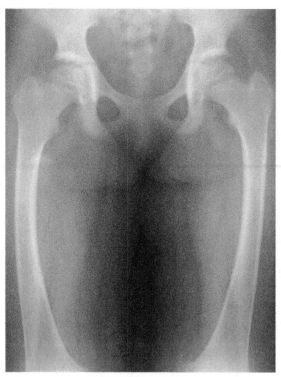

• **Figure C-42** Bowing of the femurs, broad metaphyses, and widened proximal femoral physes are seen in vitamin D resistant rickets.

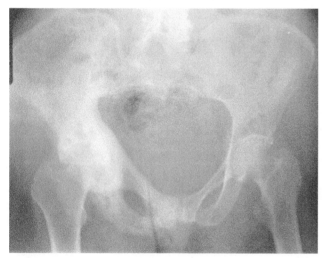

• **Figure C-43** The right pelvis is enlarged, with trabecular and cortical thickening. The right hip demonstrates secondary osteoarthritis. Paget disease.

Calcium Pyrophosphate Arthropathy

The arthropathy associated with calcium pyrophosphate crystal deposition occurs in males and females with nearly equal incidence.[2] Deposition of calcium pyrophosphate crystals produces structural damage to the cartilage and resulting in joint space narrowing, subchondral sclerosis, and osteophytes. Chondrocalcinosis of the symphysis pubis,

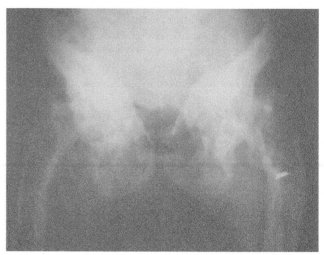

• **Figure C-44** Enlarged bones with thickened trabeculae and cortex and heterogeneous mineralization diffusely are seen in this patient with idiopathic hyperphosphatasia.

tendons, ligaments, articular cartilage, or joint capsule may be seen[60] (Fig. C-47). The hip is less commonly involved than the knee, wrist, or shoulder.[60]

Hydroxyapatite Deposition Disease

Hydroxyapatite deposition disease is characterized by deposition of calcium hydroxyapatite crystals in and around tendons, bursae, or joint capsules, with resultant local swelling and pain. Calcific tendonitis occurs less commonly in the hip than the shoulder.[61] "Toothpaste-like" calcifications of the gluteus medius and minimus tendons may be seen (Fig. C-48).

Ochronosis

Ochronosis occurs in males and females with equal incidence, as an autosomal recessive inherited condition.[62] Lack of the enzyme homogentisic acid oxidase, involved in the breakdown of amino acids phenylalanine and tyrosine, results in a build-up of homogentisic acid.[62] This leads to dystrophic calcifications in the intervertebral disks, articular cartilage, tendons, and ligaments, and formation of osteoarthritis[62] (Fig. C-49).

Dysplasias and Congenital Anomalies
Sclerosing Bone Dysplasias

The various types of sclerosing bone dysplasias occur either from excess bone production due to abnormal osteoblastic activity or from failure of bone resorption and remodeling due to defective osteoclastic activity.[63] The excess bone accumulation affects endochondral bone formation in osteopetrosis, pyknodysostosis, or osteopathia striata.[64] Intramembranous bone formation is primarily affected in progressive diaphyseal dysplasia and a few rare endosteal hyperostosis.[64] Both endochondral bone formation and intramembranous bone formation are affected in melorheostosis and metaphyseal dysplasia.[64]

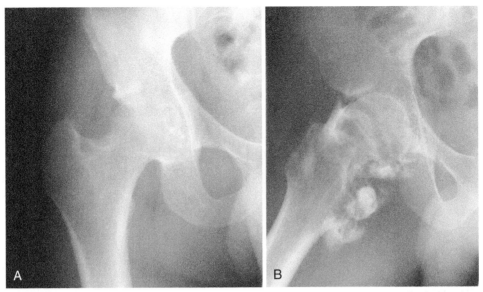

• **Figure C-45 A,** Scalloping of the femoral neck and erosions of both femoral head and acetabulum are seen in this patient with PVNS. **B,** Arthrogram demonstrates nodular-appearing filling defects.

There are three types of osteopetrosis, the infantile-malignant type, which is autosomal recessive, and the most severe form, an intermediate type, also autosomal recessive presenting typically in the first decade of life, and an autosomal dominant type with full life-expectancy.[65] In the infantile type, pancytopenia, cranial nerve dysfunction, and mental retardation occur.[65] Radiographs of the hip may demonstrate curvilinear bands of sclerosis in the ilium, with a "bone-in-bone" appearance.[2,65] The vertebrae may show similar bands of sclerosis along the vertebral endplates, with a "sandwich vertebrae" appearance. In the long bones, undertubulation, broadened metaphyses, and pathologic fractures are seen[65] (Fig. C-50).

Pyknodysostosis is a rare autosomal-recessive disorder with radiographic characteristics of both osteopetrosis and cleidocranial dysplasia.[2,66] Delayed closure of fontanelles, short stature, undertubulation of long bones, and diffuse sclerosis are seen. Bones are brittle and prone to fracture (Fig. C-51). Genetic research has demonstrated a mutation causing inactivation of the gene encoding cathepsin K, which is involved in osteoclastic function.[63]

In melorheostosis, both endochondral and intramembranous bone formation are abnormal.[64] It is characterized by hyperostosis, typically of one side of the cortex, with a lobulated, wavy appearance resembling dripping candle wax.[67] Ossifications and fibrosis in periarticular soft tissues are also common. The abnormalities may follow a dermatomal distribution (Fig. C-52). Treatment includes soft-tissue releases and excisions, and if necessary, osteotomies.[67] It commonly recurs.

In osteopoikilosis and osteopathia striata, there are localized foci of cortical bone in which resorption and remodeling fail, while in the remainder of bone, the process of endochondral ossification proceeds normally.[68] The result is numerous foci of sclerotic bone (enostoses or "bone-islands") throughout the skeleton in osteopoikilosis (Fig. C-53), or linear striations of sclerotic bone in osteopathia striata.[68] Differentiation from sclerotic metastases may at times be difficult by plain radiographs. Although radionuclide bone scan has been thought to be critical to differentiate osteopoikilosis from osteoblastic metastases, there are reports of increased radiopharmaceutical uptake in osteopoikilosis, particularly in young patients.[69] Osteopoikilosis, osteopathia striata, and/or melorheostosis can coexist in the same patient (see Fig. C-52) and probably represent a range of manifestations of the same disease process.[2]

Osteogenesis Imperfecta

Osteogenesis imperfect (OI) is a hereditary disorder characterized by abnormal type I collagen, resulting in weakened, fragile bones, ligament laxity, abnormal dentition, blue sclerae, and hearing impairment[70] (Fig. C-54). Most subtypes of OI are inherited as autosomal dominant mutations in the *COL1A1* and *COL1A2* genes that encode for the pro alpha I and pro alpha 2 chains in type 1 collagen.[70] Types I to IV, described by Sillence and co-workers, are as follows: type I, autosomal-dominant and relatively mild, with relatively normal stature, blue sclerae, and hearing impairment; type II, with subtypes described as autosomal-dominant or autosomal-recessive, the most severe form, lethal in the fetal or newborn period, with severe deformity and intrauterine growth retardation; type III, also with both autosomal-dominant and autosomal-recessive cases described, severe and progressive but with longer survival than type II; type IV, rare, autosomal dominant and mild with normal sclera and normal hearing.[71] More recently, additional types V to VII have been described, which are not associated with defects in the genes encoding type I collagen.[72] Treatment with bisphosphonates improves bone

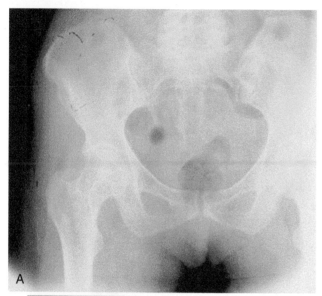

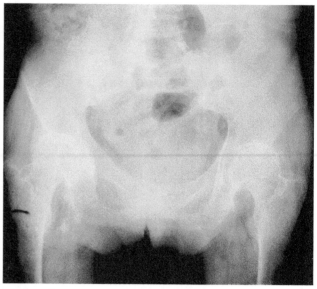

• **Figure C-47** Chondrocalcinosis of the pubic symphysis and both hips, with severe diffuse degenerative changes. Calcium pyrophosphate arthropathy.

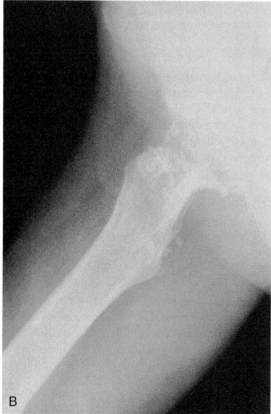

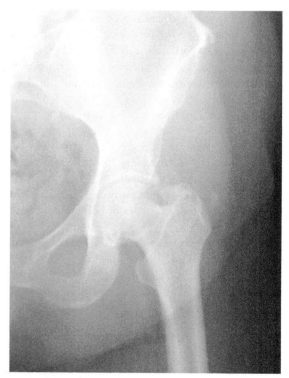

• **Figure C-46 A,** Scalloping and erosions of the femoral neck and head are seen, with ossific densities in the joint. Synovial osteochondromatosis. **B,** The same patient 4 years later demonstrates enlargement of the ossified intraarticular bodies.

• **Figure C-48** "Toothpaste"-like calcifications at the hip abductor insertion.

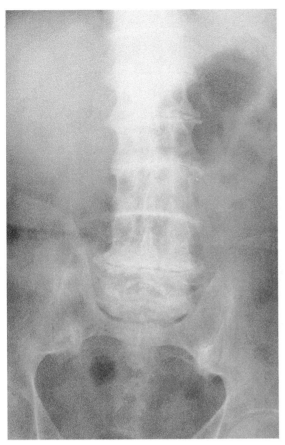

• **Figure C-49** Diffusely calcified intervertebral disks. Ochronosis.

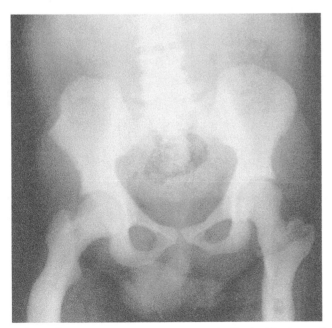

• **Figure C-50** All visualized bones are sclerotic. Previous fractures of the right femoral shaft and left femoral neck with residual deformity are visible. Osteopetrosis.

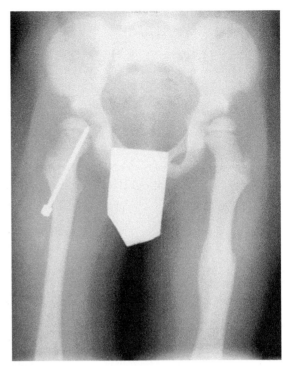

• **Figure C-51** The diffusely sclerotic bones, undertubulation, and fractures resemble osteopetrosis. Pyknodysostosis.

mass in all types, but long-term outcomes from bisphosphonate therapy are not known.[70]

Developmental Dysplasia of the Hip

The etiology of developmental dysplasia of the hip (DDH) involves both genetic and environmental factors.[73] Risk factors include oligohydramnios, breech delivery, positive family history, and certain ethnic backgrounds including Native Americans.[73] Diagnosis can be made at birth in the vast majority of cases.[73] If diagnosed at birth, the likelihood of successful nonoperative treatment such as a Pavlik harness, and the overall prognosis, is much better than with delayed diagnosis.[73,74] Ultrasound is more sensitive than radiography for diagnosis.[73] Radiographically, dislocation or subluxation of the hip can be demonstrated by discontinuity of the Shenton arc, a curvilinear line connecting the medial femoral neck with the undersurface of the superior pubic ramus[73] (Fig. C-55). With hip dislocation, the femoral head moves into the upper outer quadrant.[2] If the dislocated hip is in contact with the ilium, a pseudoacetabulum will form[73] (see Fig. C-55). Essentially all patients with hip subluxation or dislocation will develop osteoarthritis, usually in the third or fourth decade of life.[73]

Acetabular Dysplasia in Adults

Dysplasia of the acetabulum may occur without hip dislocation, and mild dysplasia may go undiagnosed until adulthood.[73] Acetabular dysplasia occurs in females more often than males and has been demonstrated to lead to development of hip joint osteoarthritis[73,75] (Fig. C-56). Evaluation for acetabular dysplasia can be performed using the

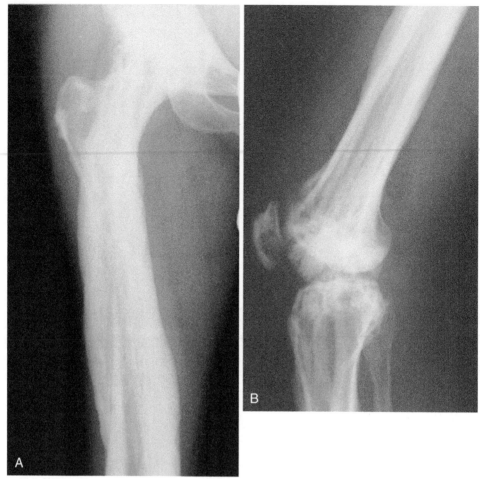

• **Figure C-52 A,** Dense sclerotic, wavy cortical thickening in the femoral shaft and superolateral acetabulum are noted. **B,** Wavy cortical thickening in the distal femoral shaft is seen, indicative of melorheostosis. Linear striations in the medullary bone are areas of osteopathia striata.

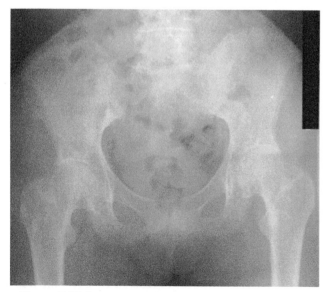

• **Figure C-53** Punctate sclerotic lesions (bone islands) scattered diffusely bilaterally. Osteopoikilosis.

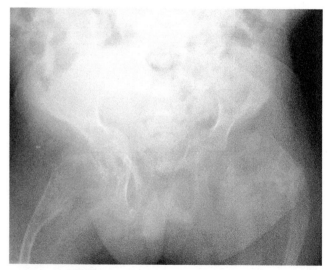

• **Figure C-54** Severe deformity and osteopenia, with multiple fractures in different stages of healing. The pelvis is deformed and narrow. Osteogenesis imperfecta.

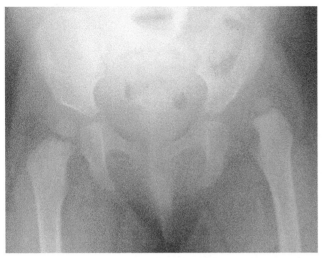

• **Figure C-55** Superior dislocation of the left hip, with pseudoacetabulum formation. Mild subluxation also of the right hip.

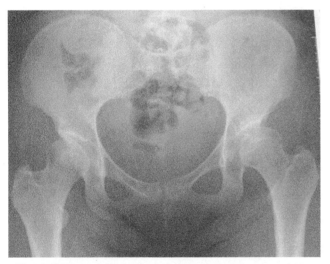

• **Figure C-56** Bilateral acetabuli are dysplastic, with only partial covering of the femoral head. On the left, early osteoarthritis has begun to develop.

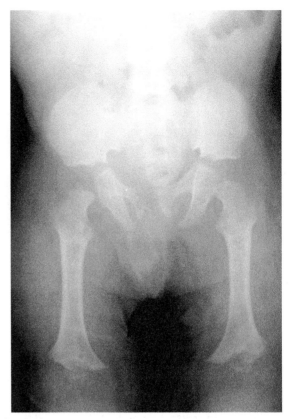

• **Figure C-57** Characteristic findings of achondroplasia—narrowing of the interpedicular distance in the lower lumbar spine, flat acetabular roofs, small greater sciatic notches, and short femurs with widened femoral metaphyses.

center-edge angle of Wiberg, performed by measuring the angle between a line drawn vertically from the center of the femoral head and a line from the center of the femoral head through the edge of the acetabulum.[75] Angle measures less than 20 degrees are dysplastic; 20 to 25 degrees are classified as borderline dysplasia, and greater than 25 degrees are normal.[75]

Femoroacetabular Impingement

The theory behind femoroacetabular impingement is that certain anatomic variations lead to impingement between the proximal femur and acetabular rim with flexion and internal rotation.[76,77] This leads to shearing and impaction of the anterior articular cartilage of the femoral head, as well as anterior labral tears.[76,77] There are two types of femoroacetabular impingement. The first is the "cam" type, thought to be caused by an enlarged femoral head or an abnormal contour of the femoral head/neck junction, which causes impingement anteriorly against a normal acetabulum (see

Fig. C-6). The second, or "pincer" type, is thought to be due to "over-coverage" of the femoral head anteriorly from either coxa profunda or a retroverted acetabulum.[76] Radiographs may demonstrate reduced offset of the femoral head-neck junction, acetabular abnormalities such as retroversion, coxa valga, coxa profunda, or protrusion acetabuli, and the eventual development of osteoarthritis. MR imaging is more sensitive to the early findings of the labral tear and cartilage injury.[76,77]

Achondroplasia

Achondroplasia is a congenital disorder of endochondral bone formation affecting fetuses in utero, transmitted as an autosomal-dominant trait.[78] The genetic defect involves an allele encoding fibroblast growth factor receptor 3, on chromosome 4p, which is the same allele implicated in both hypochondroplasia and thanatophoric dwarfism.[78] Patients have short stature, with limb shortening affecting more severely the proximal extremities. Short pedicles can predispose to spinal stenosis. Narrowing of the interpedicular width in the lower lumbar spine is seen, along with horizontally oriented acetabular roofs, small sciatic notches, and rounded, "ping-pong-paddle"-shaped iliac bones[78] (Fig. C-57). Cervicomedullary compression has been shown to be associated with sudden death in infants with achondroplasia.[79]

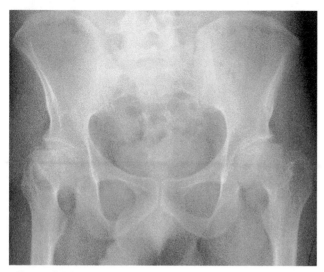

• **Figure C-58** Broad, dysplastic femoral heads, with varus angulation of the femoral necks bilaterally. Multiple epiphyseal dysplasia.

Multiple Epiphyseal Dysplasia

In multiple epiphyseal dysplasia, the abnormal growth of the femoral head epiphysis typically leads to a varus alignment of the femoral neck. This occurs due to overgrowth of the trochanteric ossification center and infundibulum, a cartilaginous connection between the femoral head and trochanteric ossification centers in the infant[73] (Fig. C-58). Secondary osteoarthritis eventually develops.

Proximal Focal Femoral Deficiency

Proximal focal femoral deficiency (PFFD) represents a congenital disorder characterized by varying severity of shortening and dysplasia of the femur and acetabulum, and varus angulation of the proximal femur[80] (Fig. C-59). A common classification system divides the disorder into types, A-D, in increasing order of severity.[80] In type A, the femur is shortened compared with the normal size, but the femoral head is present and located within the acetabulum. In type B, the femur is short with a varus angulation, and there is a gap between the femoral head, which is located within the acetabulum, and the femoral neck. In type C, the femoral head is rudimentary or absent. The femur is markedly short, and the acetabulum is dysplastic. In type D, the entire femur is rudimentary, with absent femoral head and acetabulum.

Various treatments have been used for patients with this disorder. In one recent report, patients reported similar mobility and improved satisfaction with nonoperative treatment using an extension prosthesis, compared with surgical ankle disarticulation with fitting of an above-knee prosthesis.[81]

Mucopolysaccharidoses

Mucopolysaccharidoses are a heterogeneous group of disorders characterized by accumulation of various mucopolysaccharides as a result of congenital lack of certain enzymes.[82]

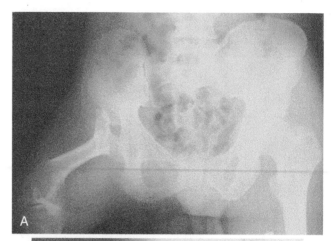

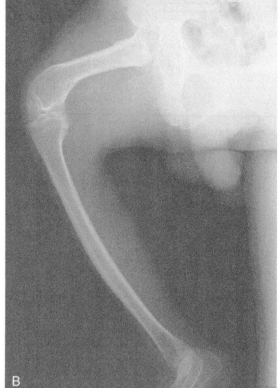

• **Figure C-59** **A** and **B,** The right femur is short and the femoral head is rudimentary. The right acetabulum is dysplastic. The fibula is absent. Proximal focal femoral deficiency type C.

Many if not all of these exhibit similar radiographic findings in the pelvis, including flared and dysplastic femoral heads, narrowed and distorted pelves, and flared iliac wings[82] (Fig. C-60).

Fibrodysplasia Ossificans Progressiva

Fibrodysplasia ossificans progressiva (FOP) represents a rare congenital disorder characterized by progressive heterotopic ossification of tendons, ligaments, muscles, and other soft tissues (Fig. C-61) with deformity of the great toe.[83] No known treatment or preventive measure exists. The typical course of the disease is progressive restriction of movement, frequent falls, and eventual respiratory difficulty from

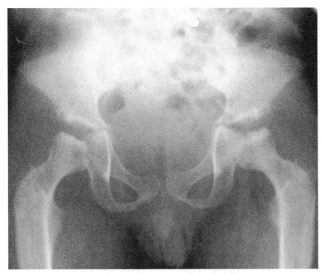

• **Figure C-60** The iliac wings are broad, the pelvis narrow, and the femoral heads dysplastic in this patient with Hurler's syndrome.

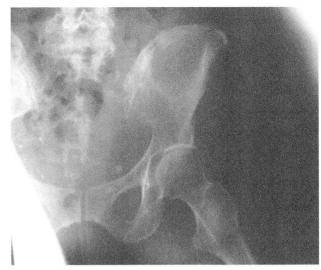

• **Figure C-62** Destructive lesion without definable borders involving the sacrum and left ilium. Myeloma.

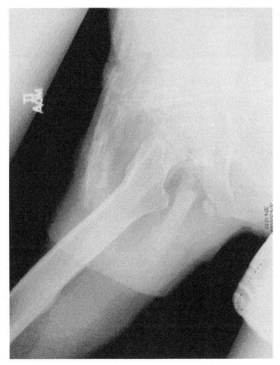

• **Figure C-61** Marked heterotopic ossification bridging the hip joint medially and laterally. Fibrodysplasia ossificans progressiva.

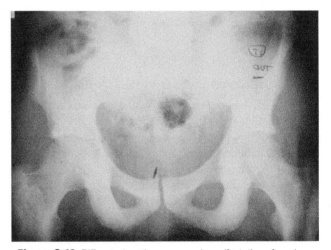

• **Figure C-63** Diffuse sclerosis, an unusual manifestation of myeloma.

involvement of the chest wall. Most patients die of pulmonary complications in their 40s or 50s.[83] Recent advances include mapping of the gene for FOP to chromosome 4q, and identification of a key protein found in lesion cells and lymphocytes.[83] These findings may prove beneficial in treating this condition in the future.

Tumors

A variety of benign and malignant tumors may affect the pelvis and proximal femur. Close inspection for the

presence of disruption or displacement of the anterior column, posterior column, cortex, sacral ala, or trabecular lines may reveal a subtle lesion. Although an in-depth discussion of all tumors that can affect the pelvis and proximal femur is beyond the scope of this article, a few common or characteristic lesions will be discussed.

Myeloma

Myeloma is the most common primary bone tumor and is a malignancy of the bone marrow.[2] Most commonly affecting males older than the age of 50 years, myeloma may be seen as a solitary plasmacytoma or multiple lesions in multiple myeloma.[2,84] The axial skeleton is most commonly affected, and the lesions are typically lytic[84] (Fig. C-62). A small minority of cases (less than 1%) may be sclerotic (Fig. C-63), with nearly half of these developing peripheral neuropathies.[2,85]

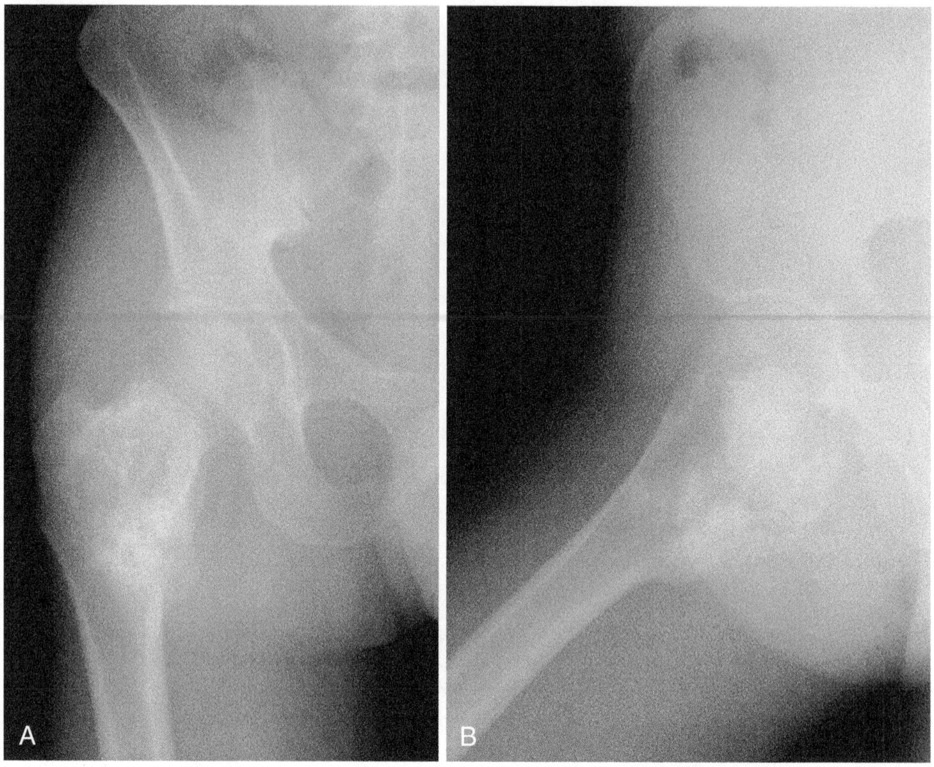

• **Figure C-64 A** and **B,** Lucent and sclerotic lesion in the femoral neck, with narrow zone of transition, but with scalloping and probable disruption of the medial cortex. Punctate and curvilinear calcifications are seen internally. Chondrosarcoma.

Chondrosarcoma

The pelvis is a common site of involvement of chondrosarcoma, a malignant cartilage-forming tumor.[86] It most commonly affects patients between ages 30 and 60 years.[86] Chondrosarcoma may be primary (of which there are several types) or may arise secondarily in the setting of the existing enchondromatosis, Paget disease, osteochondroma, or synovial chondromatosis.[2,86] Conventional chondrosarcoma appears radiographically as an expansile, lytic lesion with ring-, arc-, or popcorn-shaped internal calcifications (Fig. C-64). There may be thickening or scalloping of the cortex, and there may be a soft-tissue mass. Metastases are uncommon.

Chordoma

In the differential diagnosis for a destructive lesion of the sacrum is a chordoma, a tumor arising from notochord remnants[86] (see Fig. C-12). Typically affecting patients older than 40 years of age, the tumor is seen slightly more commonly in men. It is seen most commonly in the clivus, the sacrum, and the C2 vertebra, typically as a lytic lesion, with occasional calcifications in the matrix.[86]

Fibrous Dysplasia

Fibrous dysplasia is a benign tumor characterized by replacement of normal cancellous bone by fibroblasts and fibrous matrix, with interspersed trabeculae of immature woven bone.[87] Typically affecting patients younger than 30 years of age, the lesion is centrally located within the bone, expansile, with a narrow zone of transition and internal hazy "ground-glass" appearance (Fig. C-65). Prominent trabeculae and a sclerotic margin may or may not be seen. Fibrous dysplasia most commonly affects the proximal femur, tibia, or humerus, but is also seen in the pelvis, ribs, and craniofacial bones.[87] Cystic or cartilaginous portions of the lesions may be seen.[87,88] A minority of affected patients have polyostotic involvement, which may be accompanied by endocrine disturbances in McCune-Albright syndrome.[87]

Aneurysmal Bone Cyst

Aneurysmal bone cyst is a benign, expansile, lucent bone lesion, typically affecting patients between the ages of 10 and 30 years.[86] Believed to result from venous obstruction or vascular malformation in the bone, the internal architecture is composed of blood-filled cavities with intervening septa, although a solid variant has been described.[89] They occur most commonly about the knee, with the pelvis involved in 10% to 15% of cases.[86] They may arise from a preexisting benign or malignant lesion. Radiographically, aneurysmal bone cysts appear as lucent lesions with well-defined sclerotic borders, and often "ballooning" of the cortex (Fig. C-66). On MR, fluid-fluid levels can be seen. After curettage, they frequently recur.

Osteochondroma

The most common benign bone lesion, osteochondroma, is an abnormal projection of bone with continuity of the cortex and medullary cavity with the underlying bone.[2,86] These lesions are typically located in the metaphysis, often demonstrating continuity with the growth plate. A cartilage cap is present, and through endochondral ossification, these lesions continue to enlarge until skeletal maturity.[86]

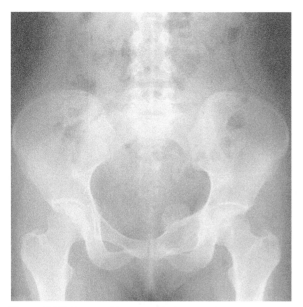

• **Figure C-65** Geographic, expansile lucent lesion in the left superior pubic ramus is noted with internal ground-glass density and septations. The exophytic portion of the tumor is an unusual appearance of fibrous dysplasia. This patient had polyostotic fibrous dysplasia with endocrinopathy (Albright syndrome).

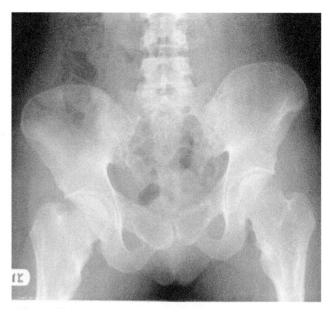

• **Figure C-67** Deformity of the proximal femur and superior pubic ramus bilaterally due to osteochondromatosis, a characteristic appearance for hereditary multiple osteochondromatosis.

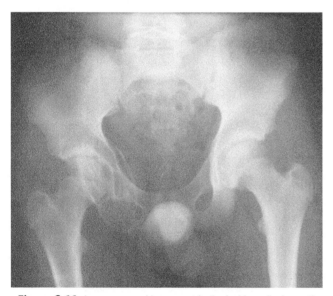

• **Figure C-66** An aneurysmal bone cyst in the ischium displaces the contour of the posterior column. The lesion is expansile and lucent, with thinning of the cortex.

Multiple lesions, often with deformity of involved bones, are seen in hereditary multiple exostoses (HME) (Fig. C-67). Malignant transformation occurs in about 1% of solitary lesions, but 5% to 15% of cases with HME.[86]

Enchondromatosis

In enchondromatosis, or Ollier disease, the pelvis femur may be involved.[86] Deformity of involved bones and expansile, irregularly shaped lesions with internal dystrophic, ring- or arc-shaped calcifications are seen[86] (Fig. C-68).

Neurofibromatosis

Neurofibromatosis is an autosomal-dominant, inherited dysplasia characterized by development of skin lesions, nerve tumors, and sarcomas.[90] Osseous involvement of the pelvis may demonstrate deformity of the pelvis or acetabulum, scoliosis, and chronic hip dislocations[90] (Fig. C-69). In long bones, such as the tibia, pseudarthroses, cortical erosions, nonossifying fibromas, and deformity may be seen.[2]

Simple Bone Cyst

Simple bone cyst is thought to be a localized disturbance of bone growth and not a true neoplasm. Most commonly affecting patients younger than 30 years of age, the etiology of simple bone cysts is unknown.[90] It affects the proximal femur and humerus most commonly, with less common sites including the ilium and calcaneus. The lesion appears as a centrally located lucent lesion with sclerotic margins (Fig. C-70). Osseous septa may be seen in the cyst. And a pathologic fracture may yield a "fallen fragment" sign of a bone fragment lying dependently in the cyst.[90]

Langerhans Cell Histiocytosis

A nonneoplastic proliferation of mononuclear cells, Langerhans cell histiocytosis most commonly affects children younger than 15 years of age.[85] Any bone can be affected, with the axial skeleton and long bones most commonly involved. A variety of radiographic appearances may be seen, varying from a sharply marginated lytic lesion to a lesion with a wide zone of transition and periosteal elevation (Fig. C-71). In the spine, vertebral involvement can lead to collapse of the vertebra, yielding a vertebra plana appearance.[85]

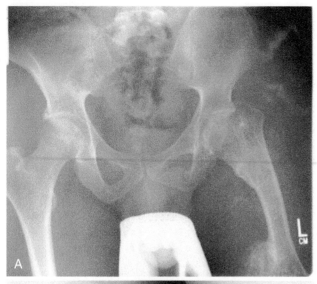

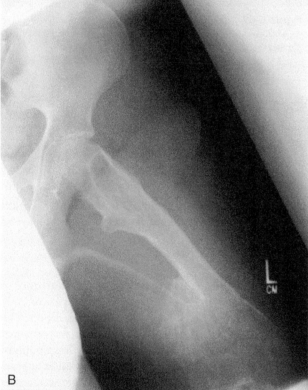

• **Figure C-68 A** and **B,** The proximal and distal femur are markedly deformed and to a lesser extent the left ischium and inferior pubic ramus. Punctate and curvilinear calcifications may be seen in the exophytic lesion in the left distal femur. Ollier disease.

Metastasis

Metastases are the most common malignant tumors of bone.[2,85] The axial skeleton is most commonly affected, as a result of hematogenous spread of malignancy. Many different radiographic appearances may be seen with metastatic disease, including sclerotic, lytic, or mixed sclerotic and lytic lesions (Fig. C-72). A high index of suspicion should be maintained when evaluating a lesion in the pelvis. MR imaging, CT, or radionuclide bone scan may be helpful to characterize a lesion, look for a primary tumor, or evaluate for other metastatic lesions.

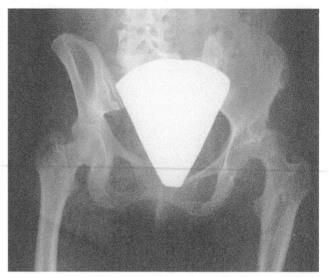

• **Figure C-69** The left hip is chronically dislocated, with pseudoacetabulum formation. Scalloping of the femoral neck is also noted. The lower lumbar spine is scoliotic and deformed in this patient with neurofibromatosis type I.

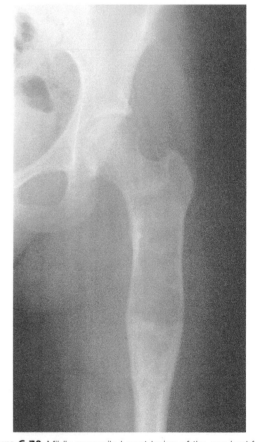

• **Figure C-70** Mildly expansile lucent lesion of the proximal femoral shaft. Simple bone cyst.

Giant Cell Tumor

Giant cell tumor is an abnormal proliferation of osteoclasts and stromal cells, typically located eccentrically in the ends of long bones (Fig. C-73). It occurs most commonly in patients 20 to 40 years of age.[91] Typically an aggressive lesion, a sclerotic border is usually absent. About 5% to

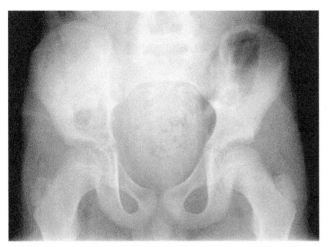

• **Figure C-71** Lucent lesion in the right superior acetabulum is associated with periosteal elevation medially. Langerhans cell histiocytosis.

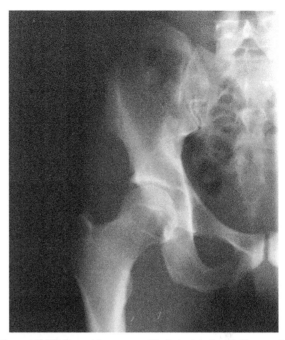

• **Figure C-73** Eccentric, geographic lucent lesion in the proximal metaphysis and epiphysis of the right femur. The lesion appears to extend nearly to the inferomedial articular surface of the femoral head. Giant cell tumor.

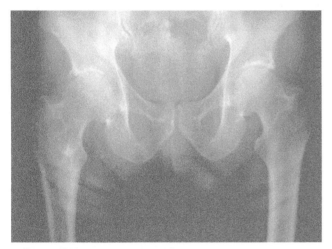

• **Figure C-72** Lucent lesion in the femoral neck and proximal shaft without sclerotic rim, nonspecific appearance. Lung cancer metastasis.

10% of cases develop metastases, generally to the lungs, though no radiographic feature reliably distinguishes benign from malignant giant cell tumors.[91]

Chondroblastoma

Chondroblastoma is a rare lesion but is in the differential diagnosis of an epiphyseal lesion in a skeletally immature patient.[92] Occurring most commonly in patients between 5 and 25 years of age, these lesions are typically found in the distal femur and proximal tibia, less commonly in the proximal femur. Radiographically, an eccentric lucent lesion with sclerotic border, at times extending through the physis into the metaphysis, may be seen[92] (Fig. C-74).

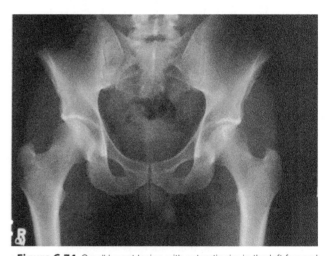

• **Figure C-74** Small lucent lesion with sclerotic rim in the left femoral head. Chondroblastoma.

disease patterns seen in the pelvis and hip improves the radiologist's ability to make the correct diagnosis.

Acknowledgement

The author expresses appreciation to the Department of Radiology and Imaging at the Hospital for Special Surgery, for the use of images from their teaching file in preparing the manuscript.

Conclusion

Conventional radiography of the hip and pelvis are useful to demonstrate a broad spectrum of inherited and acquired disease. Accurate detection and classification of these abnormalities assist the clinician in treating and counseling the patient. Understanding of the radiographic anatomy and

References

1. Bergquist TH, Coventry MB. The pelvis and hips. In: Berquist TH, ed. *Imaging of Orthopedic Trauma and Surgery*. Philadelphia: WB Saunders; 1986:181.

2. Greenspan A. Lower limb I: pelvic girdle and proximal femur. In: Greenspan A, ed. *Orthopedic Radiology: A Practical Approach*. 3rd ed. Philadelphia: Lippincott Williams & Wilkins; 2000.

3. Armbuster TG, Guerra J Jr, Resnick D, et al. The adult hip: an anatomic study. Part I: the bony landmarks. *Radiology*. 1978; 128:1-10.

4. Saks BJ. Normal acetabular anatomy for acetabular fracture assessment: CT and plain film correlation. *Radiology*. 1986;159: 139-145.

5. Johnson D, Williams A, eds. *Gray's Anatomy*. 39th ed. London: Churchill-Livingstone; 2004.

6. Ponseti IV. Growth and development of the acetabulum in the normal child. Anatomical, histological, and roentgenographic studies. *J Bone Joint Surg Am*. 1978;60:575-585.

7. Whitehouse RW. Paget's disease of bone. *Semin Musculoskelet Radiol*. 2002;6:313-322.

8. Cundy T. Idiopathic hyperphosphatasia. *Semin Musculoskelet Radiol*. 2002;6:307-312.

9. Bowerman JW, Sena JM, Chang R. The teardrop shadow of the pelvis; anatomy and clinical significance. *Radiology*. 1982;143: 659-662.

10. Deesomchok U, Tumrasvin T: Clinical comparison of patients with ankylosing spondylitis, Reiter's syndrome and psoriatic arthritis. *J Med Assoc Thai*. 1993;76:61-70.

11. Stevens MA, El-Khoury GY, Kathol MH, et al. Imaging features of avulsion injuries. *Radiographics*. 1999;19:655-672.

12. Sundar M, Carty H. Avulsion fractures of the pelvis in children: a report of 32 fractures and their outcome. *Skeletal Radiol*. 1994;23:85-90.

13. Bui-Mansfield LT, Chew FS, Lenchik L, et al. Nontraumatic avulsions of the pelvis. *AJR Am J Roentgenol*. 2002;178:423-427.

14. Dihlmann W, Tillmann B. Pericoxal fat stripes and the capsule of the hip joint. The anatomical-radiological correlations. *Rofo Fortschr Geb Rontgenstr Neuen Bildgeb Verfahr*. 1992;156:411-414.

15. Eastridge BJ, Burgess AR. Pedestrian pelvic fractures: 5-year experience of a major urban trauma center. *J Trauma*. 1997;42: 695-700.

16. Burgess AR, Eastridge BJ, Young JW, et al. Pelvic ring disruptions: effective classification system and treatment protocols. *J Trauma*. 1990;30:848-856.

17. Young JW, Burgess AR, Brumback RJ, et al. Lateral compression fractures of the pelvis: the importance of plain radiographs in the diagnosis and surgical management. *Skeletal Radiol*. 1986;15: 103-109.

18. Judet R, Judet J, Letournel E. Fractures of the acetabulum: classification and surgical approaches for open reduction. Preliminary report. *J Bone Joint Surg Am*. 1964;46:1615-1646.

19. Harris JH Jr, Coupe KJ, Lee JS, et al. Acetabular fractures revisited: part 2, a new CT-based classification. *AJR Am J Roentgenol*. 2004;182:1367-1375.

20. Hougaard K, Thomsen PB. Traumatic posterior fracture-dislocation of the hip with fracture of the femoral head or neck, or both. *J Bone Joint Surg Br*. 1988;70:233-239.

21. Oakes DA, Jackson KR, Davies MR, et al. The impact of the Garden classification on proposed operative treatment. *Clin Orthop*. 2003;409:232-240.

22. Caviglia HA, Osorio PQ, Comando D: Classification and diagnosis of intracapsular fractures of the proximal femur. *Clin Orthop*. 2002;399:17-27.

23. Blundell CM, Parker MJ, Pryor GA, et al. Assessment of the AO classification of intracapsular fractures of the proximal femur. *J Bone Joint Surg Br*. 1998;80:679-683.

24. Fox KM, Magaziner J, Hebel JR, et al. Intertrochanteric versus femoral neck hip fractures: differential characteristics, treatment, and sequelae. *J Gerontol A Biol Sci Med Sci*. 1999;54: M635-M640.

25. Daffner RH, Pavlov H. Stress fractures: current concepts. *AJR Am J Roentgenol*. 1992;159:245-252.

26. Boles CA, el-Khoury GY. Slipped capital femoral epiphysis. *Radiographics*. 1997;17:809-823.

27. Bloomberg TJ, Nuttall J, Stoker DJ. Radiology in early slipped femoral capital epiphysis. *Clin Radiol*. 1978;29:657-667.

28. Stutz G, Kuster MS, Kleinstuck F, et al. Arthroscopic management of septic arthritis: stages of infection and results. *Knee Surg Sports Traumatol Arthrosc*. 2000;8:270-274.

29. Volberg FM, Sumner TE, Abramson JS, et al. Unreliability of radiographic diagnosis of septic hip in children. *Pediatrics*. 1984;74:118-120.

30. Milgram JW, Rana NA. Resection arthroplasty for septic arthritis of the hip in ambulatory and nonambulatory adult patients. *Clin Orthop*. 1991;272:181-191.

31. Ford LS, Ellis AM, Allen HW, et al. Osteomyelitis and pyogenic sacroiliitis: a difficult diagnosis. *J Paediatr Child Health*. 2004;40: 317-319.

32. Osman AA, Govender S. Septic sacroiliitis. *Clin Orthop*. 1995;313:214-219.

33. Malaviya AN, Kotwal PP. Arthritis associated with tuberculosis. *Best Pract Res Clin Rheumatol*. 2003;17:319-343.

34. Ellis ME, el-Ramahi KM, al-Dalaan AN. Tuberculosis of peripheral joints: a dilemma in diagnosis. *Tuber Lung Dis*. 1993;74: 399-404.

35. Zvulunov A, Gal N, Segev Z. Acute hematogenous osteomyelitis of the pelvis in childhood: diagnostic clues and pitfalls. *Pediatr Emerg Care*. 2003;19:29-31.

36. Conrozier T, Tron AM, Mathieu P, et al. Quantitative assessment of radiographic normal and osteoarthritic hip joint space. *Osteoarthritis Cartilage*. 1995;3(suppl A):81-87.

37. Conrozier T, Merle-Vincent F, Mathieu P, et al. Epidemiological, clinical, biological and radiological differences between atrophic and hypertrophic patterns of hip osteoarthritis: a case-control study. *Clin Exp Rheumatol*. 2004;22:403-408.

38. Avimadje AM, Pellieux S, Goupille P, et al. Destructive hip disease complicating traumatic paraplegia. *Joint Bone Spine*. 2000;67:334-336.

39. O'Connor BL, Palmoski MJ, Brandt KD. Neurogenic acceleration of degenerative joint lesions. *J Bone Joint Surg Am*. 1985;67: 562-572.

40. Scutellari PN, Orzincolo C. Rheumatoid arthritis: sequences. *Eur J Radiol*. 1998;27(suppl 1):S31-S38.

41. Gusis SE, Riopedre AM, Penise O, et al. Protrusio acetabuli in seronegative spondyloarthropathy. *Semin Arthritis Rheum*. 1993;23:155-160.

42. Puhakka KB, Melsen F, Jurik AG, et al. MR imaging of the normal sacroiliac joint with correlation to histology. *Skeletal Radiol*. 2004;33:15-28.

43. Brower AC, Flemming DJ. *Arthritis in Black and White*. 2nd ed. Philadelphia: Saunders; 1997.

44. Pachman LM. Juvenile dermatomyositis. *Pediatr Clin North Am*. 1986;33:1097-1117.

45. Pachman LM. Juvenile dermatomyositis: immunogenetics, pathophysiology, and disease expression. *Rheum Dis Clin North Am.* 2002;28:579-602.

46. Aldridge JM 3rd, Urbaniak JR. Avascular necrosis of the femoral head: etiology, pathophysiology, classification, and current treatment guidelines. *Am J Orthop.* 2004;33:327-332.

47. Ficat RP. Idiopathic bone necrosis of the femoral head. Early diagnosis and treatment. *J Bone Joint Surg Br.* 1985;67:3-9.

48. Thompson GH, Salter RB. Legg-Calve-Perthes disease. Current concepts and controversies. *Orthop Clin North Am.* 1987;18: 617-635.

49. Singh M, Nagrath AR, Maini PS. Changes in trabecular pattern of the upper end of the femur as an index of osteoporosis. *J Bone Joint Surg Am.* 1970;52:457-467.

50. Koot VC, Kesselaer SM, Clevers GJ, et al. Evaluation of the Singh index for measuring osteoporosis. *J Bone Joint Surg Br.* 1996;78:831-834.

51. Jevtic V. Imaging of renal osteodystrophy. *Eur J Radiol.* 2003; 46:85-95.

52. Reginato AJ, Coquia JA. Musculoskeletal manifestations of osteomalacia and rickets. *Best Pract Res Clin Rheumatol.* 2003; 17:1063-1080.

53. States LJ. Imaging of metabolic bone disease and marrow disorders in children. *Radiol Clin North Am.* 2001;39:749-772.

54. Hardy DC, Murphy WA, Siegel BA, et al. X-linked hypophosphatemia in adults: prevalence of skeletal radiographic and scintigraphic features. *Radiology.* 1989;171:403-414.

55. Whitehouse RW. Paget's disease of bone. *Semin Musculoskelet Radiol.* 2002;6:313-322.

56. Rousiere M, Michou L, Cornelis F, et al. Paget's disease of bone. *Best Pract Res Clin Rheumatol.* 2003;17:1019-1041.

57. Bhimani MA, Wenz JF, Frassica FJ. Pigmented villonodular synovitis: keys to early diagnosis. *Clin Orthop.* 2001;386:197-202.

58. Crotty JM, Monu JU, Pope TL Jr. Synovial osteochondromatosis. *Radiol Clin North Am.* 1996;34:327-342.

59. Kim SH, Hong SJ, Park JS, et al. Idiopathic synovial osteochondromatosis of the hip: radiographic and MR appearances in 15 patients. *Korean J Radiol.* 2002;3:254-259.

60. Ea HK, Liote F. Calcium pyrophosphate dihydrate and basic calcium phosphate crystal-induced arthropathies: update on pathogenesis, clinical features, and therapy. *Curr Rheumatol Rep.* 2004;6:221-227.

61. Garcia GM, McCord GC, Kumar R. Hydroxyapatite crystal deposition disease. *Semin Musculoskelet Radiol.* 2003;7:187-193.

62. Phornphutkul C, Introne WJ, Perry MB, et al. Natural history of alkaptonuria. *N Engl J Med.* 2002;347:2111-2121.

63. de Vernejoul MC, Benichou O. Human osteopetrosis and other sclerosing disorders: recent genetic developments. *Calcif Tissue Int.* 2001;69:1-6.

64. Vanhoenacker FM, De Beuckeleer LH, Van Hul W, et al. Sclerosing bone dysplasias: genetic and radioclinical features. *Eur Radiol.* 2000;10:1423-1433.

65. Shapiro F. Osteopetrosis. Current clinical considerations. *Clin Orthop.* 1993;294:34-44.

66. Karkabi S, Reis ND, Linn S, et al. Pyknodysostosis: imaging and laboratory observations. *Calcif Tissue Int.* 1993;53:170-173.

67. Rozencwaig R, Wilson MR, McFarland GB Jr. Melorheostosis. *Am J Orthop.* 1997;26:83-89.

68. Lagier R, Mbakop A, Bigler A. Osteopoikilosis: a radiological and pathological study. *Skeletal Radiol.* 1984;11:161-168.

69. Mungovan JA, Tung GA, Lambiase RE, et al. Tc-99m MDP uptake in osteopoikilosis. *Clin Nucl Med.* 1994;19:6-8.

70. Rauch F, Glorieux FH. Osteogenesis imperfecta. *Lancet.* 2004;363:1377-1385.

71. Sillence DO, Senn A, Danks DM. Genetic heterogeneity in osteogenesis imperfecta. *J Med Genet.* 1979;16:101-116.

72. Roughley PJ, Rauch F, Glorieux FH. Osteogenesis imperfecta—clinical and molecular diversity. *Eur Cell Mater.* 2003;5:41-47.

73. Weinstein SL, Mubarak SJ, Wenger DR. Developmental hip dysplasia and dislocation: part I. *AAOS Instr Course Lecture.* 2004;53:523-530.

74. Weinstein SL, Mubarak SJ, Wenger DR. Developmental hip dysplasia and dislocation: part II. *AAOS Instr Course Lecture.* 2004;53:531-542.

75. Cooperman DR, Wallensten R, Stulberg SD. Acetabular dysplasia in the adult. *Clin Orthop.* 1983;175:79-85.

76. Lavigne M, Parvizi J, Beck M, et al. Anterior femoroacetabular impingement: part I. Techniques of joint preserving surgery. *Clin Orthop.* 2004;418:61-66.

77. Beck M, Leunig M, Parvizi J, et al. Anterior femoroacetabular impingement: part II. Midterm results of surgical treatment. *Clin Orthop.* 2004;418:67-73.

78. Lemyre E, Azouz EM, Teebi AS, et al. Bone dysplasia series. Achondroplasia, hypochondroplasia and thanatophoric dysplasia: review and update. *Can Assoc Radiol J.* 1999;50:185-197.

79. Keiper GL Jr, Koch B, Crone KR. Achondroplasia and cervicomedullary compression: prospective evaluation and surgical treatment. *Pediatr Neurosurg.* 1999;31:78-83.

80. Anton CG, Applegate KE, Kuivila TE, et al. Proximal femoral focal deficiency (PFFD): more than an abnormal hip. *Semin Musculoskelet Radiol.* 1999;3:215-226.

81. Kant P, Koh SH, Neumann V, et al. Treatment of longitudinal deficiency affecting the femur: comparing patient mobility and satisfaction outcomes of Syme amputation against extension prosthesis. *J Pediatr Orthop.* 2003;23:236-242.

82. Chen SJ, Li YW, Wang TR, et al. Bony changes in common mucopolysaccharidoses. *Zhonghua Min Guo Xiao Er Ke Yi Xue Hui Za Zhi.* 1996;37:178-184.

83. Mahboubi S, Glaser DL, Shore EM, et al. Fibrodysplasia ossificans progressiva. *Pediatr Radiol.* 2001;31:307-314.

84. Chang MY, Shih LY, Dunn P, et al. Solitary plasmacytoma of bone. *J Formos Med Assoc.* 1994;93:397-402.

85. Michel JL, Gaucher-Hugel AS, Reynier C, et al. POEMS syndrome: imaging of skeletal manifestations, a study of 8 cases. *J Radiol.* 2003;84:393-397.

86. Unni KK. *Dahlin's Bone Tumors: General Aspects and Data on 11,087 Cases.* 5th ed. Philadelphia: Lippincott-Raven Publishers; 1996:291-390.

87. Fitzpatrick KA, Taljanovic MS, Speer DP, et al. Imaging findings of fibrous dysplasia with histopathologic and intraoperative correlation. *AJR Am J Roentgenol.* 2004;182:1389-1398.

88. Hermann G, Klein M, Abdelwahab IF, et al. Fibrocartilaginous dysplasia. *Skeletal Radiol.* 1996;25:509-511.

89. Haga N, Nakamura S, Taniguchi K, et al. Pathologic dislocation of the hip in von Recklinghausen's disease: a report of two cases. *J Pediatr Orthop.* 1994;14:674-676.

90. Ahn JI, Park JS. Pathological fractures secondary to unicameral bone cysts. *Int Orthop.* 1994;18:20-22.

91. Tunn PU, Schlag PM. Giant cell tumor of bone. An evaluation of 87 patients. *Z Orthop Ihre Grenzgeb.* 2003;141:690-698.

92. Ramappa AJ, Lee FY, Tang P, et al. Chondroblastoma of bone. *J Bone Joint Surg Am.* 2000;82-A:1140-1145.

Index

Page numbers followed by *f* indicate figure, by *t* table, and by *b* box.

414